Sarcoidosis

A Clinician's Guide

Sarcoidosis

A Clinician's Guide

ROBERT PHILLIP BAUGHMAN, MD
Professor of Medicine
Internal Medicine
University of Cincinnati
Cincinnati, OH, United States

DOMINIQUE VALEYRE, MD
Professor of Pulmonology
Université Paris 13
AP-HP, Hôpital Avicenne
Bobigny, France

ELSEVIER

ELSEVIER

3251 Riverport Lane
St. Louis, Missouri 63043

SARCOIDOSIS: A CLINICIAN'S GUIDE ISBN: 978-0-323-54429-0

Publisher: Mica Haley
Acquisition Editor: Robin Carter
Editorial Project Manager: Jennifer Horigan
Project Manager: Kiruthika Govindaraju
Cover Designer: Alan Studholme

List of Contributors

Alejandro Aragaki, MD
Assistant Professor of Medicine
Department of Internal Medicine
University of Cincinnati Medical Center
Cincinnati, OH, United States

Zahir Amoura, MD, MSc
Service de Médecine Interne 2
Hôpital de la Pitié-Salpêtrière
Assistance Publique-Hôpitaux de Paris et Sorbonne Université
Paris, France

Robert Phillip Baughman, MD
Professor of Medicine
Internal Medicine
University of Cincinnati
Cincinnati, OH, United States

Sadia Benzaquen, MD
Director of Interventional Pulmonology
Pulmonary and Critical Care
University of Cincinnati
Cincinnati, OH, United States

Jean-François Bernaudin, MD, PhD
Professor Emeritus of Histology and Cytology
AP-HP, Hôpital Avicenne
Bobigny, France

Valérie Besnard, PhD
EA2363 Hypoxie et Poumon
Université Paris 13
Bobigny, France

Surinder S. Birring, MD
Consultant
Division of Asthma, Allergy and Lung Biology
King's College London, London
London, United Kingdom

Diane Bouvry, MD
Physician
Respiratory Disease
AP-HP, Hôpital Avicenne
Bobigny, France

Pierre-Yves Brillet, MD, PhD
Professor
Assistance Publique Hôpitaux de Paris
Avicenne Hospital
Department of Radiology
Bobigny, France

University Paris 13
COMU Sorbonne Paris Cité, EA 2363
Hypoxia and the Lung: Fibrosing Pneumonias, Ventilatory and Circulatory Modulations
Bobigny, France

Pilar Brito-Zerón, MD, PhD
Autoimmune Diseases Unit
Department of Medicine
Hospital CIMA-Sanitas
Barcelona, Spain

Laboratory of Autoimmune Diseases Josep Font
IDIBAPS-CELLEX
Department of Autoimmune Diseases
ICMiD
Hospital Clínic
University of Barcelona
Barcelona, Spain

Broos Caroline E., MD, PhD
Physician
Pulmonary Medicine
Erasmus MC
Rotterdam, The Netherlands

Thibaud Chazal, MD
Service de Médecine Interne 2
Hôpital de la Pitié-Salpêtrière
Assistance Publique-Hôpitaux de Paris et Sorbonne Université
Paris, France

Ozioma S. Chioma, PhD
Division of Infectious Diseases
Department of Medicine
Vanderbilt University School of Medicine
Nashville, TN, United States

Fleur Cohen Aubart, MD, PhD
Hôpital de la Pitié-Salpêtrière
Service de Médecine Interne 2
Sorbonne Université
Assistance Publique Hôpitaux de Paris
Paris, France

Elliott D. Crouser, MD
Professor of Medicine
Division of Pulmonary, Allergy, Critical Care, and Sleep Medicine
The Ohio State University Wexner Medical Center
Columbus, OH, United States

Daniel A. Culver, DO
Staff Physician
Pulmonary Medicine
Cleveland Clinic
Cleveland, OH, United States

Jolanda De Vries, PhD
ILD Care Foundation Research Team
Ede, The Netherlands

Dept. of Medical Psychology
Elisabeth-TweeSteden Hospital Tilburg
Tilburg, The Netherlands

Dept. of Medical and Clinical Psychology
Tilburg University
Tilburg, The Netherlands

Morgane Didier, MD
Doctor
Assistance Publique Hôpitaux de Paris
Avicenne Hospital
Department of Pneumology
Bobigny, France

University Paris 13
COMU Sorbonne Paris Cité, EA 2363
Hypoxia and the Lung: Fibrosing Pneumonias, Ventilatory and Circulatory Modulations
Bobigny, France

Wonder P. Drake, MD
Professor of Medicine
Pathology, Microbiology, and Immunology
Vanderbilt University School of Medicine
Nashville, TN, United States

Marjolein Drent, MD, PhD
Professor of Interstitial Lung Diseases
Pharmacology and Toxicology
Faculty of Health, Medicine and Life Science
Maastricht University
Maastricht, The Netherlands

Marjon Elfferich, MSc
ILD Care Foundation Research Team
Ede, The Netherlands

Joseph C. English III, MD
Professor
Department of Dermatology
University of Pittsburgh
Pittsburgh, PA, United States

Alexander Gelbard, MD
Department of Otolaryngology
Vanderbilt University
Nashville, TN, United States

Kareem Genena, MBBCH
Department of Medicine
Seton Hall University-Saint Francis Medical Center
Trenton, NJ, United States

Milanese Gianluca, MD
Division of Radiology
Department of Medicine and Surgery
University of Parma
Parma, Italy

Jan C. Grutters, MD
Pulmonologist
Department of Pulmonology and Center of Interstitial Lung Diseases
St. Antonius Hospital
Utrecht and Nieuwegein
The Netherlands

Division Heart & Lungs
University Medical Center Utrecht
Utrecht, The Netherlands

Celine Hendriks, MSc
ILD Care Foundation Research Team
Ede, The Netherlands

ILD Center of Excellence
St. Antonius Hospital
Nieuwegein, The Netherlands

Faculty of Medicine
Utrecht University
Utrecht, The Netherlands

Sotonye Imadojemu, MD, MBE
Instructor
Department of Dermatology
Brigham and Women's Hospital
Harvard University
Cambridge, MA, United States

W. Ennis James, MD
Assistant Professor
Pulmonary and Critical Care Medicine
Medical University of South Carolina
Charleston, SC, United States

Florence Jeny, MD
Pulmonology
AP-HP, Hôpital Avicenne
Bobigny, France

Marc A. Judson, MD
Chief
Division of Pulmonary and Critical Care Medicine
Albany Medical Center
Albany, NY, United States

Marianne Kambouchner, MD
Pathologist
Pathology
AP-HP, Hôpital Avicenne
Bobigny, France

R.G.M. Keijsers, MD, PhD
Nuclear Medicine Physician
Nuclear Medicine
St Antonius Hospital
Nieuwgein, The Netherlands

Belchin Kostov, PhD
Laboratory of Autoimmune Diseases Josep Font
IDIBAPS-CELLEX
Department of Autoimmune Diseases
ICMiD
Hospital Clínic
University of Barcelona
Barcelona, Spain

Primary Healthcare Transversal Research Group
IDIBAPS
Barcelona, Spain

Van Le, MD
Division of Critical Care
Pulmonary and Sleep Medicine
The Ohio State University Wexner Medical Center
Columbus, OH, United States

Raphaël Lhote, MD
Hôpital de la Pitié Salpetriere
Service de Médecine Interne 2
Assistance publique Hôpitaux de Paris
Paris, France

Huiping Li, MD
Shanghai Pulmonary Hospital
Tongji University
Department of Respiratory Medicine
School of Medicine
Shanghai, China

Elyse E. Lower, MD
Professor of Medicine
Internal Medicine
University of Cincinnati
Cincinnati, OH, United States

Silva Mario, MD, PhD
Division of Radiology
Department of Medicine and Surgery
University of Parma
Parma, Italy

Edward J. Miller, MD, PhD
Associate Professor
Medicine (Cardiology)
Yale University
New Haven, CT, United States

Kool Mirjam, PhD
Pulmonary Medicine
Erasmus MC
Rotterdam, The Netherlands

Philippe Moguelet, MD
Physician
Anatomie et Cytologie Pathologiques
Hôpital Tenon, AP-HP
Paris, France

Sverzellati Nicola, MD, PhD
Professor of Radiology
Radiology, Medicine and Surgery
University of Parma
Parma, Italy

Megan Noe, MD, MPH, MSCE
Instructor
Department of Dermatology
Perelman Center for Advanced Medicine
University of Pennsylvania
Philadelphia, PA, United States

Hilario Nunes, MD, PhD
Professor of Pulmonology
Université Paris 13
AP-HP, Hôpital Avicenne
Bobigny, France

Amit S. Patel, MD, FRCP
Physician
Respiratory Medicine
King's College London
London, United Kingdom

Manuel Ramos-Casals, MD, PhD
Physician
Servei de Malalties Autoimmunes
Hospital Clínic
Barcelona, Spain

Misha Rosenbach, MD
Associate Professor
Dermatology & Internal Medicine
Perelman Center for Advanced Medicine
University of Pennsylvania
Philadelphia, PA, United States

Nathalie Saidenberg-Kermanac'h, MD, PhD
Rheumatologist
AP-HP, Hôpital Avicenne
Bobigny, France

Milou C. Schimmelpennink, MD
Interstitial Lung Diseases Center of Excellence
Department of Pulmonology
St Antonius Hospital
Nieuwegein, Utrecht, The Netherlands

Division of Heart & Lungs
University Medical Center Utrecht
Utrecht, The Netherlands

Zartashia Shahab, MD
Yale University School of Medicine
Section of Cardiovascular Medicine
New Haven, CT, United States

Sumit Sharma, MD
Cole Eye Institute
Cleveland Clinic
Cleveland, OH, United States

Paolo Spagnolo, MD, PhD
Associate Professor
Cardiac, Thoracic and Vascular Sciences
University of Padua
Padova, Italy

Timothy Tully, MB BCH BAO MRCP
Physician
Sarcoidosis Researcher
Respiratory
Kings College Hospital
London, United Kingdom

Yurdagül Uzunhan, MD, PhD
Pneumologist
Université Paris 13
AP-HP, Hôpital Avicenne
Bobigny, France

Kouranos V, MD
Interstitial Lung Disease Unit
Royal Brompton Hospital
London, United Kingdom

Dominique Valeyre, MD
Professor of Pulmonology
Université Paris 13
AP-HP, Hôpital Avicenne
Bobigny, France

Merilyn Varghese, MD
Yale University School of Medicine
Department of Internal Medicine
New Haven, CT, United States

Adriane D.M. Vorselaars, MD, PhD
Interstitial Lung Diseases Center of Excellence
Department of Pulmonology
St Antonius Hospital
Nieuwegein, The Netherlands

Karolyn A. Wanat, MD
Associate Professor
Department of Dermatology
Medical College of Wisconsin
Milwaukee, WI, United States

Athol Wells, MD
Professor of Medicine
Royal Brompton Hospital and Imperial College
London, United Kingdom

Wim Wuyts, MD, PhD
Professor
Pulmonary Medicine Unit for Interstitial Lung Diseases
University Hospitals Leuven
Leuven, Belgium

Jonas Yserbyt, MD, PhD
Professor
Respiratory Diseases
University Hospital Leuven
Leuven, Belgium

Preface

The world of sarcoidosis is changing on many fronts. Basic and clinical research laboratories across the world have added new insights into the disease. Patient representative groups have added to these insights and helped focus research. In this book we have tried to provide the latest information regarding this multifaceted disease. Although our project was designed to help the clinician better understand the disease, we believe the book will also be useful for researchers, both clinical and basic scientist.

The book is divided into four major areas. We begin with a discussion of the epidemiology and potential cause of sarcoidosis. Dr. Ramos-Casals discusses the epidemiology of the disease, comparing the various reports from around the world and providing a sense of who gets this disease. Dr. Drake then discusses the various environmental factors associated with disease, including the potential role of one or more infectious agent as a trigger for the disease. Professor John Hutchinson who first described the disease felt it was a variant of tuberculosis. This remains an area of speculation since that time, with modern techniques providing evidence. Whatever the trigger (and there may be more than one), the immunologic response is the hallmark of the disease. Dr. Broos and her colleagues provide an updated review of the initiation of the disease, as well as the resolution or persistence of the inflammatory response. Dr. Spagnolo summarizes the insights that have come about from genetic studies of this disease. While there remains no perfect experimental model for sarcoidosis, Dr Crouser summarizes the currently available and possible new models for this disease. Finally, Dr. Bernaudin and his group provide specific information about the pathology of the granuloma, the cornerstone of sarcoidosis.

The next section deals with diagnosis of sarcoidosis. Dr. Wuyts gives an overview of the diagnostic approach to the disease. This is followed by a section by Dr. Benzaquen on bronchoscopy, the most commonly used method to make the diagnosis of sarcoidosis. The rest of the section deals with extrapulmonary manifestations of sarcoidosis, including diagnosis and outcome for the specific areas. Dr. Miller discusses cardiac sarcoidosis, an important cause of morbidity and sometimes mortality. Dr. Cohen-Aubart discusses neurosarcoidosis, a manifestation that can lead to significant long-term complications. Dr. Rosenbach and colleagues discuss the various manifestations of cutaneous sarcoidosis while Dr. Culver leads the discussion on ocular disease. While skin and eye disease are common manifestations, Dr. Li discusses some of the rarer, but still important organs. Finally, Dr. Judson has written about parasarcoidosis syndromes, which are manifestations of sarcoidosis which are not directly related to granulomatous involvement but can be quite devastating to the patient.

The next section deals with monitoring sarcoidosis. Dr. Valeyre and colleagues present an approach to monitor pulmonary disease. This is followed by chapters on specific techniques for monitoring. Dr. Sverzellati discusses conventional radiographic techniques, including computed tomography and magnetic resonance imaging. Dr. Keijsers provides information about the role of nuclear imaging, especially positron emission tomography scanning. Dr. Birring and colleagues discuss the various measures of quality of life, including several new instruments developed specifically for sarcoidosis patients. The quality of life and functional symptoms are two very important points for patients. Dr. Grutters then provides a summary of biomarkers studied in sarcoidosis, including insights about the role of these in diagnosis and management.

The last section deals with treatment and complications of the disease. Dr. Baughman and James provide evidence-based treatment recommendations. Dr. Drent and colleagues discuss management of two major parasarcoidosis symptoms, fatigue and small-fiber neuropathy. Drs. Lower and Saidenberg-Kermanac'h provide insight and direction for managing calcium and bone health in sarcoidosis patients. Dr. James discusses nonpharmaceutical treatments for sarcoidosis. Dr. Nunes and colleagues discuss the detection and management of sarcoidosis-associated pulmonary hypertension. The final chapter by Dr. Wells discusses mortality from sarcoidosis. While most patients do not die from sarcoidosis, studies have demonstrated a slow but steady rise from the disease. Whether this represents increased recognition, an aging population with disease or some other factor is not entirely clear. Dr. Wells provides evidence regarding the incidence, possible causes, and prognostic indicators.

Sarcoidosis affects people across the globe, and there are yearly international meetings of the World Association of Sarcoidosis and Other Granulomatous disease. This book reflects this international aspect of the disease. Many of the chapters reflect the input provided by the various patient groups across the world.

The editors wish to acknowledge all the hard work of the authors of the individual chapters. We also wish to thank Jennifer Horrigan of Elsevier, who was most instrumental in this project from inception to completion.

Robert Phillip Baughman, MD
Dominique Valeyre, MD

Contents

SECTION III MONITORING

SECTION IV TREATMENT AND COMPLICATIONS

CHAPTER 1

Geoepidemiology of Sarcoidosis

PILAR BRITO-ZERÓN, MD, PHD • BELCHIN KOSTOV, PHD •
ROBERT PHILLIP BAUGHMAN, MD • MANUEL RAMOS-CASALS, MD, PHD

INTRODUCTION

Sarcoidosis, a systemic disease of unknown etiology characterized by the development of noncaseating epitheloid cell granulomas, often affects young adults aged between 20 and 50 years.[1] Sarcoidosis is a systemic disease with a heterogeneous clinical presentation, although clearly dominated by thoracic involvement. Epidemiologically, sarcoidosis is a rare disease with a significant influence of ethnicity and environmental factors that play a key role in the phenotypic expression of sarcoidosis[2]; notably, the three organs most frequently affected (the lungs, skin, and eyes) are in direct contact with the external environment.[3]

The rarity of sarcoidosis, together with the key role of ethnic and geoepidemiological factors, means that the larger the population analyzed, the better the characterization of clinical expression, and the more likely the findings will reflect the real population affected by the disease. Big data–driven research is a key instrument that may help provide a high-definition picture of infrequent and heterogeneous diseases such as sarcoidosis.[4] This chapter updates the main geoepidemiological features associated with sarcoidosis using the merged data of 117,175 patients with sarcoidosis included in large series (>100 patients) reported in the PubMed library.[5–103]

PREVALENCE AND INCIDENCE

Table 1.1 summarizes the prevalence and incidence rates of sarcoidosis country per country. The highest rates are reported in Northern Europe, the United States, and India (Fig. 1.1A and B): the estimated incidence in Europe ranges between 1 and 15 cases per 100,000 inhabitants, with significantly higher rates in northern countries.[104] In the United States, sarcoidosis is more common in Black/African Americans (BAAs).[105] In the largest reported US series,[56] the highest incidence rate was reported in BAA people (17.8 per 10^6 inhabitants) compared with Whites, Hispanics, and Asians (8.1, 4.3, and 3.2, respectively). In Detroit, Rybicki et al.[106] reported an incidence rate of 35.5 in BAA versus 10.9 in Whites, while two Navy studies[107,108] reported rates of 47.8–81.8 for BAA compared with 4.4–7.6 for Whites. Similar differences are reported for the prevalence per 100,000 inhabitants in US studies (64–141 for BAAs, 7–50 for Whites, 22 for Hispanics, and 19 for Asians).[56,109,110] Out of the United States, people from India living in London or Singapore had the highest rates of incidence and those from East Asia living in the United States or Singapore the lowest rates in comparison with the other ethnicities living in the same geographical area. In multiethnic cohorts from London, with a differing ethnic distribution than the US cohorts, the highest rates were reported in West Indian (incidence of 58, prevalence of 183 cases per 10^6 inhabitants) and Irish (incidence 21, prevalence 155) people in comparison with UK-born people (incidence 4, prevalence 27).[111,112] Benatar found a prevalence among Blacks of 23.2 per 10^6 inhabitants compared with Whites (3.7) and mixed race (11.6) [113] people in Cape Town, while Anantham et al.[114] reported a yearly incidence of 0.56 per 10^6 inhabitants in Singapore, with clearly different figures for Indian (4.57), Malaysian (1.30), and Chinese (0.23) people.

AGE AND GENDER

Our big data analysis confirmed that sarcoidosis affects both sexes but with a slight predominance of females and is mainly diagnosed in the fourth and fifth decades of life, with a mean age at diagnosis of 41 years and 52% of women affected in our merged data analysis (Table 1.2). Specific analysis of cohorts from the three main geographical areas (United States, Europe, and Asia) found significant differences, especially in

Sarcoidosis. https://doi.org/10.1016/B978-0-323-54429-0.00001-X

TABLE 1.1
Worldwide Rates of Incidence and Prevalence of Sarcoidosis per 100,000 Inhabitants Ordered by Continent

First Author	Year	City/Region	Country	Incidence	Prevalence
Fletcher	1966	Kitwe	Zambia	3.1–9.7	NA
Lee	2002	Taiwan	China	NA	0.25
Wu	2016	Taiwan	China	NA	2.17
Gupta	1985	Delhi	India	NA	61.2
Gupta	1985	Calcutta	India	NA	150
Rakower	1964	–	Israel	0.5	1.6
Yigla	2006	Haifa	Israel	2	NA
Yigla	2002	Haifa	Israel	0.8	NA
Hasada	1972	–	Japan	NA	1–2
Hiraga	1974	–	Japan	1.7	NA
Hosoda & Nobechi	1964	–	Japan	NA	5.6
Hosoda	1980	–	Japan	0.5	NA
Morimoto	2008	–	Japan	1.01	NA
Nobechi	1964	Tokyo districts	Japan	0.3	NA
Pietinalho	2000	Hokkaido	Japan	1	3.7
Yamaguchi	1989	–	Japan	1.3	3
Kim	2001	Korea	Korea	0.125	NA
Al-Khouzaie	2011	Dhahran	Saudi Arabia	NA	13
Anantham	2007	Singapore	Singapore	0.56	NA
Gillman	2007	Geelong Victoria	Australia	4.4–6.3	NA
Heyworth	NA	Brisbane	Australia	10.1	NA
Marshman	1964	–	Australia	NA	9.2
Price	1980	Melbourne	Australia	8.35	NA
Reid	1964	Auckland	New Zealand	NA	6.13
Reid	1964	Wellington	New Zealand	NA	24.3
Reid	1964	Christchurch	New Zealand	NA	18.41
Thomeer	2001	Flanders	Belgium	0.26	1.94
Alilovic	2004	Croatia	Croatia	NA	4.1
Mise	2011	Split-Dalmatia County	Croatia	3.3	15.6
Kolek	1994	Moravia & Silesia	Czech	3.3–4.4	41.3–63.1
Levinsky	1964	–	Czechoslovakia	NA	10
Levinsky	1976	–	Czechoslovakia	2.3	NA
Alsbirk	1964	–	Denmark	3.4	NA
Alsbirk	1964	–	Denmark	8	NA
Byg	2003	–	Denmark	7.2	NA

TABLE 1.1
Worldwide Rates of Incidence and Prevalence of Sarcoidosis per 100,000 Inhabitants Ordered by Continent—cont'd

First Author	Year	City/Region	Country	Incidence	Prevalence
Horwitz	1964	–	Denmark	5.5	NA
Horwitz	1964	Copenhagen	Denmark	3	NA
Horwitz	1964	Zealand	Denmark	2–5.2	NA
Horwitz	1964	Bornholm	Denmark	4.1	NA
Horwitz	1964	Funen	Denmark	4–4.9	NA
Horwitz	1964	Jutland	Denmark	3.5–16.1	NA
Horwitz	1971	–	Denmark	14	NA
Horwitz	1971	–	Denmark	10.8	NA
Romer	1977	–	Denmark	5	NA
Selroos	1974	–	Denmark	9.2	NA
Patiala	1964	–	Finland	NA	8.1
Pietinalho	2000	Mjölbolsta hospital	Finland	11.4	28.2
Poukkula	1986	Northern Ostroboth-nia	Finland	15	32
Riska	1964	–	Finland	NA	5.1
Selroos	1974	–	Finland	7.5	NA
Duchemann	2017	Seine-Saint Denis (Greater Paris)	France	4.9	30.2–44.78
Turiaf	1964	–	France	NA	5.2–10.1
Behrend	1974	Marburg	Germany	NA	50
Behrend	1974	Marburg Biedenkopf distrcit	Germany	NA	98
Buss	1975	–	Germany	28	NA
Fried	1964	West Berlin	Germany	NA	14.5
Lindig	1964	Leipzig	Germany	NA	13.3
Maike	2012	–	Germany	NA	32–69
Steinbruck & Zaumseil	1974	East germany	Germany	NA	31.3
Karakatsani	2009	–	Greece	1.07	5.89
Mandi	1964	Debrecen	Hungary	NA	4–5
Donnelly	2013	Count Offaly	Ireland	NA	85
Logan	1964	Dublin	Ireland	NA	33.3
Nicholson	2010	–	Ireland	NA	28.13
Beghe	2017	Parma province	Italy	NA	49
Blasi	1974	5 northern/4 south-ern cities	Italy	3	NA
Fazzi	1992	Tuscani	Italy	1.2	NA
Muratore	1964	Puglia and Lucania	Italy	1.2–2.5	NA

Continued

TABLE 1.1
Worldwide Rates of Incidence and Prevalence of Sarcoidosis per 100,000 Inhabitants Ordered by Continent—cont'd

First Author	Year	City/Region	Country	Incidence	Prevalence
Orie	1964	–	Netherlands	21.6	NA
Riddervold	1964	–	Norway	14.4	26.7
Jaroszewicz	1964	Warsaw	Poland	NA	6.9
Jaroszewicz	1977	–	Poland	7.7	10.7
Kowalska	2014	Silesian voivodeship	Poland	3.8–4.5	NA
Villar	1964	–	Portugal	NA	0.2
Centea	1964	Nortwestern region	Romania	NA	3.3
Rabuchin	1975	Leningrad	Russia	NA	2.3
Rabuchin	1975	Moscow	Russia	NA	1.1
Rabuchin	1975	Talin	Russia	NA	3.8
Rabuchin	1975	Riga	Russia	NA	2.1
Denic-Markovic	NA	–	Serbia	NA	16.5
Pesut	2005	Serbia/Montenegro	Serbia	1.9	NA
Virsik	1974	West Slovakia	Slovakia	1	9.6
La Grasta	1964	Slovenia	Slovenia	NA	11.9
Alcoba Leza	2003	Leon	Spain	1.37	NA
Maña	1992	Barcelona	Spain	1.36	NA
Siso	2017	Catalonia	Spain	NA	25
Arkema	2016	–	Sweden	11.5	160
Bauer	1964	–	Sweden	NA	55
Bauer	1964	–	Sweden	NA	64
Hillerdal	1984	Uppsala	Sweden	14.7–23.2	NA
Wallgren	1958	–	Sweden	NA	42
Deubelbeiss	2010	–	Switzerland	7	121
Pohle	2016	–	Switzerland	NA	53.66
Sommer	1964	–	Switzerland	NA	16.3
BTTA	1969	–	UK	3.25	NA
Douglas	1964	Scotland	UK	NA	5–12
Douglas	1964	–	UK	NA	3–7
Douglas	1964	–	UK	NA	20–25
Douglas	1964	–	UK	NA	5.5–13.4
Gribbin	2006	–	UK	5	NA
James	1964	Britain	UK	NA	20
James	1964	London	UK	NA	19
Milliken	1964	North Ireland	UK	10.3	NA
Nicholson	2010	North Ireland	UK	NA	11.16

TABLE 1.1
Worldwide Rates of Incidence and Prevalence of Sarcoidosis per 100,000 Inhabitants Ordered by Continent—cont'd

First Author	Year	City/Region	Country	Incidence	Prevalence
Parkes	1985	Isle of Man	UK	14.7	NA
Parkes	1985	Isle of Man	UK	3.5	NA
Sutherland	1965	–	UK	8.3	NA
Pollak	1964	–	Canada	NA	10.5
Baughman	2016	–	US	8	60
Cragin	2009	Vermont state	US	NA	66.1
Gundelfinger	1961	–	US	NA	NA
Henke	1986	Rochester, MN	US	6.1	NA
Reich	1996	Northwest Region	US	4.8	NA
Robins	1964	New York	US	NA	39
Ungprasert	2016	Olmsted County, Minnesota	US	10	NA
Castells	1964	–	Argentina	NA	1
Purriel	1961	Buenos Aires	Argentina	1.3–2.4	NA
Rey	1964	–	Argentina	NA	5
Bethlem	1985	–	Brazil	NA	10
Certain & De Paula	1964	–	Brazil	NA	0.2
Coquart	2015	–	Guadeloupe Islands	2.28	21.09
Purriel	1961	–	Uruguay	0.4	NA

gender distribution (Fig. 1.2): the highest percentage of females was reported in Asian studies (65%) and the lowest in European (49%), while the youngest age at diagnosis was found in the US studies (39.8 years).

Ethnicity may influence the mean age at diagnosis and the gender ratio, as has been reported by US studies in BAA patients,[56] who developed the first sarcoidosis-related symptoms at an earlier age than Whites.[49,115] A classification of the reported cohorts according to the predominant ethnicity (>50%) found that the frequency of women affected was significantly higher in predominantly BAA cohorts than in Asian and White predominant cohorts (67% vs. 64% vs. 51%, respectively, $P < .001$) (Fig. 1.3); the higher the frequency of BAA patients included in a cohort, the greater the number of females, while the higher the frequency of White patients, the higher the number of males. A geographical gradient for the gender ratio is observed in studies from countries located between parallels 30 and 45 (Mediterranean countries, Japan, and Southern United States), in which two-thirds of patients with sarcoidosis are women, while in the north of Europe and India more than half the patients are men.

ETHNICITY

Although sarcoidosis affects all ethnicities, it is more frequently reported in Whites. According to our big data, ethnicity was detailed in 25,951 patients: 15,443 (59.5%) were classified as White, 6520 (25.1%) as BAA, 2985 (11.5%) as Asian, and 1003 (3.9%) as other ethnicities (Table 1.2) (Fig. 1.4). There are large ethnicity-driven variations in the frequency, epidemiological and clinical expression, and outcomes, although the differences should be always evaluated taking into account socioeconomic disparities that could modify the level of exposure to potential environmental toxins.[104]

How Ethnicity Influences the Clinical Presentation

The differing clinical expression of sarcoidosis according to ethnicity was first reported in the 1960s.[116,117] Most recent studies have been carried out in multiethnic populations and have reported a differing clinical expression when comparing between different ethnicities. The largest US studies comparing the two predominant ethnicities (BAAs vs. Whites) reported a higher frequency of advanced radiographic stages of sarcoidosis, low FVC% predictive values, and more organs involved in BAA patients, including a higher frequency of ocular, liver, bone marrow, extrathoracic lymph nodes, and skin (other than erythema nodosum) sarcoidosis, while splenic involvement and hypercalcemia were more frequent in Whites. In addition, BAA patients

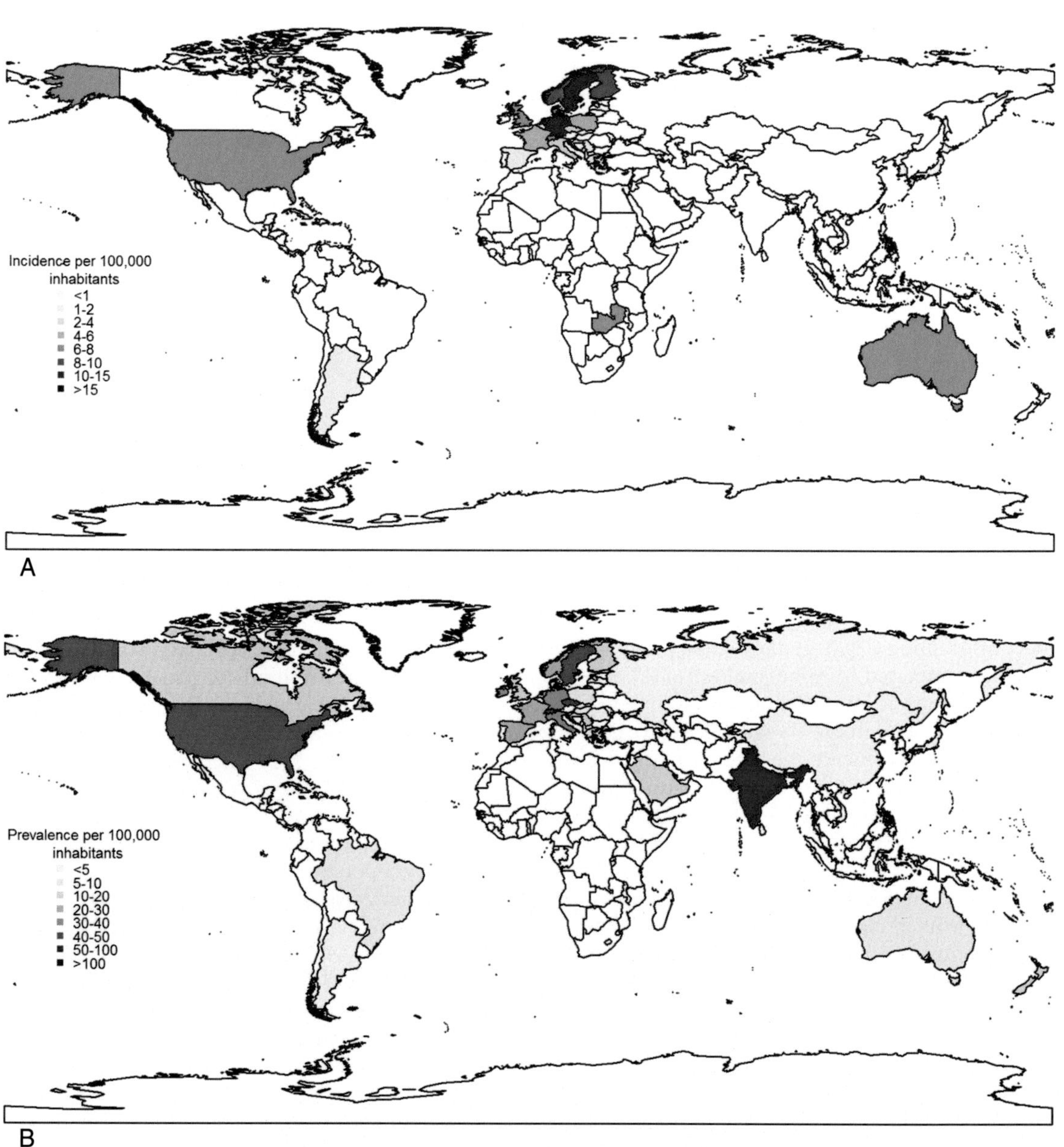

FIG. 1.1 Worldwide frequency of sarcoidosis: **(A)** incidence and **(B)** prevalence.

had a twofold higher median granuloma density,[118] had a diagnostic biopsy ($P<.0001$) approximately 10 years earlier, and more frequently required sarcoidosis-specific therapies than Whites.[7,60,119] Few studies have compared the clinical phenotype of sarcoidosis in countries with differing ethnicity distributions. Pietinalho et al.[93] carried out a comparative study of Japanese and Finnish patients and found a lower mean age at diagnosis, a higher frequency of ocular involvement and normal radiographic stage, and a lower frequency of Löfgren syndrome in Japanese patients. Studies from the Middle East reported a higher frequency of more advanced radiological stages in Arabs compared with Asians in Kuwait,[103] while radiographic stage II disease was significantly more common in Jewish patients and stage I in Arab patients in Israel.[100] In Spain, we recently reported that patients born outside Spain had a higher frequency of musculoskeletal symptomatology, pulmonary involvement, and ocular involvement compared with Spain-born patients.[12]

Our big data analysis confirms the striking clinical differences found according to the predominant ethnicity. With respect to thoracic disease, predominantly White cohorts had the highest frequency of radiological stage II, Asian cohorts the highest frequency of stage I, and BAA cohorts the highest frequency of the more severe stages (III and IV) (Fig. 1.5). Ethnicity also plays a key role in modulating the individual frequencies of the main extrathoracic involvement: Asian patients have the highest rates of the clinical clusters lymph nodes and neuro-ocular-ENT involvement, while BAA patients have the highest frequencies of the clinical clusters cardiopulmonary, skin/musculoskeletal and intraabdominal involvements (Fig. 1.6).

TABLE 1.2
Worldwide Picture of the Main Epidemiological Features of Patients With Sarcoidosis: Merged Data From Reported Series Including at Least 100 Cases

Variable	Value	Patients (n)
Age at diagnosis, mean (range)	41.5 (30.0–51.2)	50,796
GENDER		
Women	47,785 (52.4)	91,215
Men	43,430 (47.6)	91,215
Ratio W:M	1.1 (0.5–3.6)	91,215
ETHNICITY		
White	15,443 (59.5)	25,951
Black/AA	6,520 (25.1)	25,951
Asian	2,985 (11.5)	25,951
Others	1,003 (3.9)	25,951

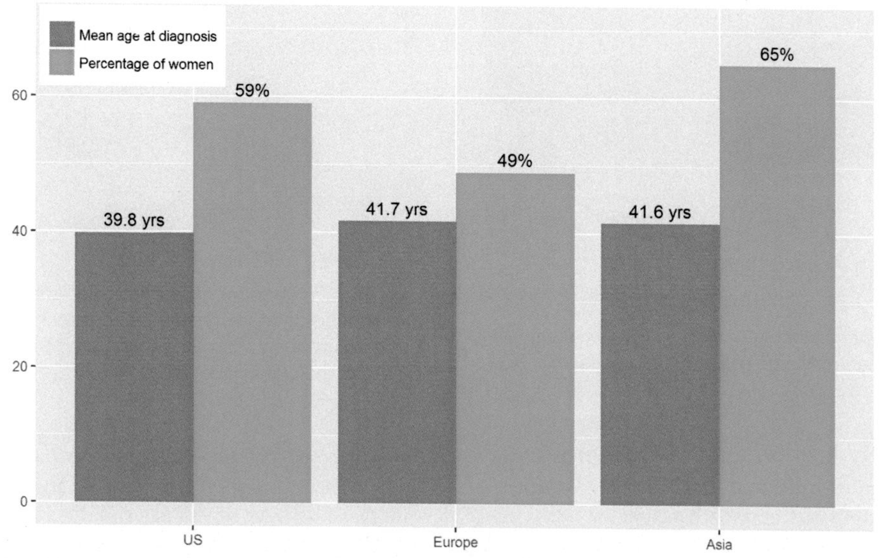

FIG. 1.2 Mean age at diagnosis and gender distribution of large series (>100 cases) reported in the Pubmed grouped according to the geographical area (United States, Europe, and Asia).

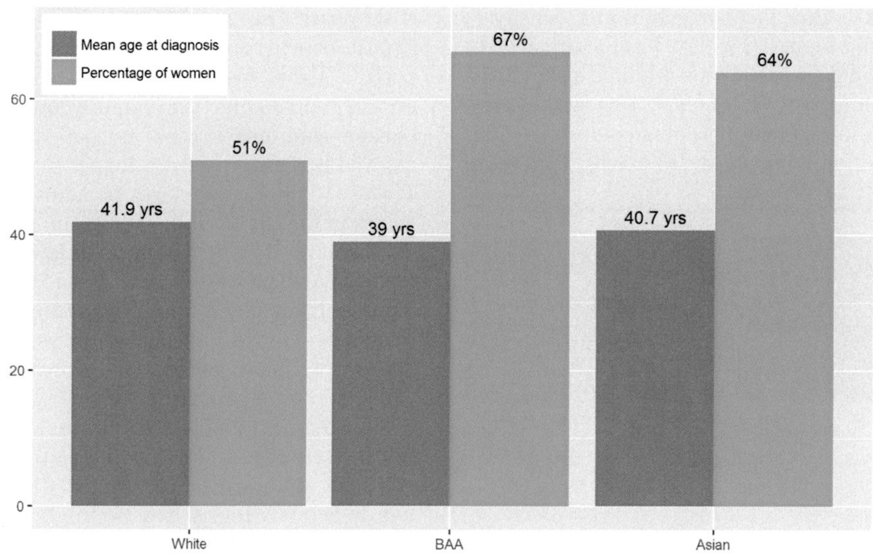

FIG. 1.3 Mean age at diagnosis and gender distribution of large series (>100 cases) reported in the Pubmed grouped according to the predominant ethnicity (>50% of included patients).

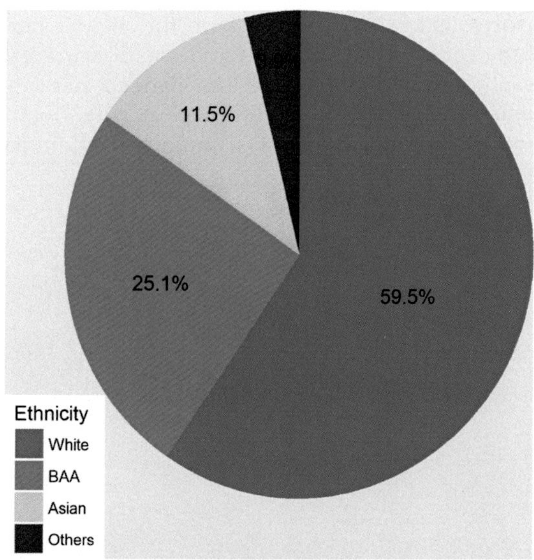

FIG. 1.4 Ethnicity distribution of 25,951 patients with sarcoidosis included in 62 large series (>100 cases) reported in the Pubmed.

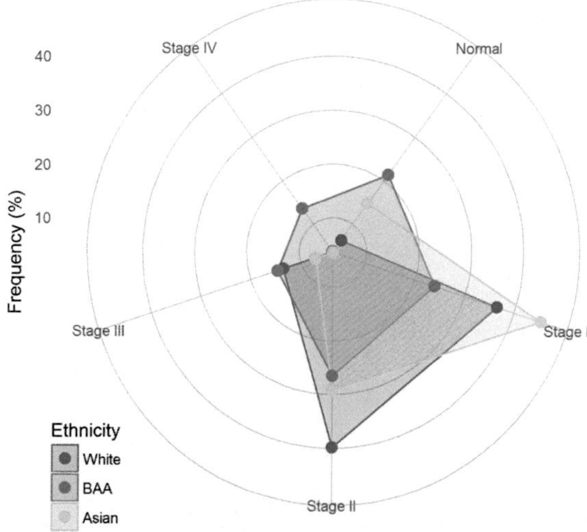

FIG. 1.5 Frequency of the Scadding radiological stages at diagnosis of large series (>100 cases) reported in the Pubmed grouped according to the predominant ethnicity (>50% of included patients).

How Ethnicity Influences the Outcome

Several US studies have reported a poor prognosis of the disease in BAA patients with respect to severity of the disease and mortality.[120–122] A study in Charleston by Kajdasz et al.[123] found an increase in sarcoidosis hospitalization rates in patients living proximal to the Atlantic coastline, especially in BAA patients compared with Whites, independently of socioeconomic status; other studies have reported similar results in BAA.[124,125] Outside the United States, Pietinalho et al.[93] reported better outcomes for pulmonary sarcoidosis in Japanese patients compared with Finnish patients. With respect

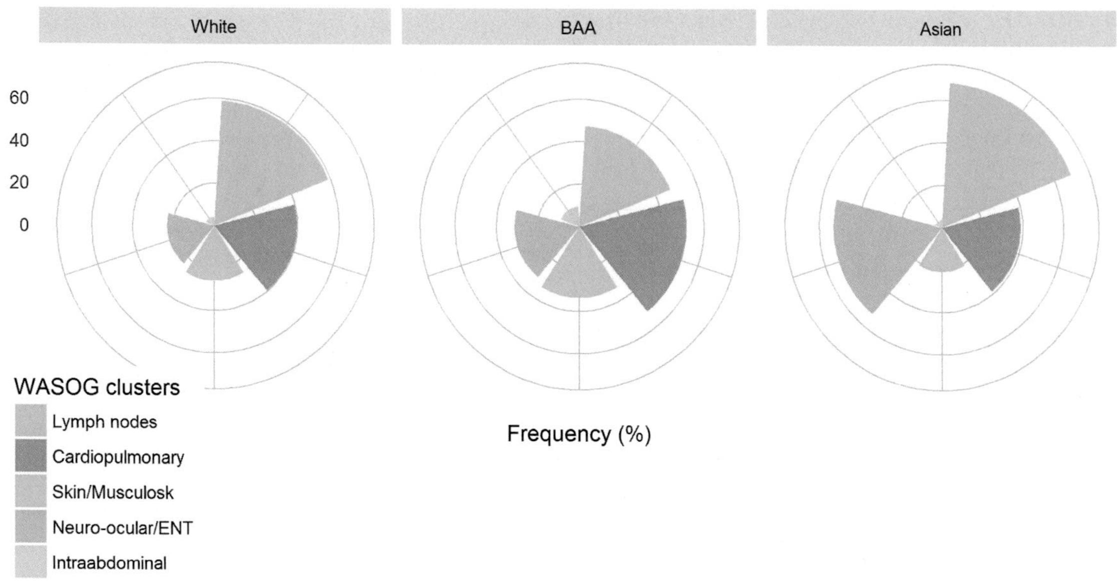

FIG. 1.6 Main organ clinical clusters (grouped according to the WASOG classification) of large series (>100 cases) reported in the Pubmed grouped according to the predominant ethnicity (>50% of included patients).

to mortality, a recent study reported a twelvefold higher age-adjusted mortality rate in BAA compared with Whites,[126] while Swigris et al.[127] (108) found the greatest increased mortality rates in BAA females.

GEOLOCATION

Geographically, sarcoidosis has overwhelmingly been reported in the Northern Hemisphere, with 96% largely reported from Northern countries. Only 458 (0.4%) of the 117,175 patients included coming from the Southern Hemisphere, a north-south ratio of reported cases of 255:1, which is 28 times higher than the population ratio of the two hemispheres. However, a potential bias about unreported figures in southern countries cannot be ruled out. By continent, there is a clear north-south gradient in the prevalence and incidence of sarcoidosis in Europe, with incidence rates being up to 15-fold higher in the north (especially in Sweden) compared with the Mediterranean countries. In addition, several studies have reported a geographical gradient within countries, with sarcoidosis being more frequent in the northern regions of Sweden,[64] Norway,[128] Italy, [129] and Japan.[130,131] In contrast, no clear gradient has been reported in studies from Switzerland[68] and Poland.[80] Other studies have reported a lower prevalence in the eastern regions of Denmark compared with the western regions,[132] while the largest US studies reported a higher prevalence in the Midwest and North East and a lower prevalence in the West.[56,133]

A specific analysis of the main series reported in the three main geographical areas (United States, Europe, and Asia) identifies significant differences in almost all clinical features. The highest frequency of thoracic involvement (stages I–IV) was reported in European cohorts (94%), and the highest frequency of pulmonary fibrosis (stage IV) in US cohorts (12%) (Fig. 1.7). With respect to extrathoracic World Association for Sarcoidosis and Other Granulomatous Disorders (WASOG) involvements, Asian cohorts have the highest rates of the clinical clusters lymph nodes and neuro-ocular-ENT involvement, while US cohorts have the highest frequencies of the clinical clusters cardiopulmonary and skin/musculoskeletal involvements (Fig. 1.8).

Regional weather is a key factor traditionally linked to the yearly variation in the frequency of sarcoidosis. Analysis of 16 studies in which the seasonal occurrence of sarcoidosis was detailed shows that the seasonal peaks of cases may be influenced by geolocation[16,17,38,55,63,71,105,128,134–138] (Fig. 1.9); several of these studies have been centered on Löfgren syndrome,[55,71,128,135–137] which seems to be one of the clinical presentations with the greatest seasonal influence. The further the area is from the Equator, the more frequent the peak of disease occurrence in winter months

(Northern US, Northern Europe, New Zealand). The lowest incidence by far is reported in autumn.[38,49,136]

Several studies have evaluated the influence of living in rural areas, often linking low-density population and predominantly agricultural activities. An inverse significant association was found between population density and the regional frequency of sarcoidosis in Switzerland,[68] while in Sweden, the highest prevalence rates were reported in the less-densely populated areas of the Northwest.[64] In the United States, the ACCESS study found a reduced risk in people who lived in suburbia within the three previous years.[90] In contrast, no significant association with population density has been found in other studies.[55,139-142] In India,[142] patients with sarcoidosis were more frequently reported from urban centers.

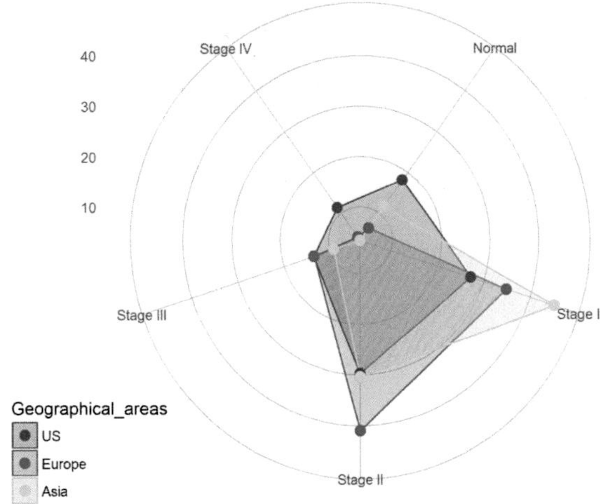

FIG. 1.7 Frequency of the Scadding radiological stages at diagnosis of large series (>100 cases) reported in the Pubmed grouped according to the geographical area (United States, Europe, and Asia).

ENVIRONMENTAL EXPOSURES

The personal environment seems to drive a differentiated frequency and clinical expression of sarcoidosis. The main epidemiological studies suggest a key influence of environmental exposures linked to the area of residence, the workplace, household, lifestyle, and socioeconomic status.

Area of Residence

Recent studies have examined the relationship between the risk of sarcoidosis and local/regional industries. A Swiss study[68] reports an enhanced frequency of the disease in people living in areas with high rates of agriculture and metallurgy and in those living in areas with a high density of water supply

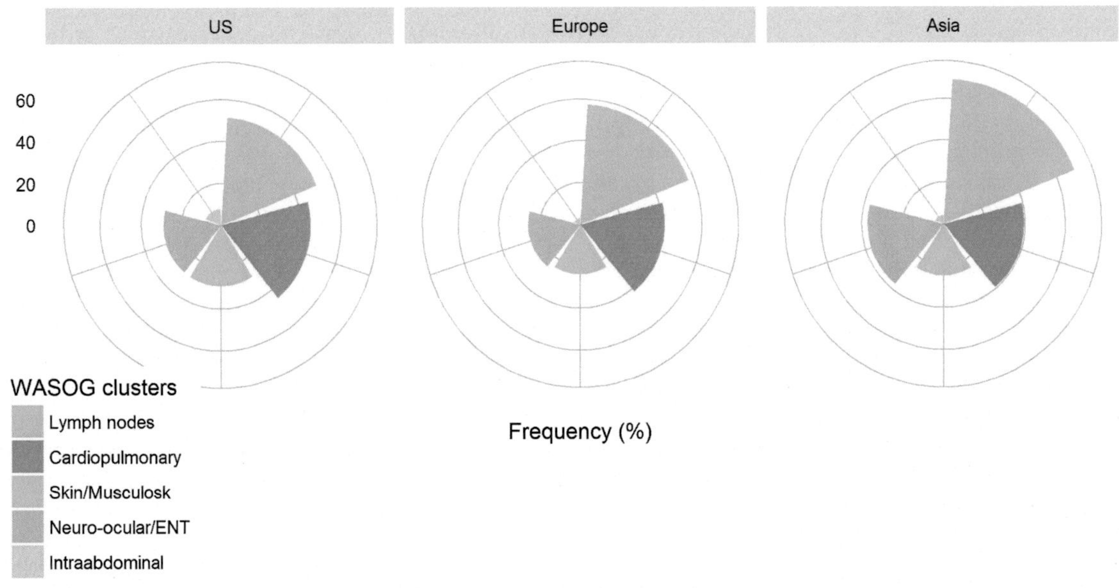

FIG. 1.8 Main organ clinical clusters (grouped according to the WASOG classification) of large series (>100 cases) reported in the Pubmed grouped according to the geographical area (United States, Europe, and Asia).

companies and air transport factories. Other environmental factors, such as air quality and pollution, have been little studied. One study found no significant association between air quality and the frequency of sarcoidosis,[68] while a study in South Carolina reported a higher incidence in people living near to the Atlantic Ocean.[123]

Occupational Exposure

The first reports of a potential influence of the workplace in modifying the risk of sarcoidosis came in the 1960s.[143–145] All but one of the main recent epidemiological studies have been carried out in the United States, mostly as part of the ACCESS project.[55,90,125,146–153] The jobs mainly associated with a significant modification in the risk of developing the disease are centered on occupations related to agriculture, the water industry, construction, metallurgy, education, and healthcare activities (Table 1.3).

Agriculture

Several studies have reported a close association between sarcoidosis and agriculture-related occupations, including farmworkers,[55,90,147] persons involved in raising birds[90] or cotton ginning,[90] and those exposed to organic/vegetable dust or insecticides.[55,90,146] The list of potential exposures in agricultural workers is long, including chemicals and aerosolized particulates such as grains, bedding materials, silicates, animal proteins, insect proteins, fungi, bacteria, mycotoxins, endotoxins, and, especially, insecticides and pesticides.[90] The risk is also enhanced in people working in industries related to organic dust exposures,[146,149] rubber factories,[146] gardening materials,[149] and pesticide-using industries.[90] Ethnicity may modulate the risk (enhanced in Caucasians)[149] and the disease severity (lower risk of extrathoracic disease in BAA workers exposed to organic dust),[149] as well as gender (higher risk in men exposed to industrial organic dust)[149] and some HLA markers (higher risk in DRB1*1101/1501 carriers exposed to insecticides).[146]

Water-related jobs

Another solid association reported by most studies is the high risk found in occupations with direct or indirect contact with water, including jobs in moldy/musty work environments,[55,90,146,148] indoor exposure to high humidity,[148] exposure to water damage[148] and firefighters.[153] Newman et al.[90] hypothesized that exposure to high-humidity environments may favor the production of bioaerosols that could enhance the risk of sarcoidosis. Since some microorganisms involved in the etiopathogenesis of sarcoidosis-like diseases grow readily in standing water[90]; some cases of granulomatous pneumonitis have been reported in people working in the automotive/metal machining industry exposed to microbially contaminated metalworking fluids.[90]

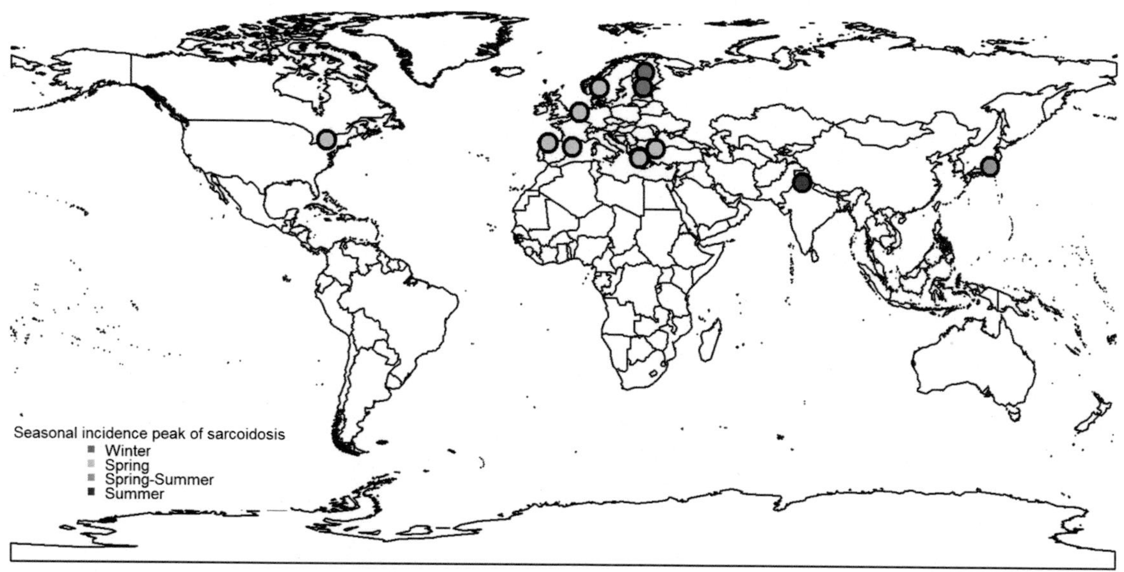

FIG. 1.9 Worldwide seasonal peak of incidence of new diagnosed cases of sarcoidosis: North-to-South geographical pattern.

TABLE 1.3
Risk of Development of Sarcoidosis According to Occupational Exposures and Jobs

Area	Enhanced Risk of Disease (Specific Subpopulations at Risk)	Lower Risk of Disease (Specific Subpopulations at Risk)
Agriculture	Industrial organic/vegetable dust exposures	
	Job in cotton ginning	
	Raising birds	
	Gardening materials workers	
	Rubber factory	
	Insecticides exposure	
	Pesticide-using industry	
Water	Bioaerosol exposure to moldy, musty environments	
	Indoor exposure high humidity (BAA)	
	Exposures water damage (BAA)	
Construction	Suppliers of building materials/garden supplies/ mobile homes	
	Hardware workers	
	WTC debris pile	
	Firefighters	
	Real estate (women)	
	Manual jobs (men)	
Metal	Automotive manufacturing/fitters	
	Metal dust/metal fume exposures (BAA)	Metal dust/metal fume exposures (White, men)
	Metal machining (BAA)	Exposure to welding
	Metalworking fluids (BAA)	
	Titanium exposure: paint, plastics, papers, inks (BAA)	
Military	Ship's servicemen US Navy (BAA)	Ship's servicemen US Navy (Women)
	Aviation structural mechanics US Navy (BAA)	National security (Women)
	Mess management specialists US Navy (White)	
Transportation/electricity	Transportation services industry (BAA)	Electric energy
	Drivers (BAA)	
Education	Educators	
	Elementary/secondary schools	
	Colleges/universities (White)	
Health	Physician	
	Radiation exposure	
	Job in animal laboratory	

TABLE 1.3
Risk of Development of Sarcoidosis According to Occupational Exposures and Jobs—cont'd

Area	Enhanced Risk of Disease (Specific Subpopulations at Risk)	Lower Risk of Disease (Specific Subpopulations at Risk)
Services	Retail trade industry (Women)	Retail trade industry (BAA)
	Supervisors sales/retail (women)	General merchandise stores (BAA)
	Dusty trades with crustal dust (BAA)	Personal service
		Waiter/waitress
Business/government	Executive, legislative and general government (BAA)	Data processor, typist, computer programmer
		Information clerks
		Business services (BAA)
People care		Exposure to children at work
		Work providing childcare
		Social and rehabilitation services

Construction-related occupations

Jobs related to construction are also associated with a higher risk of sarcoidosis, including hardware workers;[149] suppliers of building materials, garden supplies, and mobile homes;[146,149] firefighters; [153] and others dealing with debris piles such as those involved in the World Trade Center (WTC) response.[154] Jordan et al.[151] reported an enhanced risk in people working in the WTC debris pile, but not in those exposed to the dust cloud. Gender may modulate the risk, which is enhanced in men doing manual construction jobs.[55]

Metal-related jobs

The risk of sarcoidosis in people occupationally exposed to metals is Janus-faced. On the one hand, several studies have reported an enhanced risk in people working in metal machining and[148] automotive manufacturing/fitters[55,90] or those exposed to metalworking fluids,[148] with a higher rate of sarcoidosis-related mortality reported in workers involved in metal machining.[152] Titanium exposure (paint, plastics, inks) has also been related to a higher risk.[148] An enhanced ethnically driven risk was reported in BAA workers exposed to metalworking fluids [149] and a reduced risk in White workers exposed to metal dust/fumes.[149] On the other hand, a reduced risk has been reported in workers exposed to metal dust, fumes, or welding,[90,146,149] who also have a low risk of extrapulmonary disease.[150]

Education and health occupations

Working as educators has been linked to a higher risk of developing sarcoidosis,[148,149] especially in elementary/secondary schools[90,146,149] and colleges/universities, but only for Whites.[149] An analysis of US death certificates found a higher rate of sarcoidosis-related mortality in teachers and healthcare workers.[152] A higher risk of sarcoidosis has also been reported in healthcare workers, including physicians,[90] people exposed to radiation,[90] and people working in laboratories in contact with animals.[90]

Services and caring occupations

Several studies have reported a reduced risk of developing sarcoidosis in people exposed to children,[90] providing childcare,[149] working in social and rehabilitation services,[146,149] or being hospital volunteers.[90] In addition, service jobs have also been associated with a low risk of sarcoidosis, including waiters,[90] retail/general trade workers,[148] and people working in business services like banking and administration.[149] Other service jobs not involving personal contact, such as data processing, typists and computer programmers,[90,146] and people working in the electrical supply industry [149] also have a lower risk. Other studies have reported a higher risk in male drivers and transportation workers,[55,148] especially in BAA people.[149]

Household Exposures

The influence of exposures to potential household toxins has been evaluated by some studies. A higher risk of sarcoidosis has been reported in people living with central air conditioning[90,146] and in those using coal/wood stoves, fireplaces, humidifiers, or nonpublic water supplies.[146,147] In contrast to occupational exposure, domestic use of insecticides does not enhance the risk.[90,147] Other household exposures are associated with reduced risk, including domestic exposure to children (including people involved in home childcare of their own or other children), feather/down pillow stuffing, and household pets (cats, fish tanks, or animal dust)[90,146,148]; the risk is also reduced in people with passive household exposure to smoking.[90]

LIFESTYLE AND SOCIOECONOMIC FACTORS

Lifestyle

Smoking

Lifestyle determinants may also influence the frequency and clinical expression of sarcoidosis, with smoking being the most frequently investigated factor. However, the association with smoking seems to be influenced by geographical factors. An inverse relationship between smoking and the rate of sarcoidosis has been consistently reported by most US and European case-control studies, including the Netherlands,[11,135] France,[155–157] the United Kingdom,[158] and the United States.[49,90,146] However, the results are quite different in Asia, with no significant differences found in India,[159] while a higher prevalence of smoking was reported in all age groups (except men in their 30s) in Japanese patients with sarcoidosis.[75] Some studies have reported an influence of smoking on the clinical expression of sarcoidosis, contributing to a higher frequency of extrathoracic involvement in US studies.[27,77]

Obesity

Two recent US case-control studies have reported a close association between sarcoidosis and obesity. Ungprasert et al[49] reported that the odds ratio of having sarcoidosis was 2.54-fold higher in obese subjects (BMI ≥ 30 kg/m^2) than in those with normal/low BMI, while Cozier et al.[160] reported an increased incidence of sarcoidosis in BAA women with BMI >30 kg/m^2. Outside the United States, Gvozdenovic et al.[161] reported a higher frequency of people with BMI ≥25 kg/m^2 in patients with sarcoidosis compared with healthy volunteers (78% vs. 47%, $P < .01$) in Serbia.

Leisure activities

The main epidemiological studies have reported some leisure activities as protective factors including having fish tanks or cats in the household, bird watching/keeping, exposure to indoor pools/hot tubs, exposure to auto/truck repair or to printing as a hobby, or being hospital volunteers.[90,146]

Other

No studies have analyzed the influence of other lifestyle factors (exercise, diet). Only one study has evaluated the association between alcohol consumption and the risk of sarcoidosis, with negative results.[11]

Socioeconomic Factors

Several studies have studied the relationship between socioeconomic factors and the risk of sarcoidosis. The influence of the educational levels on the risk of developing sarcoidosis varies country by country. In Sweden, the lowest incidence rates were reported among the best educated people,[64] in India[142] sarcoidosis was reported more frequently in people with higher levels of education and incomes, and in Brazil no association between educational levels and sarcoidosis was found.[88] A US study carried out by telephone interview by Rabin et al.[95] found impairment of forced vital capacity in people with a lower educational level. Rabin et al.[95] also reported a more advanced radiographic stage in people with lower incomes, and a worse health status and more severe dyspnea in people with low socioeconomic status and no or only public insurance; the same authors[119] linked low income and low FEV1 predicted values, and the absence of private or Medicare health insurance with low FVC% predicted values.

COMBINING GEOEPIDEMIOLOGICAL RISK FACTORS

A specific exposure may not always have the same influence on the risk, suggesting the need to consider additional factors (both personal and environmental) in different combinations and/or at different levels of exposure; in addition, occupational exposure to a specific toxin might be a surrogate for workplace exposures to additional antigens not investigated.[90] Several studies have reported a differentiated risk for some epidemiological subsets of people working in jobs with a potential common exposure, including exposure to construction/building materials (enhanced risk in workers in the WTC debris pile but not for those exposed to the dust cloud), metals (enhanced risk for machining, manufacturing, and exposure to metalworking fluids and reduced risks for exposure to metal dust, fumes, or welding), childcare (enhanced risk for educators, reduced risk for childcare), or health-related occupations (enhanced risk for physicians, reduced risk for social and rehabilitation services). In addition, the risk may differ according to the location of the exposure, as has been reported for insecticides (enhanced risk for occupational exposure, no influence for home use), animals (enhanced risk for occupational exposure, reduced risk for pets in the household), children (enhanced risk for educators, reduced risk for domestic exposure to children), water-related environments (enhanced risk for occupational/household exposures, reduced risk for leisure exposures in indoor pools/hot tubs), metal (enhanced risk for vehicle manufacturing/fitters, reduced risk for auto/truck repair as a hobby), and health-related environments (enhanced risk for physicians, reduced risk for hospital volunteers).

The heterogeneous nature of how environmental and personal factors are combined in a specific person may help to explain why the same factor enhances or reduces the risk under the influence of personal epidemiological features (gender and ethnicity). Thus, men (but not women) with occupational exposure to organic industrial dust, manual construction jobs, and those working as drivers or in transportation services have an enhanced risk of developing sarcoidosis, while women (but not men) working in the retail trade or real estate have a reduced risk. With respect to ethnicity, only White people have an enhanced risk when exposed to organic industrial dust or work in colleges/universities, and have a reduced risk when they are exposed to metal dust/fumes, while BAA people have an enhanced risk if working as drivers or in transportation services and a reduced risk when working in trading occupations.

CONCLUSIONS

Sarcoidosis is one of the systemic diseases with the greatest influence of geoepidemiological factors on the frequency and phenotypic expression. Ethnicity contributes to explain the significant variations in the frequency, epidemiological and clinical expression, and outcomes of sarcoidosis reported across the different countries. In addition to ethnicity, it would be of interest to investigate the influence of ancestry, since there is a significant variation in Europe according to geographical genetic differences between northern and southern people,[162] and also in US people, in whom a Scandinavian ancestry is predominantly reported in White people from the North and West. Geographically, 96% of the reported cohorts including at least 100 cases are from countries located in the Northern Hemisphere countries, with a clear north-south gradient in the incidence and prevalence of the disease in Europe, with incidence rates being up to 15-fold higher in the north. Personal risk factors should be added to geolocation and ethnicity as key players in modulating the epidemiology and clinical expression of sarcoidosis. One of the more solid personal factors reported is the influence of jobs potentially linked to specific occupational exposures. The risk of sarcoidosis is enhanced in people working in jobs directly related to agriculture, water, construction, metal machining, education, and health and reduced in those working in jobs centered on people care. The influence of the local/regional environment, including climate and predominant local industries, may also be a modulating factor. Various studies have confirmed seasonal-related peaks of sarcoidosis incidence according to a geographical west-east distribution pattern, and high rates of new cases have been reported in people living in areas in which agriculture, metal, water-related, and transport facilities are the predominant industries, following a similar pattern to that reported for occupational associations; people living on a farm and those living on the coast also have higher disease rates. Other personal factors associated with a low risk of developing sarcoidosis include smoking exposure (except in Asian people), personal household exposures, and some leisure activities.

Future geoepidemiological research should focus on evaluating the combined effects of environmental exposures and genetic factors (some studies have started this approach by identifying the fact that carriers of specific HLA markers have enhanced risks for some occupational exposures),[146] the identification of clusters of geographically driven exposures, and the quantification of all personal exposures (degree of combination, length, and level of exposure). A new era in the collection, management, and interpretation of large amounts of geoepidemiological medical data are opening up for diseases that, like sarcoidosis, are both rare and have a complex etiopathogenic scenario. The use of big data–based approaches will be essential to analyze both the huge number of factors potentially involved and their complex relationships (different exposures in different geographical locations). Geoepidemiological studies enhanced by big data could yield important clues to a better understanding of the etiopathogenesis of sarcoidosis, helping to design strategies able to reduce not only the development of the disease but also its severity and mortality.

REFERENCES

1. Baughman RP, Lower EE, du Bois RM. Sarcoidosis. *Lancet*. 2003;361(9363):1111–1118. https://doi.org/10.1016/S0140-6736(03)12888-7.
2. Pereira CAC, Dornfeld MC, Baughman R, Judson MA. Clinical phenotypes in sarcoidosis. *Curr Opin Pulm Med*. 2014;20(5):496–502. https://doi.org/10.1097/MCP.0000000000000077.
3. Rybicki BA, Iannuzzi MC. Epidemiology of sarcoidosis: recent advances and future prospects. *Semin Respir Crit Care Med*. 2007;28(1):22–35. https://doi.org/10.1055/s-2007-970331.
4. Birnbaum AD, Rifkin LM. Sarcoidosis: sex-dependent variations in presentation and management. *J Ophthalmol*. 2014;2014:236905. https://doi.org/10.1155/2014/236905.
5. Antonelli A, Fazzi P, Fallahi P, Ferrari SM, Ferrannini E. Prevalence of hypothyroidism and Graves disease in sarcoidosis. *Chest*. 2006;130(2):526–532. https://doi.org/10.1378/chest.130.2.526.
6. Askling J, Grunewald J, Eklund A, Hillerdal G, Ekbom A. Increased risk for cancer following sarcoidosis. *Am J Respir Crit Care Med*. 1999;160(5 Pt 1):1668–1672. https://doi.org/10.1164/ajrccm.160.5.9904045.
7. Baughman RP, Teirstein AS, Judson MA, et al. Clinical characteristics of patients in a case control study of sarcoidosis. *Am J Respir Crit Care Med*. 2001;164(10 Pt 1):1885–1889. https://doi.org/10.1164/ajrccm.164.10.2104046.
8. Baughman RP, Drent M, Kavuru M, et al. Infliximab therapy in patients with chronic sarcoidosis and pulmonary involvement. *Am J Respir Crit Care Med*. 2006;174(7):795–802. https://doi.org/10.1164/rccm.200603-402OC.
9. Baughman RP, Sparkman BK, Lower EE. Six-minute walk test and health status assessment in sarcoidosis. *Chest*. 2007;132(1):207–213. https://doi.org/10.1378/chest.06-2822.
10. Bourbonnais JM, Samavati L. Clinical predictors of pulmonary hypertension in sarcoidosis. *Eur Respir J*. 2008;32(2):296–302. https://doi.org/10.1183/09031936.00175907.
11. Bours S, de Vries F, van den Bergh JPW, et al. Risk of vertebral and non-vertebral fractures in patients with sarcoidosis: a population-based cohort. *Osteoporos Int*. 2016;27(4):1603–1610. https://doi.org/10.1007/s00198-015-3426-1.
12. Brito-Zeron P, Sellares J, Bosch X, et al. Epidemiologic patterns of disease expression in sarcoidosis: age, gender and ethnicity-related differences. *Clin Exp Rheumatol*. 2016;34(3):380–388.
13. Cox CE, Donohue JF, Brown CD, Kataria YP, Judson MA. The Sarcoidosis Health Questionnaire: a new measure of health-related quality of life. *Am J Respir Crit Care Med*. 2003;168(3):323–329. https://doi.org/10.1164/rccm.200211-1343OC.
14. Christoforidis GA, Spickler EM, Recio MV, Mehta BM. MR of CNS sarcoidosis: correlation of imaging features to clinical symptoms and response to treatment. *AJNR Am J Neuroradiol*. 1999;20(4):655–669.
15. Darlington P, Gabrielsen A, Sorensson P, Cederlund K, Eklund A, Grunewald J. Cardiac involvement in Caucasian patients with pulmonary sarcoidosis. *Respir Res*. 2014;15:15. https://doi.org/10.1186/1465-9921-15-15.
16. Demirkok SS, Basaranoglu M, Akbilgic O. Seasonal variation of the onset of presentations in stage 1 sarcoidosis. *Int J Clin Pract*. 2006;60(11):1443–1450. https://doi.org/10.1111/j.1742-1241.2005.00773.x.
17. Gerke AK, Tangh F, Yang M, Cavanaugh JE, Polgreen PM. An analysis of seasonality of sarcoidosis in the United States veteran population: 2000–2007. *Sarcoidosis, Vasc Diffus lung Dis Off J WASOG/World Assoc Sarcoidosis Other Granulomatous Disord*. 2012;29(2):155–158.
18. Gottlieb JE, Israel HL, Steiner RM, Triolo J, Patrick H. Outcome in sarcoidosis. The relationship of relapse to corticosteroid therapy. *Chest*. 1997;111(3):623–631.
19. Handa T, Nagai S, Miki S, et al. Incidence of pulmonary hypertension and its clinical relevance in patients with sarcoidosis. *Chest*. 2006;129(5):1246–1252. https://doi.org/10.1378/chest.129.5.1246.
20. Heiligenhaus A, Wefelmeyer D, Wefelmeyer E, Rosel M, Schrenk M. The eye as a common site for the early clinical manifestation of sarcoidosis. *Ophthalmic Res*. 2011;46(1):9–12. https://doi.org/10.1159/000321947.
21. Hermans C, Petrek M, Kolek V, et al. Serum Clara cell protein (CC16), a marker of the integrity of the air-blood barrier in sarcoidosis. *Eur Respir J*. 2001;18(3):507–514.
22. Huggins JT, Doelken P, Sahn SA, King L, Judson MA. Pleural effusions in a series of 181 outpatients with sarcoidosis. *Chest*. 2006;129(6):1599–1604. https://doi.org/10.1378/chest.129.6.1599.
23. Joyce E, Ninaber MK, Katsanos S, et al. Subclinical left ventricular dysfunction by echocardiographic speckle-tracking strain analysis relates to outcome in sarcoidosis. *Eur J Heart Fail*. 2015;17(1):51–62. https://doi.org/10.1002/ejhf.205.
24. Judson MA, Chaudhry H, Louis A, Lee K, Yucel R. The effect of corticosteroids on quality of life in a sarcoidosis clinic: the results of a propensity analysis. *Respir Med*. 2015;109(4):526–531. https://doi.org/10.1016/j.rmed.2015.01.019.
25. Kiter G, Musellim B, Cetinkaya E, et al. Clinical presentations and diagnostic work-up in sarcoidosis: a series of Turkish cases (clinics and diagnosis of sarcoidosis). *Tuberk Toraks*. 2011;59(3):248–258.
26. Kollert F, Geck B, Suchy R, et al. The impact of gas exchange measurement during exercise in pulmonary sarcoidosis. *Respir Med*. 2011;105(1):122–129. https://doi.org/10.1016/j.rmed.2010.09.007.
27. Krell W, Bourbonnais JM, Kapoor R, Samavati L. Effect of smoking and gender on pulmonary function and clinical features in sarcoidosis. *Lung*. 2012;190(5):529–536. https://doi.org/10.1007/s00408-012-9406-8.
28. Le Jeune I, Gribbin J, West J, Smith C, Cullinan P, Hubbard R. The incidence of cancer in patients with idiopathic pulmonary fibrosis and sarcoidosis in the UK. *Respir Med*. 2007;101(12):2534–2540. https://doi.org/10.1016/j.rmed.2007.07.012.

29. Maimon N, Salz L, Shershevsky Y, Matveychuk A, Guber A, Shitrit D. Sarcoidosis-associated pulmonary hypertension in patients with near-normal lung function. *Int J Tuberc Lung Dis*. 2013;17(3):406–411. https://doi.org/10.5588/ijtld.12.0428.
30. Mana J, Salazar A, Manresa F. Clinical factors predicting persistence of activity in sarcoidosis: a multivariate analysis of 193 cases. *Respiration*. 1994;61(4):219–225.
31. Martusewicz-Boros MM, Boros PW, Wiatr E, Roszkowski-Sliz K. What comorbidities accompany sarcoidosis? A large cohort (n=1779) patients analysis. *Sarcoidosis, Vasc Diffus lung Dis Off J WASOG/World Assoc Sarcoidosis Other Granulomatous Disord*. 2015;32(2):115–120.
32. Maver A, Medica I, Salobir B, Tercelj M, Peterlin B. Genetic variation in osteopontin gene is associated with susceptibility to sarcoidosis in Slovenian population. *Dis Markers*. 2009;27(6):295–302. https://doi.org/10.3233/DMA-2009-0675.
33. Morais A, Lima B, Peixoto MJ, Alves H, Marques A, Delgado L. BTNL2 gene polymorphism associations with susceptibility and phenotype expression in sarcoidosis. *Respir Med*. 2012;106(12):1771–1777. https://doi.org/10.1016/j.rmed.2012.08.009.
34. Morimoto T, Azuma A, Abe S, et al. Epidemiology of sarcoidosis in Japan. *Eur Respir J*. 2008;31(2):372–379. https://doi.org/10.1183/09031936.00075307.
35. Nowinski A, Puscinska E, Goljan A, et al. The influence of comorbidities on mortality in sarcoidosis: a observational prospective cohort study. *Clin Respir J*. October 2015. https://doi.org/10.1111/crj.12398.
36. Patel AS, Siegert RJ, Creamer D, et al. The development and validation of the King's Sarcoidosis Questionnaire for the assessment of health status. *Thorax*. 2013;68(1):57–65. https://doi.org/10.1136/thoraxjnl-2012-201962.
37. Piotrowski WJ, Gorski P, Pietras T, Fendler W, Szemraj J. The selected genetic polymorphisms of metalloproteinases MMP2, 7, 9 and MMP inhibitor TIMP2 in sarcoidosis. *Med Sci Monit*. 2011;17(10):CR598–CR607.
38. Pohle S, Baty F, Brutsche M. In-hospital disease burden of sarcoidosis in Switzerland from 2002 to 2012. *PLoS One*. 2016;11(3):e0151940. https://doi.org/10.1371/journal.pone.0151940.
39. Prasse A, Katic C, Germann M, Buchwald A, Zissel G, Muller-Quernheim J. Phenotyping sarcoidosis from a pulmonary perspective. *Am J Respir Crit Care Med*. 2008;177(3):330–336. https://doi.org/10.1164/rccm.200705-742OC.
40. Rajoriya N, Wotton CJ, Yeates DGR, Travis SPL, Goldacre MJ. Immune-mediated and chronic inflammatory disease in people with sarcoidosis: disease associations in a large UK database. *Postgrad Med J*. 2009;85(1003):233–237. https://doi.org/10.1136/pgmj.2008.067769.
41. Saidenberg-Kermanac'h N, Semerano L, Nunes H, et al. Bone fragility in sarcoidosis and relationships with calcium metabolism disorders: a cross sectional study on 142 patients. *Arthritis Res Ther*. 2014;16(2):R78. https://doi.org/10.1186/ar4519.
42. Saremi F, Saremi A, Hassani C, et al. Computed tomographic diagnosis of myocardial fat deposits in sarcoidosis. *J Comput Assist Tomogr*. 2015;39(4):578–583. https://doi.org/10.1097/RCT.0000000000000235.
43. Sharma SK, Soneja M, Sharma A, Sharma MC, Hari S. Rare manifestations of sarcoidosis in modern era of new diagnostic tools. *Indian J Med Res*. 2012;135(5):621–629.
44. Takada K, Ina Y, Noda M, Sato T, Yamamoto M, Morishita M.The clinical course and prognosis of patients with severe, moderate or mild sarcoidosis. *J Clin Epidemiol*. 1993;46(4):359–366.
45. Takada T, Suzuki E, Morohashi K, Omori K, Gejyo F. MCP-1 and MIP-1A gene polymorphisms in Japanese patients with sarcoidosis. *Intern Med*. 2002;41(10):813–818.
46. Teirstein AS, Machac J, Almeida O, Lu P, Padilla ML, Iannuzzi MC. Results of 188 whole-body fluorodeoxyglucose positron emission tomography scans in 137 patients with sarcoidosis. *Chest*. 2007;132(6):1949–1953. https://doi.org/10.1378/chest.07-1178.
47. Tomita H, Ina Y, Sugiura Y, et al. Polymorphism in the angiotensin-converting enzyme (ACE) gene and sarcoidosis. *Am J Respir Crit Care Med*. 1997;156(1):255–259. https://doi.org/10.1164/ajrccm.156.1.9612011.
48. Torrington KG, Shorr AF, Parker JW. Endobronchial disease and racial differences in pulmonary sarcoidosis. *Chest*. 1997;111(3):619–622.
49. Ungprasert P, Carmona EM, Utz JP, Ryu JH, Crowson CS, Matteson EL. Epidemiology of sarcoidosis 1946-2013: a population-based study. *Mayo Clin Proc*. 2016;91(2):183–188. https://doi.org/10.1016/j.mayocp.2015.10.024.
50. Valentonyte R, Hampe J, Huse K, et al. Sarcoidosis is associated with a truncating splice site mutation in BTNL2. *Nat Genet*. 2005;37(4):357–364. https://doi.org/10.1038/ng1519.
51. Veltkamp M, Van Moorsel CHM, Rijkers GT, Ruven HJT, Van Den Bosch JMM, Grutters JC. Toll-like receptor (TLR)-9 genetics and function in sarcoidosis. *Clin Exp Immunol*. 2010;162(1):68–74. https://doi.org/10.1111/j.1365-2249.2010.04205.x.
52. Walsh SL, Wells AU, Sverzellati N, et al. An integrated clinicoradiological staging system for pulmonary sarcoidosis: a case-cohort study. *Lancet Respir Med*. 2014;2(2):123–130. https://doi.org/10.1016/S2213-2600(13)70276-5.
53. Wijnen PA, Nelemans PJ, Verschakelen JA, Bekers O, Voorter CE, Drent M. The role of tumor necrosis factor alpha G-308A polymorphisms in the course of pulmonary sarcoidosis. *Tissue Antigens*. 2010;75(3):262–268. https://doi.org/10.1111/j.1399-0039.2009.01437.x.
54. Yanardag H, Pamuk ON. Bone cysts in sarcoidosis: what is their clinical significance? *Rheumatol Int*. 2004;24(5):294–296. https://doi.org/10.1007/s00296-003-0370-8.

55. Alilovic M, Peros-Golubicic T, Tekavec-Trkanjec J, Smojver-Jezek S, Liscic R. Epidemiological characteristics of sarcoidosis patients hospitalized in the university hospital for lung diseases "Jordanovac" (Zagreb, Croatia) in the 1997–2002 period. *Coll Antropol*. 2006;30(3):513–517.
56. Baughman RP, Field S, Costabel U, et al. Sarcoidosis in America. Analysis based on health care use. *Ann Am Thorac Soc*. 2016;13(8):1244–1252. https://doi.org/10.1513/AnnalsATS.201511-760OC.
57. Cremers JP, Drent M, Bast A, et al. Multinational evidence-based World Association of Sarcoidosis and Other Granulomatous Disorders recommendations for the use of methotrexate in sarcoidosis: integrating systematic literature research and expert opinion of sarcoidologists worldwide. *Curr Opin Pulm Med*. 2013;19(5):545–561. https://doi.org/10.1097/MCP.0b013e3283642a7a.
58. Demirkok SS, Basaranoglu M, Akinci ED, Karayel T. Analysis of 275 patients with sarcoidosis over a 38 year period; a single-institution experience. *Respir Med*. 2007;101(6):1147–1154. https://doi.org/10.1016/j.rmed.2006.11.013.
59. Gupta D, Agarwal R, Aggarwal AN. Seasonality of sarcoidosis: the "heat" is on.... *Sarcoidosis, Vasc Diffus lung Dis Off J WASOG*. 2013;30(3):241–243.
60. Judson MA, Boan AD, Lackland DT. The clinical course of sarcoidosis: presentation, diagnosis, and treatment in a large white and black cohort in the United States. *Sarcoidosis, Vasc Diffus lung Dis Off J WASOG/World Assoc Sarcoidosis Other Granulomatous Disord*. 2012;29(2):119–127.
61. Sogaard KK, Svaerke C, Thomsen RW, Norgaard M. Sarcoidosis and subsequent cancer risk: a Danish nationwide cohort study. *Eur Respir J*. 2015;45(1):269–272. https://doi.org/10.1183/09031936.00084414.
62. Nardi A, Brillet P-Y, Letoumelin P, et al. Stage IV sarcoidosis: comparison of survival with the general population and causes of death. *Eur Respir J*. 2011;38(6):1368–1373. https://doi.org/10.1183/09031936.00187410.
63. Foumani AA, Akhoundzadeh N, Karkan MF. Sarcoidosis, a report from Guilan (an Iranian northern province) (2001–09). *Sarcoidosis, Vasc Diffus lung Dis Off J WASOG*. 2015;31(4):282–288.
64. Arkema EV, Grunewald J, Kullberg S, Eklund A, Askling J. Sarcoidosis incidence and prevalence: a nationwide register-based assessment in Sweden. *Eur Respir J*. 2016;48(6):1690–1699. https://doi.org/10.1183/13993003.00477-2016.
65. Baughman RP, Lower EE. Medical therapy of sarcoidosis. *Semin Respir Crit Care Med*. 2014;35(3):391–406. https://doi.org/10.1055/s-0034-1376401.
66. Cragin LA, Laney AS, Lohff CJ, Martin B, Pandiani JA, Blevins LZ. Use of insurance claims data to determine prevalence and confirm a cluster of sarcoidosis cases in Vermont. *Public Health Rep*. 2009;124(3):442–446. https://doi.org/10.1177/003335490912400314.
67. de Kleijn WPE, Elfferich MDP, De Vries J, et al. Fatigue in sarcoidosis: American versus Dutch patients. *Sarcoidosis, Vasc Diffus lung Dis Off J WASOG*. 2009;26(2):92–97.
68. Deubelbeiss U, Gemperli A, Schindler C, Baty F, Brutsche MH. Prevalence of sarcoidosis in Switzerland is associated with environmental factors. *Eur Respir J*. 2010;35(5):1088–1097. https://doi.org/10.1183/09031936.00197808.
69. Dudvarski-Ilic A, Mihailovic-Vucinic V, Gvozdenovic B, Zugic V, Milenkovic B, Ilic V. Health related quality of life regarding to gender in sarcoidosis. *Coll Antropol*. 2009;33(3):837–840.
70. Erdal BS, Clymer BD, Yildiz VO, Julian MW, Crouser ED. Unexpectedly high prevalence of sarcoidosis in a representative U.S. Metropolitan population. *Respir Med*. 2012;106(6):893–899. https://doi.org/10.1016/j.rmed.2012.02.007.
71. Fernandez Gonzalez S, Lopez Gonzalez R. Epidemiology, presentation forms, radiological stage and diagnostic methods of sarcoidosis in the area of Leon (2001–2008). *Rev Clin Esp*. 2011;211(6):291–297. https://doi.org/10.1016/j.rce.2011.03.001.
72. Gillman A, Steinfort C. Sarcoidosis in Australia. *Intern Med J*. 2007;37(6):356–359. https://doi.org/10.1111/j.1445-5994.2007.01365.x.
73. Gribbin J, Hubbard RB, Le Jeune I, Smith CJP, West J, Tata LJ. Incidence and mortality of idiopathic pulmonary fibrosis and sarcoidosis in the UK. *Thorax*. 2006;61(11):980–985. https://doi.org/10.1136/thx.2006.062836.
74. Grunewald J, Brynedal B, Darlington P, et al. Different HLA-DRB1 allele distributions in distinct clinical subgroups of sarcoidosis patients. *Respir Res*. 2010;11:25. https://doi.org/10.1186/1465-9921-11-25.
75. Hattori T, Konno S, Shijubo N, Ohmichi M, Nishimura M. Increased prevalence of cigarette smoking in Japanese patients with sarcoidosis. *Respirology*. 2013;18(7):1152–1157. https://doi.org/10.1111/resp.12153.
76. Hinz A, Fleischer M, Brahler E, Wirtz H, Bosse-Henck A. Fatigue in patients with sarcoidosis, compared with the general population. *Gen Hosp Psychiat*. 2011;33(5):462–468. https://doi.org/10.1016/j.genhosppsych.2011.05.009.
77. Janot AC, Huscher D, Walker M, et al. Cigarette smoking and male sex are independent and age concomitant risk factors for the development of ocular sarcoidosis in a New Orleans sarcoidosis population. *Sarcoidosis, Vasc Diffus lung Dis Off J WASOG*. 2015;32(2):138–143.
78. Kalkanis A, Yucel RM, Judson MA. The internal consistency of PRO fatigue instruments in sarcoidosis: superiority of the PFI over the FAS. *Sarcoidosis, Vasc Diffus lung Dis Off J WASOG*. 2013;30(1):60–64.
79. Kieszko R, Krawczyk P, Chocholska S, Dmoszynska A, Milanowski J. TNF-alpha and TNF-beta gene polymorphisms in Polish patients with sarcoidosis. Connection with the susceptibility and prognosis. *Sarcoidosis, Vasc Diffus lung Dis Off J WASOG*. 2010;27(2):131–137.
80. Kowalska M, Niewiadomska E, Zejda JE. Epidemiology of sarcoidosis recorded in 2006-2010 in the Silesian voivodeship on the basis of routine medical reporting. *Ann Agric Environ Med*. 2014;21(1):55–58.

81. Kuroda H, Saijo Y, Fujiuchi S, Takeda H, Ohsaki Y, Hasebe N. Relationship between cytokine single nucleotide polymorphisms and sarcoidosis among Japanese subjects. *Sarcoidosis, Vasc Diffus lung Dis Off J WASOG.* 2013;30(1):36–42.
82. Lemos-Silva V, Araujo PB, Lopes C, Rufino R, da Costa CH. Epidemiological characteristics of sarcoidosis patients in the city of Rio de Janeiro, Brazil. *J Bras Pneumol publicacao Of da Soc Bras Pneumol e Tisilogia.* 2011;37(4):438–445.
83. Lill H, Kliiman K, Altraja A. Factors signifying gender differences in clinical presentation of sarcoidosis among Estonian population. *Clin Respir J.* 2016;10(3):282–290. https://doi.org/10.1111/crj.12213.
84. Louzir B, Cherif J, Mehiri N, et al. Sarcoidosis in Tunisia: epidemiologic and clinical study. *Tunis Med.* 2011;89(4):332–335.
85. Matsuo T, Fujiwara N, Nakata Y. First presenting signs or symptoms of sarcoidosis in a Japanese population. *Jpn J Ophthalmol.* 2005;49(2):149–152. https://doi.org/10.1007/s10384-004-0154-z.
86. Mihailovic-Vucinic V, Gvozdenovic B, Stjepanovic M, et al. Administering the sarcoidosis health questionnaire to sarcoidosis patients in Serbia. *J Bras Pneumol publicacao Of da Soc Bras Pneumol e Tisilogia.* 2016;42(2):99–105. https://doi.org/10.1590/S1806-37562015000000063.
87. Mirsaeidi M, Omar HR, Baughman R, Machado R, Sweiss N. The association between BNP, 6MWD test, DLCO% and pulmonary hypertension in sarcoidosis. *Sarcoidosis, Vasc Diffus lung Dis Off J WASOG.* 2016;33(4):317–320.
88. Rodrigues MM, Coletta ENAM, Ferreira RG, Pereira CA de C. Delayed diagnosis of sarcoidosis is common in Brazil. *J Bras Pneumol publicacao Of da Soc Bras Pneumol e Tisilogia.* 2013;39(5):539–546. https://doi.org/10.1590/S1806-37132013000500003.
89. Musellim B, Kumbasar OO, Ongen G, et al. Epidemiological features of Turkish patients with sarcoidosis. *Respir Med.* 2009;103(6):907–912. https://doi.org/10.1016/j.rmed.2008.12.011.
90. Newman LS, Rose CS, Bresnitz EA, et al. A case control etiologic study of sarcoidosis: environmental and occupational risk factors. *Am J Respir Crit Care Med.* 2004;170(12):1324–1330. https://doi.org/10.1164/rccm.200402-249OC.
91. Okumus G, Musellim B, Cetinkaya E, et al. Extrapulmonary involvement in patients with sarcoidosis in Turkey. *Respirology.* 2011;16(3):446–450. https://doi.org/10.1111/j.1440-1843.2010.01878.x.
92. Pabst S, Hammerstingl C, Grau N, et al. Pulmonary arterial hypertension in patients with sarcoidosis: the Pulsar single center experience. *Adv Exp Med Biol.* 2013;755:299–305. https://doi.org/10.1007/978-94-007-4546-9_38.
93. Pietinalho A, Ohmichi M, Hirasawa M, Hiraga Y, Lofroos AB, Selroos O. Familial sarcoidosis in Finland and Hokkaido, Japan–a comparative study. *Respir Med.* 1999;93(6):408–412. https://doi.org/10.1053/rmed.1999.0579.
94. Pizarro C, Goebel A, Dabir D, et al. Cardiovascular magnetic resonance-guided diagnosis of cardiac affection in a Caucasian sarcoidosis population. *Sarcoidosis, Vasc Diffus lung Dis Off J WASOG.* 2016;32(4):325–335.
95. Rabin DL, Richardson MS, Stein SR, Yeager HJ. Sarcoidosis severity and socioeconomic status. *Eur Respir J.* 2001;18(3):499–506.
96. Rapti A, Kouranos V, Gialafos E, et al. Elevated pulmonary arterial systolic pressure in patients with sarcoidosis: prevalence and risk factors. *Lung.* 2013;191(1):61–67. https://doi.org/10.1007/s00408-012-9442-4.
97. Strookappe B, De Vries J, Elfferich M, Kuijpers P, Knevel T, Drent M. Predictors of fatigue in sarcoidosis: the value of exercise testing. *Respir Med.* 2016;116:49–54. https://doi.org/10.1016/j.rmed.2016.05.010.
98. Uygun S, Yanardag H, Karter Y, Demirci S. Course and prognosis of sarcoidosis in a referral setting in Turkey; analysis of 166 patients. *Acta medica.* 2006;49(1):51–57.
99. Wilsher M, Hopkins R, Zeng I, Cornere M, Douglas R. Prevalence of asthma and atopy in sarcoidosis. *Respirology.* 2012;17(2):285–290. https://doi.org/10.1111/j.1440-1843.2011.02066.x.
100. Yigla M, Badarna-Abu-Ria N, Goralnik L, Rubin A-HE, Weiler-Ravell D. Sarcoidosis in residents of northern Israel of Arabic and Jewish origin: a comparative study. *Respirology.* 2006;11(5):586–591. https://doi.org/10.1111/j.1440-1843.2006.00891.x.
101. Zappala CJ, Desai SR, Copley SJ, et al. Optimal scoring of serial change on chest radiography in sarcoidosis. *Sarcoidosis, Vasc Diffus lung Dis Off J WASOG.* 2011;28(2):130–138.
102. Zurkova M, Kolek V, Tomankova T, Kriegova E. Extrapulmonary involvement in patients with sarcoidosis and comparison of routine laboratory and clinical data to pulmonary involvement. *Biomed Pap Med Fac Univ Palacky Olomouc Czech Repub.* 2014;158(4):613–620. https://doi.org/10.5507/bp.2014.026.
103. Behbehani N, JayKrishnan B, Khadadah M, Hawa H, Farah Y. Clinical presentation of sarcoidosis in a mixed population in the middle east. *Respir Med.* 2007;101(11):2284–2288. https://doi.org/10.1016/j.rmed.2007.06.025.
104. Dubrey S, Shah S, Hardman T, Sharma R. Sarcoidosis: the links between epidemiology and aetiology. *Postgrad Med J.* 2014;90(1068):582–589. https://doi.org/10.1136/postgradmedj-2014-132584.
105. Henke CE, Henke G, Elveback LR, Beard CM, Ballard DJ, Kurland LT. The epidemiology of sarcoidosis in Rochester, Minnesota: a population-based study of incidence and survival. *Am J Epidemiol.* 1986;123(5):840–845.
106. Rybicki BA, Major M, Popovich JJ, Maliarik MJ, Iannuzzi MC. Racial differences in sarcoidosis incidence: a 5-year study in a health maintenance organization. *Am J Epidemiol.* 1997;145(3):234–241.
107. Gundelfinger BF, Britten SA. Sarcoidosis in the United States Navy. *Am Rev Respir Dis.* 1961;84(5)Pt(2):109–115. https://doi.org/10.1164/arrd.1961.84.1.109a.

108. Sartwell PE, Edwards LB. Epidemiology of sarcoidosis in the U.S. Navy. *Am J Epidemiol*. 1974;99(4):250–257.
109. Robins AB, Abeles H, Chaves AD. Prevalence and demographic characteristics of sarcoidosis in New York City. *Acta Med Scand Suppl*. 1964;425:149–151.
110. Siltzbach LE, James DG, Neville E, et al. Course and prognosis of sarcoidosis around the world. *Am J Med*. 1974;57(6):847–852.
111. McNicol MW, Luce PJ. Sarcoidosis in a racially mixed community. *J R Coll Physicians Lond*. 1985;19(3):179–183.
112. Brett GZ. Epidemiological trends in tuberculosis and sarcoidosis in a district of London between 1958 and 1963. *Tubercle*. 1965;46(4):413–416.
113. Benatar SR. Sarcoidosis in South Africa. A comparative study in Whites, Blacks and coloureds. *S Afr Med J*. 1977;52(15):602–606.
114. Anantham D, Ong SJ, Chuah KL, Fook-Chong S, Hsu A, Eng P. Sarcoidosis in Singapore: epidemiology, clinical presentation and ethnic differences. *Respirology*. 2007;12(3):355–360. https://doi.org/10.1111/j.1440-1843.2007.01074.x.
115. Sawahata M, Sugiyama Y, Nakamura Y, et al. Age-related and historical changes in the clinical characteristics of sarcoidosis in Japan. *Respir Med*. 2015;109(2):272–278. https://doi.org/10.1016/j.rmed.2014.12.012.
116. Hsing CT, Han FC, Liu HC, Chu BY. Sarcoidosis among Chinese. *Am Rev Respir Dis*. 1964;89:917–922. https://doi.org/10.1164/arrd.1964.89.6.917.
117. Labow TA, Atwood WG, Nelson CT. Sarcoidosis in the American Negro. *Arch Dermatol*. 1964;89:682–689.
118. Burke RR, Stone CH, Havstad S, Rybicki BA. Racial differences in sarcoidosis granuloma density. *Lung*. 2009;187(1):1–7. https://doi.org/10.1007/s00408-008-9111-9.
119. Rabin DL, Thompson B, Brown KM, et al. Sarcoidosis: social predictors of severity at presentation. *Eur Respir J*. 2004;24(4):601–608. https://doi.org/10.1183/09031936.04.00070503.
120. Israel HL, Karlin P, Menduke H, DeLisser OG. Factors affecting outcome of sarcoidosis. Influence of race, extrathoracic involvement, and initial radiologic lung lesions. *Ann N Y Acad Sci*. 1986;465:609–618.
121. Gillum RF. Sarcoidosis in the United States–1968 to 1984. Hospitalization and death. *J Natl Med Assoc*. 1988;80(11):1179–1184.
122. Gideon NM, Mannino DM. Sarcoidosis mortality in the United States 1979–1991: an analysis of multiple-cause mortality data. *Am J Med*. 1996;100(4):423–427. https://doi.org/10.1016/S0002-9343(97)89518-6.
123. Kajdasz DK, Judson MA, Mohr LCJ, Lackland DT. Geographic variation in sarcoidosis in South Carolina: its relation to socioeconomic status and health care indicators. *Am J Epidemiol*. 1999;150(3):271–278.
124. Gerke AK, Yang M, Tang F, Cavanaugh JE, Polgreen PM. Increased hospitalizations among sarcoidosis patients from 1998 to 2008: a population-based cohort study. *BMC Pulm Med*. 2012;12:19. https://doi.org/10.1186/1471-2466-12-19.
125. Gorham ED, Garland CF, Garland FC, Kaiser K, Travis WD, Centeno JA. Trends and occupational associations in incidence of hospitalized pulmonary sarcoidosis and other lung diseases in Navy personnel: a 27-year historical prospective study, 1975–2001. *Chest*. 2004;126(5):1431–1438. https://doi.org/10.1378/chest.126.5.1431.
126. Mirsaeidi M, Machado RF, Schraufnagel D, Sweiss NJ, Baughman RP. Racial difference in sarcoidosis mortality in the United States. *Chest*. 2015;147(2):438–449. https://doi.org/10.1378/chest.14-1120.
127. Swigris JJ, Olson AL, Huie TJ, et al. Sarcoidosis-related mortality in the United States from 1988 to 2007. *Am J Respir Crit Care Med*. 2011;183(11):1524–1530. https://doi.org/10.1164/rccm.201010-1679OC.
128. Glennas A, Kvien TK, Melby K, et al. Acute sarcoid arthritis: occurrence, seasonal onset, clinical features and outcome. *Br J Rheumatol*. 1995;34(1):45–50.
129. Blasi A, Pezza A. Epidemiology of sarcoidosis in Italy. *Sarcoidosis*. 1989;6(1):55–56.
130. Hosoda Y, Hiraga Y, Odaka M, et al. A cooperative study of sarcoidosis in Asia and Africa: analytic epidemiology. *Ann N Y Acad Sci*. 1976;278:355–367.
131. Yamaguchi M, Hosoda Y, Sasaki R, Aoki K. Epidemiological study on sarcoidosis in Japan. Recent trends in incidence and prevalence rates and changes in epidemiological features. *Sarcoidosis*. 1989;6(2):138–146.
132. Byg K-E, Milman N, Hansen S. Sarcoidosis in Denmark 1980–1994. A registry-based incidence study comprising 5536 patients. *Sarcoidosis, Vasc Diffus lung Dis Off J WASOG*. 2003;20(1):46–52.
133. Dumas O, Abramovitz L, Wiley AS, Cozier YC, Camargo CAJ. Epidemiology of sarcoidosis in a prospective cohort study of U.S. Women. *Ann Am Thorac Soc*. 2016;13(1):67–71. https://doi.org/10.1513/AnnalsATS.201508-568BC.
134. Ungprasert P, Crowson CS, Matteson EL. Seasonal variation in incidence of sarcoidosis: a population-based study, 1976-2013. *Thorax*. August 2016. https://doi.org/10.1136/thoraxjnl-2016-209032.
135. Visser H, Vos K, Zanelli E, et al. Sarcoid arthritis: clinical characteristics, diagnostic aspects, and risk factors. *Ann Rheum Dis*. 2002;61(6):499–504.
136. Demirkok SS, Basaranoglu M, Coker E, Karayel T. Seasonality of the onset of symptoms, tuberculin test anergy and Kveim positive reaction in a large cohort of patients with sarcoidosis. *Respirology*. 2007;12(4):591–593. https://doi.org/10.1111/j.1440-1843.2007.01062.x.
137. Wilsher ML. Seasonal clustering of sarcoidosis presenting with erythema nodosum. *Eur Respir J*. 1998;12(5):1197–1199.
138. Hosoda Y, Yamaguchi M, Hiraga Y. Global epidemiology of sarcoidosis. What story do prevalence and incidence tell us? *Clin Chest Med*. 1997;18(4):681–694.
139. Kieszko R, Krawczyk P, Powrozek T, et al. The impact of ACE gene polymorphism on the incidence and phenotype of sarcoidosis in rural and urban settings. *Arch Med Sci*. 2016;12(6):1263–1272. https://doi.org/10.5114/aoms.2015.48966.

140. Alcoba Leza M, Perez-Simon MR, Guerra Laso JM, et al. Sarcoidosis in a sanitary area at Leon (Spain). Epidemiology and clinical features. *An Med Interna.* 2003;20(12):617–620.
141. Buxbaum L, Judson H, Mohr. Geographic patterns of pulmonary disease in South Carolina. *Ann Epidemiol.* 2000;10(7):460–461.
142. Gupta D, Vinay N, Agarwal R, Agarwal AN. Socio-demographic profile of patients with sarcoidosis vis-a-vis tuberculosis. *Sarcoidosis, Vasc Diffus lung Dis Off J WASOG.* 2013;30(3):186–193.
143. Werner E. Boeck's disease as an occupational disease. *Tuberkulosearzt.* 1959;13:780–785.
144. Seiler E. On the epidemiology of sarcoidosis (Boeck's disease) in Switzerland. Statistical research on the geographical and occupational distribution of 108 military patients with sarcoidosis. *Schweizerische Zeitschrift fur Tuberkulose und Pneumonol Rev suisse la Tuberc Pneumonol Riv Svizz della Tuberc e della Pneumonol.* 1960;17:205–228.
145. Newman KL, Newman LS. Occupational causes of sarcoidosis. *Curr Opin Allergy Clin Immunol.* 2012;12(2):145–150. https://doi.org/10.1097/ACI.0b013e3283515173.
146. Rossman MD, Thompson B, Frederick M, et al. HLA and environmental interactions in sarcoidosis. *Sarcoidosis, Vasc Diffus lung Dis Off J WASOG.* 2008;25(2):125–132.
147. Kajdasz DK, Lackland DT, Mohr LC, Judson MA. A current assessment of rurally linked exposures as potential risk factors for sarcoidosis. *Ann Epidemiol.* 2001;11(2):111–117.
148. Kucera GP, Rybicki BA, Kirkey KL, et al. Occupational risk factors for sarcoidosis in African-American siblings. *Chest.* 2003;123(5):1527–1535.
149. Barnard J, Rose C, Newman L, et al. Job and industry classifications associated with sarcoidosis in A case-control etiologic study of sarcoidosis (ACCESS). *J Occup Environ Med.* 2005;47(3):226–234.
150. Kreider ME, Christie JD, Thompson B, et al. Relationship of environmental exposures to the clinical phenotype of sarcoidosis. *Chest.* 2005;128(1):207–215. https://doi.org/10.1378/chest.128.1.207.
151. Jordan HT, Stellman SD, Prezant D, Teirstein A, Osahan SS, Cone JE. Sarcoidosis diagnosed after September 11, 2001, among adults exposed to the World Trade Center disaster. *J Occup Environ Med.* 2011;53(9):966–974. https://doi.org/10.1097/JOM.0b013e31822a3596.
152. Liu H, Patel D, Welch AM, et al. Association between occupational exposures and sarcoidosis: an analysis from death certificates in the United States, 1988–1999. *Chest.* 2016;150(2):289–298. https://doi.org/10.1016/j.chest.2016.01.020.
153. Prezant DJ, Dhala A, Goldstein A, et al. The incidence, prevalence, and severity of sarcoidosis in New York City firefighters. *Chest.* 1999;116(5):1183–1193.
154. Crowley LE, Herbert R, Moline JM, et al. "Sarcoid like" granulomatous pulmonary disease in World Trade Center disaster responders. *Am J Ind Med.* 2011;54(3):175–184. https://doi.org/10.1002/ajim.20924.
155. Valeyre D, Soler P, Clerici C, et al. Smoking and pulmonary sarcoidosis: effect of cigarette smoking on prevalence, clinical manifestations, alveolitis, and evolution of the disease. *Thorax.* 1988;43(7):516–524.
156. Hance AJ, Basset F, Saumon G, et al. Smoking and interstitial lung disease. The effect of cigarette smoking on the incidence of pulmonary histiocytosis X and sarcoidosis. *Ann N Y Acad Sci.* 1986;465:643–656.
157. Harf RA, Ethevenaux C, Gleize J, Perrin-Fayolle M, Guerin JC, Ollagnier C. Reduced prevalence of smokers in sarcoidosis. Results of a case-control study. *Ann N Y Acad Sci.* 1986;465:625–631.
158. Douglas JG, Middleton WG, Gaddie J, et al. Sarcoidosis: a disorder commoner in non-smokers? *Thorax.* 1986;41(10):787–791.
159. Gupta D, Singh AD, Agarwal R, Aggarwal AN, Joshi K, Jindal SK. Is tobacco smoking protective for sarcoidosis? A case-control study from North India. *Sarcoidosis, Vasc Diffus lung Dis Off J WASOG.* 2010;27(1):19–26.
160. Cozier YC, Berman JS, Palmer JR, Boggs DA, Serlin DM, Rosenberg L. Sarcoidosis in black women in the United States: data from the black women's health study. *Chest.* 2011;139(1):144–150. https://doi.org/10.1378/chest.10-0413.
161. Gvozdenovic BS, Mihailovic-Vucinic V, Vukovic M, et al. Effect of obesity on patient-reported outcomes in sarcoidosis. *Int J Tuberc Lung Dis.* 2013;17(4):559–564. https://doi.org/10.5588/ijtld.12.0665.
162. Moskvina V, Smith M, Ivanov D, et al. Genetic differences between five European populations. *Hum Hered.* 2010;70(2):141–149. https://doi.org/10.1159/000313854.

CHAPTER 2

Environmental and Infectious Causes of Sarcoidosis

OZIOMA S. CHIOMA, PHD • ALEXANDER GELBARD, MD • WONDER P. DRAKE, MD

ABBREVIATION

BAL Bronchoalveolar lavage

INTRODUCTION

Sarcoidosis is a systemic multiorgan inflammatory disease of unknown etiology, characterized by the presence of noncaseating epithelioid granulomas most commonly involving the lungs and lymph nodes.[1,2] While two-thirds of sarcoidosis patients spontaneously resolve the disease, one-third of patients experience persistent and recurring disease. Twenty percent of Sarcoidosis patients progress to pulmonary fibrosis, which can be highly fatal.[3,4]

The immunopathogenesis of pulmonary sarcoidosis involves antigen-driven CD4+ T-cell activation, due to exposure to putative inhaled antigen(s) in genetically susceptible individuals. Dendritic cells present these antigens to CD4+ T cells, which leads to their activation and proliferation. This is followed by chemokine-orchestrated recruitment of activated T cells to the lung. Proinflammatory cytokines such as IL-2, interferon γ (IFN-γ), as well as tumor necrosis factor α (TNF-α), transforming growth factor β (TGF-β), interleukin 5 and 17 (IL-5 and IL-17) are released, which aid the recruitment of other immune cells. This carefully orchestrated recruitment results in granuloma formation.

Sarcoidosis is a worldwide disease that affects all races and ages. In the United States, the annual incidence varies widely by races/ethnicities: 11 per 100,000 in US Caucasian subjects and 36 per 100,000 in US African American subjects.[5,6] African Americans are three times more likely than Caucasian Americans to develop sarcoidosis, and African American women are the most affected group with a 3% lifetime risk of getting the inflammatory disease, which often remains untreated.[5,7] Sarcoidosis in African Americans is more likely to be chronic, involves multiple organs, and leads to death.[8]

Although the etiology of the disease remains unknown, evidence from immunologic, microbiologic, genetic, and epidemiological studies suggests that exposure to certain environmental factors in genetically susceptible individuals may play a role in the etiology of the disease. In this chapter, we will focus on the environmental triggers, such as exposure to infectious agents, as well as organic and inorganic particulate matter.

Fig. 2.1 highlights the different environmental and infectious causes of sarcoidosis based on a systematic review of the current literature research.

Environmental Triggers

Seasonal clustering in the northern (United Kingdom, Norway, Greece, Spain, Finland, and Japan) and southern (New Zealand) hemisphere provided one of the earliest evidence of a link between the environment and incidence of sarcoidosis.[9–16]

Badrinas and colleagues reviewed the records of 423 cases of sarcoidosis diagnosed between 1972 and 1986 in three University Hospitals in Barcelona and reported that all cases were resident in the same geographical location, and symptoms were first noticed in spring season.[13] Other researchers have also shown evidence of temporal and spatial clustering of sarcoidosis cases[17–19] as well as familial cases of sarcoidosis.[20,21] These observations support the possibility of a shared environmental exposure or a transmissible agent in the etiology of sarcoidosis. Furthermore, because sarcoidosis most commonly involves the lungs, exposure to airborne agents in susceptible individuals has been suspected. Assessment of occupations associated with the development of pulmonary sarcoidosis implicates work environments associated with aerosolization.[22] Environmental triggers of sarcoidosis such as organic matter, inorganic particulate matter, or infectious agents are among the leading suspects.[22]

Sarcoidosis. https://doi.org/10.1016/B978-0-323-54429-0.00002-1

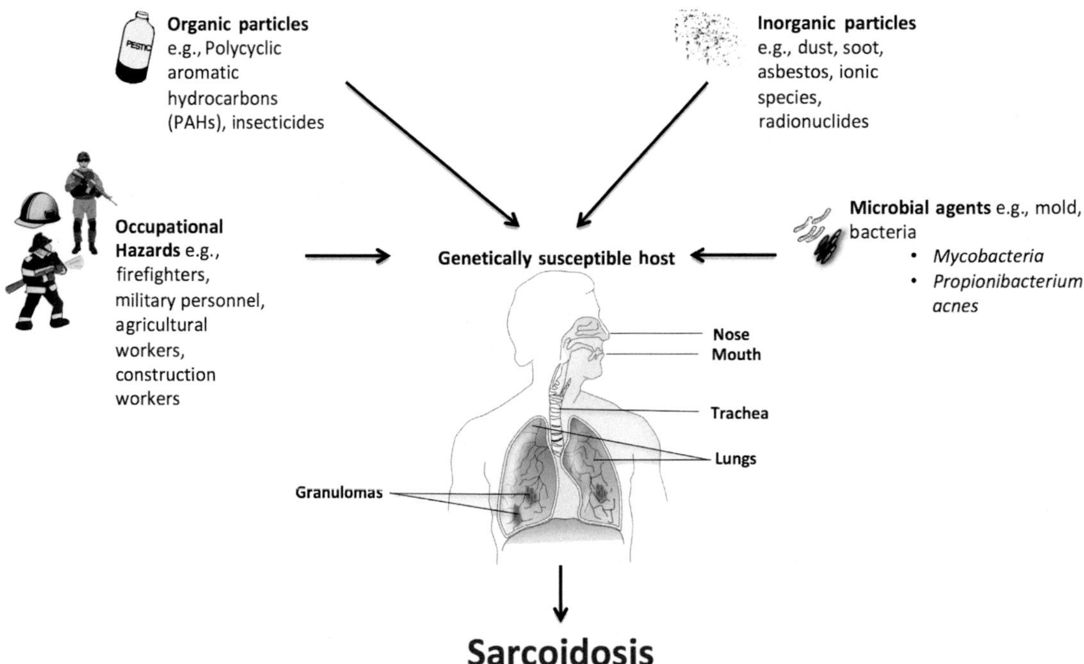

FIG. 2.1 **Environmental and Infectious Causes of Sarcoidosis.** Based on research studies, sarcoidosis has been associated with exposure to environmental and infectious agents, which increase the risk factors of sarcoidosis in genetically susceptible hosts. These factors include exposure to organic particles, inorganic particulate matter, and certain microbial agents. In addition, some occupations increase the risk of sarcoidosis by increased exposure to inorganic, organic, or microbial agents. The lungs are the organs most affected by sarcoidosis, and formation of granulomas in the affected organ is typical of the disease.

A Case Control Etiologic Study of Sarcoidosis (ACCESS) was conducted across 10 centers with 706 newly diagnosed sarcoidosis patients to evaluate the environmental and occupational risk factors of sarcoidosis.[22] Although the study did not recognize a single, predominant cause of sarcoidosis, positive associations were observed between sarcoidosis and specific occupations such as agricultural employments (exposure to insecticides at work) and work environments with mold/mildew exposures.[22] These observations strengthen the possibility of a shared environmental exposure or a transmissible agent in the etiology of sarcoidosis.

Currently, the focus is on infectious agents, especially species of *Mycobacterium* and *Propionibacterium*. Metaanalyses of Mycobacteria and Propionibacteria studies show the involvement of these bacteria in sarcoidosis.[23,24] Other infectious agents have been investigated with inconclusive or conflicting results, such as *Borrelia burgdorferi, Rickettsia helvetica, Chlamydia pneumoniae,* viruses (Human Herpesvirus 6, 8), fungal infections, and *Leishmania* species.[25–33]

Bacteria

There is increasing evidence that points to bacterial involvement in the etiology of sarcoidosis. Over the past decade, propionibacteria[34,35] and mycobacteria[36] have been the two organisms of interest in the disease. Both organisms can exist in macrophages, owing to the high lipid contents of their cell wall, Although meta-analysis shows a strong correlation between both mycobacteria and propionibacteria[24] with sarcoidosis,[23,37] there is no consensus as to which of the two organisms is the major culprit primarily due to the absence of histologic or culture evidence of a replicating organism. Limited heterogeneity in the T-cell receptors suggests antigenic stimulation with limited repertoire of pathogenic antigen(s). Defining the microbial community within sarcoidosis granulomas using culture-independent mechanisms will greatly aid the efforts to identify possible infectious agents.

Mycobacteria

One of the earliest evidences of the presence of mycobacteria in sarcoidosis tissue was reported by Hanngren and colleagues in 1987, when they detected the mycobacterial saturated fatty acid, tuberculostearic acid, in the lymph nodes of sarcoidosis patients by gas chromatography and mass spectrometry.[38]

Mycobacteria are aerobic bacteria that are typically acid fast.[39] The distinguishing feature is its cell wall, which is mycolic acid–rich, and a polysaccharide, arabinogalactan, that holds the peptidoglycan layer in place. This characteristic cell wall contributes to its hardiness. The high lipid contents of their cell wall allow this organism to exist in host macrophages.

Several studies have since emerged that report evidence of mycobacterial constituents from sarcoidosis tissues. Various researchers have documented the presence of Mycobacterial antigens from nucleic acid,[40–43] protein,[44] and immunologic evidence.[36,41,45–50]

A metaanalysis conducted by Gupta and colleagues to evaluate the available molecular evidence on the possible role of mycobacteria in the etiology of sarcoidosis showed demonstrable mycobacterial presence in sarcoidosis lesions, suggesting an association between mycobacteria and some cases of sarcoidosis.[23]

Drake and colleagues have shown the presence of mycobacterial DNA in sarcoidosis tissues by amplification of mycobacterial genes such as 16srRNA and rpoB,[51] and the detection of Th-1 immune response to mycobacterial antigens such as early-secreted antigenic target protein (E-SAT-6), catalase-peroxidase (KatG).[36,41] Furthermore, Carlisle and associates also showed that mycobacterial antigens such as mycobacterial superoxide dismutase A (sodA), katG, and ESAT-6 induce IFN-ϒ production, [47] while others show T-cell response to *Mycobacterium tuberculosis* catalase peroxidase [48] and superoxide dismutase (SodA).[45]

There are limited therapeutic options available for the treatment of sarcoidosis; therefore the success of broad-spectrum antimycobacterial therapies in several cases of sarcoidosis[52–54] is an indication that mycobacteria may play a role in this disease. Drake and colleagues showed that the use of broad-spectrum antimycobacterial therapy, levofloxacin, ethambutol, azithromycin, and rifampin (the CLEAR regimen) for treatment of chronic, pulmonary sarcoidosis, is associated with improved absolute forced vital capacities, as well as increased functional capacity and quality of life in selected chronic pulmonary sarcoidosis patients.[52] Another randomized, placebo-controlled study by the Drake group using the CLEAR regimen revealed significant reductions in chronic cutaneous sarcoidosis lesion diameter and reversal of pathways associated with disease severity and enhanced T-cell function following T-cell receptor stimulation.[53]

The use of experimental disease models in research has dramatically improved our understanding of the etiology and progression of human diseases and has proven to be a useful tool for discovering targets for therapeutic interventions. Several disease models have been established that show Th-1 and Th-17 immune responses directed against mycobacterial or propionibacterial antigens.[55–57] Chen and colleagues showed the effects of serum amyloid A on regulating helper T-cell type 1 (Th1) granulomatous inflammation using *M. tuberculosis* catalase-peroxidase murine model of sarcoidosis,[58] while Swaisgood and associates showed that mycobacterial superoxide dismutase A (SodA) in murine model of sarcoidosis induced increased levels of Th1 cytokines (especially IL-2 and IFN-γ).[55]

Furthermore, similarities in the transcriptome profile of sarcoidosis to tuberculosis infection support common immunologic pathway and a possible link with mycobacteria.[59–62] Maertzdorf and colleagues investigated the transcriptomes of peripheral blood cells from active tuberculosis and sarcoidosis patients with the transcriptomes of healthy individuals as controls, and they found a highly similar upregulation of IFN-signaling and IFN-inducible genes in blood expression profiles between tuberculosis and sarcoidosis.[59] Koth and colleagues also analyzed transcriptomic data from blood and lung biopsies in sarcoidosis and compared these profiles with blood transcriptomic data from tuberculosis and other diseases. They found that there is shared overlap between sarcoidosis and tuberculosis in blood gene expression compared with other diseases.[62]

Despite multiple studies showing the involvement of mycobacteria in sarcoidosis, the mechanism of pathogenesis remains unclear. This is primarily due to the lack of evidence of actively replicating mycobacteria from sarcoidosis tissues.[63] Furthermore, injection of homogenates of lymph node and skin biopsy specimens and lymphocyte suspensions from patients with sarcoidosis and control subjects into the footpads of CBA/J mice failed to confirm previous reports of a "transmissible agent" as granulomas developed in both groups.[64] Others have demonstrated that inoculation of mice with BAL homogenates or sputum from sarcoidosis patients failed to induce granulomas and resulted in mild and local inflammation.[65]

Conflicting reports from other experimental models of sarcoidosis[66] show that organisms not related to sarcoidosis have been reported to induce sarcoid-like granulomas in murine disease models. Such microorganisms include *Cryptococcus neoformans*[67] and

Schistosoma mansoni[68]; however, the granuloma histology and immunologic responses in both cases are different from that observed in cases of sarcoidosis.

Propionibacteria

Propionibacterium is another genus of bacteria implicated in the etiology of sarcoidosis primarily because it can be cultured from sarcoidosis tissue.[35,69–71] Other experimental findings from nucleic acids,[72–78] immune response,[34,57,79–86] and experimental disease models[87,88] of sarcoidosis also support the association of this bacteria with sarcoidosis.

Propionibacterium acnes is the prionibacterial species mostly associated with sarcoidosis, although *Propionibacterium granulosum is present in some cases.*[72,73,77] *P. acnes* is a Gram-positive, rod-shaped anaerobic-aerotolerant bacillus, largely commensal and commonly found in the skin flora, ear, oral cavity, and intestinal tract.[89–91] Homma and colleagues reported *P. acnes* could be isolated from sarcoidosis biopsy specimens, primarily lymph nodes.[71] Since then, numerous studies have been done to elucidate the role of propionibacteria in sarcoidosis. Several experimental models of sarcoidosis report host immune response to live, heat-killed, or microbial constituents of *P. acnes.*[87,88,92,93]

Antibiotics have also been successfully used as therapeutic interventions in cases of *P. acnes*–associated sarcoidosis. Takemori and colleagues report success of the antimicrobial clarithromycin in improving *P. acnes*–associated sarcoidosis, possible due to the induction of apoptosis induced in sarcoid granulomas.[94] It is noteworthy that clarithromycin also possesses immunosuppressive and immunomodulatory properties in addition to its antimycobacterial effects. These properties cannot be ruled out as contributors of the improvement in *P. acnes*–associated sarcoidosis following administration of this drug. Bachelez and colleagues also reported that the tetracyclines, minocycline, and doxycycline may be beneficial for the treatment of cutaneous sarcoidosis.[95] The tetracyclines also have antimicrobial as well as antiinflammatory properties, therefore it is controversial as to which mechanism (or both) is employed in tetracycline-induced killing of microbes in sarcoid granulomas.

An international collaborative effort conducted by Ishige and colleagues to evaluate the etiological link between sarcoidosis and suspected bacterial species from paraffin-embedded lymph nodes of sarcoidosis patients, collected from two institutes in Japan and three institutes in Italy, Germany, and England, resulted in detection of genomes of *P. acnes, P. granulosum, M. tuberculosis,* and *Mycobacterium avium* subsp. Paratuberculosis.[73] However, the investigators report higher total genome numbers *of P. acnes, P. granulosum* in sarcoidosis lymph nodes compared with the mycobacterial strains, and thus conclude that Propionibacteria is more likely to cause sarcoidosis.

Sarcoidosis is characterized by the accumulation of immune cells, i.e., macrophages and lymphocytes in the alveoli,[96] and an increase in proinflammatory cytokines.[1,97] Several studies have shown host immune response on *P. acnes* exposure in sarcoidosis disease models. Mori and colleagues report *P. acnes*–induced production of interleukin-2 (IL-2), a proinflammatory cytokine, produced by alveolar lymphocytes.[83] This observation is also corroborated by Furusawa and colleagues in the peripheral blood mononuclear cell (PBMC) obtained from sarcoidosis patients.[57] Secretion of other proinflammatory cytokines has also been reported in other studies after BAL or PBMCs from sarcoidosis patients were stimulated with *P. acnes.*[79,80] While *P. acnes* is implicated in sarcoidosis, little is known about the mechanism of pathogenesis in this disease. *P. acnes* is known to be cutaneous and pulmonary normal flora. One postulation by Eishi and colleagues is that *P. acnes* may exist in the lymph nodes and lungs in a latent form, which gets reactivated in certain susceptible hosts, i.e., patients with *P. acnes* hypersensitivity. In these patients, the reactivated infection could then go on to cause systemic sarcoidosis.[98]

Although metaanalysis shows a strong correlation between sarcoidosis and propionibacteria,[24] there is currently no consensus on the etiology of sarcoidosis owing to the fact that *P. acnes* are the most common commensal bacteria in the lungs and lymph nodes; therefore it can also be detected in healthy individuals. Some have argued that it is found in greater amounts in sarcoidosis patients than in healthy controls, but this could be as a result of the immunocompromised state of the hosts.

Fungi: Indoor Air and Mold

There is increasing evidence that exposure to molds (fungi) may influence the development of sarcoidosis[99–102] and the effectiveness of antifungal therapy in the treatment of sarcoidosis.[103–105] Tercelj and colleagues investigated the homes of patients with active and recurrent sarcoidosis for fungal presence using the enzyme *N*-acetylhexosaminidase (NAHA) as a marker of fungal cell biomass to detect the presence of fungal cells. They reported higher activities of NAHA enzyme in homes of sarcoidosis patients, suggesting that exposure to fungi is related to increased risk of sarcoidosis.[99] Laney and colleagues also reported that sarcoidosis developed in a group of individuals working in a water-damaged and mold-infested building.[102]

While the detection of mold in the environment may not directly mean the presence of an infection, findings indicate that fungi in the environment could play a role in the development of sarcoidosis, as several components of the fungal cell wall such as β-glucan or chitin can stimulate immune reactions leading to a late hypersensitivity reaction, resulting in the formation of granulomas.[101]

A recent study by Clarke and colleagues employed metagenomics DNA sequencing of two distinct sets of paraffin-embedded sarcoidosis specimens, as well as nonsarcoidosis controls and various environmental cohorts. Sarcoidosis specimens consisted of two independent sets of formalin-fixed, paraffin-embedded lymph node biopsies, BAL, Kveim reagent, and fresh granulomatous spleen from a patient with sarcoidosis. All specimens were analyzed by bacterial 16S and fungal internal transcribed spacer ribosomal RNA gene sequencing. In one tissue set, fungi in the Cladosporiaceae family were enriched in sarcoidosis compared with nonsarcoidosis tissues; in the other tissue set, we detected enrichment of several bacterial lineages in sarcoidosis but not Cladosporiaceae. BAL showed limited enrichment of Aspergillus fungi. Several microbial lineages were detected in Kveim and spleen, including Cladosporium. Most notable was the identification of the Cladosporiaceae fungal family and *Corynebacterium* bacterial taxa. No microbial lineage was enriched in more than one sample type after correction for multiple comparisons.[106]

OTHER MICROBIAL AGENTS

Other microbial agents have been investigated with inconclusive or conflicting results, such as *B. burgdorferi*,[26] *R. helvetica*,[25,27] *C. pneumoniae*,[29,30,107] viruses and *Leishmania* species.[25–33] While there is lack of microbiologic and clinical data for the association of viruses, lymphotropic viruses such as *Cytomegalovirus*,[108,109] Human Herpesvirus 6[31] and 8[28,110] (HHV6, HHV8), Human T-lymphotropic virus-1 (HTLV1)[111,112] with sarcoidosis, immunologic evidence, in the form of high circulating antibody titers, has been observed in sarcoidosis patients.

Occupational Hazard and Exposure to Organic/Inorganic Particulate Matter

Several studies have explored occupational risk factors for sarcoidosis. Sarcoidosis can occur in workplace settings where individuals are exposed to foreign antigens and inorganic particulate matter, which then triggers inflammation and an exuberant granulomatous immune response.

Firefighters/rescue workers (exposure to heavy dust, nanoparticles, carbon exposure),[113–115] military personnel (organic dust, wood dust, metal dust, wood burning),[116–118] construction workers (inorganic dust),[119] mining and agricultural workers (silicates, insecticides, pesticides, mold/mildew)[22,120] have an increased risk of sarcoidosis.

A 7-year study on sarcoidosis in the Isle of Man during 1962–83 showed that healthcare workers (particularly nurses) had an increased incidence of sarcoidosis (18.8%) compared with control group (4.2% incidence),[18,121] and other studies have supported this finding.[122,123]

In 1985, The New York City Fire Department (FDNY) started a program to monitor the incidence, prevalence, and severity of biopsy-proven sarcoidosis in firefighters. Studies conducted by Prezant and colleagues between 1985 and 1998, showed 4 prior cases and 21 new cases of sarcoidosis among FDNY firefighters, resulting in a significantly higher annual incidence of sarcoidosis than FDNY Emergency Medical Services workers and other control subjects.[113] While the average yearly rate of sarcoidosis in firefighters was at 12.9 per 100,000, following the World Trade Center (WTC) attack on September 11, 2001, the incidence of sarcoidosis in WTC-exposed FDNY rescue workers increased to 25 per 100,000. Some of the potential culprits include inorganic antigens such as metals, fibers (glass and asbestos), organic pollutants (polychlorinated biphenyls, pesticides, and polycyclic aromatic hydrocarbons), and particulate matter (calcium carbonate and silica).[114]

Epidemiological and experimental studies support the link between nanoparticles and sarcoidosis,[124–127] and with the increasing production of nanomaterials the impact on health is worrisome.[128–131] Huizar and colleagues demonstrated using a murine model of carbon nanoparticles that nanoparticles can induce granuloma-like lesions resembling chronic human lung granulomatous inflammation.[132] Another group showed that exposure to cadmium-based nanoparticle, quantum dot 75, induced chronic inflammation and granuloma formation in the lungs of mice.[133]

Table 2.1 provides evidence of different environmental, infectious, and occupational factors associated with sarcoidosis.

Until now, no single environmental, infectious, or genetic factor is on its own linked to the etiology of sarcoidosis. A combined role of these factors in genetically susceptible individuals is the current understanding. Most of these findings on occupations that expose an individual to the risk of sarcoidosis are based on epidemiological data solely. More robust studies that combine clinical, microbiologic, and immunologic evidence is needed to delineate the link between environmental agents and sarcoidosis.

TABLE 2.1
Evidence of Environmental and Infectious Factors Implicated in the Etiology of Sarcoidosis

Environmental Factors	Evidence	References
1. INFECTIOUS AGENTS		
Bacteria		
a. Mycobacteria	• Nucleic acid	40, 42, 43, 45, 51
	• Cell constituent	38
	• Immune response and circulating antibodies	36,41,46–50,134–138
	• Success of Antimycobacterial therapy	52–54
	• Experimental disease models	55,58,68,139–149
	• Proteomics	44
	• Metaanalysis	23, 37
	• *Mycobacterium tuberculosis* infection triggered	150
	• Similarities in transcriptome profile of sarcoidosis to tuberculosis infection	59–62
b. Propionibacteria	• Bacterial culture	35,69–71
	• Immune response, immunohistochemistry	34,57,79–87,151,152
	• Microbial components	72, 73
	• Nucleic acid	72–78,153
	• Success of antibiotics	94, 95, 154, 155
	• Experimental disease models	87,88,92,93,156–160
	• Metaanalysis	24
c. *Chlamydia pneumoniae*	• Immune response	29, 30, 107
Viruses		
Epstein-Barr virus (EBV)	• Antibodies, immunosuppression therapy may contribute to an increased risk for the development of EBV in sarcoidosis patients	161, 162, 163
Human herpesvirus 6 (HHV6)	• Antibodies	31
Human herpesvirus 8 (HHV8)	• Antibodies	28
Human T-lymphotropic virus 1 (HTLV1)	• Antibodies	112, 164
Cytomegalovirus (CMV)	• Antibodies	108, 109
Fungi		
Molds	• Immune response and elevated N-acetylhexosaminidase (NAHA) in homes of sarcoidosis patients	33,99–101
	• Success of antifungal therapy	103–105
Borrelia burgdorferi	• Nucleic acid and immunohistochemistry	26
Rickettsia helvetica	• Nucleic acid	25, 27
Leishmania species	• Nucleic acid	32

TABLE 2.1
Evidence of Environmental and Infectious Factors Implicated in the Etiology of Sarcoidosis—cont'd

Environmental Factors	Evidence	References
2. INORGANIC PARTICLES		
Construction materials, soot, paint (leaded and unleaded), fibers (e.g., mineral wool, fiberglass, asbestos, wood, paper, and cotton), metals, radionuclides, and ionic species	• Data from World Trade Center attacks	114
Nanoparticles	• Experimental models of sarcoidosis	132, 133, 165, 166
	• Saroid-like granulomas developing after exposure to nanoparticles	124–127
	• Immune response	167, 168
3. ORGANIC PARTICLES		
	• Polycyclic aromatic hydrocarbons (PAHs), polychlorinated biphenyls, polychlorinated dibenzodioxins, polychlorinated dibenzofurans, pesticides, phthalate esters, brominated diphenyl ethers, and other hydrocarbons	114
4. OCCUPATIONAL HAZARD		
Fire/rescue workers, heavy dust exposure, nanoparticles, carbon	• Epidemiologic evidence	113–115
Agricultural workers	• Epidemiologic evidence, insecticides, pesticides, mold/mildew, silicates	22, 120, 169
Military/navy personnel	• Organic dust, wood dust, metal dust, wood burning	117, 118, 170, 171
Mining silicates	• Epidemiologic evidence	172
Metal industries, metal dust, metal-working fluid, aerosols	• Epidemiologic evidence	173–175
Construction inorganic dust	• Epidemiologic evidence	119, 126
Office jobs		
Indoor air (molds, bacteria, microbial contaminant)	• Immunologic and epidemiologic evidence	22, 102
Healthcare workers	• Epidemiological evidence	18, 122, 123

REFERENCES

1. Statement on sarcoidosis. Joint Statement of the American Thoracic Society (ATS), the European Respiratory Society (ERS) and the World association of sarcoidosis and other granulomatous disorders (WASOG) adopted by the ATS board of Directors and by the ERS Executive Committee, February 1999. *Am J Respir Crit Care Med.* 1999;160(2):736–755.
2. Iwai K, Tachibana T, Takemura T, Matsui Y, Kitaichi M, Kawabata Y. Pathological studies on sarcoidosis autopsy. I. Epidemiological features of 320 cases in Japan. *Acta Pathol Jpn.* 1993;43(7–8):372–376.
3. Bonham CA, Strek ME, Patterson KC. From granuloma to fibrosis: sarcoidosis associated pulmonary fibrosis. *Curr Opin Pulm Med.* 2016;22(5):484–491.
4. Patterson KC, Strek ME. Pulmonary fibrosis in sarcoidosis. Clinical features and outcomes. *Ann Am Thorac Soc.* 2013;10(4):362–370.
5. Rybicki BA, Major M, Popovich Jr J, Maliarik MJ, Iannuzzi MC. Racial differences in sarcoidosis incidence: a 5-year study in a health maintenance organization. *Am J Epidemiol.* 1997;145(3):234–241.
6. Rybicki BA, Maliarik MJ, Major M, Popovich Jr J, Iannuzzi MC. Epidemiology, demographics, and genetics of sarcoidosis. *Semin Respir Infect.* 1998;13(3):166–173.

7. Tukey MH, Berman JS, Boggs DA, White LF, Rosenberg L, Cozier YC. Mortality among African American women with sarcoidosis: data from the Black Women's health study. *Sarcoidosis Vasc Dif.* 2013;30(2):128–133.
8. Israel HL, Karlin P, Menduke H, DeLisser OG. Factors affecting outcome of sarcoidosis. Influence of race, extrathoracic involvement, and initial radiologic lung lesions. *Ann N Y Acad Sci.* 1986;465:609–618.
9. Glennas A, Kvien TK, Melby K, et al. Acute sarcoid arthritis: occurrence, seasonal onset, clinical features and outcome. *Br J Rheumatol.* 1995;34(1):45–50.
10. Panayeas S, Theodorakopoulos P, Bouras A, Constantopoulos S. Seasonal occurrence of sarcoidosis in Greece. *Lancet.* 1991;338(8765):510–511.
11. Jawad AS, Hamour AA, Wenley WG, Scott DG. An outbreak of acute sarcoidosis with arthropathy in Norfolk. *Br J Rheumatol.* 1989;28(2):178.
12. James DG. Erythema nodosum. *Br Med J.* 1961;1(5229): 853–857.
13. Bardinas F, Morera J, Fite E, Plasencia A. Seasonal clustering of sarcoidosis. *Lancet.* 1989;2(8660):455–456.
14. Poukkula A, Huhti E, Lilja M, Saloheimo M. Incidence and clinical picture of sarcoidosis in a circumscribed geographical area. *Br J Dis Chest.* 1986;80(2):138–147.
15. Hosoda Y, Hiraga Y, Odaka M, et al. A cooperative study of sarcoidosis in Asia and Africa: analytic epidemiology. *Ann N Y Acad Sci.* 1976;278:355–367.
16. Wilsher ML. Seasonal clustering of sarcoidosis presenting with erythema nodosum. *Eur Respir J.* 1998;12(5):1197–1199.
17. Henke CE, Henke G, Elveback LR, Beard CM, Ballard DJ, Kurland LT. The epidemiology of sarcoidosis in Rochester, Minnesota: a population-based study of incidence and survival. *Am J Epidemiol.* 1986;123(5):840–845.
18. Parkes SA, Baker SB, Bourdillon RE, Murray CR, Rakshit M. Epidemiology of sarcoidosis in the Isle of Man–1: a case controlled study. *Thorax.* 1987;42(6):420–426.
19. Hills SE, Parkes SA, Baker SB. Epidemiology of sarcoidosis in the Isle of Man–2: evidence for space-time clustering. *Thorax.* 1987;42(6):427–430.
20. Rybicki BA, Iannuzzi MC, Frederick MM, et al. Familial aggregation of sarcoidosis. A case-control etiologic study of sarcoidosis (ACCESS). *Am J Respir Crit Care Med.* 2001;164(11):2085–2091.
21. McGrath DS, Daniil Z, Foley P, et al. Epidemiology of familial sarcoidosis in the UK. *Thorax.* 2000;55(9):751–754.
22. Newman LS, Rose CS, Bresnitz EA, et al. A case control etiologic study of sarcoidosis: environmental and occupational risk factors. *Am J Respir Crit Care Med.* 2004;170(12):1324–1330.
23. Gupta D, Agarwal R, Aggarwal AN, Jindal SK. Molecular evidence for the role of mycobacteria in sarcoidosis: a meta-analysis. *Eur Respir J.* 2007;30(3):508–516.
24. Zhou Y, Hu Y, Li H. Role of *Propionibacterium acnes* in sarcoidosis: a meta-analysis. *Sarcoidosis Vasc Diffuse Lung Dis.* 2013;30(4):262–267.
25. Svendsen CB, Milman N, Nielsen HW, Krogfelt KA, Larsen KR. A prospective study evaluating the presence of Rickettsia in Danish patients with sarcoidosis. *Scand J Infect Dis.* 2009;41(10):745–752.
26. Derler AM, Eisendle K, Baltaci M, Obermoser G, Zelger B. High prevalence of 'Borrelia-like' organisms in skin biopsies of sarcoidosis patients from Western Austria. *J Cutan Pathol.* 2009;36(12):1262–1268.
27. Planck A, Eklund A, Grunewald J, Vene S. No serological evidence of *Rickettsia helvetica* infection in Scandinavian sarcoidosis patients. *Eur Respir J.* 2004;24(5):811–813.
28. Lebbe C, Agbalika F, Flageul B, et al. No evidence for a role of human herpesvirus type 8 in sarcoidosis: molecular and serological analysis. *Br J Dermatol.* 1999;141(3):492–496.
29. Mills GD, Allen RK, Timms P. *Chlamydia pneumoniae* DNA is not detectable within sarcoidosis tissue. *Pathology.* 1998;30(3):295–298.
30. Blasi F, Rizzato G, Gambacorta M, et al. Failure to detect the presence of *Chlamydia pneumoniae* in sarcoid pathology specimens. *Eur Respir J.* 1997;10(11):2609–2611.
31. Biberfeld P, Petren AL, Eklund A, et al. Human herpesvirus-6 (HHV-6, HBLV) in sarcoidosis and lymphoproliferative disorders. *J Virol Methods.* 1988;21(1–4):49–59.
32. Moravvej H, Vesal P, Abolhasani E, Nahidi S, Mahboudi F. Comorbidity of leishmania major with cutaneous sarcoidosis. *Indian J Dermatol.* 2014;59(3):316.
33. Suchankova M, Paulovicova E, Paulovicova L, et al. Increased antifungal antibodies in bronchoalveolar lavage fluid and serum in pulmonary sarcoidosis. *Scand J Immunol.* 2015;81(4):259–264.
34. Negi M, Takemura T, Guzman J, et al. Localization of *propionibacterium acnes* in granulomas supports a possible etiologic link between sarcoidosis and the bacterium. *Mod Pathol.* 2012;25(9):1284–1297.
35. Ishige I, Eishi Y, Takemura T, et al. *Propionibacterium acnes* is the most common bacterium commensal in peripheral lung tissue and mediastinal lymph nodes from subjects without sarcoidosis. *Sarcoidosis Vasc Diffuse Lung Dis.* 2005;22(1):33–42.
36. Oswald-Richter KA, Beachboard DC, Zhan X, et al. Multiple mycobacterial antigens are targets of the adaptive immune response in pulmonary sarcoidosis. *Respir Res.* 2010;11:161.
37. Fang C, Huang H, Xu Z. Immunological evidence for the role of mycobacteria in sarcoidosis: a meta-analysis. *PLoS One.* 2016;11(8):e0154716.
38. Hanngren A, Odham G, Eklund A, Hoffner S, Stjernberg N, Westerdahl G. Tuberculostearic acid in lymph nodes from patients with sarcoidosis. *Sarcoidosis.* 1987;4(2):101–104.
39. Ryan KJ, Ray C. *Sherris Medical Microbiology.* 4th ed. McGraw Hill; 2004.
40. Ding XL, Cai L, Zhang JZ. Detection and identification of mycobacterial gene in skin lesions and lymph nodes in patients with sarcoidosis. *Zhongguo Yi Xue Ke Xue Yuan Xue Bao.* 2009;31(1):20–23.

41. Drake WP, Dhason MS, Nadaf M, et al. Cellular recognition of *Mycobacterium tuberculosis* ESAT-6 and KatG peptides in systemic sarcoidosis. *Infect Immun.* 2007;75(1):527–530.
42. Dubaniewicz A, Dubaniewicz-Wybieralska M, Sternau A, et al. *Mycobacterium tuberculosis* complex and mycobacterial heat shock proteins in lymph node tissue from patients with pulmonary sarcoidosis. *J Clin Microbiol.* 2006;44(9):3448–3451.
43. Li N, Bajoghli A, Kubba A, Bhawan J. Identification of mycobacterial DNA in cutaneous lesions of sarcoidosis. *J Cutan Pathol.* 1999;26(6):271–278.
44. Song Z, Marzilli L, Greenlee BM, et al. Mycobacterial catalase-peroxidase is a tissue antigen and target of the adaptive immune response in systemic sarcoidosis. *J Exp Med.* 2005;201(5):755–767.
45. Allen SS, Evans W, Carlisle J, et al. Superoxide dismutase A antigens derived from molecular analysis of sarcoidosis granulomas elicit systemic Th-1 immune responses. *Respir Res.* 2008;9:36.
46. Hajizadeh R, Sato H, Carlisle J, et al. *Mycobacterium tuberculosis* Antigen 85A induces Th-1 immune responses in systemic sarcoidosis. *J Clin Immunol.* 2007;27(4):445–454.
47. Carlisle J, Evans W, Hajizadeh R, et al. Multiple Mycobacterium antigens induce interferon-gamma production from sarcoidosis peripheral blood mononuclear cells. *Clin Exp Immunol.* 2007;150(3):460–468.
48. Chen ES, Wahlstrom J, Song Z, et al. T cell responses to mycobacterial catalase-peroxidase profile a pathogenic antigen in systemic sarcoidosis. *J Immunol.* 2008;181(12):8784–8796.
49. Oswald-Richter KA, Culver DA, Hawkins C, et al. Cellular responses to mycobacterial antigens are present in bronchoalveolar lavage fluid used in the diagnosis of sarcoidosis. *Infect Immun.* 2009;77(9):3740–3748.
50. Oswald-Richter KA, Beachboard DC, Seeley EH, et al. Dual analysis for mycobacteria and propionibacteria in sarcoidosis BAL. *J Clin Immunol.* 2012;32(5):1129–1140.
51. Drake WP, Pei Z, Pride DT, Collins RD, Cover TL, Blaser MJ. Molecular analysis of sarcoidosis tissues for mycobacterium species DNA. *Emerg Infect Dis.* 2002;8(11):1334–1341.
52. Drake WP, Richmond BW, Oswald-Richter K, et al. Effects of broad-spectrum antimycobacterial therapy on chronic pulmonary sarcoidosis. *Sarcoidosis Vasc Diffuse Lung Dis.* 2013;30(3):201–211.
53. Drake WP, Oswald-Richter K, Richmond BW, et al. Oral antimycobacterial therapy in chronic cutaneous sarcoidosis: a randomized, single-masked, placebo-controlled study. *JAMA Dermatol.* 2013;149(9):1040–1049.
54. Richmond BW, Richter K, King LE, Drake WP. Resolution of chronic ocular sarcoidosis with antimycobacterial therapy. *Case Rep Intern Med.* 2014;1(2).
55. Swaisgood CM, Oswald-Richter K, Moeller SD, et al. Development of a sarcoidosis murine lung granuloma model using Mycobacterium superoxide dismutase A peptide. *Am J Respir Cell Mol Biol.* 2011;44(2):166–174.
56. Hu Y, Yibrehu B, Zabini D, Kuebler WM. Animal models of sarcoidosis. *Cell Tissue Res.* 2017;367(3):651–661.
57. Furusawa H, Suzuki Y, Miyazaki Y, Inase N, Eishi Y. Th1 and Th17 immune responses to viable *Propionibacterium acnes* in patients with sarcoidosis. *Respir Investig.* 2012;50(3):104–109.
58. Chen ES, Song Z, Willett MH, et al. Serum amyloid A regulates granulomatous inflammation in sarcoidosis through Toll-like receptor-2. *Am J Respir Crit Care Med.* 2010;181(4):360–373.
59. Maertzdorf J, Weiner 3rd J, Mollenkopf HJ, et al. Common patterns and disease-related signatures in tuberculosis and sarcoidosis. *Proc Natl Acad Sci U S A.* 2012;109(20):7853–7858.
60. Zhou T, Zhang W, Sweiss NJ, et al. Peripheral blood gene expression as a novel genomic biomarker in complicated sarcoidosis. *PLoS One.* 2012;7(9):e44818.
61. Thillai M, Eberhardt C, Lewin AM, et al. Sarcoidosis and tuberculosis cytokine profiles: indistinguishable in bronchoalveolar lavage but different in blood. *PLoS One.* 2012;7(7):e38083.
62. Koth LL, Solberg OD, Peng JC, Bhakta NR, Nguyen CP, Woodruff PG. Sarcoidosis blood transcriptome reflects lung inflammation and overlaps with tuberculosis. *Am J Respir Crit Care Med.* 2011;184(10):1153–1163.
63. Milman N, Lisby G, Friis S, Kemp L. Prolonged culture for mycobacteria in mediastinal lymph nodes from patients with pulmonary sarcoidosis. A negative study. *Sarcoidosis Vasc Diffuse Lung Dis.* 2004;21(1):25–28.
64. Belcher RW, Reid JD. Sarcoid granulomas in CBA/J mice. Histologic response after inoculation with sarcoid and nonsarcoid tissue homogenates. *Arch Pathol.* 1975;99(5):283–285.
65. Ikonomopoulos J, Gazouli M, Dontas I, et al. The infectivity of sarcoid clinical material and its bacterial content inoculated in CBA mice. *In Vivo.* 2006;20(6B):807–813.
66. Chen ES, Moller DR. Etiologies of sarcoidosis. *Clin Rev Allergy Immunol.* 2015;49(1):6–18.
67. Farnoud AM, Bryan AM, Kechichian T, Luberto C, Del Poeta M. The granuloma response controlling cryptococcosis in mice depends on the sphingosine kinase 1-sphingosine 1-phosphate pathway. *Infect Immun.* 2015;83(7):2705–2713.
68. Chensue SW, Warmington K, Ruth J, Lincoln P, Kuo MC, Kunkel SL. Cytokine responses during mycobacterial and schistosomal antigen-induced pulmonary granuloma formation. Production of Th1 and Th2 cytokines and relative contribution of tumor necrosis factor. *Am J Pathol.* 1994;145(5):1105–1113.
69. Abe C, Iwai K, Mikami R, Hosoda Y. Frequent isolation of *Propionibacterium acnes* from sarcoidosis lymph nodes. *Zentralbl Bakteriol Mikrobiol Hyg.* 1984;256(4):541–547.
70. de Brouwer B, Veltkamp M, Wauters CA, Grutters JC, Janssen R. Propionibacterium acnes isolated from lymph nodes of patients with sarcoidosis. *Sarcoidosis Vasc Diffuse Lung Dis.* 2015;32(3):271–274.

71. Homma JY, Abe C, Chosa H, et al. Bacteriological investigation on biopsy specimens from patients with sarcoidosis. *Jpn J Exp Med*. 1978;48(3):251–255.
72. Ishige I, Usui Y, Takemura T, Eishi Y. Quantitative PCR of mycobacterial and propionibacterial DNA in lymph nodes of Japanese patients with sarcoidosis. *Lancet*. 1999;354(9173):120–123.
73. Eishi Y, Suga M, Ishige I, et al. Quantitative analysis of mycobacterial and propionibacterial DNA in lymph nodes of Japanese and European patients with sarcoidosis. *J Clin Microbiol*. 2002;40(1):198–204.
74. Yamada T, Eishi Y, Ikeda S, et al. In situ localization of *Propionibacterium acnes* DNA in lymph nodes from sarcoidosis patients by signal amplification with catalysed reporter deposition. *J Pathol*. 2002;198(4):541–547.
75. Hiramatsu J, Kataoka M, Nakata Y, et al. *Propionibacterium acnes* DNA detected in bronchoalveolar lavage cells from patients with sarcoidosis. *Sarcoidosis Vasc Diffuse Lung Dis*. 2003;20(3):197–203.
76. Ichikawa H, Kataoka M, Hiramatsu J, et al. Quantitative analysis of propionibacterial DNA in bronchoalveolar lavage cells from patients with sarcoidosis. *Sarcoidosis Vasc Diffuse Lung Dis*. 2008;25(1):15–20.
77. Zhou Y, Wei YR, Zhang Y, Du SS, Baughman RP, Li HP. Real-time quantitative reverse transcription-polymerase chain reaction to detect propionibacterial ribosomal RNA in the lymph nodes of Chinese patients with sarcoidosis. *Clin Exp Immunol*. 2015;181(3):511–517.
78. Zhao MM, Du SS, Li QH, et al. High throughput 16SrRNA gene sequencing reveals the correlation between *Propionibacterium acnes* and sarcoidosis. *Resp Res*. 2017;18.
79. Schupp JC, Tchaptchet S, Lutzen N, et al. Immune response to *Propionibacterium acnes* in patients with sarcoidosis–in vivo and in vitro. *BMC Pulm Med*. 2015;15:75.
80. Yorozu P, Furukawa A, Uchida K, et al. *Propionibacterium acnes* catalase induces increased Th1 immune response in sarcoidosis patients. *Respir Investig*. 2015;53(4):161–169.
81. Ebe Y, Ikushima S, Yamaguchi T, et al. Proliferative response of peripheral blood mononuclear cells and levels of antibody to recombinant protein from Propionibacterium acnes DNA expression library in Japanese patients with sarcoidosis. *Sarcoidosis Vasc Diffuse Lung Dis*. 2000;17(3):256–265.
82. Akimoto J, Nagai K, Ogasawara D, et al. Solitary tentorial sarcoid granuloma associated with *Propionibacterium acnes* infection: case report. *J Neurosurg*. 2017;127(3):687–690.
83. Mori Y, Nakata Y, Kataoka M, et al. Interleukin-2 production and receptor expression of alveolar lymphocytes stimulated by *Propionibacterium acnes* in sarcoidosis. *Nihon Kyobu Shikkan Gakkai Zasshi*. 1989;27(1):42–50.
84. Nagata K, Eishi Y, Uchida K, et al. Immunohistochemical detection of *Propionibacterium acnes* in the retinal granulomas in patients with ocular sarcoidosis. *Sci Rep*. 2017;7(1):15226.
85. Yang G, Eishi Y, Raza A, et al. *Propionibacterium acnes*-associated neurosarcoidosis: a case report with review of the literature. *Neuropathology*. 2017.
86. Goto H, Usui Y, Umazume A, Uchida K, Eishi Y. *Propionibacterium acnes* as a possible pathogen of granuloma in patients with ocular sarcoidosis. *Brit J Ophthalmol*. 2017;101(11):1510–1513.
87. McCaskill JG, Chason KD, Hua X, et al. Pulmonary immune responses to *Propionibacterium acnes* in C57BL/6 and BALB/c mice. *Am J Respir Cell Mol Biol*. 2006;35(3):347–356.
88. Kishi J, Nishioka Y, Kuwahara T, et al. Blockade of Th1 chemokine receptors ameliorates pulmonary granulomatosis in mice. *Eur Respir J*. 2011;38(2):415–424.
89. Delgado S, Suarez A, Mayo B. Identification, typing and characterisation of Propionibacterium strains from healthy mucosa of the human stomach. *Int J Food Microbiol*. 2011;149(1):65–72.
90. Grice EA, Segre JA. The skin microbiome. *Nat Rev Microbiol*. 2011;9(4):244–253.
91. Bruggemann H, Henne A, Hoster F, et al. The complete genome sequence of *Propionibacterium acnes*, a commensal of human skin. *Science*. 2004;305(5684):671–673.
92. Nishiwaki T, Yoneyama H, Eishi Y, et al. Indigenous pulmonary *Propionibacterium acnes* primes the host in the development of sarcoid-like pulmonary granulomatosis in mice. *Am J Pathol*. 2004;165(2):631–639.
93. Kamata M, Tada Y, Mitsui A, et al. ICAM-1 deficiency exacerbates sarcoid-like granulomatosis induced by *Propionibacterium acnes* through impaired IL-10 production by regulatory T cells. *Am J Pathol*. 2013;183(6):1731–1739.
94. Takemori N, Nakamura M, Kojima M, Eishi Y. Successful treatment in a case of Propionibacterium acnes-associated sarcoidosis with clarithromycin administration: a case report. *J Med Case Rep*. 2014;8:15.
95. Bachelez H, Senet P, Cadranel J, Kaoukhov A, Dubertret L. The use of tetracyclines for the treatment of sarcoidosis. *Arch Dermatol*. 2001;137(1):69–73.
96. Nakata Y, Ejiri T, Kishi T, et al. Alveolar lymphocyte proliferation induced by *Propionibacterium acnes* in sarcoidosis patients. *Acta Med Okayama*. 1986;40(5):257–264.
97. Valeyre D, Prasse A, Nunes H, Uzunhan Y, Brillet PY, Muller-Quernheim J. Sarcoidosis. *Lancet*. 2014;383(9923):1155–1167.
98. Eishi Y. Etiologic link between sarcoidosis and Propionibacterium acnes. *Respir Investig*. 2013;51(2):56–68.
99. Tercelj M, Salobir B, Harlander M, Rylander R. Fungal exposure in homes of patients with sarcoidosis - an environmental exposure study. *Environ Health*. 2011;10(1):8.
100. Tercelj M, Stopinsek S, Ihan A, et al. In vitro and in vivo reactivity to fungal cell wall agents in sarcoidosis. *Clin Exp Immunol*. 2011;166(1):87–93.
101. Tercelj M, Salobir B, Rylander R. Microbial antigen treatment in sarcoidosis–a new paradigm? *Med Hypotheses*. 2008;70(4):831–834.

102. Laney AS, Cragin LA, Blevins LZ, et al. Sarcoidosis, asthma, and asthma-like symptoms among occupants of a historically water-damaged office building. *Indoor Air.* 2009;19(1):83–90.
103. Tercelj M, Salobir B, Zupancic M, Rylander R. Antifungal medication is efficient in the treatment of sarcoidosis. *Ther Adv Respir Dis.* 2011;5(3):157–162.
104. Tercelj M, Rott T, Rylander R. Antifungal treatment in sarcoidosis–a pilot intervention trial. *Respir Med.* 2007;101(4):774–778.
105. Tercelj M, Salobir B, Zupancic M, Rylander R. Sarcoidosis treatment with antifungal medication: a follow-up. *Pulm Med.* 2014;2014:739673.
106. Clarke EL, Lauder AP, Hofstaedter CE, et al. Microbial lineages in sarcoidosis. A metagenomic analysis tailored for low-microbial content samples. *Am J Respir Crit Care Med.* 2018;197(2):225–234.
107. Puolakkainen M, Campbell LA, Kuo CC, Leinonen M, Gronhagen-Riska C, Saikku P. Serological response to *Chlamydia pneumoniae* in patients with sarcoidosis. *J Infect.* 1996;33(3):199–205.
108. Yonemaru M, Ustumi K, Kasuga I, et al. A case of pulmonary fibrosis associated with CMV inclusion body. *Nihon Kyobu Shikkan Gakkai Zasshi.* 1994;32(2):184–188.
109. Yonemaru M, Kasuga I, Kusumoto H, et al. Elevation of antibodies to cytomegalovirus and other herpes viruses in pulmonary fibrosis. *Eur Respir J.* 1997;10(9):2040–2045.
110. Di Alberti L, Piattelli A, Artese L, et al. Human herpesvirus 8 variants in sarcoid tissues. *Lancet.* 1997;350(9092):1655–1661.
111. Rottoli P, Bianchi Bandinelli ML, Rottoli L, Zazzi M, Panzardi G, Valensin PE. Sarcoidosis and infections by human lymphotropic viruses. *Sarcoidosis.* 1990;7(1):31–33.
112. McKee DH, Young AC, Haeney M. Sarcoidosis and HTLV-1 infection. *J Clin Pathol.* 2005;58(9):996–997.
113. Prezant DJ, Dhala A, Goldstein A, et al. The incidence, prevalence, and severity of sarcoidosis in New York City firefighters. *Chest.* 1999;116(5):1183–1193.
114. Lioy PJ, Weisel CP, Millette JR, et al. Characterization of the dust/smoke aerosol that settled east of the World Trade Center (WTC) in lower Manhattan after the collapse of the WTC 11 September 2001. *Environ Health Perspect.* 2002;110(7):703–714.
115. Kern DG, Neill MA, Wrenn DS, Varone JC. Investigation of a unique time-space cluster of sarcoidosis in firefighters. *Am Rev Respir Dis.* 1993;148(4 Pt 1):974–980.
116. Jajosky P. Sarcoidosis diagnoses among U.S. military personnel: trends and ship assignment associations. *Am J Prev Med.* 1998;14(3):176–183.
117. Guzman D, Broderick B, Sotolongo A, Osinubi O, Helmer D. A case of sarcoidosis in a veteran with military-related environmental and occupational exposure. *Chest.* 2017;152(4):A830.
118. Sartwell PE, Edwards LB. Epidemiology of sarcoidosis in the U.S. Navy. *Am J Epidemiol.* 1974;99(4):250–257.
119. Chubineh S, Katona K. A rare case of peritoneal sarcoidosis in a 36-year-old construction worker. *Case Rep Gastroenterol.* 2008;2(3):369–372.
120. Deubelbeiss U, Gemperli A, Schindler C, Baty F, Brutsche MH. Prevalence of sarcoidosis in Switzerland is associated with environmental factors. *Eur Respir J.* 2010;35(5):1088–1097.
121. Parkes SA, Baker SB, Bourdillon RE, et al. Incidence of sarcoidosis in the Isle of Man. *Thorax.* 1985;40(4):284–287.
122. Edmondstone WM. Sarcoidosis in nurses: is there an association? *Thorax.* 1988;43(4):342–343.
123. Bresnitz EA, Stolley PD, Israel HL, Soper K. Possible risk factors for sarcoidosis. A case-control study. *Ann N Y Acad Sci.* 1986;465:632–642.
124. Perlman SE, Friedman S, Galea S, et al. Short-term and medium-term health effects of 9/11. *Lancet.* 2011;378(9794):925–934.
125. Izbicki G, Chavko R, Banauch GI, et al. World Trade Center "sarcoid-like" granulomatous pulmonary disease in New York City Fire Department rescue workers. *Chest.* 2007;131(5):1414–1423.
126. Crowley LE, Herbert R, Moline JM, et al. Sarcoid like" granulomatous pulmonary disease in World Trade Center disaster responders. *Am J Ind Med.* 2011;54(3):175–184.
127. Wu M, Gordon RE, Herbert R, et al. Case report: lung disease in World Trade Center responders exposed to dust and smoke: carbon nanotubes found in the lungs of World Trade Center patients and dust samples. *Environ Health Perspect.* 2010;118(4):499–504.
128. Song Y, Li X, Wang L, et al. Nanomaterials in humans: identification, characteristics, and potential damage. *Toxicol Pathol.* 2011;39(5):841–849.
129. Tamagawa E, Bai N, Morimoto K, et al. Particulate matter exposure induces persistent lung inflammation and endothelial dysfunction. *Am J Physiol Lung Cell Mol Physiol.* 2008;295(1):L79–L85.
130. Morimoto Y, Izumi H, Kuroda E. Significance of persistent inflammation in respiratory disorders induced by nanoparticles. *J Immunol Res.* 2014;2014:962871.
131. Dumortier H. When carbon nanotubes encounter the immune system: desirable and undesirable effects. *Adv Drug Deliv Rev.* 2013;65(15):2120–2126.
132. Huizar I, Malur A, Midgette YA, et al. Novel murine model of chronic granulomatous lung inflammation elicited by carbon nanotubes. *Am J Respir Cell Mol Biol.* 2011;45(4):858–866.
133. Ho CC, Chang H, Tsai HT, et al. Quantum dot 705, a cadmium-based nanoparticle, induces persistent inflammation and granuloma formation in the mouse lung. *Nanotoxicology.* 2013;7(1):105–115.
134. Chapman JS. Mycobacterial and mycotic antibodies in sera of patients with sarcoidosis. Results of studies using agar double-diffusion technique. *Ann Intern Med.* 1961;55:918–924.
135. Reid JD, Chiodini RJ. Serologic reactivity against *Mycobacterium paratuberculosis* antigens in patients with sarcoidosis. *Sarcoidosis.* 1993;10(1):32–35.

136. Ahmadzai H, Cameron B, Chui JJ, Lloyd A, Wakefield D, Thomas PS. Peripheral blood responses to specific antigens and CD28 in sarcoidosis. *Respir Med.* 2012;106(5):701–709.
137. Inui N, Suda T, Chida K. Use of the QuantiFERON-TB Gold test in Japanese patients with sarcoidosis. *Respir Med.* 2008;102(2):313–315.
138. Horster R, Kirsten D, Gaede KI, et al. Antimycobacterial immune responses in patients with pulmonary sarcoidosis. *Clin Respir J.* 2009;3(4):229–238.
139. Kobayashi K, Yamazaki J, Kasama T, et al. Interleukin (IL)-12 deficiency in susceptible mice infected with *Mycobacterium avium* and amelioration of established infection by IL-12 replacement therapy. *J Infect Dis.* 1996;174(3):564–573.
140. Zhao S, Kuge Y, Kohanawa M, et al. Extensive FDG uptake and its modification with corticosteroid in a granuloma rat model: an experimental study for differentiating granuloma from tumors. *Eur J Nucl Med Mol Imag.* 2007;34(12):2096–2105.
141. Birkness KA, Guarner J, Sable SB, et al. An in vitro model of the leukocyte interactions associated with granuloma formation in *Mycobacterium tuberculosis* infection. *Immunol Cell Biol.* 2007;85(2):160–168.
142. Kapoor N, Pawar S, Sirakova TD, Deb C, Warren WL, Kolattukudy PE. Human granuloma in vitro model, for TB dormancy and resuscitation. *PLoS One.* 2013; 8(1):e53657.
143. Puissegur MP, Botanch C, Duteyrat JL, Delsol G, Caratero C, Altare F. An in vitro dual model of mycobacterial granulomas to investigate the molecular interactions between mycobacteria and human host cells. *Cell Microbiol.* 2004;6(5):423–433.
144. Seitzer U, Gerdes J. Generation and characterization of multicellular heterospheroids formed by human peripheral blood mononuclear cells. *Cells Tissues Organs.* 2003;174(3):110–116.
145. Wang H, Maeda Y, Fukutomi Y, Makino M. An in vitro model of *Mycobacterium leprae* induced granuloma formation. *BMC Infect Dis.* 2013;13:279.
146. Bentley AG, Phillips SM, Kaner RJ, Theodorides VJ, Linette GP, Doughty BL. In vitro delayed hypersensitivity granuloma formation: development of an antigen-coated bead model. *J Immunol.* 1985;134(6):4163–4169.
147. Shikama Y, Kobayashi K, Kasahara K, et al. Granuloma formation by artificial microparticles in vitro. Macrophages and monokines play a critical role in granuloma formation. *Am J Pathol.* 1989;134(6):1189–1199.
148. Reyes N, Bettin A, Reyes I, Geliebter J. Microarray analysis of the in vitro granulomatous response to *Mycobacterium tuberculosis* H37Ra. *Colomb Méd.* 2015;46(1):26–32.
149. Taflin C, Miyara M, Nochy D, et al. FoxP3+ regulatory T cells suppress early stages of granuloma formation but have little impact on sarcoidosis lesions. *Am J Pathol.* 2009;174(2):497–508.
150. Piotrowski WJ, Gorski P, Duda-Szymanska J, Kwiatkowska S. *Mycobacterium tuberculosis* as a sarcoid factor? A case report of family sarcoidosis. *Am J Case Rep.* 2014;15:216–220.
151. Igarashi R, Inatomi K. *Propionibacterium acnes* in the biopsied lymph nodes of sarcoidosis patients demonstrated by an immunofluorescence and immunoperoxidase staining technics. *Nihon Kyobu Shikkan Gakkai Zasshi.* 1988;26(5):507–511.
152. Asakawa N, Uchida K, Sakakibara M, et al. Immunohistochemical identification of *Propionibacterium acnes* in granuloma and inflammatory cells of myocardial tissues obtained from cardiac sarcoidosis patients. *PLoS One.* 2017;12(7).
153. Miura Y, Ishige I, Soejima N, et al. Quantitative PCR of *Propionibacterium acnes* DNA in samples aspirated from sebaceous follicles on the normal skin of subjects with or without acne. *J Med Dent Sci.* 2010;57(1):65–74.
154. Baba K, Yamaguchi E, Matsui S, et al. A case of sarcoidosis with multiple endobronchial mass lesions that disappeared with antibiotics. *Sarcoidosis Vasc Diffuse Lung Dis.* 2006;23(1):78–79.
155. Park DJ, Woog JJ, Pulido JS, Cameron JD. Minocycline for the treatment of ocular and ocular adnexal sarcoidosis. *Arch Ophthalmol.* 2007;125(5):705–709.
156. Minami J, Eishi Y, Ishige Y, et al. Pulmonary granulomas caused experimentally in mice by a recombinant trigger-factor protein of Propionibacterium acnes. *J Med Dent Sci.* 2003;50(4):265–274.
157. Werner JL, Escolero SG, Hewlett JT, et al. Induction of pulmonary granuloma formation by *Propionibacterium acnes* is regulated by MyD88 and Nox2. *Am J Respir Cell Mol Biol.* 2017;56(1):121–130.
158. Ichiyasu H, Suga M, Iyonaga K, Ando M. Role of monocyte chemoattractant protein-1 in *Propionibacterium acnes*-induced pulmonary granulomatosis. *Microsc Res Tech.* 2001;53(4):288–297.
159. Iio K, Iio TU, Okui Y, et al. Experimental pulmonary granuloma mimicking sarcoidosis induced by *Propionibacterium acnes* in mice. *Acta Med Okayama.* 2010;64(2):75–83.
160. Itakura M, Tokuda A, Kimura H, et al. Blockade of secondary lymphoid tissue chemokine exacerbates *Propionibacterium acnes*-induced acute lung inflammation. *J Immunol.* 2001;166(3):2071–2079.
161. Nikoskelainen J, Hannuksela M, Palva T. Antibodies to Epstein-Barr virus and some other herpesviruses in patients with sarcoidosis, pulmonary tuberculosis and erythema nodosum. *Scand J Infect Dis.* 1974;6(3):209–216.
162. Theate I, Michaux L, Dardenne S, et al. Epstein-Barr virus-associated lymphoproliferative disease occurring in a patient with sarcoidosis treated by methotrexate and methylprednisolone. *Eur J Haematol.* 2002;69(4):248–253.
163. Bassoe CF, Hausken T, Bostad L, Kristoffersen EK. Co-occurrence of Epstein-Barr virus infection and ascites in sarcoidosis. *Scand J Infect Dis.* 2004;36(3):232–234.

164. Saghafi M, Rezaieyazdi Z, Nabavi S, Mirfeizi Z, Sahebari M, Salari M. HTLV-1 seroprevalance in sarcoidosis. A clinical and laboratory study in northeast of Iran. *Int J Rheum Dis*. 2017.
165. Blum JL, Rosenblum LK, Grunig G, Beasley MB, Xiong JQ, Zelikoff JT. Short-term inhalation of cadmium oxide nanoparticles alters pulmonary dynamics associated with lung injury, inflammation, and repair in a mouse model. *Inhal Toxicol*. 2014;26(1):48–58.
166. Lebecque S, Renno T, Bentaher A, et al. Characterisation of an experimental mouse model of exposure to nanoparticles. Relevance to human sarcoidosis. *Eur Respir J*. 2015;46.
167. Nishi K, Morimoto Y, Ogami A, et al. Expression of cytokine-induced neutrophil chemoattractant in rat lungs by intratracheal instillation of nickel oxide nanoparticles. *Inhal Toxicol*. 2009;21(12):1030–1039.
168. Morimoto Y, Hirohashi M, Ogami A, et al. Expression of cytokine-induced neutrophil chemoattractant in rat lungs following an intratracheal instillation of micron-sized nickel oxide nanoparticle agglomerates. *Toxicol Ind Health*. 2014;30(9):851–860.
169. Zuskin E, Mustajbegovic J, Schachter EN, et al. Respiratory function in pesticide workers. *J Occup Environ Med*. 2008;50(11):1299–1305.
170. McDonough C, Gray GC. Risk factors for sarcoidosis hospitalization among U.S. Navy and Marine Corps personnel, 1981 to 1995. *Mil Med*. 2000;165(8):630–632.
171. Cooch JW. Sarcoidosis in the United States army, 1952 through 1956. *Am Rev Respir Dis*. 1961;84(5)Pt(2):103–108.
172. Rafnsson V, Ingimarsson O, Hjalmarsson I, Gunnarsdottir H. Association between exposure to crystalline silica and risk of sarcoidosis. *Occup Environ Med*. 1998;55(10):657–660.
173. Redline S, Barna BP, Tomashefski Jr JF, Abraham JL. Granulomatous disease associated with pulmonary deposition of titanium. *Br J Ind Med*. 1986;43(10):652–656.
174. De Vuyst P, Dumortier P, Schandene L, Estenne M, Verhest A, Yernault JC. Sarcoid-like lung granulomatosis induced by aluminum dusts. *Am Rev Respir Dis*. 1987;135(2):493–497.
175. Skelton 3rd HG, Smith KJ, Johnson FB, Cooper CR, Tyler WF, Lupton GP. Zirconium granuloma resulting from an aluminum zirconium complex: a previously unrecognized agent in the development of hypersensitivity granulomas. *J Am Acad Dermatol*. 1993;28(5 Pt 2):874–876.

CHAPTER 3

Immunological Manifestations in Sarcoidosis

KOOL MIRJAM, PHD • BROOS CAROLINE E., MD, PHD

INTRODUCTION

Sarcoidosis is an intriguingly complex disease. Unraveling the immunological response that takes place in sarcoidosis faces some problems, withholding our understanding of this disease for already a few decades. Like in many other inflammatory diseases and cancer, it is not a single trigger that causes sarcoidosis pathology. Environmental exposure, genetic background, ethnicity, infections, hormones, and epigenetic changes contribute to disease susceptibility. Sarcoidosis is thought to result from both genetic susceptibility and specific environmental triggers or infections, which all can contribute to the induction of sarcoidosis signature cytokines, interferon gamma (IFNγ) and tumor necrosis factor alpha (TNFα). From an immunological angle, it is highly unlikely that a single cell of our immune system is responsible for the development of sarcoidosis. Over the last decades, researchers have examined several cell types from the innate and adaptive immune system in sarcoidosis patients. As the "architectural" construction of a granuloma also contains both innate and adaptive immune cells, in this chapter we will systematically discuss all immune cells contributing to the enhanced immune response observed in sarcoidosis.

INNATE AND ADAPTIVE IMMUNE RESPONSES

Granulomas found in sarcoidosis patients are characterized by an accumulation of macrophages, dendritic cells (DCs), T-cells, a few B-cells, and fibroblasts (Fig. 3.1). Although the order of the immunological cascade in granuloma formation is still unknown, it is generally accepted that the innate immune response precedes the adaptive immune response. These immune reactions involve a plethora of cytokines and chemokines, found in increased amounts released by diverse immune cells from sarcoidosis patients, together with an enhanced activation status of these cells. These features are most prominently found in affected organs, thereby demonstrating that granuloma formation is induced by a strong interplay between several cell types and cytokines/chemokines. Although the exact trigger(s) remains unknown, a network of cells of the innate and adaptive immune system and their mediators drive the immunopathogenesis of sarcoidosis.

INNATE RESPONSE IN SARCOIDOSIS

Macrophages

The formation of granulomas is an immunological process that serves to protect our body from unwanted invaders. Initiation of an immune response warrants identification of invading pathogens that are recognized by ancient receptors, including pattern recognition receptors (PRRs) that are expressed by sentinel cells such as macrophages and DCs.[1] Macrophages are widely found in the lung alveoli, both supraepithelial and subepithelial. At least two macrophage populations are present in the healthy lung, alveolar macrophages and interstitial macrophages. These two populations can be distinguished based on their unique combination of surface markers and are long-lived cells that are derived from embryonic precursors. During inflammatory responses a third population of monocyte-derived macrophages may be recruited to the lung[2,3].

Bronchoalveolar lavage fluid (BALF), which is commonly gathered during the diagnostic workup of pulmonary sarcoidosis, is thought to contain the immune cells found in lung alveoli and can therefore provide important information regarding the immunological response that takes place. Indeed, human BALF contains mostly macrophages. Macrophages are thought to contribute to granuloma formation because they are the predominant cell type present in early granulomas found in interstitial pneumonitis patients.[4] Alveolar macrophages from sarcoidosis patients show an enhanced activation status, indicated by an increase in key signaling molecules, such as p38 and interleukin receptor–associated kinase (IRAK),[5] enhanced

Sarcoidosis. https://doi.org/10.1016/B978-0-323-54429-0.00003-3

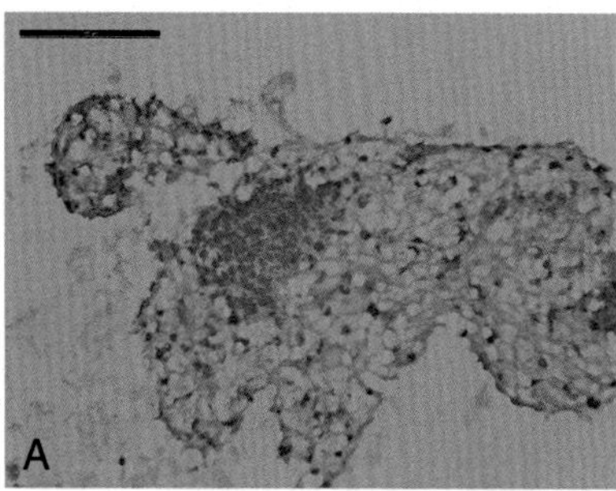

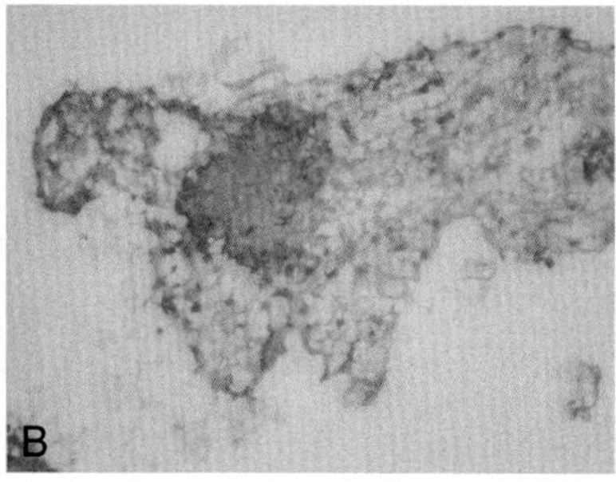

FIG. 3.1 **Histological View of a Sarcoid Granuloma.** Histological slide of a lymph node puncture [biopsy using Endobronchial ultrasound (EBUS)] revealing a granuloma (**A**) with surrounding T cells (**B**) stained with anti-CD3 antibodies in red. Scale bar in A represents 100 μm.

proinflammatory cytokine production (e.g., TNFα), and higher costimulatory molecule expression, such as CD80 and CD86,[6,7] than control macrophages.

Macrophage activation is mediated via membrane-bound PRRs, such as toll-like receptors (TLRs) and C-type lectin receptors (CLR), or intracellular PRRS including nucleotide-binding oligomerization domain protein (NOD)-like receptors (NLRs) and certain TLRs. These PRRs are capable of recognizing pathogen-associated molecular patterns (PAMPs) and damage-associated molecular patterns (DAMPs).[8] DAMPs are associated with components of the host's cells that are released during cell damage or death. The specific PAMP or DAMP that is recognized by macrophages can therefore provide information regarding the initiating antigen. Interestingly the expression of several PRRs is altered in sarcoidosis (or sarcoid-like disease). TLR2, TLR9, dectin-1, and NOD2 are highly expressed by sarcoidosis macrophages compared with controls,[7,9,10] and NOD2 is associated with early-onset sarcoidosis (e.g., Blau syndrome).[11] Proteins/peptides involved in sarcoidosis, namely serum amyloid A (SAA) or mycobacterial derived peptide (ESAT-6) activate TLR2 and thereby induce increased production of proinflammatory cytokines, such as TNFα, interleukin (IL)-1β, IL-6, IL-10, and IL-18 by sarcoidosis macrophages.[7,12,13]

Strikingly, specific TLR9 triggering with CpG-rich DNA, predominantly present in viral or bacterial DNA in contrast to human DNA, did not provoke proinflammatory cytokine production by alveolar macrophages of sarcoidosis patients.[9] However, chemokines, like the chemokine C-X-C motif chemokine ligand 10 (CXCL10) was produced especially by macrophages of Scadding stage II patients.[9] Several other chemokines, including CXCL9 and CXCL11, are also spontaneously produced by *in vitro* cultured alveolar macrophages from sarcoidosis patients and found in elevated amounts in BALF and serum.[14] Interestingly, all of these chemokines are induced by a key sarcoidosis cytokine IFNγ.[15] CXCL9, CXCL10, and CXCL11 are ligands for the cell surface receptor CXCR3 and can attract monocytes, macrophages, T-cells, and DCs to the lungs/granuloma.[15] Increased mRNA expression of CXCL9, CXCL10, and CXCL11 was also observed in these macrophages, but this finding could not be confirmed by others.[7] The discrepancy may be caused not only by differences in the procedures (e.g., direct mRNA isolation or after overnight culture) but also by the presence of Löfgren's syndrome (LS) patients in the latter study, which comprises a clinically favorable subgroup of sarcoidosis patients.[7] The presence of CXCL9, CXCL10, or CXCL11 in BALF correlated with Scadding stage and/or presence of LS versus non-LS symptoms,[16] and sustained increased serum CXCL10 concentrations were found over time in chronic progressive patients.[17] However, CXCL10 did not show an association with disease prognosis after 2 years follow-up.[16] Another T-cell–attracting chemokine, C–C motif chemokine ligand 18 (CCL18), was also produced in high amounts by sarcoidosis macrophages.[7] CCL18 is associated with fibrosis as BALF cells of Scadding stage IV patients produced more CCL18, and enhanced CCL18 was observed in other fibrosing lung diseases.[7] Complementarily, CCL18 provokes collagen production in fibroblasts.[18]

Next to activation of macrophages via PRR, cytokines can also trigger macrophage activation. The sarcoidosis key cytokine IFNγ stimulates macrophages to produce TNFα and induces their fusion into multinucleated giant cells (MGCs)[19] found in the center of sarcoid granulomas (Fig. 3.2).

Macrophages are heterogeneous, and the microenvironment regulates their phenotype and function.

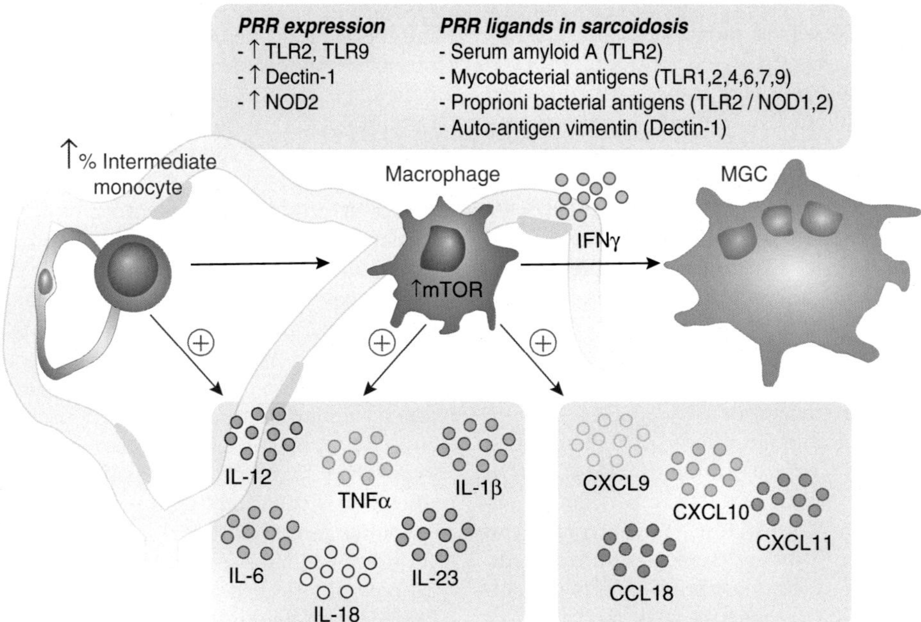

FIG. 3.2 **Alterations in Innate Immune Cells in Sarcoidosis.** Monocytes and macrophages are altered in sarcoidosis. Intermediate monocytes are elevated in peripheral blood and produced enhance amounts of cytokines. Macrophages express higher levels of PRRs and secrete increased amounts of cytokines and chemokines. Under the influence of IFNγ, macrophages can form multinucleated giant cells. *IFN*, interferon; *IL*, interleukin; *MGC*, multinucleated giant cell; *PRR*, pattern recognition receptors; *TNF*, tumor necrosis factor.

Next to their innate function in controlling infections, macrophages also possess a variety of functions in tissue development, homeostasis, repair, and immunity.[20] Macrophages can come in two flavors, (1) M1 or classically activated macrophages and (2) M2 or alternatively activated macrophages. M1 macrophages are triggered by TLR4 stimulation [lipopolysaccharide (LPS)] and/or IFNγ and harbor a proinflammatory phenotype and antimicrobial activity. On the other hand, M2 macrophages are induced by Th2-cell cytokines (e.g., IL-4 and IL-13), IL-10, and corticosteroids and have an antiinflammatory function; they are involved in tissue repair and wound healing. It is becoming more and more evident that the M1/M2 paradigm lacks usefulness when considering disease states in the lung, as macrophages often coexpress markers of M1/M2 activation. This indicates that these cells are highly plastic and may represent a sliding scale of activation states rather than being terminally differentiated distinct lineages.[3] In different sarcoidosis studies examining macrophages for M1 and M2 markers, different results are obtained. The enhanced cytokine and chemokine production by macrophages described previously is suggestive for an M1 phenotype. In contrast, increased CD163 expression specific for M2 macrophages was observed inside granulomas in sarcoidosis lymph node (LN) compared with tuberculosis LN.[21] Also, cytokines secreted by M2 macrophages, such as IL-10 and IL-1ra, are present in high amounts in BALF of sarcoidosis patients.[22–24]

In conclusion, it is highly possible that the phenotype and function of pulmonary macrophages in sarcoidosis depend on disease phase, Scadding stage, and/or progression of the disease. Additionally, macrophages present in sarcoidosis patients could harbor a mixed phenotype; however, in most sarcoidosis studies they appear to play a proinflammatory role.

Monocytes

Monocytes originate in the bone marrow and travel through the blood stream to peripheral tissues. They sense the environment and replenish the pool of tissue macrophages and DCs. Distinct populations of monocytes can be identified based on CD14 and CD16 expression including CD14⁺⁺ classical monocytes, CD14⁺CD16⁺ intermediate monocytes, and CD16⁺⁺ nonclassical monocytes.[25]

Classical monocytes, also called inflammatory monocytes, can infiltrate tissues, produce inflammatory cytokines, and differentiate into inflammatory macrophages.[26] Classical monocytes express several PRRs and are involved in removing microorganisms and dying cells via phagocytosis. Strikingly, blood monocytes of sarcoidosis patients have increased expression of Fc receptors (FcRs) and complement receptors (CRs), both of which enhance their phagocytic activity.[27] $CD14^+$ cells can be observed within sarcoidosis granulomas, which could be monocytes, monocytes differentiated into macrophages, or DCs.[21] $CD14^+$ cells in the center of granulomas most likely are macrophages; however, a detailed characterization of $CD14^+$ cells at the rim of the granuloma has not been performed.[21] In approximately 50% of sarcoidosis patients, peripheral $CD14^+$ monocytes, including classical and intermediate monocytes, have a reduced expression of the inhibitory receptor CD200R, which is associated with an increased capacity to produce TNFα and IL-6.[28]

Intermediate monocytes also have proinflammatory functions, producing high amounts of IL-1β, IL-6, IL-12, and TNFα, upon stimulation.[29] Their gene expression signature indicates their ability to present antigens and induce T-cell activation.[30] Intermediate monocytes specifically promote proinflammatory Th17-cell responses,[31] which also contribute to alveolar granulomas and fibrotic processes in sarcoidosis,[32] as discussed in the following paragraphs. In sarcoidosis, specifically in male patients, significantly higher proportions of circulating intermediate monocytes are found than in healthy controls[28,33,34] (Fig. 3.2). Interestingly, sarcoidosis patients who responded to infliximab (anti-TNFα) therapy harbored more intermediate monocytes at baseline than nonresponders,[35] which could suggest that intermediate monocytes are an important source of serum TNFα.

Nonclassical or antiinflammatory monocytes patrol the vasculature for DAMPs and differentiate into tissue-resident macrophages in steady state or into antiinflammatory macrophages during inflammation to repair damaged tissues. High proportions of CD16-expressing monocytes were also found in sarcoidosis patients than in controls;[36,37] however, these studies did not discriminate between intermediate and nonclassical monocytes. It is crucial to monitor monocytes in untreated sarcoidosis patients as intermediate and nonclassical monocytes undergo apoptosis during corticosteroid treatment.[38]

Trained Innate Immunity

Immunological memory is a distinct characteristic of our immune system, and it relates to its ability to remember antigens from pathogens and mount an immunological response of greater magnitude and with faster kinetics upon reencounter of the same antigens. Specifically, cells of our adaptive immune system, such as T cells and B cells, can mount specificity for the antigen, and these adaptive cells provide memory that lasts up to several decades in the body. Classically, innate immune cells have been thought to lack immunological memory. However, recently this dogma has been challenged as cells of the innate immune system can adapt features of the adaptive response called trained innate immunity.[39] Macrophages, monocytes, and natural killer cells show an enhanced responsiveness when they encounter pathogens for a second time. Epigenetic modifications occurring after the first encounter largely drive trained immunity,[40,41] which is short lived and less specific than classical immunological memory. Trained innate immunity is most likely a host defense method contributing to the maturation of innate cells and mediating protection after certain infections. However, when induced inappropriately by endogenous stimuli, trained innate immunity may play a role in the pathogenesis of autoinflammatory and/or autoimmune diseases.[42,43]

The increased responsiveness of sarcoidosis macrophages and monocytes to produce proinflammatory mediators could be a consequence of "training," e.g., priming after a primary activation stimulus. Several lines of evidence point toward similarities found in trained innate immunity and sarcoidosis. First, trained immunity can be induced by NOD2 and dectin-1 triggering;[44,45] ligands for both PRRs are found in sarcoidosis and trigger macrophage activation (Fig. 3.2). Interestingly, both NOD2 and dectin-1 were increased on sarcoidosis macrophages.[9,10] Second, trained immunity was first observed in patients after Bacille Calmette-Guerin (BCG) vaccination used for protection against *Mycobacterium tuberculosis* (Mtb) infections.[46] Mycobacterial-derived antigens, such as mKatG and ESAT-6, are speculated to be antigens within sarcoidosis pathology as mKatG and ESAT-6 are recognized by sarcoidosis $CD4^+$ T cells.[47–49] Third, the mammalian target of rapamycin (mTOR)/glycolysis pathway is important for training monocytes.[41,49,50] The mTOR pathway is initiated by metabolic demanding processes, which are triggered after activation of innate cells.[51] These processes include translation and protein synthesis, cell growth, metabolism, and anabolic processes. Recently, increased mTOR activity was observed in sarcoid granulomas.[52] When mTOR activity was specifically increased in myeloid cells through deletion of tuberous sclerosis 2 (TSC2), mice developed cellular conglomerates, resembling granulomas observed in sarcoidosis patients.[52] TSC2 controlled macrophage quiescence, and uncontrolled mTOR activation resulted in macrophage proliferation and hypertrophy (Fig. 3.2). Interestingly, genes associated with mTOR activity were enhanced in active progressive sarcoidosis patients compared with self-limiting patients.[52] Finally, to promote cellular effector responses, the mTOR pathway regulates energy metabolism processes, such as glycolysis and mitochondrial metabolism. Within sarcoid granulomas, a strong metabolic activity was observed, including increased glycolysis.[53] Also, the glycolysis gene set was enriched in active progressive sarcoidosis patients compared with self-limiting patients.[52]

Whether "training" of innate immune cells occurs in sarcoidosis is unknown at present. Examination of epigenetic marks and metabolic profiles of sarcoid monocytes could provide insight into whether these processes take place in sarcoidosis.

BRIDGING INNATE-ADAPTIVE IN SARCOIDOSIS

Dendritic Cells

Initiation of the adaptive immune response requires an (auto)antigen that is presented by antigen-presenting cells (APCs). Within our immune system, dendritic cells (DCs) are the most potent APCs, and they bridge innate and adaptive immune responses. DCs, similar to macrophages, harbor several PRRs on their cell surface, enabling them to quickly respond to invading pathogens or cell damage. Additionally, they are strategically positioned just below the lung epithelial lining to sample their environment for these danger signals. Involvement of DCs in granuloma formation in sarcoidosis is also plausible as subcutaneous injection of the elusive Kveim reagent into patients with sarcoidosis induces granulomas containing twofold more DCs than granulomas in foreign body reactions.[54] Also, successful immunotherapy by DC injections in melanoma patients provoked sarcoid-like granulomas.[55] Although this does not prove that DCs drive granuloma formation, it is highly suggestive of DC involvement.

In the human lung, three different DC subsets can be found: plasmacytoid DCs (pDCs) and conventional DCs (cDCs, also called myeloid DCs), subdivided into type 1 cDCs (cDC1s) and type 2 cDCs (cDC2s).[56] Unfortunately, there is no single marker that discriminates human DCs from monocytes and macrophages, and a descriptive set of markers is needed to identify DCs and subsequently DC subsets.[56,57] From mouse studies it is known that lung DC subsets are distinctively distributed. During steady state, cDC1s are closely associated with the airway epithelium and extend processes into the airway lumen, whereas cDC2s mainly reside beneath the airway basement membrane. During inflammatory conditions, monocytes can also give rise to the number of DCs, termed monocyte-derived DCs (mo-DCs).

Unfortunately, most studies that investigated human DC function compared pDCs to cDCs that include both cDC1s and cDC2s or evaluated *in vitro* generated mo-DCs. Both pDC and total cDC frequencies were increased in BALF of sarcoidosis patients,[58] and a specific increase of $CD1a^+$ cDCs was also reported.[59] Within cDCs, the proportion of $CD1c^+$ cDC2s was reduced in sarcoidosis BALF compared with healthy control BALF[59] (Fig. 3.3A). Conventional $CD11c^+$ DCs are localized in the T-cell area of granulomas in lung and LNs of sarcoidosis patients, suggesting that T-cell (re)activation can also occur within the granuloma.[58,60] DCs are also found within lymphatic vessels surrounding granulomas; it could very well be that they are positioned here to migrate to the draining LN or to sample for antigens.[61] Interestingly, highly characteristic for sarcoid granulomas is the distinct lymphatic distribution surrounding the granulomas,[62] again suggesting that DCs might be of great importance in sarcoidosis pathology. It would be of great value to investigate which cDC subset is present in sarcoid granulomas as cDC1s are known to cross-present antigens and produce chemokines favorable for Th1-cell differentiation,[63,64] whereas cDC2s produce many proinflammatory cytokines, including IL-23, and thus are potent Th17-cell inducers.[65] Because increased numbers of both of these Th-cell subsets are found in sarcoidosis, it is conceivable that both DC subsets are involved in sarcoid immunopathology.

Excessive DC activation/function may play a major role in disease processes of several chronic disorders. In sarcoidosis lung, cDCs in the lung parenchyma and inside the T-cell area of sarcoid granulomas harbor an activated phenotype, e.g., CD86 expression[58] (Fig. 3.3C), in contrast to BALF cDCs that either show a similar or reduced activation status compared with controls.[58,59] Similar to macrophage activation, DCs can be activated through PRR stimulation and/or cytokines. IFNγ induce DC maturation and cytokine production, including the major Th1-polarizing cytokine, IL-12. Both IFNγ and IL-12 levels are elevated in sarcoidosis BALF,[66,67] suggesting an ongoing

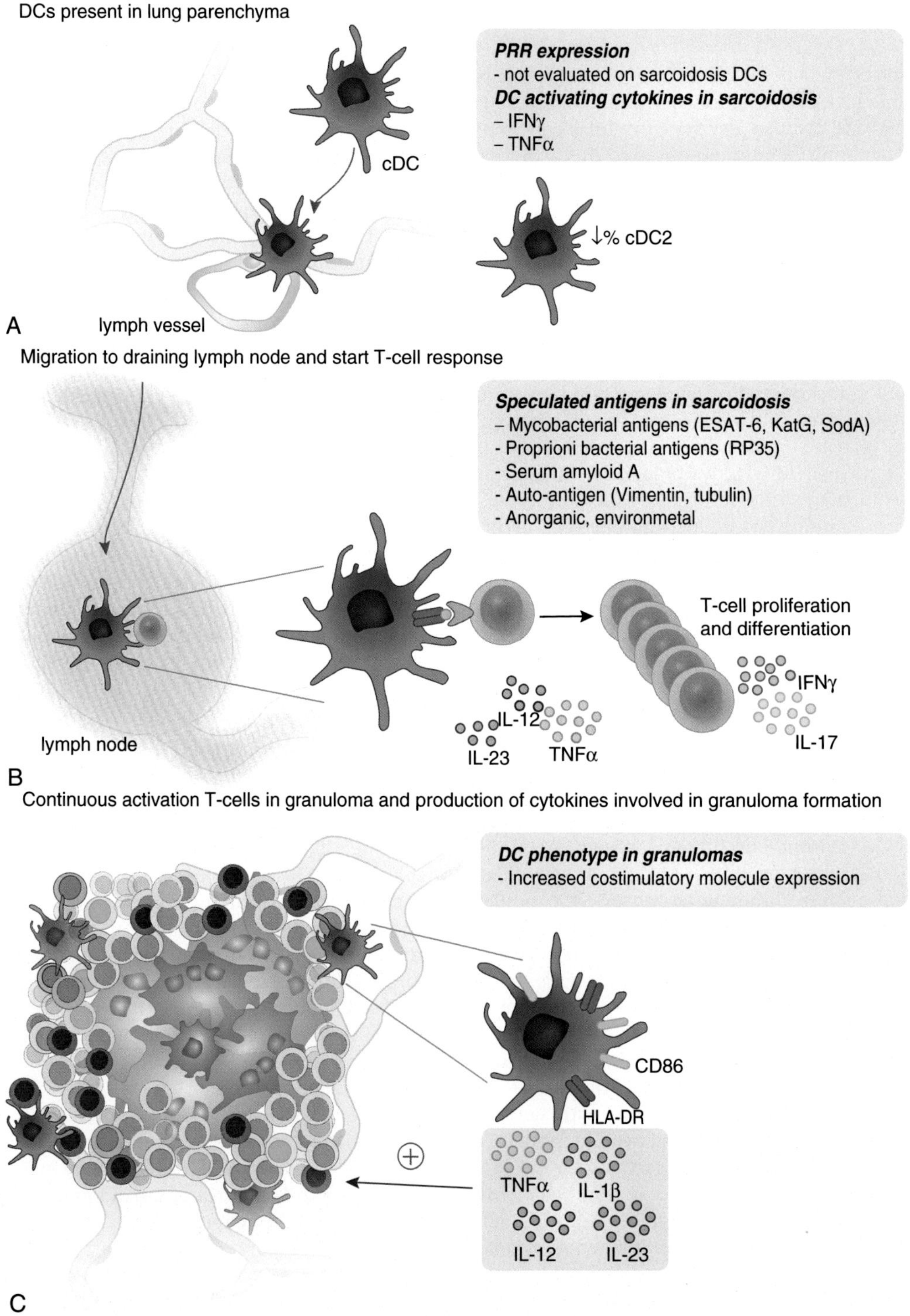

DCs present in lung parenchyma

PRR expression
- not evaluated on sarcoidosis DCs

DC activating cytokines in sarcoidosis
– IFNγ
– TNFα

cDC

↓% cDC2

A

lymph vessel

Migration to draining lymph node and start T-cell response

Speculated antigens in sarcoidosis
– Mycobacterial antigens (ESAT-6, KatG, SodA)
- Proprioni bacterial antigens (RP35)
- Serum amyloid A
- Auto-antigen (Vimentin, tubulin)
- Anorganic, environmetal

T-cell proliferation and differentiation

IFNγ

IL-17

IL-12

IL-23

TNFα

lymph node

B

Continuous activation T-cells in granuloma and production of cytokines involved in granuloma formation

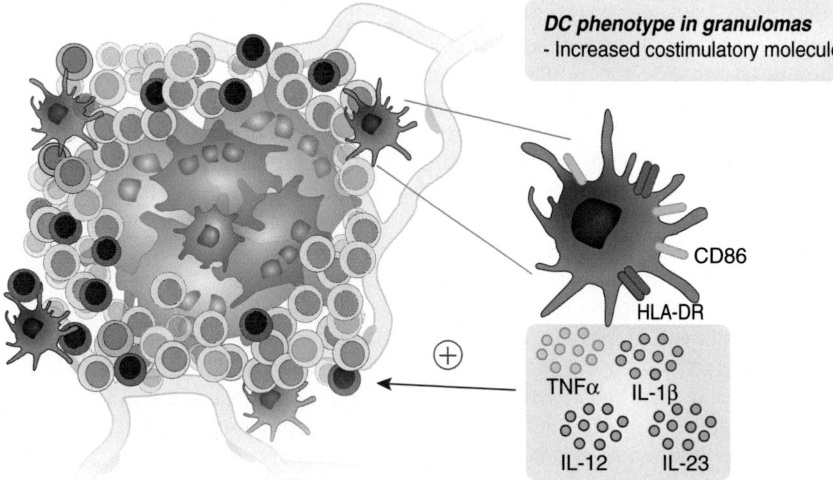

C

FIG. 3.3 **Dendritic Cell Function in Innate and Adaptive Immunity in Sarcoidosis.** (**A**) Dendritic cells (DCs) can be activated sarcoidosis key cytokines IFNγ and TNFα. (**B**) After activation, DCs migrate towards the draining lymph node to initiate T-cell responses. After HLA-DR-peptide complex recognition by the T-cell receptor (TCR) on T cells, T cells will proliferate. Speculated antigens involved in sarcoidosis pathology are shown. Under the influence of IL-12, IL-23, and TNFα, Th-cell can differentiate into IFNγ/IL-17A–producing Th-cells. (**C**) DCs present in the rim of the granuloma harbors an activated phenotype, and BALF DCs can secrete increased amounts of TNFα, IL-1β, IL-12, and possibly IL-23. *DC*, dendritic cell; *IFN*, interferon; *IL*, interleukin; *TNF*, tumor necrosis factor.

feed-forward loop. Several cytokines produced by activated DCs, such as IL-1β, IL-6, IL-12, IL-23, and TNFα, will activate T cells and contribute to granuloma formation.[58,68,69] Upon activation, DCs migrate to the lung-draining mediastinal LN (MLN), where they initiate antigen-specific T-cell responses by inducing T-cell proliferation and differentiation (Fig. 3.3B). Little is known about the phenotype LN-DCs in sarcoidosis, although they are present in LN granulomas.[60] In the T-cell area of the LN, DCs promote T-cell proliferation through presentation of antigens on HLA-DR to the T-cell receptor (TCR). Many HLA haplotypes exist, and disease prognosis is associated with specific HLA-DR alleles in sarcoidosis.[70] For instance, prognosis is favorable in patients positive for the HLA-DRB1*0301 allele, whereas HLA-DRB1*15 and HLA-DRB1*14 are associated with development of chronic disease.[71,72] Additionally, HLA-DRB1*0301^{+} patients also present with clonal expansion of Vα2.3/Vβ22 TCR T-cells, indicative of an ongoing antigen-specific response.[73] Molecular modeling of this HLA-TCR complex revealed an ideal fit for a peptide of vimentin,[74] one of the postulated auto-antigens in sarcoidosis. Vimentin was also found in the Kveim reagent,[75] eluted from HLA molecules from BALF macrophages from sarcoidosis patients,[76,77] and promoted IFNγ production in sarcoidosis BALF T-cells.[78] Interestingly, vimentin can also trigger dectin-1 activation,[79] one of the PRRs increased in sarcoidosis PBMCs.[10]

Although it is very likely that LN-specific DC-T-cell interactions are responsible for the initial T-cell activation in sarcoidosis, direct evidence is still lacking. In combination with antigen presentation by DCs to T cells, T cells must receive signals for proliferation, survival, and/or differentiation, which will be discussed in the following paragraph.

ADAPTIVE IMMUNE RESPONSE IN SARCOIDOSIS

Adaptive immune response creates immunological memory after an initial response to a specific pathogen and leads to an enhanced response to subsequent encounters with that pathogen. As a consequence, the adaptive immune response is highly specific to a particular pathogen and can provide long-lasting protection. Cells of the adaptive immune system are T cells and B cells. B cells are part of the humoral immune response, whereas T cells are intimately involved in cell-mediated immune responses. Within the T-cell compartment, CD8^{+} T cells and CD4^{+} helper T (Th) cells exist. Initiation of adaptive immunity occurs within the draining LN, where antigen presentation by DCs activates naïve T cells, and subsequently B cells are activated by specialized T cells.

Th-Cell Response

CD4^{+} Th-cells are abundantly present in sarcoid granulomas. Naïve Th-cells are activated by APCs, such as DCs, through TCR-peptide-HLA interaction, after which T-cell proliferation occurs before differentiation (Fig. 3.3B). Surrounding T-cell–skewing cytokines will influence differentiation of Th-cells by induction of lineage-specific transcription factors and epigenetic alterations of cytokine loci, resulting in subset-specific cytokine production. Sarcoidosis has long been considered a Th1-mediated disease, defined by a typical increase in IFNγ production by Th-cells in BALF,[80] as well as the presence of Th1-skewing cytokines IL-12 and IL-18 in both granulomatous tissue and BALF.[81,82]

However, during the past 10 years, new findings have altered our perception of sarcoidosis as a purely Th1-cell–driven disease to a general understanding that both Th1-cells and Th17-cells contribute to disease progression and outcome. Th17-cells are classically defined as IL-17–producing Th-cells, and IL-17–positive cells are found inside and in the vicinity of sarcoid granulomas.[32,83] Surprisingly, especially HLA-DRB1*0301^{+} LS patients showed enhanced IL-17 concentrations in BALF compared with healthy controls and non-LS sarcoidosis patients,[84] suggestive that IL-17 contributes to a favorable disease outcome. Th17-cell proportions correlated with neutrophil frequencies;[84] however, neutrophils are not implicated in sarcoidosis pathology.

A prominent role for IL-23/Th17-signaling pathway in the genetic etiology of sarcoidosis was also identified by functional prediction and protein network analyses.[85] More and more, it is becoming evident that Th-cells show plasticity to change subset or to increase the range of cytokines they produce.[86] Thus mixed phenotypes can be present in one Th-cell of two opposing differentiation programs.[87,88] Of all Th-subsets, especially Th17-cells are highly plastic, and stimulation through IL-12[89] and/or IL-23[90] induces their differentiation into IFNγ/IL-17A double-producing cells called Th1/Th17-cells. Enhanced IL-23 receptor (IL-23R) expression has been found on sarcoidosis IL-17–producing Th-cells in BALF and blood compared with controls,[32] suggestive of higher susceptibility for this transdifferentiation. Indeed, during chronic inflammation in mice, IL-23R expression on Th17-cells contributed to conversion toward Th1/Th17-cells.[91,92] Increased proportions of Th1/Th17-cells are observed in BALF and peripheral blood of sarcoidosis patients,[32,83,93–95] and their proportions increased with Scadding stage.[95] Probably these hybrid Th1/Th17-cells are pathogenic in sarcoidosis pathogenesis as this has also been described for other (granulomatous) inflammatory disorders, including Crohn's disease, multiple sclerosis, and rheumatoid arthritis.[89,92,96] Under the influence of Th1-skewing cytokines such as IFNγ, IL-12, and TNFα, Th1/Th17-cells can further develop into IFNγ-single-producing Th17-cells, also called nonclassical Th1-cells.[89,97,98] High expression of TNF receptor II (TNFRII) on Th17-cells promotes their switch to nonclassical Th1-cells, which have a low TNFRII expression.[98] In juvenile idiopathic arthritis, anti-TNFα treatment blocked the development of nonclassical Th1-cells from Th17-cells,[98] which could also translate to the success of anti-TNFα treatment in sarcoidosis patients.

IFNγ-producing Th17-cells, including both IFNγ/IL-17A double-positive (Th1/Th17-cells) and IFNγ-single positive cells (nonclassical Th1-cells), can be discriminated based on their chemokine expression and called Th17.1-cells.[93,96,99] Chemokine receptors that identify Th17.1-cells are CCR6 (Th17-lineage) together with CXCR3 (Th1-lineage). In three independent patient cohorts, both treatment naïve and cross-sectional, the majority of Th-cells in sarcoidosis BALF coexpressed CXCR3 and CCR6, suggesting the lung microenvironment to promote a Th17.1-cell phenotype that is augmented in sarcoidosis[93,100] (Fig. 3.4). Importantly however, increased proportions of Th17.1-cells in BALF were observed in sarcoidosis patients compared with healthy controls,[93] and even a more pronounced increase of the proportions of Th17.1-cells at the time of diagnosis was observed in patients who develop chronic sarcoidosis compared to those undergoing resolution.[99] Additionally, a sarcoidosis population that included progressive patients who are on first-, second- and/or third-line therapy also showed increased BALF Th17.1-cells proportions.[93] Somewhat unexpected, increased proportions of Th17.1-cells were also observed LS patients compared with non-LS chronic sarcoidosis patients.[100] However, a broader range of cytokines was found in BALF T-cells from LS than in non-LS patients, including IL-17A, IL-10, IL-22, and IL-2.[100] In contrast, in non-LS sarcoidosis, >90% of total BALF Th-cells produced IFNγ, and of all Th17-lineage cells, ~60% were IFNγ producers, whereas only 5% produced IL-17A, and <2% produced both cytokines.[93,100] These findings could suggest that potentially separate immune pathways are involved in the pathogenesis of LS and non-LS sarcoidosis. The dominant IFNγ signature strongly argues for a pathogenic role for Th17.1-cells in the development and progression of non-LS pulmonary sarcoidosis.[99] The presence of IL-17A, IL-10, and IL-22 could favor a good prognosis observed in LS patients as these all these cytokines are involved in immune regulation and maintenance of immune homeostasis.[101] However, whether this cytokine cocktail influences disease course is unknown, as in another cohort including stage I and II sarcoidosis patients, the proportions of cytokine-producing Th-cells were more in line with those found in LS patients (~60% IFNγ$^+$, ~25% IL-17A$^+$, and ~15% IFNγ/IL17A-double positive of total effector memory Th-cells).[83]

As written previously, activation and polarization of Th-cells is initiated in the draining LNs. In sarcoidosis LNs, granulomas are found that include a rim of activated Th-cells.[102] Within the MLN of sarcoidosis patients, the fraction of CCR6$^+$ Th17-lineage cells, including Th17-cells and Th17.1-cells, was increased compared with control MLN.[99] In contrast to sarcoidosis BALF, sarcoidosis MLN contained enhanced proportions of a Th17/Th17.1-intermediate Th-cell, named CCR6$^+$CXCR3$^+$CCR4$^+$ Th-cells or CCR6$^+$ double-positive (DP) Th-cells.[99,103–105] Especially those CCR6$^+$ DP Th-cells and Th17-cells were highly proliferative, both in BALF and MLN, whereas Th17.1-cells were not.[99] Together, these findings suggest that differentiation of Th17-cells is induced within T-cell areas of the sarcoidosis MLN and display plasticity toward pathogenic Th17.1-cells at chronically inflamed sites such as sarcoidosis lungs and also granulomatous parts of the MLN. Importantly, Th17.1-cells are refractory to glucocorticoids as they express high levels of the multidrug-resistant type 1 membrane transporter (MDR1),[96] contributing to their pathogenic signature.

Collectively, insight into the phenotype and effector function of Th17-lineage cells could reveal potential therapeutic targets, and possibly Th17.1-cell proportions could serve as a diagnostic and/or prognostic marker in clinical practice.

Th-Cell Suppressive Mechanisms in Sarcoidosis

Immunological changes observed in sarcoidosis are characteristic for an exaggerated antigen-driven immune response. Over the last years, some pieces of the puzzle of the underlying mechanisms leading to the amplified Th-cell response in sarcoidosis have been uncovered. Both regulatory mechanisms within T-cells (e.g., by checkpoint molecules) and the balance between proinflammatory Th-cells and suppressive regulatory Th-cells (Tregs) are critical to maintain tolerance. Not only Treg numbers but also their suppressive capacity is important to prevent inappropriate immune activation.[106]

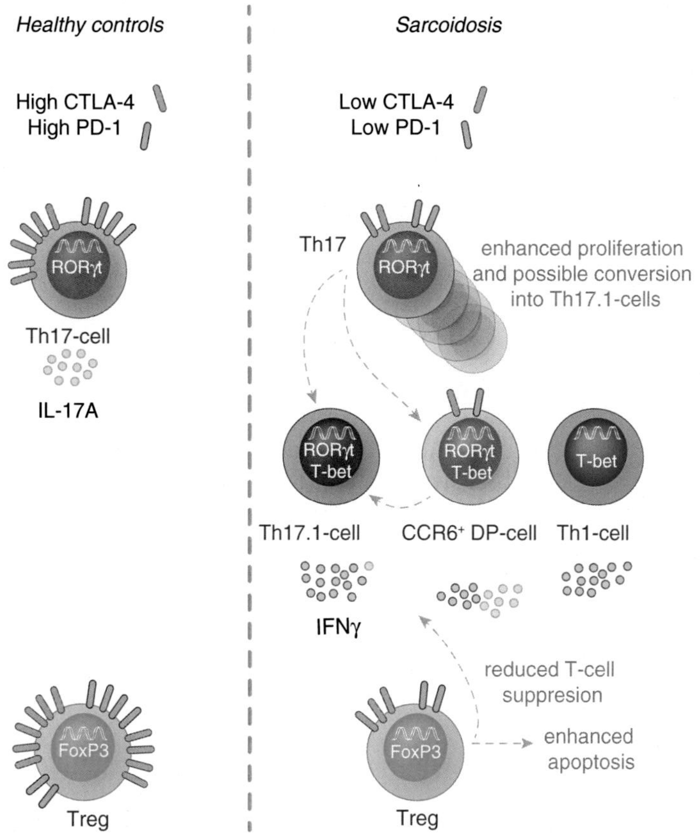

FIG. 3.4 **Alteration in the T-cell Compartment Promoting an Exaggerated Immune Response in Sarcoidosis.** Th17-cells in sarcoidosis express low levels of CTLA-4 and PD-1 compared with Th17-cells of healthy controls. This reduced expression of CTLA-4 and PD-1 can contribute to the development of Th17.1-cells. Regulatory Th-cells (Tregs) also express reduces amounts of CTLA-4 and PD-1 and harbor a proapoptotic phenotype, both contributing to a reduced immune-regulatory phenotype of these cells in sarcoidosis. For clarity, only Th17-cell subsets based on chemokine receptor expression are shown. *CTLA-4*, cytotoxic T-lymphocyte–associated antigen 4; *IFN*, interferon; *IL*, interleukin; *PD-1*, programmed death-1; *Th-cell*, T helper cell; *Treg*, regulatory T-cell.

Not surprisingly, Tregs are involved in sarcoidosis pathogenesis. Although inconsistent results are obtained regarding Treg numbers in BALF and blood,[107–115] a decreased immunosuppressive capacity of both BALF and blood Tregs has been consistently reported[108,111–114] (Fig. 3.4). They fail to restrain proliferation and cytokine production, such as IFNγ, TNFα, and IL-2, contributing to granuloma formation.[107,112,114] The defective suppression of sarcoidosis Tregs is due to intrinsic defects as sarcoid-derived effector Th-cells are suppressed by healthy Tregs.[112] Localization should be taken into account when evaluating the phenotype of Tregs in sarcoidosis patients. Tregs in granulomatous organs of sarcoidosis patients, e.g., LN and BALF, clearly show a different phenotype than those in peripheral blood (PB). When focusing on Tregs from BALF or lung-draining LN, these intrinsic defects could be mediated by reduced cytotoxic T-lymphocyte antigen 4 (CTLA-4) expression in LN and BALF,[116] one of the pathways used by Tregs to suppress T-cell activation.[117] In contrast, in PB Tregs harbor a highly differentiated effector phenotype illustrated by increased CD15s, CD25, and CTLA-4 expression and enhanced CD45RO proportion.[108,118] After activation and during suppression, effector Tregs are generally susceptible to apoptosis.[119–121] Indeed, apoptosis susceptibility and increased expression of CD95, the apoptosis signal receptor of sarcoidosis PB Tregs, were observed, which could contribute to the impaired immunosuppressive function found in sarcoidosis[108] (Fig. 3.4). In sarcoidosis patients treated with VIP, next to controlling macrophage activation, the fraction of BALF Tregs as well as their suppressive capacity increased.[113] This is in line with increased CTLA-4 expression on Tregs after VIP treatment *in vitro.*[113]

Coinhibitory receptors on T cells play a pivotal immune-regulatory role as they determine the functional outcome of TCR signaling and therefore proliferation and cytokine production by T cells. Alterations in the expression of coinhibitory receptors, such as CTLA-4, butyrophilin-like 2 (BTNL2), and programmed death-1 (PD-1), are speculated to contribute to the exaggerated immune response observed in sarcoidosis. CTLA-4 is constitutively highly expressed on Tregs and can be upregulated on activated Th-cells. Consequently, CTLA-4 harbors both cell-extrinsic and cell-intrinsic properties to control Th-cell responses.[122] CTLA-4 has a >10-fold higher affinity than CD28 for CD80/86 on APCs, thereby able to outcompete the costimulatory CD28 and leading to T-cell suppression.[122] Interestingly, of all human effector Th-cell subsets, Th17-cells display the highest expression of CTLA-4.[116] In sarcoidosis-affected organs, such as lung and LN, especially Tregs, Th17-cells, and CCR6+ DP Th-cells display reduced protein levels of CTLA-4[99,116] (Fig. 3.4). In healthy controls, CCR6+ DP Th-cells show an intermediate CTLA-4 expression in comparison to Th17-cells (high expression) and Th17.1-cells (low expression), which would be consistent with the notion that the conversion of Th17-cells into Th17.1-cells goes via intermediate CCR6+ DP Th-cells.[99] The decrease of CTLA-4 on both Th17-cells and Tregs can cause "double trouble"[116] as reduced CTLA-4 on Tregs will lead to a reduced regulation of T-cell activation[117] and low CTLA-4 on Th17-cells and CCR6+ DP Th-cells will increase their proliferation and activation state.[123] Indeed, CCR6+ DP Th-cells are highly proliferative in sarcoidosis LN.[99] Downregulated *CTLA4* mRNA expression was observed on whole-blood mRNA expression in sarcoidosis compared with controls.[124] Interestingly, Th-cells of LS patients have a relatively higher degree of CTLA-4 expression than non-LS sarcoidosis,[125] possibly contributing to the self-limiting disease course observed in this patient group.

Several other lines of evidence also support a crucial role for CTLA-4 expression in the exaggerated immune response observed in sarcoidosis. First, heterozygous *CTLA4* gene mutations have been identified in four unrelated families with common variable immunodeficiency (CVID), including granulomatous lung disease.[126] These mutations lead to one dysfunctional allele and reduced, but not absent, CTLA-4 expression on Tregs;[126] however, those *CTLA4* gene mutations have yet not been linked to sarcoidosis. This is also shown by the dissimilarity of CTLA-4 expression of Tregs in blood and tissue, being high and low, respectively, compared with controls.[108,116] Second, sarcoid-like granulomas can also be observed with anti-CTLA-4 immunotherapy used to treat various cancers. As a consequence, immune tolerance against the tumor will be broken[127] and as immune-related adverse event sarcoid-like granulomas were observed in a proportion of patients.[128–130] CTLA-4 also controls the number and proportion of Th17-cells, as in a patient with anti-CTLA-4 treatment-associated sarcoid-like reactions, increased numbers and proportions of Th17-cells were found during therapy compared with baseline.[129]

Next to CTLA-4, the coinhibitory receptor PD-1 also appears crucial in control of Th17-cell (plasticity), as melanoma patients with anti-PD-1–induced sarcoid-like disease presented with elevated peripheral Th17.1-cells before the first dose of treatment, compared with patients who did not develop granulomas and healthy controls.[131] This further strengthens the notion of an amplified immune response in sarcoidosis and the relationship between pathogenic Th17(.1)-cells and sarcoidosis. Th17-cells and Treg in MLN of sarcoidosis patients show a reduced PD-1 expression compared with those cells in control MLN (*Broos et al. unpublished data*). BALF Th-cells of LS patients also have higher PD-1 expression alongside CTLA-4 than non-LS sarcoidosis,[125] again possibly contributing to the self-limiting phenotype. However, no comparison of CTLA-4 and PD-1 expression on Th-cells from healthy controls was made.[125] In contrast, also during active disease, increased proportions of PD-1-expressing cells have been found within Th-cells in sarcoidosis BALF and PB compared with healthy controls. Especially IL-17–producing Th-cells highly expressed PD-1.[132,133] Whether the high PD-1 expression on IL-17+ Th-cells in BALF is specific for sarcoidosis or also occurs on IL-17+ Th-cells from healthy controls is yet unknown. These contradicting findings are puzzling; however as several patients receiving anti-PD1 treatment developed sarcoid-like granulomas in MLN and skin,[131,134,135] it favors the notion that sarcoidosis occurs due to an overwhelming immune response. The discrepancy may be related to the immune paradox observed in sarcoidosis patients, e.g., extensive local granulomatous inflammation versus peripheral anergy.[107]

The role of BTNL2, a B7 family member thought to function as a negative costimulatory molecule, in immune regulation remains largely unknown.[136] Its function has mainly been investigated in in vitro studies, in which an inhibitory effect of membrane-bound BTNL2 has been observed on Th-cell proliferation and cytokine production.[137,138] BTNL2 negatively influenced CD80-CD86/TCR-dependent activation of Th-cells, along with induction of FoxP3 expression, the Treg signature transcription factor.[139] These induced FoxP3+ Th-cells also harbored suppressive capacities.[139] Interestingly, polymorphisms of BTNL2 have been associated with (chronic) sarcoidosis.[140–143] The sarcoidosis-associated truncating splice site polymorphism (rs2076530 (G/A)) within the BTNL2 gene leads to disruption of the membrane localization of the BTNL2 molecule[140] and may thus contribute to dysregulated ongoing T-cell activation,[137] which is also seen in sarcoidosis.

Taken together, several immune inhibitory mechanisms are hampered in sarcoidosis, especially in affected organs. Defects in several of these control mechanisms can lead to an increase in pathogenic Th17(.1)-cells, possibly propagating a chronic inflammatory state.

B-Cell Responses in Sarcoidosis

Although Th-cells are critically involved in sarcoidosis immunopathology and show predominance in the rim surrounding granulomas, B cells and plasma cells are also present[144] and can contribute to disease pathogenesis.

In PB, sarcoidosis patients with active disease showed increased naive B cells and IgA^{+}CD27^{neg} memory B cells with decrease in CD27^{+} memory B cells and plasmablasts.[144–146] Specifically, IgA-positive plasma cells were observed around granulomas.[144] This could be of interest as IgA-producing plasma cells produce TNFα; however, increased TNFα production was not observed. The role of IgA^{+} memory B cells and IgA-producing plasma cells in sarcoidosis remains unclear; however, IgA is produced in a TGFβ-rich environment,[147] which also stimulates Th17-cell differentiation.

Increased serum levels of B-cell–activating factor (BAFF), also known as BlyS, a B-cell survival factor, are observed in (active) sarcoidosis for B cells.[145,146] Specifically, peripheral sarcoidosis monocytes produced increased amounts of BAFF.[145,146] Interestingly, BAFF production by monocytes is provoked by IFNγ,[148] and BAFF is also needed for APC-driven Th17-cell differentiation in RA.[149] This process could contribute to a feed-forward loop in sarcoidosis and continues immune activation. B-cell maturation and function depends on BAFF;[145,146] therefore its aberrant expression can also initiate defective selection of B cells, leading to autoantibody production. In sarcoidosis, some reports show that approximately 30%–60% of the patients exhibit antinuclear antibody (ANA) positivity,[145] and also increased anti-*M. tuberculosis*-antigen and antifungal antibodies are observed in BALF and/or serum.[150,151] It is currently unclear whether increased BAFF levels in sarcoidosis affect B-cell selection or activity or whether antigen-specific antibodies influence disease pathogenesis. There are case reports showing successful use of B-cell depletion using rituximab in refractory sarcoidosis with lung, eye, heart, and/or skin involvement, which could suggest that B cells are involved in disease progression.[152] Importantly, care should be taken as a refractory pemphigus vulgari patient treated with rituximab developed sarcoid-like granulomas.[153]

Altogether, these data suggest that B-cell immunity might be involved in sarcoidosis pathology; however, more knowledge about their role is needed.

TIPPING THE BALANCE TOWARD PROINFLAMMATORY IMMUNE RESPONSES IN SARCOIDOSIS

It is clear that immune cells of both the innate and adaptive system are involved in the enhanced proinflammatory response in sarcoidosis pathogenesis. The harmony between proinflammatory and antiinflammatory pathway is disturbed. For instance, an imbalance between M1 and in M2 macrophages could promote inflammation on one side and excessive would healing and/or fibrosis on the other side.[3]

The decrease in immune inhibitory checkpoint molecules, being CTLA-4 and PD-1, on both Tregs and Th17-cells can cause double trouble for the immune response in sarcoidosis, e.g., impairing Treg-mediated suppression[117] and contributing to Th17-cell proliferation[123] (Fig. 3.4).

Also, a disturbance in Th17-cell and Treg proportion is important in sarcoidosis immunopathology as a decreased Treg/Th17 ratio in BALF and PB is observed in active sarcoidosis patients compared with healthy controls.[154] Within sarcoidosis patients, the Treg/Th17 ratio in PB was higher in sarcoidosis patients who remained stable after steroid withdrawal than in relapsing patients.[154] Comparing Treg/Th17 ratios of relapsing sarcoidosis patients, before and 12 weeks after starting prednisone showed that the Treg/Th17 ratios increased due to treatment.[154] Because Treg/Th17 ratios were also inversely correlated with serum angiotensin-converting enzyme levels and positively correlated with lung function parameters, these data highlight that proinflammatory responses are key in sarcoidosis pathogenesis.

CLINICAL IMPLICATIONS

As multiple immune cells are involved in the pathogenesis of granuloma formation and sarcoidosis, it is only logical that interventions to treat sarcoidosis patients should aim at influencing several cell types. Most likely, this is why the main stay of sarcoidosis therapy, prednisone, is highly successful[155,156] as it targets survival and function of several cell types involved in granuloma maintenance, including macrophages and T cells. However, unfortunately, prednisone has several side effects, such as weight gain,[157] and this is why research into sarcoidosis immune responses is highly needed. New interventions should aim at influencing function, induction, localization, and/or survival of multiple immune cells in the sarcoid granuloma.[105] This can be achieved by a given drug that affects many pathways or by combining specific treatment strategies, with the least side effects. Only then are we able to control the exaggerated immune response leading to granulomas and possibly the detrimental fibrosis in sarcoidosis patients.

REFERENCES

1. Medzhitov R, Janeway CA. Innate immunity: the virtues of a nonclonal system of recognition. *Cell.* 1997;91(3):295–298.
2. Baharom F, Rankin G, Blomberg A, Smed-Sörensen A. Human lung mononuclear phagocytes in health and disease. *Front Immunol.* 2017;8. https://doi.org/10.3389/fimmu.2017.00499. 121–16.
3. Byrne AJ, Maher TM, Lloyd CM. Pulmonary macrophages: a new therapeutic pathway in fibrosing lung disease? *Trends Mol Med.* 2016;22(4):303–316. https://doi.org/10.1016/j.molmed.2016.02.004.
4. Rosen Y, Athanassiades TJ, Moon S, Lyons HA. Nongranulomatous interstitial pneumonitis in sarcoidosis. *Chest.* 1978;74(2):122–125. https://doi.org/10.1378/chest.74.2.122.
5. Talreja J, Talwar H, Ahmad N, Rastogi R, Samavati L. Dual inhibition of Rip2 and IRAK1/4 regulates IL-1β and IL-6 in sarcoidosis alveolar macrophages and peripheral blood mononuclear cells. *J Immunol.* 2016;197(4):1368–1378. https://doi.org/10.4049/jimmunol.1600258.
6. Nicod LP, Isler P. Alveolar macrophages in sarcoidosis coexpress high levels of CD86 (B7.2), CD40, and CD30L. *Am J Respir Cell Mol Biol.* 1997;17(1):91–96. https://doi.org/10.1165/ajrcmb.17.1.2781.
7. Wikén M, Idali F, Hayja Al MA, Grunewald J, Eklund A, Wahlström J. No evidence of altered alveolar macrophage polarization, but reduced expression of TLR2, in bronchoalveolar lavage cells in sarcoidosis. *Respir Res.* 2010;11(1):121. https://doi.org/10.1186/1465-9921-11-121.
8. Bianchi ME. DAMPs, PAMPs and alarmins: all we need to know about danger. *J Leukoc Biol.* 2007;81(1):1–5. https://doi.org/10.1189/jlb.0306164.
9. Schnerch J, Prasse A, Vlachakis D, et al. Functional toll-like receptor 9 expression and CXCR3 ligand release in pulmonary sarcoidosis. *Am J Respir Cell Mol Biol.* 2016;55(5):749–757. https://doi.org/10.1165/rcmb.2015-0278OC.
10. Stopinšek S, Ihan A, Salobir B, Terčelj M, Simčič S. Fungal cell wall agents and bacterial lipopolysaccharide in organic dust as possible risk factors for pulmonary sarcoidosis. *J Occup Med Toxicol.* 2016;11(1):46. https://doi.org/10.1186/s12995-016-0135-4.
11. Kanazawa N, Okafuji I, Kambe N, et al. Early-onset sarcoidosis and CARD15 mutations with constitutive nuclear factor-kappaB activation: common genetic etiology with Blau syndrome. *Blood.* 2005;105(3):1195–1197. https://doi.org/10.1182/blood-2004-07-2972.
12. Chen ES, Song Z, Willett MH, et al. Serum amyloid a regulates granulomatous inflammation in sarcoidosis through toll-like Receptor-2. *Am J Respir Crit Care Med.* 2010;181(4):360–373. https://doi.org/10.1164/rccm.200905-0696OC.
13. Chatterjee S, Dwivedi VP, Singh Y, et al. Early secreted antigen ESAT-6 of *Mycobacterium tuberculosis* promotes protective T helper 17 cell responses in a toll-like receptor-2-dependent manner. Bishai Jr WR, ed. *PLoS Pathog.* 2011;7(11):e1002378. https://doi.org/10.1371/journal.ppat.1002378.
14. Nishioka Y, Manabe K, Kishi J, et al. CXCL9 and 11 in patients with pulmonary sarcoidosis: a role of alveolar macrophages. *Clin Exp Immunol.* 2007;149(2):317–326. https://doi.org/10.1111/j.1365-2249.2007.03423.x.
15. Groom JR, Luster AD. CXCR3 ligands: redundant, collaborative and antagonistic functions. *Immunol Cell Biol.* 2011;89(2):207–215. https://doi.org/10.1038/icb.2010.158.
16. Piotrowski WJ, Młynarski W, Fendler W, et al. Chemokine receptor CXCR3 ligands in bronchoalveolar lavage fluid: associations with radiological pattern, clinical course, and prognosis in sarcoidosis. *Pol Arch Med Wewn.* 2014;124(7–8):395–402.
17. Su R, Nguyen M-LT, Agarwal MR, et al. Interferon-inducible chemokines reflect severity and progression in sarcoidosis. *Respir Res.* 2013;14(1):121. https://doi.org/10.1186/1465-9921-14-121.
18. Atamas SP, Luzina IG, Choi J, et al. Pulmonary and activation-regulated chemokine stimulates collagen production in lung fibroblasts. *Am J Respir Cell Mol Biol.* 2003;29(6):743–749. https://doi.org/10.1165/rcmb.2003-0078OC.

19. Nagasawa H, Miyaura C, Abe E, Horiguchi M, Suda T. Fusion and activation of human alveolar macrophages induced by recombinant interferon-gamma and their suppression by dexamethasone. *Am Rev Respir Dis.* 1987;136(4):916–921. https://doi.org/10.1164/ajrccm/136.4.916.
20. Wynn TA, Chawla A, Pollard JW. Macrophage biology in development, homeostasis and disease. *Nature.* 2013;496(7446):445–455. https://doi.org/10.1038/nature12034.
21. Shamaei M, Mortaz E, Pourabdollah M, et al. Evidence for M2 macrophages in granulomas from pulmonary sarcoidosis: a new aspect of macrophage heterogeneity. *Hum Immunol.* 2018;79(1):63–69. https://doi.org/10.1016/j.humimm.2017.10.009.
22. Oltmanns U, Schmidt B, Hoernig S, Witt C, John M. Increased spontaneous interleukin-10 release from alveolar macrophages in active pulmonary sarcoidosis. *Exp Lung Res.* 2003;29(5):315–328.
23. John M, Oltmanns U, Fietze I, Witt C, Jung K. Increased production of matrix metalloproteinase-2 in alveolar macrophages and regulation by interleukin-10 in patients with acute pulmonary sarcoidosis. *Exp Lung Res.* 2002;28(1):55–68.
24. Kline JN, Schwartz DA, Monick MM, Floerchinger CS, Hunninghake GM. Relative release of interleukin-1 beta and interleukin-1 receptor antagonist by alveolar macrophages. A study in asbestos-induced lung disease, sarcoidosis, and idiopathic pulmonary fibrosis. *Chest.* 1993;104(1):47–53. https://doi.org/10.1378/chest.104.1.47.
25. Ziegler-Heitbrock L, Ancuta P, Crowe S, et al. Nomenclature of monocytes and dendritic cells in blood. *Blood.* 2010;116(16):e74–e80. https://doi.org/10.1182/blood-2010-02-258558.
26. Jakubzick CV, Randolph GJ, Henson PM. Monocyte differentiation and antigen-presenting functions. *Nat Rev Immunol.* May 2017:1–14. https://doi.org/10.1038/nri.2017.28.
27. Dubaniewicz A, Typiak M, Wybieralska M, et al. Changed phagocytic activity and pattern of Fcγ and complement receptors on blood monocytes in sarcoidosis. *Hum Immunol.* 2012;73(8):788–794. https://doi.org/10.1016/j.humimm.2012.05.005.
28. Fraser SD, Sadofsky LR, Kaye PM, Hart SP. Reduced expression of monocyte CD200R is associated with enhanced proinflammatory cytokine production in sarcoidosis. *Sci Rep.* 2016;6(1):38689. https://doi.org/10.1038/srep38689.
29. Murray PJ. Immune regulation by monocytes. *Semin Immunol.* December 2017. https://doi.org/10.1016/j.smim.2017.12.005.
30. Wong KL, Tai JJ-Y, Wong W-C, et al. Gene expression profiling reveals the defining features of the classical, intermediate, and nonclassical human monocyte subsets. *Blood.* 2011;118(5):e16–e31. https://doi.org/10.1182/blood-2010-12-326355.
31. Rossol M, Kraus S, Pierer M, Baerwald C, Wagner U. The CD14(bright) CD16+ monocyte subset is expanded in rheumatoid arthritis and promotes expansion of the Th17 cell population. *Arthritis Rheum.* 2012;64(3):671–677. https://doi.org/10.1002/art.33418.
32. Facco M, Cabrelle A, Teramo A, et al. Sarcoidosis is a Th1/Th17 multisystem disorder. *Thorax.* 2011;66(2):144–150. https://doi.org/10.1136/thx.2010.140319.
33. Hijdra D, Vorselaars AD, Grutters JC, Claessen AM, Rijkers GT. Differential expression of TNFR1 (CD120a) and TNFR2 (CD120b) on subpopulations of human monocytes. *J Inflamm.* 2012;9(1):38. https://doi.org/10.1186/1476-9255-9-38.
34. Hofer TPJ, Zawada AM, Frankenberger M, et al. Slan-defined subsets of CD16-positive monocytes: impact of granulomatous inflammation and M-CSF receptor mutation. *Blood.* 2015;126(24):2601–2610. https://doi.org/10.1182/blood-2015-06-651331.
35. Hijdra D, Vorselaars ADM, Crommelin HA, et al. Can intermediate monocytes predict response to infliximab therapy in sarcoidosis? *Eur Respir J.* 2016;48(4):1242–1245. https://doi.org/10.1183/13993003.00709-2016.
36. Heron M, Grutters JC, van Velzen-Blad H, Veltkamp M, Claessen AME, van den Bosch JMM. Increased expression of CD16, CD69, and very late antigen-1 on blood monocytes in active sarcoidosis. *Chest.* 2008;134(5):1001–1008. https://doi.org/10.1378/chest.08-0443.
37. Okamoto H, Mizuno K, Horio T. Circulating CD14+ CD16+ monocytes are expanded in sarcoidosis patients. *J Dermatol.* 2003;30(7):503–509.
38. Fingerle-Rowson G, Angstwurm M, Andreesen R, Ziegler-Heitbrock HW. Selective depletion of CD14+ CD16+ monocytes by glucocorticoid therapy. *Clin Exp Immunol.* 1998;112(3):501–506. https://doi.org/10.1046/j.1365-2249.1998.00617.x.
39. Netea MG, Quintin J, van der Meer JWM. Trained immunity: a memory for innate host defense. *Cell Host Microbe.* 2011;9(5):355–361. https://doi.org/10.1016/j.chom.2011.04.006.
40. Kleinnijenhuis J, Quintin J, Preijers F, et al. Bacille Calmette-Guerin induces NOD2-dependent nonspecific protection from reinfection via epigenetic reprogramming of monocytes. *Proc Natl Acad Sci USA.* 2012;109(43):17537–17542. https://doi.org/10.1073/pnas.1202870109.
41. Saeed S, Quintin J, Kerstens HHD, et al. Epigenetic programming of monocyte-to-macrophage differentiation and trained innate immunity. *Science.* 2014;345(6204):1251086. https://doi.org/10.1126/science.1251086.
42. Netea MG, Joosten LAB, Latz E, et al. Trained immunity: a program of innate immune memory in health and disease. *Science.* 2016;352(6284):aaf1098. https://doi.org/10.1126/science.aaf1098.
43. Bekkering S, Joosten LAB, van der Meer JWM, Netea MG, Riksen NP. Trained innate immunity and atherosclerosis. *Curr Opin Lipidol.* 2013;24(6):487–492. https://doi.org/10.1097/MOL.0000000000000023.

44. Ifrim DC, Quintin J, Joosten LAB, et al. Trained immunity or tolerance: opposing functional programs induced in human monocytes after engagement of various pattern recognition receptors. Papasian CJ, ed. *Clin Vaccine Immunol.* 2014;21(4):534–545. https://doi.org/10.1128/CVI.00688-13.
45. Domínguez-Andrés J, Arts RJW, Horst ter R, et al. Rewiring monocyte glucose metabolism via C-type lectin signaling protects against disseminated candidiasis. *PLoS Pathog.* 2017;13(9):e1006632. https://doi.org/10.1371/journal.ppat.1006632.
46. Arts RJW, Carvalho A, La Rocca C, et al. Immunometabolic pathways in BCG-induced trained immunity. *Cell Rep.* 2016;17(10):2562–2571. https://doi.org/10.1016/j.celrep.2016.11.011.
47. Oswald-Richter KA, Sato H, Hajizadeh R, et al. Mycobacterial ESAT-6 and katG are recognized by sarcoidosis CD4+ T cells when presented by the American sarcoidosis susceptibility allele, DRB1*1101. *J Clin Immunol.* 2010;30(1):157–166. https://doi.org/10.1007/s10875-009-9311-y.
48. Drake W, Dhason MS, Nadaf M, et al. Cellular recognition of *Mycobacterium tuberculosis* ESAT-6 and KatG peptides in systemic sarcoidosis. *Infect Immun.* 2007;75(1):527–530. https://doi.org/10.1128/IAI.00732-06.
49. Chen ES, Wahlström J, Song Z, et al. T cell responses to mycobacterial catalase-peroxidase profile a pathogenic antigen in systemic sarcoidosis. *J Immunol.* 2008;181(12):8784–8796.
50. Cheng S-C, Quintin J, Cramer RA, et al. mTOR- and HIF-1α-mediated aerobic glycolysis as metabolic basis for trained immunity. *Science.* 2014;345(6204):1250684. https://doi.org/10.1126/science.1250684.
51. Weichhart T, Hengstschläger M, Linke M. Regulation of innate immune cell function by mTOR. *Nat Rev Immunol.* 2015;15(10):599–614. https://doi.org/10.1038/nri3901. Nature Publishing Group.
52. Linke M, Pham HTT, Katholnig K, et al. Chronic signaling via the metabolic checkpoint kinase mTORC1 induces macrophage granuloma formation and marks sarcoidosis progression. *Nat Immunol.* 2017;18(3):293–302. https://doi.org/10.1038/ni.3655.
53. Eckert H, Zaumseil I, Sehrt I. The value of modern morphological methods (histochemistry, immunopathology) in sarcoidosis. *Z Erkr Atmungsorgane.* 1977;149(1):94–95.
54. Shaw PA, Fletcher A. Counts of S-100 positive epidermal dendritic cells in Kveim test skin biopsies. *Histopathology.* 1991;18(2):149–153.
55. Uslu U, Erdmann M, Schliep S, et al. Sarcoidosis under dendritic cell vaccination immunotherapy in long-term responding patients with metastatic melanoma. *Anticancer Res.* 2017;37(6):3243–3248. https://doi.org/10.21873/anticanres.11687.
56. Guilliams M, Dutertre C-A, Scott CL, et al. Unsupervised high-dimensional analysis aligns dendritic cells across tissues and species. *Immunity.* 2016;45(3):669–684. https://doi.org/10.1016/j.immuni.2016.08.015.
57. Liu H, Jakubzick CV, Osterburg AR, et al. Dendritic cell trafficking and function in rare lung diseases. *Am J Respir Cell Mol Biol.* 2017;57(4):393–402. https://doi.org/10.1165/rcmb.2017-0051PS.
58. Berge Ten B, KleinJan A, Muskens F, et al. Evidence for local dendritic cell activation in pulmonary sarcoidosis. *Respir Res.* 2012;13(1):33. https://doi.org/10.1186/1465-9921-13-33.
59. Lommatzsch M, Bratke K, Bier A, et al. Airway dendritic cell phenotypes in inflammatory diseases of the human lung. *Eur Respir J.* 2007;30(5):878–886. https://doi.org/10.1183/09031936.00036307.
60. Ota M, Amakawa R, Uehira K, et al. Involvement of dendritic cells in sarcoidosis. *Thorax.* 2004;59(5):408–413. https://doi.org/10.1136/thx.2003.006049.
61. Yamashita M, Mouri T, Niisato M, et al. Heterogeneous characteristics of lymphatic microvasculatures associated with pulmonary sarcoid granulomas. *Ann Am Thorac Soc.* 2013;10(2):90–97. https://doi.org/10.1513/AnnalsATS.201209-078OC.
62. Kambouchner M, Pirici D, Uhl J-F, Mogoanta L, Valeyre D, Bernaudin J-F. Lymphatic and blood microvasculature organisation in pulmonary sarcoid granulomas. *Eur Respir J.* 2011;37(4):835–840. https://doi.org/10.1183/09031936.00086410.
63. Hemont C, Neel A, Heslan M, Braudeau C, Josien R. Human blood mDC subsets exhibit distinct TLR repertoire and responsiveness. *J Leukoc Biol.* 2013;93(4):599–609. https://doi.org/10.1189/jlb.0912452.
64. Jongbloed SL, Kassianos AJ, McDonald KJ, et al. Human CD141+ (BDCA-3)+ dendritic cells (DCs) represent a unique myeloid DC subset that cross-presents necrotic cell antigens. *J Exp Med.* 2010;207(6):1247–1260. https://doi.org/10.1084/jem.20092140.
65. Schlitzer A, McGovern N, Teo P, et al. IRF4 transcription factor-dependent CD11b+ dendritic cells in human and mouse control mucosal IL-17 cytokine responses. *Immunity.* 2013;38(5):970–983. https://doi.org/10.1016/j.immuni.2013.04.011.
66. Moller DR, Forman JD, Liu MC, et al. Enhanced expression of IL-12 associated with Th1 cytokine profiles in active pulmonary sarcoidosis. *J Immunol.* 1996;156(12):4952–4960.
67. Wahlström J, Berlin M, Sköld CM, Wigzell H, Eklund A, Grunewald J. Phenotypic analysis of lymphocytes and monocytes/macrophages in peripheral blood and bronchoalveolar lavage fluid from patients with pulmonary sarcoidosis. *Thorax.* 1999;54(4):339–346.
68. Tristão FSM, Rocha FA, Carlos D, et al. Th17-Inducing cytokines IL-6 and IL-23 are crucial for granuloma formation during experimental paracoccidioidomycosis. *Front Immunol.* 2017;8:949. https://doi.org/10.3389/fimmu.2017.00949.
69. Mihret A. The role of dendritic cells in *Mycobacterium tuberculosis* infection. *Virulence.* 2012;3(7):654–659. https://doi.org/10.4161/viru.22586.

70. Grunewald J, Spagnolo P, Wahlström J, Eklund A. Immunogenetics of disease-causing inflammation in sarcoidosis. *Clin Rev Allergy Immunol.* 2015;49(1):19–35. https://doi.org/10.1007/s12016-015-8477-8.
71. Grunewald J, Eklund A. Löfgren's syndrome: human leukocyte antigen strongly influences the disease course. *Am J Respir Crit Care Med.* 2009;179(4):307–312. https://doi.org/10.1164/rccm.200807-1082OC.
72. Grunewald J, Brynedal B, Darlington P, et al. Different HLA-DRB1 allele distributions in distinct clinical subgroups of sarcoidosis patients. *Respir Res.* 2010;11(1):25. https://doi.org/10.1186/1465-9921-11-25.
73. Grunewald J, Wahlström J, Berlin M, Wigzell H, Eklund A, Olerup O. Lung restricted T cell receptor AV2S3+ CD4+ T cell expansions in sarcoidosis patients with a shared HLA-DRbeta chain conformation. *Thorax.* 2002;57(4):348–352. https://doi.org/10.1136/thorax.57.4.348.
74. Grunewald J, Kaiser Y, Ostadkarampour M, et al. T-cell receptor-HLA-DRB1 associations suggest specific antigens in pulmonary sarcoidosis. *Eur Respir J.* 2016;47(3):898–909. https://doi.org/10.1183/13993003.01209-2015.
75. Eberhardt C, Thillai M, Parker R, et al. Proteomic analysis of Kveim reagent identifies targets of cellular immunity in sarcoidosis. *PLoS One.* 2017;12(1):e0170285. https://doi.org/10.1371/journal.pone.0170285.
76. Heyder T, Kohler M, Tarasova NK, et al. Approach for identifying human leukocyte antigen (HLA)-DR bound peptides from scarce clinical samples. *Mol Cell Proteomics.* 2016;15(9):3017–3029. https://doi.org/10.1074/mcp.M116.060764.
77. Wahlström J, Dengjel J, Persson B, et al. Identification of HLA-DR-bound peptides presented by human bronchoalveolar lavage cells in sarcoidosis. *J Clin Investig.* 2007;117(11):3576–3582. https://doi.org/10.1172/JCI32401.
78. Wahlström J, Dengjel J, Winqvist O, et al. Autoimmune T cell responses to antigenic peptides presented by bronchoalveolar lavage cell HLA-DR molecules in sarcoidosis. *Clin Immunol.* 2009;133(3):353–363. https://doi.org/10.1016/j.clim.2009.08.008.
79. Thiagarajan PS, Yakubenko VP, Elsori DH, et al. Vimentin is an endogenous ligand for the pattern recognition receptor Dectin-1. *Cardiovasc Res.* 2013;99(3):494–504. https://doi.org/10.1093/cvr/cvt117.
80. Robinson BW, McLemore TL, Crystal RG. Gamma interferon is spontaneously released by alveolar macrophages and lung T lymphocytes in patients with pulmonary sarcoidosis. *J Clin Investig.* 1985;75(5):1488–1495. https://doi.org/10.1172/JCI111852.
81. Shigehara K, Shijubo N, Ohmichi M, et al. IL-12 and IL-18 are increased and stimulate IFN-gamma production in sarcoid lungs. *J Immunol.* 2001;166(1):642–649.
82. Antoniou KM, Tzouvelekis A, Alexandrakis MG, et al. Upregulation of Th1 cytokine profile (IL-12, IL-18) in bronchoalveolar lavage fluid in patients with pulmonary sarcoidosis. *J Interferon Cytokine Res.* 2006;26(6):400–405. https://doi.org/10.1089/jir.2006.26.400.
83. Berge Ten B, Paats MS, Bergen IM, et al. Increased IL-17A expression in granulomas and in circulating memory T cells in sarcoidosis. *Rheumatology (Oxf).* 2012;51(1):37–46. https://doi.org/10.1093/rheumatology/ker316.
84. Ostadkarampour M, Eklund A, Moller DR, et al. Higher levels of interleukin IL-17 and antigen-specific IL-17 responses in pulmonary sarcoidosis patients with Löfgren's syndrome. *Clin Exp Immunol.* 2014;178(2):342–352. https://doi.org/10.1111/cei.12403.
85. Fischer A, Ellinghaus D, Nutsua M, et al. Identification of immune-relevant factors conferring sarcoidosis genetic risk. *Am J Respir Crit Care Med.* 2015;192(6):727–736. https://doi.org/10.1164/rccm.201503-0418OC.
86. Stadhouders R, Lubberts E, Hendriks RW. A cellular and molecular view of T helper 17 cell plasticity in autoimmunity. *J Autoimmun.* 2018;87:1–15. https://doi.org/10.1016/j.jaut.2017.12.007.
87. Fang D, Zhu J. Dynamic balance between master transcription factors determines the fates and functions of CD4 T cell and innate lymphoid cell subsets. *J Exp Med.* 2017;214(7):1861–1876. https://doi.org/10.1084/jem.20170494.
88. Antebi YE, Reich-Zeliger S, Hart Y, et al. Mapping differentiation under mixed culture conditions reveals a tunable continuum of T cell fates. Bhandoola A, ed. *PLoS Biol.* 2013;11(7):e1001616. https://doi.org/10.1371/journal.pbio.1001616.
89. Annunziato F, Cosmi L, Santarlasci V, et al. Phenotypic and functional features of human Th17 cells. *J Exp Med.* 2007;204(8):1849–1861. https://doi.org/10.1084/jem.20070663.
90. Duhen R, Glatigny S, Arbelaez CA, Blair TC, Oukka M, Bettelli E. Cutting edge: the pathogenicity of IFN-γ-producing Th17 cells is independent of T-bet. *J Immunol.* 2013;190(9):4478–4482. https://doi.org/10.4049/jimmunol.1203172.
91. Awasthi A, Riol-Blanco L, Jäger A, et al. Cutting edge: IL-23 receptor gfp reporter mice reveal distinct populations of IL-17-producing cells. *J Immunol.* 2009;182(10):5904–5908. https://doi.org/10.4049/jimmunol.0900732.
92. Gaublomme JT, Yosef N, Lee Y, et al. Single-cell genomics unveils critical regulators of Th17 cell pathogenicity. *Cell.* 2015;163(6):1400–1412. https://doi.org/10.1016/j.cell.2015.11.009.
93. Ramstein J, Broos CE, Simpson LJ, et al. IFN-γ–producing T-helper 17.1 cells are increased in sarcoidosis and are more prevalent than T-helper type 1 cells. *Am J Respir Crit Care Med.* 2016;193(11):1281–1291. https://doi.org/10.1164/rccm.201507-1499OC.
94. Richmond BW, Ploetze K, Isom J, et al. Sarcoidosis Th17 cells are ESAT-6 antigen specific but demonstrate reduced IFN-γ expression. *J Clin Immunol.* 2013;33(2):446–455. https://doi.org/10.1007/s10875-012-9817-6.

95. Tøndell A, Moen T, Børset M, Salvesen Ø, Rø AD, Sue-Chu M. Bronchoalveolar lavage fluid IFN-γ+ Th17 cells and regulatory T cells in pulmonary sarcoidosis. *Mediat Inflamm.* 2014;2014(2):438070–438079. https://doi.org/10.1155/2014/438070.
96. Ramesh R, Kozhaya L, McKevitt K, et al. Pro-inflammatory human Th17 cells selectively express P-glycoprotein and are refractory to glucocorticoids. *J Exp Med.* 2014;211(1):89–104. https://doi.org/10.1084/jem.20130301.
97. Lexberg MH, Taubner A, Albrecht I, et al. IFN-γ and IL-12 synergize to convert in vivo generated Th17 into Th1/Th17 cells. *Eur J Immunol.* 2010;40(11):3017–3027. https://doi.org/10.1002/eji.201040539.
98. Maggi L, Cimaz R, Capone M, et al. Brief report: etanercept inhibits the tumor necrosis factor α-driven shift of Th17 lymphocytes toward a nonclassic Th1 phenotype in juvenile idiopathic arthritis. *Arthritis Rheumatol.* 2014;66(5):1372–1377. https://doi.org/10.1002/art.38355.
99. Broos CE, Koth LL, van Nimwegen M, et al. Increased T-helper 17.1 cells in sarcoidosis mediastinal lymph nodes. *Eur Respir J.* 2018;51(3):1701124. https://doi.org/10.1183/13993003.01124-2017.
100. Kaiser Y, Lepzien R, Kullberg S, Eklund A, Smed-Sörensen A, Grunewald J. Expanded lung T-bet+RORγT+ CD4+ T-cells in sarcoidosis patients with a favourable disease phenotype. *Eur Respir J.* 2016;48(2):484–494. https://doi.org/10.1183/13993003.00092-2016.
101. Littman DR, Rudensky AY. Th17 and regulatory T cells in mediating and restraining inflammation. *Cell.* 2010;140(6):845–858. https://doi.org/10.1016/j.cell.2010.02.021.
102. Kita S, Tsuda T, Sugisaki K, Miyazaki E, Matsumoto T. Characterization of distribution of T lymphocyte subsets and activated T lymphocytes infiltrating into sarcoid lesions. *Intern Med.* 1995;34(9):847–855.
103. Paulissen SMJ, van Hamburg JP, Dankers W, Lubberts E. The role and modulation of CCR6+ Th17 cell populations in rheumatoid arthritis. *Cytokine.* 2015;74(1):43–53. https://doi.org/10.1016/j.cyto.2015.02.002.
104. Lubberts E. The IL-23-IL-17 axis in inflammatory arthritis. *Nat Rev Rheumatol.* 2015;11(7):415–429. https://doi.org/10.1038/nrrheum.2015.53.
105. Miedema JR, Kaiser Y, Broos CE, Wijsenbeek MS, Grunewald J, Kool M. Th17-lineage cells in pulmonary sarcoidosis and Löfgren's syndrome: friend or foe? *J Autoimmun.* 2018;87:82–96. https://doi.org/10.1016/j.jaut.2017.12.012.
106. Miyara M, Gorochov G, Ehrenstein M, Musset L, Sakaguchi S, Amoura Z. Human FoxP3+ regulatory T cells in systemic autoimmune diseases. *Autoimmun Rev.* 2011;10(12):744–755. https://doi.org/10.1016/j.autrev.2011.05.004.
107. Miyara M, Amoura Z, Parizot C, et al. The immune paradox of sarcoidosis and regulatory T cells. *J Exp Med.* 2006;203(2):359–370. https://doi.org/10.1084/jem.20050648.
108. Broos CE, van Nimwegen M, KleinJan A, et al. Impaired survival of regulatory T cells in pulmonary sarcoidosis. *Respir Res.* 2015;16(1):108. https://doi.org/10.1186/s12931-015-0265-8.
109. Idali F, Wahlström J, Müller-Suur C, Eklund A, Grunewald J. Analysis of regulatory T cell associated forkhead box P3 expression in the lungs of patients with sarcoidosis. *Clin Exp Immunol.* 2008;152(1):127–137. https://doi.org/10.1111/j.1365-2249.2008.03609.x.
110. Wikén M, Grunewald J, Eklund A, Wahlström J. Multiparameter phenotyping of T-cell subsets in distinct subgroups of patients with pulmonary sarcoidosis. *J Intern Med.* 2012;271(1):90–103. https://doi.org/10.1111/j.1365-2796.2011.02414.x.
111. Rappl G, Pabst S, Riemann D, et al. Regulatory T cells with reduced repressor capacities are extensively amplified in pulmonary sarcoid lesions and sustain granuloma formation. *Clin Immunol.* 2011;140(1):71–83. https://doi.org/10.1016/j.clim.2011.03.015.
112. Oswald-Richter KA, Richmond BW, Braun NA, et al. Reversal of global CD4+ subset dysfunction is associated with spontaneous clinical resolution of pulmonary sarcoidosis. *J Immunol.* 2013;190(11):5446–5453. https://doi.org/10.4049/jimmunol.1202891.
113. Prasse A, Zissel G, Lützen N, et al. Inhaled vasoactive intestinal peptide exerts immunoregulatory effects in sarcoidosis. *Am J Respir Crit Care Med.* 2010;182(4):540–548. https://doi.org/10.1164/rccm.200909-1451OC.
114. Taflin C, Miyara M, Nochy D, et al. FoxP3+ regulatory T cells suppress early stages of granuloma formation but have little impact on sarcoidosis lesions. *Am J Pathol.* 2009;174(2):497–508. https://doi.org/10.2353/ajpath.2009.080580.
115. Sakthivel P, Grunewald J, Eklund A, Bruder D, Wahlström J. Pulmonary sarcoidosis is associated with high-level inducible co-stimulator (ICOS) expression on lung regulatory T cells - possible implications for the ICOS/ICOS-ligand axis in disease course and resolution. *Clin Exp Immunol.* 2016;183(2):294–306. https://doi.org/10.1111/cei.12715.
116. Broos CE, van Nimwegen M, In 't Veen JCCM, et al. Decreased cytotoxic T-lymphocyte antigen 4 expression on regulatory T cells and Th17 cells in sarcoidosis: double trouble? *Am J Respir Crit Care Med.* 2015;192(6):763–765. https://doi.org/10.1164/rccm.201503-0635LE.
117. Walker LSK, Sansom DM. The emerging role of CTLA4 as a cell-extrinsic regulator of T cell responses. *Nat Rev Immunol.* 2011;11(12):852–863. https://doi.org/10.1038/nri3108.
118. Miyara M, Chader D, Sage E, et al. Sialyl Lewis x (CD15s) identifies highly differentiated and most suppressive FOXP3high regulatory T cells in humans. *Proc Natl Acad Sci USA.* 2015;112(23):7225–7230. https://doi.org/10.1073/pnas.1508224112.
119. Sakaguchi S, Miyara M, Costantino CM, Hafler DA. FOXP3+ regulatory T cells in the human immune system. *Nat Rev Immunol.* 2010;10(7):490–500. https://doi.org/10.1038/nri2785.

120. Miyara M, Yoshioka Y, Kitoh A, et al. Functional delineation and differentiation dynamics of human CD4+ T cells expressing the FoxP3 transcription factor. *Immunity*. 2009;30(6):899–911. https://doi.org/10.1016/j.immuni.2009.03.019.
121. Fritzsching B, Oberle N, Pauly E, et al. Naive regulatory T cells: a novel subpopulation defined by resistance toward CD95L-mediated cell death. *Blood*. 2006;108(10):3371–3378. https://doi.org/10.1182/blood-2006-02-005660.
122. Walker LSK. EFIS Lecture: understanding the CTLA-4 checkpoint in the maintenance of immune homeostasis. *Immunol Lett*. 2017;184:43–50. https://doi.org/10.1016/j.imlet.2017.02.007.
123. Ying H, Yang L, Qiao G, et al. Cutting edge: CTLA-4–B7 interaction suppresses Th17 cell differentiation. *J Immunol*. 2010;185(3):1375–1378. https://doi.org/10.4049/jimmunol.0903369.
124. Monast CS, Li K, Judson MA, et al. Sarcoidosis extent relates to molecular variability. *Clin Exp Immunol*. 2017;188(3):444–454. https://doi.org/10.1111/cei.12942.
125. Kaiser Y, Lakshmikanth T, Chen Y, et al. Mass cytometry identifies distinct lung CD4+T cell patterns in Löfgren's syndrome and non-Löfgren's syndrome sarcoidosis. *Front Immunol*. 2017;8:1130. https://doi.org/10.3389/fimmu.2017.01130.
126. Schubert D, Bode C, Kenefeck R, et al. Autosomal dominant immune dysregulation syndrome in humans with CTLA4 mutations. *Nat Med*. 2014;20(12):1410–1416. https://doi.org/10.1038/nm.3746.
127. Hodi FS, O'Day SJ, McDermott DF, et al. Improved survival with ipilimumab in patients with metastatic melanoma. *N Engl J Med*. 2010;363(8):711–723. https://doi.org/10.1056/NEJMoa1003466.
128. Eckert A, Schoeffler A, Dalle S, Phan A, Kiakouama L, Thomas L. Anti-CTLA4 monoclonal antibody induced sarcoidosis in a metastatic melanoma patient. *Dermatology (Basel)*. 2009;218(1):69–70. https://doi.org/10.1159/000161122.
129. Vogel WV, Guislain A, Kvistborg P, Schumacher TNM, Haanen JBAG, Blank CU. Ipilimumab-induced sarcoidosis in a patient with metastatic melanoma undergoing complete remission. *J Clin Oncol*. 2012;30(2):e7–e10. https://doi.org/10.1200/JCO.2011.37.9693.
130. Suozzi KC, Stahl M, Ko CJ, et al. Immune-related sarcoidosis observed in combination ipilimumab and nivolumab therapy. *JAAD Case Rep*. 2016;2(3):264–268. https://doi.org/10.1016/j.jdcr.2016.05.002.
131. Lomax AJ, McGuire HM, McNeil C, et al. Immunotherapy-induced sarcoidosis in patients with melanoma treated with PD-1 checkpoint inhibitors: case series and immunophenotypic analysis. *Int J Rheum Dis*. 2017;372(1):2521–2529. https://doi.org/10.1111/1756-185X.13076.
132. Braun NA, Celada LJ, Herazo-Maya JD, et al. Blockade of the programmed death-1 pathway restores sarcoidosis CD4(+) T-cell proliferative capacity. *Am J Respir Crit Care Med*. 2014;190(5):560–571. https://doi.org/10.1164/rccm.201401-0188OC.
133. Celada LJ, Rotsinger JE, Young A, et al. Programmed death-1 inhibition of phosphatidylinositol 3-kinase/AKT/mechanistic target of rapamycin signaling impairs sarcoidosis CD4+ T cell proliferation. *Am J Respir Cell Mol Biol*. 2017;56(1):74–82. https://doi.org/10.1165/rcmb.2016-0037OC.
134. Danlos F-X, Pagès C, Baroudjian B, et al. Nivolumab-induced sarcoid-like granulomatous reaction in a patient with advanced melanoma. *Chest*. 2016;149(5):e133–e136. https://doi.org/10.1016/j.chest.2015.10.082.
135. Birnbaum MR, Ma MW, Fleisig S, et al. Nivolumab-related cutaneous sarcoidosis in a patient with lung adenocarcinoma. *JAAD Case Rep*. 2017;3(3):208–211. https://doi.org/10.1016/j.jdcr.2017.02.015.
136. Rhodes DA, Reith W, Trowsdale J. Regulation of immunity by butyrophilins. *Annu Rev Immunol*. 2016;34(1):151–172. https://doi.org/10.1146/annurev-immunol-041015-055435.
137. Nguyen T, Liu XK, Zhang Y, Dong C. BTNL2, a butyrophilin-like molecule that functions to inhibit T cell activation. *J Immunol*. 2006;176(12):7354–7360.
138. Arnett HA, Escobar SS, Gonzalez-Suarez E, et al. BTNL2, a butyrophilin/B7-like molecule, is a negative costimulatory molecule modulated in intestinal inflammation. *J Immunol*. 2007;178(3):1523–1533.
139. Swanson RM, Gavin MA, Escobar SS, et al. Butyrophilin-like 2 modulates B7 costimulation to induce Foxp3 expression and regulatory T cell development in mature T cells. *J Immunol*. 2013;190(5):2027–2035. https://doi.org/10.4049/jimmunol.1201760.
140. Valentonyte R, Hampe J, Huse K, et al. Sarcoidosis is associated with a truncating splice site mutation in BTNL2. *Nat Genet*. 2005;37(4):357–364. https://doi.org/10.1038/ng1519.
141. Li Y, Wollnik B, Pabst S, et al. BTNL2 gene variant and sarcoidosis. *Thorax*. 2006;61(3):273–274. https://doi.org/10.1136/thx.2005.056564.
142. Morais A, Lima B, Peixoto MJ, Alves H, Marques A, Delgado L. BTNL2 gene polymorphism associations with susceptibility and phenotype expression in sarcoidosis. *Respir Med*. 2012;106(12):1771–1777. https://doi.org/10.1016/j.rmed.2012.08.009.
143. Pacheco Y, Calender A, Israel-Biet D, et al. Familial vs. sporadic sarcoidosis: BTNL2 polymorphisms, clinical presentations, and outcomes in a French cohort. *Orphanet J Rare Dis*. 2016;11(1):165. https://doi.org/10.1186/s13023-016-0546-4.
144. Kamphuis LS, van Zelm MC, Lam KH, et al. Perigranuloma localization and abnormal maturation of B cells: emerging key players in sarcoidosis? *Am J Respir Crit Care Med*. 2013;187(4):406–416. https://doi.org/10.1164/rccm.201206-1024OC.
145. Ueda-Hayakawa I, Tanimura H, Osawa M, et al. Elevated serum BAFF levels in patients with sarcoidosis: association with disease activity. *Rheumatology (Oxf)*. 2013;52(9):1658–1666. https://doi.org/10.1093/rheumatology/ket186.

146. Saussine A, Tazi A, Feuillet S, et al. Active chronic sarcoidosis is characterized by increased transitional blood B cells, increased IL-10-producing regulatory B cells and high BAFF levels. Hoshino Y, ed. *PLoS One*. 2012;7(8):e43588. https://doi.org/10.1371/journal.pone.0043588.
147. Cazac BB, Roes J. TGF-beta receptor controls B cell responsiveness and induction of IgA in vivo. *Immunity*. 2000;13(4):443–451.
148. Nardelli B, Belvedere O, Roschke V, et al. Synthesis and release of B-lymphocyte stimulator from myeloid cells. *Blood*. 2001;97(1):198–204.
149. Lai Kwan Lam Q, King Hung Ko O, Zheng B-J, Lu L. Local BAFF gene silencing suppresses Th17-cell generation and ameliorates autoimmune arthritis. *Proc Natl Acad Sci USA*. 2008;105(39):14993–14998. https://doi.org/10.1073/pnas.0806044105.
150. Ferrara G, Valentini D, Rao M, et al. Humoral immune profiling of mycobacterial antigen recognition in sarcoidosis and Löfgren's syndrome using high-content peptide microarrays. *Int J Infect Dis*. 2017;56:167–175. https://doi.org/10.1016/j.ijid.2017.01.021.
151. Suchankova M, Paulovicova E, Paulovicova L, et al. Increased antifungal antibodies in bronchoalveolar lavage fluid and serum in pulmonary sarcoidosis. *Scand J Immunol*. 2015;81(4):259–264. https://doi.org/10.1111/sji.12273.
152. Saketkoo LA, Baughman RP. Biologic therapies in the treatment of sarcoidosis. *Expert Rev Clin Immunol*. 2016;12(8):817–825. https://doi.org/10.1080/1744666X.2016.1175301.
153. Galimberti F, Fernandez AP. Sarcoidosis following successful treatment of pemphigus vulgaris with rituximab: a rituximab-induced reaction further supporting B-cell contribution to sarcoidosis pathogenesis? *Clin Exp Dermatol*. 2016;41(4):413–416. https://doi.org/10.1111/ced.12793.
154. Liu Y, Qiu L, Wang Y, et al. The circulating Treg/Th17 cell ratio is correlated with relapse and treatment response in pulmonary sarcoidosis patients after corticosteroid withdrawal. *PLoS One*. 2016;11(2):e0148207. https://doi.org/10.1371/journal.pone.0148207.
155. Broos CE, Wapenaar M, Looman CWN, et al. Daily home spirometry to detect early steroid treatment effects in newly treated pulmonary sarcoidosis. *Eur Respir J*. 2018;51(1):1702089. https://doi.org/10.1183/13993003.02089-2017.
156. Baughman RP, Lower EE. Treatment of sarcoidosis. *Clin Rev Allergy Immunol*. 2015;49(1):79–92. https://doi.org/10.1007/s12016-015-8492-9.
157. Broos CE, Poell LHC, Looman CWN, et al. No evidence found for an association between prednisone dose and FVC change in newly-treated pulmonary sarcoidosis. *Respir Med*. October 2017. https://doi.org/10.1016/j.rmed.2017.10.022.

CHAPTER 4

Genetics of Sarcoidosis

PAOLO SPAGNOLO, MD, PHD

EVIDENCE FOR A GENETIC PREDISPOSITION TO SARCOIDOSIS

Sarcoidosis (SA) is a systemic, immune-mediated disease of unknown origin. A number of epidemiological and clinical observations support the existence of a genetic susceptibility to develop SA.[1,2] For instance, prevalence, incidence, and presentation of the disease vary greatly between different ethnic groups, and familial clustering and increased concordance of the disease in monozygotic twins are well described. In addition, the severity of SA may range from a radiographic or laboratory abnormality detected in asymptomatic patients to a relentlessly progressive and potentially life-threatening disease. Studies have revealed several human leukocyte antigen (HLA) and non-HLA alleles consistently associated with SA susceptibility. However, SA is not due to defects in a single major gene or molecular pathway; instead, it results from a complex interaction of multiple genes—some with a major disease effect, but many with a relatively minor effect—with contributing environmental factors that determine not only the development of the disease but also its protean clinical manifestations.[3] Phenotypic heterogeneity is such that some believe SA represents a "family" of diseases, including Löfgren's syndrome, non-resolving/progressive lung disease, and granulomatous uveitis, among others, each with potentially distinct genetic associations.[4,5] In this respect, berylliosis could also be considered as a subset of the broad grouping "sarcoidosis" and almost certainly was historically.[6]

Familial Clustering

Familial clustering of SA has been described in several populations. It was first reported by Marteinstein in two German sisters in 1923,[7] and since then, studies across Europe and US have confirmed that family members of SA patients have a several-fold increased risk of disease compared with the general population.[8–10] The main limitation of these original reports, however, was the lack of a comparison group, which makes it difficult determining whether variations in familial SA are due to variation in familial aggregation of disease risk, disease prevalence, or both. Rybicki et al. estimated familial relative risk of SA using data on disease occurrence in 10,862 first- and 17,047 second-degree relatives of 706 age-, sex-, race-, and geographically matched cases and controls who participated to the multicenter ACCESS (A Case-Control Etiology Study of Sarcoidosis). They showed that siblings of the affected patients had the highest relative risk (odds ratio = 5.8), while the odds ratio for the parents was 3.8.[10] Moreover, white cases had a significantly higher familial relative risk than African American cases (18.0 vs. 2.8). A registry-based study of Danish and Finnish twins showed that cotwins of affected monozygotic brothers or sisters have an 80-fold increased risk of developing SA compared with the general population, whereas the increased risk in dizygotic twins was only sevenfold.[11]

GENETIC STUDIES

Linkage studies, candidate-gene studies, and genome-wide association studies (GWAS) have been performed in SA. *Linkage studies* are performed in closely related patients—often including unaffected family members—and are based on the assumption that genetic markers and the disease of interest cosegregate. This approach may allow the identification of rare risk variants with strong effects. In general, however, the identified chromosomal regions are large, which makes it difficult to precisely localize the underlying risk gene. The *candidate-gene case-control* approach relies on predicting the correct gene/s based on biological plausibility (or the location of the candidate gene within a previously identified region). As such, when the fundamental defects underlying a given disease are unknown, as with SA, this approach may be inadequate to uncover the genetic basis of the disease.[12] Association studies are based on the investigation of unrelated patients and unaffected controls by comparing the frequency of a genetic variant in the two groups. The power of association studies increases with the frequency of the genetic

Sarcoidosis. https://doi.org/10.1016/B978-0-323-54429-0.00004-5

variant in the general population; thus this approach favors the discovery of high-frequency risk variants of small effects. Conversely, GWAS are independent of any prior knowledge and thus have the potential to identify risk loci in (or near) genes not previously suspected of being involved in disease pathobiology or within noncoding regions. Sufficiently large sample size and careful marker selection are crucial for successful GWAS, although they are unable to detect rare risk alleles (e.g., mutations).

SCANNING THE GENOME

Genome-Wide Studies in Caucasians

In an early genome-wide study, Schürmann et al. genotyped 122 affected siblings from 55 German families for seven DNA markers flanking and covering HLA region.[13] Multipoint nonparametric linkage analysis revealed linkage for the entire class III region with the highest score observed at marker locus D6S1666. In a follow-up study, the same group investigated an expanded cohort of 63 German families with affected siblings by using 225 microsatellite markers.[14] Linkage was confirmed with the HLA region with the most prominent peak mapping nearer the class II loci. Further refinement of the area and a single nucleotide polymorphisms (SNP) scan of 16.4 Mb linkage peak centered at chromosome 6p21 led to the identification of a 15-kb disease-associated region containing the butyrophilin-like 2 (BTNL2) gene in the HLA class II region.[15] In a German cohort including familial and sporadic SA cases, Valentonyte et al. found that the BTNL2 rs2076530 A allele was associated with increased risk for SA in both the familial and case-control samples. The authors also demonstrated that the risk allele causes a functional change (e.g., the lack of the C-terminal IgC domain and transmembrane helix), which disrupts the membrane localization and hence function of the protein. BTNL2 is a member of the B7 family of cell receptors that suppress activation of T cells by antigen-presenting cells.[15] Nonfunctional BTNL2 could theoretically result in an exaggerated T-lymphocyte activation, compatible with the hypothesized pathogenesis of SA. Notably, BTNL2 rs2076530 A was reported to confer risk for SA independent of HLA class II alleles, despite almost complete linkage disequilibrium (LD; e.g., the nonrandom association of alleles at different loci located close to each other on the same chromosome) with HLA-DRB1. Rybicki et al. investigated the same BTNL2 polymorphism as well as a further nine variants in an African American family cohort and in two case-control cohorts, one African American and one white, but confirmed the rs2076530 A association with SA risk only in their white population.[16] Two recent metaanalyses have confirmed the association between rs2076530 A and increased risk for SA.[17,18] A recent study of 256 sporadic and 207 familial SA cases from 140 families replicated the association between rs2076530 A and disease risk but found no differences between sporadic and familial cases.[19] Similarly, no association was found with disease severity or outcome. Li et al. sequenced six coding exons within BTNL2 and identified a previously unknown one–base pair deletion (c.450delC) in exon 3, which could cause a frameshift at amino acid position 150, thus introducing 96 additional amino acids.[20] However, the c.450delC genotype frequencies do not differ between SA cases (n = 210) and controls (n = 201).

Although the BTNL2 association with SA is well established, uncertainty remains on whether the BTNL2 effect is independent on HLA-DRB1.[21] Indeed, BTNL2 rs2076530 A associations with diseases such as ulcerative colitis, multiple sclerosis, type 1 diabetes, rheumatoid arthritis (RA), systemic lupus erythematosus (SLE), Graves' disease, tuberculosis, leprosy, and Crohn's disease (CD) [22–26] appear to be driven by LD with various HLA-DRB1 alleles. Similarly, a genome-wide study of African and European American SA patients confirmed the BTNL2 association but not its independency of HLA class II alleles.[27] Moreover, in the combined African American data set, the strongest BTNL2 signal was at rs9268480 (a coding but synonymous SNP), emphasizing the difficulties in pinpointing the causal variant/s when HLA genes and nearby loci in tight LD are considered simultaneously.[27] More extensive genotyping across HLA class I and II regions would be needed to define haplotypes accurately. However, at present, this genomic area is too complex for the current generation of microarray or DNA chips to genotype.

Franke et al. performed a 100 k GWAS using 83,360 SNPs on 382 CD patients, 398 SA patients, and 394 healthy controls.[28] Twenty-four SNPs most strongly associated with the combined CD/SA phenotype were selected for verification in an independent sample of 1317 patients (660 CD and 657 SA) and 1091 controls. The most significant association was observed on chromosome 10p12.2 (rs1398024 A allele) with an odds ratio for both diseases of 0.81. Finer mapping of the 10p12.2 locus pointed to yet unidentified variant/s in the C10ORF67 gene region as the most likely underlying risk factors. In the first complete GWAS in SA, Hofmann et al. looked at 440,000 SNPs in 499 German patients and 490 controls. The strongest association signal mapped to the annexin A11 (ANXA11) gene on chromosome 10q22.3 and was validated in an independent cohort of 1649 cases and 1832 controls. Finer mapping of the region identified a common nonsynonymous SNP (rs1049550, R230C) residing in the first of four annexin core domains within ANXA11 as the variant most strongly associated with SA.[29] The ANXA11 rs1049550 association with SA has been independently confirmed in two different European populations[30,31] as well as in African Americans and European Americans.[27,32] Levin et al. genotyped a large sample of African Americans (1242 cases and 899 controls) and a smaller sample of European Americans (447 cases and 353 controls) for 209 SNPs spanning 100 kb including the 5′ promoter, coding, and 3′ untranslated regions of ANXA11.[32] After adjustment for rs1049550, two novel ANXA11 SA associations were identified (e.g., rs61860052 and rs4377299), although only in African Americans. These associations were stronger in patients with radiographic stage IV disease. A recent metaanalysis comprising 4567 cases and 4278 controls from six studies found that patients homozygous for the ANXA11 rs1049550 C allele (CC) have a nearly 50% increased risk of developing the disease compared with individuals carrying the T allele (TT or TC)[33]; however, not unsurprisingly, the authors observed significant heterogeneity across the studies, consistent with population-specific effects. Annexin A11 belongs to a family of calcium-dependent, phospholipid-binding proteins involved in cell proliferation and apoptosis[34] and has been implicated in the pathogenesis of several autoimmune disorders, including RA, SLE, and Sjögren's syndrome.[35] In SA, dysfunctional annexin A11 might affect the apoptosis pathway, hence modifying the balance between apoptosis and survival of activated inflammatory cells. However, the role of rs1049550 in disease pathogenesis, if any, remains to be elucidated.

In a linkage study of German families (n = 181), Fischer et al. genotyped 528 affected members for 3882 SNPs and observed the two most prominent peaks at 12p13.31 and 9q33.1.[36] Linkage to 9q33.1 had already been observed in a previous study of African American SA families.[37] A genome scan in 381 German patients and 392 controls using 97,000 SNPs revealed a novel SA risk locus on chromosome 6p12.1.[38] Fine-mapping of the region around rs10484410—the only marker associated with SA after correction for multiple testing—pointed to RAB23 as the most likely risk factor. A subsequent GWAS including 1.3 million markers identified a novel SA risk locus on 11q13.1.[39] This association was consistent across three independent case-control populations from Germany, Sweden, and Czech Republic. Fine-mapping of the region surrounding the lead marker (rs479777) suggested CCDC88B as the most promising candidate, although its role in disease pathogenesis, if any, is unknown. Interestingly this locus has been associated with CD, primary biliary cirrhosis, and psoriasis, among others, thus suggesting a shared genetic background.[40–42] An independent susceptibility locus was also identified at 12q13.3-q14.1 with the Osteosarcoma amplified 9 (OS9) representing the most likely candidate risk factor. This association has been validated in an independent German population and replicated in a metaanalysis of three independent cohorts of SA patients from Germany, Czech Republic, and Sweden.[43]

Fischer et al. recently applied the Illumina Immunochip SNP array containing 128,705 SNPs to a cohort of 1726 European patients with SA and 5482 healthy controls and validated their findings in multiple additional European cohorts and one African American cohort, using other methods.[44] Overall they genotyped more than 19,000 individuals, making this the largest SA case-control study ever performed. In the European case-control populations, they identified four novel susceptibility loci, located on chromosomes 12q24.12 (rs653178; ATXN2/SH2B3), 5q33.3 (rs4921492; IL12B), 4q24 (rs223498; MANBA/NFKB1), and 2q33.2 (rs6748088; FAM117B). In addition, they found three independent associations in the HLA region—peaking in the BTNL2 promoter region (rs5007259), at HLA-B (rs4143332/HLA-B*0801), and at HLA-DPB1 (rs9277542)—and an additional independent signal near IL23R (rs12069782) on chromosome 1p31.3. Notably, and consistent with the hypothesis that SA may share part of its genetic background with other immune-related diseases,[45] the novel susceptibility loci identified are located near genes previously associated with psoriasis and inflammatory bowel disease.[46] However, none of the associations with SA patients of European origin were identified in patients of African descent, despite inclusion of a large cohort. This apparent paradox is likely to be inherent with the use of Immunochip assays, which were designed based on SNPs identified in individuals of European origin and may not cover adequately variations present in populations of non-European origin.[47]

Genome-Wide Studies in Non-Caucasians

An initial genome-wide, sib pair multipoint linkage analysis in 229 African American families (Sarcoidosis Genetic Analysis [SAGA] study) revealed a number of statistically significant peaks (but no positive signal within the HLA region), the most prominent one being located at D5S2500 on chromosome 5q11 ($P = .0005$).[37]

Notably the agreement for linkage between the scans performed in the European and African American populations was only modest. In a follow-up study on the same patient population using additional microsatellite markers to refine regions with significant linkage, SA susceptibility alleles were identified on chromosome 5p15.2 and protective alleles on chromosome 5q11.2.[48] A further linkage analysis of the SAGA sample stratified by genetically determined ancestry to reduce ethnic confounding confirmed the peaks on chromosome five and revealed additional associated loci.[49]

Studies in African Americans suggest that focusing on genes of African ancestry may uncover ethnicity-specific risk variants. Rybicki et al. conducted a genome-wide scan using a panel of highly ancestry markers in a large sample of African American SA cases (n = 1357) and healthy controls (n = 703) and observed the most significant association at 6p22.3 (rs11966463).[50] Other markers that demonstrated suggestive ancestry associations with SA mapped on chromosome 8p12, which had the most significant association with European ancestry, 5p13 and 5q31, which correspond to regions previously identified through sib pair linkage analyses. More recently, Adrianto et al. performed a GWAS in African and European Americans patients evaluating >6 million SNPs.[27] They identified a novel SA risk locus—NOTCH4—independent of neighboring HLA genes as well multiple independent signals within the HLA class II region. NOTCH4, which encodes a member of the NOTCH family that is involved in the control of cell fate decision during developmental processes and regulation of T cell response, has been associated with immune-related disorders, such as SLE and systemic sclerosis.[43,51] In this same study, some associations were shared between ethnicities, whereas others were unique to either African Americans or European Americans, confirming the existence of ethnicity-specific genetic effects.[27]

HLA GENES

The HLA complex on chromosome six contains over 200 genes, more than 40 of which encode leukocyte antigens. The rest are a variety of genes that are not evolutionarily related to the HLA genes themselves, although some are involved with them functionally.[52,53] Many genes within this complex are not related to immunity. The HLA genes that are involved in the immune response fall into two classes, I and II, which are structurally and functionally different.[52,53] The HLA class III region, which is located between the class I and class II regions, contains genes encoding tumor necrosis factor (TNF)-α, TNF-β, the complement proteins (C4A, C4B, C2 and Bf), enzymes involved in steroid synthesis (CYP21A and CYP21B), and heat-shock proteins (HSPA1A, HSPA1B, and HSPA1L).

Several studies have shown the HLA genes to be associated with SA, suggesting a functional role for antigen-presenting molecules and immune mediators in disease pathogenesis.

HLA Class I

HLA association studies began more than 30 years ago and concentrated on HLA class I alleles (HLA-A, HLA-B, and HLA-C) using serological typing. Varying and often controversial results were obtained, depending on the cohort and the ethnicity studied; however, HLA-B7 and HLA-B8 were most commonly linked to SA. The role of HLA-B7 is somehow controversial as the frequency of this allele is increased among SA patients of African American ancestry (a population with a high disease prevalence)[54] but significantly decreased in Japanese patients (a population with a low disease prevalence)[55] and unchanged in Moravian Czechs.[56] The HLA-B8 allele association is more robust. Indeed a number of studies across racial boundaries have reported an association between this allele and SA of acute onset and short duration.[57–61] Interestingly, as more studies of SA and HLA-B8 were published, it was noted that HLA-B8/DR3 genes were inherited as a unique disease risk haplotype in Caucasians, suggesting that disease associations with class I genes may be simply due to LD with class II genes.[59,61–63] However, a study of Scandinavian patients showed that HLA-B7 and HLA-B8 increased the risk for SA independently of class II genes.[64] Therefore HLA class I alleles might have more influence on disease susceptibility and prognosis than previously thought.

HLA Class II

HLA class II genes have been extensively studied in SA based on the pathogenetic hypothesis of the disease being triggered by exogenous antigen/s. Indeed, several HLA class II associations with SA have been reported to date, supporting the hypothesis that HLA alleles—acting either in concert or independently—predispose to SA. However, the high and variable LD within the HLA region makes it difficult to determine which specific genes confer SA risk. For instance, Grunewald et al. showed in their Scandinavian patients with SA that the associations of HLA-DRB1*15 with chronic disease and HLA-DRB1*03 with mild disease were synonymous with the HLA-DQB1*0602-chronic disease and HLA-DQB1*0201-mild disease associations.[64]

The associations of SA with HLA class II genes vary greatly by ethnicity and race. In Japanese patients, HLA-DR5, HLA-DR6, HLA-DR8, and HLA-DR9 have been associated with increased disease risk,[65,66] whereas in Germans, HLA-DR5 has been linked with chronic disease and HLA-DR3 with acute and benign disease.[67,68] This pattern of differential linkage according to clinical phenotypes has been confirmed in Scandinavian patients with HLA-DR14 and HLA-DR15 being associated with persistent disease and HLA-DR17 (DR3) predisposing to an acute and self-limiting form of SA.[69] HLA-DR9 has been associated with disease risk in Japanese patients but with disease protection in Scandinavians.[69] Interestingly, in African Americans, HLA-DQB1 and not HLA-DRB1 represents the strongest association with SA.[70]

Genetic studies in SA have often produced conflicting results. Sato et al. applied consistent clinical definitions and HLA genotyping across three independent patient populations (from UK, The Netherlands, and Japan) to test the hypothesis that inconsistencies across genetic studies may (also) be accounted for by interethnic differences in SA susceptibility and disease manifestations.[71] Despite clear differences in the frequency of various disease phenotypes between the cohorts, they found that a number of HLA associations were similar across their ethnically different study populations. Specifically, DRB1*01 was consistently associated with disease protection, DRB1*12 with disease risk, and DRB1*1401/2 with lung-predominant SA, whereas DRB1*0803 conferred disease risk only in Japanese patients—particularly in those with uveitis. Conversely, DRB1*0301 and DQB1*0201 were absent among Japanese. In addition, DRB1*0401-DQB1*0301 was found to be protective for disease overall in British but a clear risk factor in Japanese patients. Notably this study did not confirm the previously reported association between HLA-DRB1*11 and disease risk in white American patients.[72]

HLA-DRB1*0301 is associated with increased susceptibility to SA but also with disease resolution in Europeans.[73] Conversely, the HLA-DRB1 associations with disease risk and course are not as well established. Levin et al. evaluated associations between genotyped and imputed HLA-DRB1 alleles and disease susceptibility/resolution in 1277 African American SA patients and 1467 controls.[74] Carriage of HLA-DRB1*1201 and *1101 was associated with increased disease risk (OR 2.11 and 1.69, respectively), whereas the strongest protective association was found with HLA-DRB1*0301 (OR 0.56). Moreover, DRB1*1501 was associated with increased risk for persistent disease, similar to what had been previously reported in patients of European ancestry.[64,75,76]

West African ancestry confers a higher risk for SA than European ancestry. Levin et al. performed fine-mapping of four previously identified ancestry-associated regions—6p24.3-p12.1, 17p13.3-13.1, 2p13.3-q12.1, and 6q23.3-q25.2[77]—in 2727 African Americans.[78] Fine-mapping was performed by imputation, based on a previous GWAS,[50] and significant variants were validated by direct genotyping. Within the 6p24.3-p12.1 locus, the most significant ancestry-adjusted SNP was rs74318745 ($P = 9.4 \times 10^{-11}$), an intronic SNP within the HLA-DRA gene. In addition, the locus on chromosome 17p13.3-13.1 revealed a novel SA risk variant (rs6502976), within intron five of the gene X-linked inhibitor of apoptosis-associated factor 1 (XAF1) that accounted for the majority of the admixture linkage signal. XAF1 is a negative regulator of X-linked inhibitor of apoptosis (XIAP), and dysfunctional XIAP/XAF1 pathway may potentially result in inhibition of apoptosis, thus influencing granuloma formation and maintenance in SA.

HLA Class III

Wolin et al. used tag-SNPs to study four genes in the HLA class III region (lymphotoxin alpha [LTA], TNF, advanced glycosylation end product–specific receptor [AGER], and BTNL2) and HLA-DRA in a combined population of 805 SA patients and 870 healthy controls from four study cohorts (Finnish, Swedish, Dutch, and Czech).[79] They found eight SNPs to be associated with Löfgren's syndrome (LS) and seven with non-LS SA. Five additional SNPs were associated with SA disease course. However, when LD between the associated SNPs and HLA-DRB1 was taken into account, independent associations were observed for four SNPs in the HLA-DRA/BTNL2 region: rs3135365 (non-LS; $P = .015$), rs3177928 (non-LS; $P < P$ .001), rs6937545 (LS; $P = .012$), and rs5007259 (disease activity; $P = .002$). These findings confirm that polymorphisms within HLA-DRA and BTNL2 are involved in SA susceptibility and demonstrate that some of these associations are independent of HLA-DRB1.

Löfgren's Syndrome

LS is a form of acute and usually self-limiting SA presenting with fever, erythema nodosum, arthralgia, and bilateral hilar lymphadenopathy.[80] Grunewald and Eklund characterized and typed for HLA-DRB1 301 patients with LS.[73] They not only confirmed the strong association between carriage of DRB1*03 and LS but also showed that while 95% of DRB1*03^{positive} patients had a resolving disease (defined as disease duration <2 years), disease resolved in only approximately half of DRB1*03^{negative} patients. A clustering of disease onset in January, April, and May was also observed only in DRB1*03^{positive} patients, suggesting a putative role for season-specific antigens in the development of LS.[73] The mechanisms through which DRB1*03 influences disease prognosis in LS is unknown; however, these patients display a less pronounced T helper one-type immune response with reduced level of IFN-γ and TNF-α.[81]

Genetic variants other than HLA alleles have also been associated with LS. Carriage of a particular combination of variants (e.g., haplotype) within CC chemokine receptor 2 (CCR2) gene increases the risk for LS independently of HLA-DRB1*03.[82] This association has been validated in two independent patient populations, [83] but not replicated in a German case-control and family-based study, which however noted a positive linkage at 3p21 (where CCR2 lies), indicating a susceptibility gene in the surrounding chromosomal area.[84] Whether the discrepancies are due to inconsistent case definition, subset ascertainment or true ethnic variation is unclear. Polymorphisms within class II major histocompatibility complex transactivator (MHC2TA) gene, which encodes a positive regulator of class II HLA gene transcription, have also been associated with LS but not with non-LS SA.[85] Importantly, this association appears to be independent of HLA-DRB1*03, which is in line with the hypothesis that LS is a separate disease entity.[5]

Rivera et al. performed a fine-mapping (Immunochip) analysis of 384 Swedish patients with LS, 664 with non-LS SA, and 2086 controls.[86] Four independent cohorts, three of white European ancestry (Germany, n = 4975; the Netherlands, n = 613; and Czech Republic, n = 521) and one of black African origin (n = 1657) served as validation cohorts. The authors identified and confirmed 727 variants associated with LS expanding throughout the extended HLA region and 68 non-LS-associated variants located in the HLA class II region. Notably the genetic overlap between LS and non-LS SA was only modest consisting of 17 variants located in the HLA class II region. Outside the HLA region, two loci—one in ADCY3 (2p23.3) and one between CSMD1 and MCPH1 (8p23.1 - 8p23.2)—were found to be consistently associated with LS. This comprehensive and integrative analysis of genetics and pathway modeling indicates that LS and non-LS SA have different genetic susceptibility and genomic distributions and limited genetic overlap, suggesting the existence of distinct underlying pathogenetic mechanisms. Notably the higher presence of HLA genes in LS suggests that this phenotype may result from HLA genes and gene x factor (a *factor* is defined as a gene, regulatory/epigenetic element, or protein) interactions located within one chromosome. Conversely, the higher presence of non-HLA genes in non-LS SA raises the possibility for gene x factor interactions across chromosomes, consistent with a polygenic phenotype.

ASSOCIATIONS WITH ORGAN-SPECIFIC MANIFESTATIONS AND DISEASE BEHAVIOR

The genetics of organ-specific manifestations of SA remains poorly defined due to the small size of the cohorts studied and the lack of clear associations from GWAS. Examples of association with specific disease subsets include HLA-DRB1*04/*15 with extrapulmonary disease,[87] HLA-DQB1*0601 with cardiac SA,[88] HLA-DQB1*0602—which is in strong LD with DRB1*1501—with splenomegaly[89] and with small fiber neuropathy, and HLA-DRB1*04 with uveitis.[71,72,90] More recently a variant in a zinc finger gene (ZNF592) has been associated with neurosarcoidosis in African Americans and European Americans.[91] Moreover, polymorphisms within TAK1-binding protein 2 (TAB2) and within TAB2, mitogen-activated protein kinase 13 (MAPK13) and TAB1 have been associated with skin and bone/joint involvement in SA patients of European American and African American origin, respectively.[92] Finally, a recent study showed a strong association between HLA-DRB1*04 and Caucasian SA patients presenting with Heerfordt's syndrome, which is characterized by the combination of uveitis (the most common symptom), fever, cranial nerve palsy (most often the facial nerve), and parotid or salivary gland enlargement.[93]

ADDITIONAL GENES ASSOCIATED WITH SA

The HLA-DRB1 associations predominate in the SA genetic literature. However, in roughly half of the patients, the HLA genes do not seem to play any role.

Solute carrier family 11 member 1 (SLC11A1). SLC11A1 (formerly Human natural resistance–associated macrophage protein 1 (NRAMP1)) has been associated with susceptibility to tuberculosis.[94] The importance of SLC11A1 in animal models of granulomatous disorders and its putative role in macrophage activation make it an attractive candidate gene in SA. Maliarik et al. analyzed several polymorphisms within SLC11A1 in a case-control study including individuals of African American origin and found that a (CA)(n) repeat in the 5′ region of the gene was protective against SA.[95] The SLC11A1 association with risk of SA has been replicated in patients from Poland and Turkey,[96,97] although the role of SLC11A1 in disease pathogenesis, if any, remains to be elucidated.

Caspase recruitment domain 15 (CARD15)/nucleotide-binding oligomerization domain protein 2 (NOD2). CARD15/NOD2 codes for a leukocyte receptor of the innate immune system that recognizes intracellular bacterial lipopolysaccharides and activates nuclear factor-kappa B (NF-kB).[98] CARD15/NOD2 is also implicated in the pathogenesis of granulomatous diseases such as Blau syndrome and CD.[99,100] Polymorphisms within CARD15/NOD2 have been also investigated in SA with conflicting results. Schürmann et al. evaluated the four main CARD15/NOD2 variants and found no association with SA among German patients.[101] Similarly, Milman et al. found no association between CARD15/NOD2 variants and SA risk in Danish patients.[102] However, Sato et al. reported an association between the CARD15/NOD2 functional polymorphism 2104T (702W) and severe pulmonary SA, as assessed by radiographic stage of disease and pulmonary function test.

Tumor necrosis factor (TNF). The TNF gene complex is located within the MHC region between the complement cluster region and the HLA-B locus and includes TNF-α and lymphotoxin-α (LT-α, previously known as TNF-β). TNF-α is known to play a crucial role in granuloma formation and persistence,[3] as demonstrated by the significantly increased TNF-α production by alveolar macrophages from patients with SA.[103] A number of SNPs have been identified within TNF-α and LT-α, but a G-to-A variant at position −308 in the promoter region of TNF-α (rs1800629) and an A-to-G variant in the first intron of LT-α (rs909253, NcoI) have been studied more extensively. These studies, however, have often provided mixed results due to small sample size of the cohorts studied. An association between the rarer allele of TNF-α −308, which leads to increased TNF-α production (TNFA2) (Allen RD 1999), and LS has been initially reported.[68,104] The same association has been confirmed in a cohort of British and Dutch patients.[105] This latter study also showed that another rare allele of the TNF-α promoter, −857T, was associated with risk of SA in both populations. Notably, SA patients who carry the G allele in either heterozygous (AG) or homozygous (GG) form display a significantly higher response to TNF inhibitors (infliximab or adalimumab).[106] Song et al. performed a metaanalysis including 1396 patients and 2344 controls to verify the association between TNF-α −308 A/G and LT-α +252 A/G polymorphisms and SA.[107] The metaanalysis revealed significant associations between the TNF-α −308 A and the LT-α +252 G alleles with SA (odds ratio = 1.480, P = .002, and odds ratio = 1.266, P = .014, respectively). However, stratification by ethnicity indicated that both associations were statistically significant in European but not in Asian patients. A metaanalysis by Feng et al. investigating the association of six polymorphisms in TNF-α and LT-α genes with SA and including 1584 patients and 2636 controls from 13 studies found similar findings.[108]

Interleukin-1 (IL-1). Hutyrova et al. investigated a number of polymorphisms within the IL-1α and IL-1β genes as well as an 86-bp variable number tandem repeat polymorphism in intron two of the interleukin-1 receptor antagonist (IL-1Ra) gene. They found the IL-1α −889 C/C genotype to be significantly overrepresented among SA patients (n = 95) compared with healthy controls (n = 199), both from Czech Republic.[109] The association between IL-1α and SA had been previously reported by Rybicki et al. in patients of African American ancestry.[110] They observed that patients carrying both the IL-1α*137 and F13A*188 alleles had a sixfold increased risk of disease, which raised to a 15-fold increase in patients with a family history of SA. However, a subsequent study from two different European countries failed to reproduce this association in either population.[111]

Interleukin 7 receptor-alpha (IL7R-α). Interleukin seven receptor-alpha (IL7R-α) gene encodes a receptor highly expressed on both naïve and memory T cells. Heron et al. genotyped 475 SA patients and 465 healthy controls for six SNPs within IL7R and found the variant rs10213865 to be significantly associated with SA.[112] They subsequently validated this association in an independent cohort of patients. Notably, rs10213865 is in complete LD with a functional nonsynonymous coding variant in exon 6 (rs6897932, T244I).

Prostaglandin-endoperoxide synthase 2 (PTGS2). Prostaglandin-endoperoxide synthase 2 (PTGS2), also known as cyclooxygenase 2 (COX-2), is involved in the enzymatic conversion of arachidonic acid to prostanoids, which provide an essential homeostatic control in normal tissues and regulate inflammation. Hill et al. investigated the frequency of a G to C promoter polymorphism at position −765 in 198 SA patients and 166 controls.[113] Of note, the −765 variant appears to be functional, with the C allele displaying lower promoter activity. Carriage of the -765C allele conferred increased risk of developing both SA and persistent pulmonary disease. The authors were able to replicate the -765C association with SA in a smaller independent data set.

Vascular endothelial growth factor (VEGF). VEGF is a potent mediator of vascular permeability and angiogenesis that acts through two high-affinity receptor tyrosine kinases: VEGF receptor 1 (VEGFR-1) and VEFG receptor 2 (VEGFR-2). In a study of 103 Japanese patients and 146 healthy controls, Morohashi et al. observed that SA patients were significantly less likely than controls to carry the rs3025039 T allele, suggesting a protective effect from the disease.[114] In a subsequent study of 300 Caucasian patients and 381 matched controls, Pabst et al. observed several genetic associations: between VEGFR-1 variants and SA susceptibility, between VEGF variants and acute disease, and between different VEGFR-2 variants and both acute and chronic SA.[115] While VEGF and its receptors appear plausible candidate genes in SA predisposition and prognosis, the reported associations have not been validated yet in larger populations or different ethnic groups.

Factor 2 receptor (F2R). The minor allele of the rs2227744 G>A SNP, which is located in the promoter region of the *F2R* gene (chromosome 5q13.3), has been shown to confer higher promoter activity, and hence higher proteinase-activated receptor-1 (*PAR-1*) expression levels.[116] In a case-control study of 184 individuals with SA and 368 controls, Platé et al. observed that carriage of the rs2227744A allele confers protection from SA (P=.003, OR=0.68).[117] At present, the mechanism through which dysfunctional *F2R* may protect from the development of SA is unknown, although the authors speculate this can be related to increased PAR-1 expression. In addition, because the study did not include a replication cohort, the F2R association with SA needs to be validated in larger cohorts and different populations.

GENE EXPRESSION STUDIES

Gene expression analysis has been used to identify potential gene signatures to serve as biomarkers for the presence of SA as well as for the susceptibility to develop complicated disease. A gene expression study on tissues obtained from untreated patients with active SA (n=6) compared with normal lung tissue (n=6) identified overexpression of two gene networks.[118] One network included genes engaged in Th1-type responses (i.e., IL-7, which was not previously reported in the context of SA, IL-15, the transcription factor family STAT1, and lymphocyte chemoattractant genes); the second network included the proteases MMP-12 and ADAMDEC1. MMP-12 and ADAMDEC1 transcripts were most highly expressed (>25-fold) in SA lung tissues, corresponding with increased protein expression by immunohistochemistry. MMP-12 and ADAMDEC1 gene and protein expression were also increased in bronchoalveolar lavage samples from patients with SA, correlating with disease severity. Lockstone et al. examined microarray expression of 26,626 genes in transbronchial biopsies from SA patients with active but self-limiting (n=8) versus those with active, progressive (± fibrotic) pulmonary disease (n=7).[119] Three hundred thirty-four genes were differentially expressed between the two groups. In particular, genes related to host immune activation, proliferation, and defense were upregulated in the progressive fibrotic group. Notably the authors observed similarity in gene expression profiles between progressive fibrotic pulmonary SA and hypersensitivity pneumonitis but not idiopathic pulmonary fibrosis. In a separate study using genome-wide peripheral blood gene expression analysis, an unbiased gene signature comprised of 20 autosomal genes was identified that appears to distinguish patients with complicated SA from patients with uncomplicated disease.[120]

CONCLUSIONS

We are just beginning to unravel the complex mix of genes that determine the genetic susceptibility to SA. However, considering the phenotypic heterogeneity and the variable presentation and course and outcome of the disease, genes that predispose to specific disease phenotypes are likely to be largely separate from those underlying disease susceptibility. If this is the case, further refinement of SA phenotypes will facilitate the identification of additional novel genetic associations with specific disease manifestations. Yet, the identification of genetic associations with SA does not imply causation, and functional studies are required to determine the role of the associated variants in disease pathogenesis. Much work remains to be carried out, but a fuller understanding of the genetic basis of SA is likely to open up new therapeutic avenues for the treatment of both SA and other granulomatous disorders.

REFERENCES

1. McGrath DS, Goh N, Foley PJ, du Bois RM. Sarcoidosis: genes and microbes: soil or seed? *Sarcoidosis Vasc Diffuse Lung Dis*. 2001;18:149–164.
2. Grunewald J. Genetics of sarcoidosis. *Curr Opin Pulm Med*. 2008;14:434–439.
3. Spagnolo P, Rossi G, Trisolini R, et al. Pulmonary sarcoidosis. *Lancet Respir Med*. 2018;123:245–253.

4. Schupp JC, Freitag-Wolf S, Bargagli E, et al. Phenotypes of organ involvement in sarcoidosis. *Eur Respir J*. 2018;51(1) pii: 1700991. https://doi.org/10.1183/13993003.00991-2017.
5. Spagnolo P, Grunewald J. Recent advances in the genetics of sarcoidosis. *J Med Genet*. 2013;50:290–297.
6. Grutters JC, Sato H, Welsh KI, du Bois RM. The importance of sarcoidosis genotype to lung phenotype. *Am J Respir Cell Mol Biol*. 2003;29:59–S62.
7. Martenstein H. Knochveranderungen bei lupus pernio. *Zentralbl Haut und Geschlechts-krankheiten sowie deren Grenzgebiete*. 1923;7:208.
8. McGrath DS, Daniil Z, Foley P, et al. Epidemiology of familial sarcoidosis in the UK. *Thorax*. 2000;55:51–54.
9. Pietinalho A, Ohmichi M, Hirasawa M, et al. Familial sarcoidosis in Finland and Hokkaido, Japan: a comparative study. *Respir Med*. 1999;93:408–412.
10. Rybicki BA, Kirkey KL, Major M, et al. Familial risk ratio of sarcoidosis in African-American sibs and parents. *Am J Epidemiol*. 2001;153:188–193.
11. Sverrild A, Backer V, Kyvik KO, et al. Heredity in sarcoidosis: a registry-based twin study. *Thorax*. 2008;63:894–896.
12. Hirschhorn JN, Daly MJ. Genome-wide association studies for common diseases and complex traits. *Nat Rev Genet*. 2005;6:95–108.
13. Schurmann M, Lympany PA, Reichel P, et al. Familial sarcoidosis is linked to the major histocompatibility complex region. *Am J Respir Crit Care Med*. 2000;162:861–864.
14. Schurmann M, Reichel P, Muller-Myhsok B, et al. Results from a genome-wide search for predisposing genes in sarcoidosis. *Am J Respir Crit Care Med*. 2001;164:840–846.
15. Valentonyte R, Hampe J, Huse K, et al. Sarcoidosis is associated with a truncating splice site mutation in BTNL2. *Nat Genet*. 2005;37:357–364.
16. Rybicki BA, Walewski JL, Maliarik MJ, et al. The BTNL2 gene and sarcoidosis susceptibility in African Americans and Whites. *Am J Hum Genet*. 2005;77:491–499.
17. Tong X, Ma Y, Niu X. The BTNL2 G16071A gene polymorphism increases granulomatous disease susceptibility: a meta-analysis including FPRP test of 8710 participants. *Medicine (Baltim)*. 2016;95:e4325.
18. Lin Y, Wei J, Fan L, et al. BTNL2 gene polymorphism and sarcoidosis susceptibility: a meta-analysis. *PLoS One*. 2015;10:e0122639.
19. Pacheco Y, Calender A, Israël-Biet D. Familial vs. sporadic sarcoidosis: BTNL2 polymorphisms, clinical presentations, and outcomes in a French cohort. *Orphanet J Rare Dis*. 2016;11:165.
20. Li Y, Pabst S, Lokhande S, et al. Extended genetic analysis of BTNL2 in sarcoidosis. *Tissue Antigens*. 2009;73:59–61.
21. Spagnolo P, Sato H, Grutters JC, et al. Analysis of BTNL2 genetic polymorphisms in British and Dutch patients with sarcoidosis. *Tissue Antigens*. 2007;70:219–227.
22. Mochida A, Kinouchi Y, Negoro K, et al. Butyrophilin-like 2 gene is associated with ulcerative colitis in the Japanese under strong linkage disequilibrium with HLA-DRB1*1502. *Tissue Antigens*. 2007;70:128–135.
23. Traherne JA, Barcellos LF, Sawcer SJ, et al. Association of the truncating splice site mutation in BTNL2 with multiple sclerosis is secondary to HLA-DRB1*15. *Hum Mol Genet*. 2006;15:155–161.
24. Orozco G, Eerligh P, Sanchez E, et al. Analysis of a functional BTNL2 polymorphism in type 1 diabetes, rheumatoid arthritis, and systemic lupus erythematosus. *Hum Immunol*. 2005;66:1235–1241.
25. Simmonds MJ, Heward JM, Barrett JC, Franklyn JA, Gough SC. Association of the BTNL2 rs2076530 single nucleotide polymorphism with Graves' disease appears to be secondary to DRB1 exon 2 position beta74. *Clin Endocrinol (Oxf)*. 2006;65:429–432.
26. Johnson CM, Traherne JA, Jamieson SE, et al. Analysis of the BTNL2 truncating splice site mutation in tuberculosis, leprosy and Crohn's disease. *Tissue Antigens*. 2007;69:23–41.
27. Adrianto I, Lin CP, Hale JJ, et al. Genome-wide association study of African and European Americans implicates multiple shared and ethnic specific loci in sarcoidosis susceptibility. *PLoS One*. 2012;7:e43907.
28. Franke A, Fischer A, Nothnagel M, et al. Genome-Wide Association analysis in sarcoidosis and Crohn's disease unravels a common susceptibility locus on 10p12.2. *Gastroenterology*. 2008;135:1207–1215.
29. Hofmann S, Franke A, Fischer A, et al. Genome-wide association study identifies ANXA11 as a new susceptibility locus for sarcoidosis. *Nat Genet*. 2008;40:1103–1106.
30. Li Y, Pabst S, Kubisch C, et al. First independent replication study confirms the strong genetic association of ANXA11 with sarcoidosis. *Thorax*. 2010;65:939–940.
31. Mrazek F, Stahelova A, Kriegova E, et al. Functional variant ANXA11 R230C: true marker of protection and candidate disease modifier in sarcoidosis. *Genes Immun*. 2011;12:490–494.
32. Levin AM, Iannuzzi MC, Montgomery CG, et al. Association of ANXA11 genetic variation with sarcoidosis in African Americans and European Americans. *Genes Immun*. 2013;14:13–18.
33. Zhou H, Diao M, Zhang M. The association between ANXA11 gene polymorphisms and sarcoidosis: a meta-analysis and systematic review. *Sarcoidosis Vasc Diffuse Lung Dis*. 2016;33:102–111.
34. Moss S, Morgan R. The annexins. *Genome Biol*. 2004;5:219.
35. Perucci LO, Sugimoto MA, Gomes KB, et al. Annexin A1 and specialized proresolving lipid mediators: promoting resolution as a therapeutic strategy in human inflammatory diseases. *Expert Opin Ther Targets*. 2017;21:879–896.
36. Fischer A, Nothnagel M, Schürmann M, Müller-Quernheim J, Schreiber S, Hofmann S. A genome-wide linkage analysis in 181 German sarcoidosis families using clustered biallelic markers. *Chest*. 2010;138:151–157.
37. Iannuzzi MC, Iyengar SK, Gray-McGuire C, et al. Genome-wide search for sarcoidosis susceptibility genes in African Americans. *Genes Immun*. 2005;6:509–518.

38. Hofmann S, Fischer A, Till A, et al. A genome-wide association study reveals evidence of association with sarcoidosis at 6p12.1. *Eur Respir J*. 2011;38:1127–1135.
39. Fischer A, Schmid B, Ellinghaus D, et al. A novel sarcoidosis risk locus for Europeans on chromosome 11q13.1. *Am J Respir Crit Care Med*. 2012;186:877–885.
40. Franke A, McGovern DP, Barrett JC, et al. Genome-wide meta-analysis increases to 71 the number of confirmed Crohn's disease susceptibility loci. *Nat Genet*. 2010;42:1118–1125.
41. Mells GF, Floyd JA, Morley KI, et al. Genome-wide association study identifies 12 new susceptibility loci for primary biliary cirrhosis. *Nat Genet*. 2011;43:329–332.
42. Ellinghaus D, Ellinghaus E, Nair RP, et al. Combined analysis of genome-wide association studies for Crohn disease and psoriasis identifies seven shared susceptibility loci. *Am J Hum Genet*. 2012;90:636–647.
43. Hofmann S, Fischer A, Nothnagel M, et al. A genome-wide association analysis reveals chromosome 12q13.3-q14.1 as a new risk locus for sarcoidosis. *Eur Respir J*. 2013;41:888–900.
44. Fischer A, Ellinghaus D, Nutsua M, et al. Identification of immune-relevant factors conferring sarcoidosis genetic risk. *Am J Respir Crit Care Med*. 2015;192:727–736.
45. Lareau CA, DeWeese CF, Adrianto I, et al. Polygenic risk assessment reveals pleiotropy between sarcoidosis and inflammatory disorders in the context of genetic ancestry. *Genes Immun*. 2017;18:88–94.
46. Fischer A, Nothnagel M, Franke A, et al. Association of inflammatory bowel disease risk loci with sarcoidosis, and its acute and chronic subphenotypes. *Eur Respir J*. 2011;37:610–616.
47. Parkes M, Cortes A, van Heel DA, et al. Genetic insights into common pathways and complex relationships among immune-mediated diseases. *Nat Rev Genet*. 2013;14:661–673.
48. Gray-McGuire C, Sinha R, Iyengar S, et al. Genetic characterization and fine mapping of susceptibility loci for sarcoidosis in African Americans on chromosome 5. *Hum Genet*. 2006;120:420–430.
49. Thompson CL, Rybicki BA, Iannuzzi MC, Elston RC, Iyengar SK, Gray-McGuire C, Sarcoidosis Genetic Analysis Consortium (SAGA). Reduction of sample heterogeneity through use of population substructure: an example from a population of African American families with sarcoidosis. *Am J Hum Genet*. 2006;79:606–613.
50. Rybicki BA, Levin AM, McKeigue P, et al. A genome-wide admixture scan for ancestry-linked genes predisposing to sarcoidosis in African-Americans. *Genes Immun*. 2011;12:67–77.
51. Barcellos LF, May SL, Ramsay PP, et al. High-density SNP screening of the major histocompatibility complex in systemic lupus erythematosus demonstrates strong evidence for independent susceptibility regions. *PLoS Genet*. 2009;5:e1000696.
52. Klein J, Sato A. The HLA system. First of two parts. *N Engl J Med*. 2000;343:702–709.
53. Klein J, Sato A. The HLA system. Second of two parts. *N Engl J Med*. 2000;343:782–786.
54. Mcntyre JA, McKee KT, Loadholt CB, et al. Increased HLA-B7 antigen frequency in South Carolina blacks in association with sarcoidosis. *Transplant Proc*. 1977;9:173–176.
55. Ina Y, Takada K, Yamamoto M, et al. HLA and sarcoidosis in the Japanese. *Chest*. 1989;95:1257–1261.
56. Lenhart K, Kolek V, Bartova A. HLA antigens associated with sarcoidosis. *Dis Markers*. 1990;8:23–29.
57. Smith MJ, Turton CW, Mitchell DN, et al. Association of HLA B8 with spontaneous resolution in sarcoidosis. *Thorax*. 1981;36:296–298.
58. Olenchock SA, Heise ER, Marx JJ, et al. HLA-B8 in sarcoidosis. *Ann Allergy*. 1981;47:151.
59. Hedfors E, Lindstrom F. HLA-B8/DR3 in sarcoidosis. Correlation to acute onset disease with arthritis. *Tissue Antigens*. 1983;22:200–203.
60. Guyatt GH, Bensen WG, Stolmon LP, et al. HLA-B8 and erythema nodosum. *Can Med Assoc J*. 1982;127:1005–1006.
61. Gardner J, Kennedy HG, Hamblin A, Jones E. HLA associations in sarcoidosis: a study of two ethnic groups. *Thorax*. 1984;39:19–22.
62. Krause A, Goebel KM. Class II MHC antigen (HLA-DR3) predisposes to sarcoid arthritis. *J Clin Lab Immunol*. 1987;24:25–27.
63. Kremer JM. Histologic findings in siblings with acute sarcoid arthritis: association with the B8, DR3 phenotype. *J Rheumatol*. 1986;13:593–597.
64. Grunewald J, Eklund A, Olerup O. Human leukocyte antigen class I alleles and the disease course in sarcoidosis patients. *Am J Respir Crit Care Med*. 2004;169:696–702.
65. Ishihara M, Ishida T, Inoko H, et al. HLA serological and class II genotyping in sarcoidosis patients in Japan. *Jpn J Ophthalmol*. 1996;40:86–94.
66. Ishihara M, Inoko H, Suzuki K, et al. HLA class II genotyping of sarcoidosis patients in Hokkaido by PCR-RFLP. *Jpn J Ophthalmol*. 1996;40:540–543.
67. Nowack D, Goebel KM. Genetic aspects of sarcoidosis. Class II histocompatibility antigens and a family study. *Arch Intern Med*. 1987;147:481–483.
68. Swider C, Schnittger L, Bogunia-Kubik K, et al. TNF-alpha and HLA-DR genotyping as potential prognostic markers in pulmonary sarcoidosis. *Eur Cytokine Netw*. 1999;10:143–146.
69. Berlin M, Fogdell-Hahn A, Olerup O, et al. HLA-DR predicts the prognosis in Scandinavian patients with pulmonary sarcoidosis. *Am J Respir Crit Care Med*. 1997;156:1601–1605.
70. Iannuzzi MC, Maliarik MJ, Poisson LM, Rybicki BA. Sarcoidosis susceptibility and resistance HLA-DQB1 alleles in African Americans. *Am J Respir Crit Care Med*. 2003;167:1225–1231.
71. Sato H, Woodhead FA, Ahmad T, et al. Sarcoidosis HLA class II genotyping distinguishes differences of clinical phenotype across ethnic groups. *Hum Mol Genet*. 2010;19:4100–4111.

72. Rossman MD, Thompson B, Frederick M, et al. HLA-DRB1*1101: a significant risk factor for sarcoidosis in blacks and whites. *Am J Hum Genet*. 2003;73:720–735.
73. Grunewald J, Eklund A. Löfgren's syndrome: human leukocyte antigen strongly influences the disease course. *Am J Respir Crit Care Med*. 2009;179:307–312.
74. Levin AM, Adrianto I, Datta I, et al. Association of HLA-DRB1 with sarcoidosis susceptibility and progression in African Americans. *Am J Respir Cell Mol Biol*. 2015;53:206–216.
75. Grunewald J, Brynedal B, Darlington P, et al. Different HLA-DRB1 allele distributions in distinct clinical subgroups of sarcoidosis patients. *Respir Res*. 2010;11:25.
76. Voorter CE, Drent M, van den Berg-Loonen EM. Severe pulmonary sarcoidosis is strongly associated with the haplotype HLADQB1*0602-DRB1*150101. *Hum Immunol*. 2005;66:826–835.
77. McKeigue P, Colombo M, Agakov F, et al. Extending admixture mapping to nuclear pedigrees: application to sarcoidosis. *Genet Epidemiol*. 2013;37:256–266.
78. Levin AM, Iannuzzi MC, Montgomery CG, et al. Admixture fine-mapping in African Americans implicates XAF1 as a possible sarcoidosis risk gene. *PLoS One*. 2014;9:e92646.
79. Wolin A, Lahtela EL, Anttila V, et al. SNP variants in major histocompatibility complex are associated with sarcoidosis susceptibility-a joint analysis in four European populations. *Front Immunol*. 2017;8:422.
80. Lofgren S, Lundback H. The bilateral hilar lymphoma syndrome; a study of the relation to tuberculosis and sarcoidosis in 212 cases. *Acta Med Scand*. 1952;142:265–273.
81. Idali F, Wikén M, Wahlström J, et al. Reduced Th1 response in the lungs of HLA-DRB1*0301 patients with pulmonary sarcoidosis. *Eur Respir J*. 2006;27:451–459.
82. Spagnolo P, Renzoni EA, Wells AU, et al. C-C chemokine receptor 2 and sarcoidosis: association with Lofgren's syndrome. *Am J Respir Crit Care Med*. 2003;168:1162–1166.
83. Spagnolo P, Sato H, Grunewald J, et al. A common haplotype of the C-C chemokine receptor 2 gene and HLA-DRB1*0301 are independent genetic risk factors for Löfgren's syndrome. *J Intern Med*. 2008;264:433–441.
84. Valentonyte R, Hampe J, Croucher PJ, et al. Study of C-C chemokine receptor 2 alleles in sarcoidosis, with emphasis on family-based analysis. *Am J Respir Crit Care Med*. 2005;171:1136–1141.
85. Grunewald J, Idali F, Kockum I, et al. MHC class II transactivator gene polymorphism in sarcoidosis: specific associations with Löfgren´s syndrome. *Tissue Antigens*. 2010;76:96–101.
86. Rivera NV, Ronninger M, Shchetynsky K, et al. High-Density genetic mapping identifies new susceptibility variants in sarcoidosis phenotypes and shows genomic-driven phenotypic differences. *Am J Respir Crit Care Med*. 2016;193:1008–1022.
87. Darlington P, Gabrielsen A, Sörensson P, et al. HLA-alleles associated with increased risk for extrapulmonary involvement in sarcoidosis. *Tissue Antigens*. 2014;83:267–272.
88. Naruse TK, Matsuzawa Y, Ota M, et al. HLA-DQB1*0601 is primarily associated with the susceptibility to cardiac sarcoidosis. *Tissue Antigens*. 2000;56:52–57.
89. Sato H, Nagai S, du Bois RM, et al. HLA-DQB1 0602 allele is associated with splenomegaly in Japanese sarcoidosis. *J Intern Med*. 2007;262:449–457.
90. Darlington P, Haugom-Olsen H, von Sivers K, et al. T-cell phenotypes in bronchoalveolar lavage fluid, blood and lymph nodes in pulmonary sarcoidosis - indication for an airborne antigen as the triggering factor in sarcoidosis. *J Intern Med*. 2012;272:465–471.
91. Lareau CA, Adrianto I, Levin AM, et al. Fine mapping of chromosome 15q25 implicates ZNF592 in neurosarcoidosis patients. *Ann Clin Transl Neurol*. 2015;2:972–977.
92. Bello GA, Adrianto I, Dumancas GG, et al. Role of NOD2 pathway genes in sarcoidosis cases with clinical characteristics of Blau syndrome. *Am J Respir Crit Care Med*. 2015;192:1133–1135.
93. Darlington P, Tallstedt L, Padyukov L, et al. HLA-DRB1* alleles and symptoms associated with Heerfordt's syndrome in Sarcoidosis. *Eur Respir J*. 2011;38:1151–1157.
94. Bellamy R, Ruwende C, Corrah T, et al. Variations in the NRAMP1 gene and susceptibility to tuberculosis in West Africans. *N Engl J Med*. 1998;338:640–644.
95. Maliarik MJ, Chen KM, Sheffer RG, et al. The natural resistance-associated macrophage protein gene in African Americans with sarcoidosis. *Am J Respir Cell Mol Biol*. 2000;22:672–675.
96. Dubaniewicz A, Jamieson SE, Dubaniewicz-Wybieralska M, Fakiola M, Nancy Miller E, Blackwell JM. Association between SLC11A1 (formerly NRAMP1) and the risk of sarcoidosis in Poland. *Eur J Hum Genet*. 2005;13:829–834.
97. Akçakaya P, Azeroglu B, Even I, et al. The functional SLC11A1 gene polymorphisms are associated with sarcoidosis in Turkish population. *Mol Biol Rep*. 2012;39:5009–5016.
98. Girardin SE, Boneca IG, Viala J, et al. Nod2 is a general sensor of peptidoglycan through muramyl dipeptide (MDP) detection. *J Biol Chem*. 2003;278:8869–8872.
99. Miceli-Richard C, Lesage S, Rybojad M, et al. CARD15 mutations in Blau syndrome. *Nat Genet*. 2001;29:19–20.
100. Hugot JP, Chamaillard M, Zouali H, et al. Association of NOD2 leucine-rich repeat variants with susceptibility to Crohn's disease. *Nature*. 2001;411:599–603.
101. Schurmann M, Valentonyte R, Hampe J, et al. CARD15 gene mutations in sarcoidosis. *Eur Respir J*. 2003;22:748–754.
102. Milman N, Nielsen OH, Hviid TV, Fenger K. CARD15 single nucleotide polymorphisms 8, 12 and 13 are not increased in ethnic Danes with sarcoidosis. *Respiration*. 2007;74:76–79.

103. Fehrenbach H, Zissel G, Goldmann T, et al. Alveolar macrophages are the main source for tumour necrosis factor-α in patients with sarcoidosis. *Eur Respir J.* 2003;21:421–428.
104. Seitzer U, Swider C, Stuber F, et al. Tumour necrosis factor alpha promoter gene polymorphism in sarcoidosis. *Cytokine.* 1997;9:787–790.
105. Grutters JC, Sato H, Pantelidis P, et al. Increased frequency of the uncommon tumor necrosis factor -857T allele in British and Dutch patients with sarcoidosis. *Am J Respir Crit Care Med.* 2002;165:1119–1124.
106. Wijnen PA, Cremers JP, Nelemans PJ, et al. Association of the TNF-α G-308A polymorphism with TNF-inhibitor response in sarcoidosis. *Eur Respir J.* 2014;43:1730–1739.
107. Song GG, Kim JH, Lee YH. Associations between TNF-α -308 A/G and lymphotoxin-α +252 A/G polymorphisms and susceptibility to sarcoidosis: a meta-analysis. *Mol Biol Rep.* 2014;41:259–267.
108. Feng Y, Zhou J, Gu C, et al. Association of six well-characterized polymorphisms in TNF-α and TNF-β genes with sarcoidosis: a meta-analysis. *PLoS One.* 2013;8:e80150. https://doi.org/10.1371/annotation/679667f2-b4aa-42e8-8c59-511f60256420. Erratum in: *PLoS One.* 2013;8.
109. Hutyrova B, Pantelidis P, Drabek J, et al. Interleukin-1 gene cluster polymorphisms in sarcoidosis and idiopathic pulmonary fibrosis. *Am J Respir Crit Care Med.* 2002;165:148–151.
110. Rybicki BA, Maliarik MJ, Malvitz E, et al. The influence of T cell receptor and cytokine genes on sarcoidosis susceptibility in African Americans. *Hum Immunol.* 1999;60:867–874.
111. Grutters JC, Sato H, Pantelidis P, et al. Analysis of IL6 and IL1A gene polymorphisms in UK and Dutch patients with sarcoidosis. *Sarcoidosis Vasc Diffuse Lung Dis.* 2003;20:20–27.
112. Heron M, Grutters JC, van Moorsel CH, et al. Variation in IL7R predisposes to sarcoid inflammation. *Genes Immun.* 2009;10:647–653.
113. Hill MR, Papafili A, Booth H, et al. Functional prostaglandin-endoperoxide synthase 2 polymorphism predicts poor outcome in sarcoidosis. *Am J Respir Crit Care Med.* 2006;174:915–922.
114. Morohashi K, Takada T, Omori K, et al. Vascular endothelial growth factor gene polymorphisms in Japanese patients with sarcoidosis. *Chest.* 2003;123:520–526.
115. Pabst S, Karpushova A, Diaz-Lacava A, et al. VEGF gene haplotypes are associated with sarcoidosis. *Chest.* 2010;137:156–163.
116. Platé M, Lawson PJ, Hill MR, et al. Impact of a functional polymorphism in the PAR-1 gene promoter in COPD and COPD exacerbations. *Am J Physiol Lung Cell Mol Physiol.* 2014;307:L311–L316.
117. Platé M, Lawson PJ, Hill MR. Role of a functional polymorphism in the F2R gene promoter in sarcoidosis. *Respirology.* 2015;20:1285–1287.
118. Crouser ED, Culver DA, Knox KS, et al. Gene expression profiling identifies MMP-12 and ADAMDEC1 as potential pathogenic mediators of pulmonary sarcoidosis. *Am J Respir Crit Care Med.* 2009;179:929–938.
119. Lockstone HE, Sanderson S, Kulakova N, et al. Gene-set analysis of lung samples provides insight into pathogenesis of progressive, fibrotic pulmonary sarcoidosis. *Am J Respir Crit Care Med.* 2010;181:1367–1375.
120. Zhou T, Zhang W, Sweiss NJ, et al. Peripheral blood gene expression as a novel genomic biomarker in complicated sarcoidosis. *PLoS One.* 2012;7:e44818.

CHAPTER 5

Sarcoidosis Models: Past, Present, and Future

VAN LE, MD • ELLIOTT D. CROUSER, MD

INTRODUCTION

Sarcoidosis is defined as a granulomatous disease of the lungs, and in many cases, it involves other organs, the etiology of which is unknown. Recent studies have documented increasing disease prevalence and serious disease complications, particularly among African Americans and women.[1,2] Presumably, the observed increase in sarcoidosis prevalence is related in part to improved disease detection,[3] highlighting the need for better biomarkers and treatments, the development of which is greatly impeded by the lack of appropriate disease models. Consequently, organizations such as the National Institutes of Health and Foundation for Sarcoidosis Research have prioritized initiatives to improve upon current sarcoidosis research models.[4]

One of the more daunting challenges confronted by sarcoidosis researchers relates to the highly variable nature of the disease, including disparities relating to race and gender.[4] There are numerous knowledge gaps in this regard, including the independent contributions of environmental exposures and host factors, including complex and poorly understood genetic and epigenetic variables. The situation is further complicated by the nature of granuloma formation, which involves dynamic interactions among diverse immune cell populations, the immunological features of which change over time. Conventional research approaches, such as molecular manipulation of isolated cell lines or genetically altered mice, are unable to account for the phenotypic diversity and the molecular complexity of the disease. Analyses of diseased human tissues and genome-wide association studies have been informative but provide minimal insight into early mechanisms of granuloma formation or the subsequent progression of inflammation to tissue fibrosis, the direst consequence of the disease. Further elucidation of disease mechanisms awaits the development of highly relevant disease models that will expedite the discovery of biomarkers and novel therapeutic targets to facilitate the early detection and more effective treatment of severe sarcoidosis phenotypes.

What are the features of the ideal research model for sarcoidosis? First and foremost, the model should reliably replicate the essential molecular and morphological features of human sarcoidosis granulomas, including manifestations of diverse disease phenotypes. Second, the model would accurately reflect the various stages of granuloma evolution, including initiation and propagation by putative disease-causing and/or disease-modifying antigens, and the progression to fibrosis or to harmless granuloma resolution. Third, the model would be convenient in terms of reproducibility, low cost, and ease of use. Fourth, the model would provide high-throughput, so as to accelerate the pace of research and to facilitate the preclinical evaluation of novel therapies or determine the most effective therapies on a personalized basis (Table 5.1).

MECHANISMS

Sarcoidosis immunopathogenesis is complex and is only partially understood. It is believed that individuals with genetic susceptibilities develop uncontrolled immune responses when exposed to as yet unidentified antigens. These antigens classically activate undifferentiated macrophages into M1 (classically activated) phenotype through various receptors, including signaling lymphocyte-activation molecule family,[5] Toll-like receptors (TLRs), and nucleotide oligomerization domain (NOD)-like receptors, subsequently promoting T effector cell responses via major histocompatibility complex (MHC) class II antigen presentation. M1 macrophages further produce proinflammatory cytokines such as tumor necrosis factor alpha (TNF-α) and interleukin (IL)-12. TNF-α contributes to granuloma formation by recruiting naïve T cells, promoting pro-inflammatory CD4+ T helper cell (Th1) polarization (i.e., interferon gamma production), and by promoting

Sarcoidosis. https://doi.org/10.1016/B978-0-323-54429-0.00005-7

TABLE 5.1
Criteria for Optimal Sarcoidosis Model

1. Replicate human molecular and morphological features of granulomas with high fidelity
2. Ability to model diverse disease phenotypes
3. Reflect the various stages of granuloma evolution including initiation, propagation, and progression to fibrosis or to harmless granuloma resolution
4. Ability to test putative disease-causing antigens and therapeutics
5. Reproduce easily with low cost to facilitate high-throughput

immune cell aggregation.[6] Activated Th1 cells oligoclonally expand and produce interferon-gamma (INF-γ) to promote further M1 activation. Accordingly, the earliest stages of granulomatous inflammation are thought to be Th1/M1 mediated and driven by state of exaggerated TNF-α and INF-γ. Once the process is initiated, other cells, such as natural killer (NK) cells, Th17 cells, and B cells, engage in innate and adaptive immune responses that promote sustained granulomatous inflammation in patients with sarcoidosis.[7,8] The mechanisms by which granuloma formation and resolution are dysregulated in sarcoidosis patients are unclear and likely differ depending on the disease phenotype.

Sarcoidosis has a highly variable disease course as the tissue granulomas may resolve, persist, or, in the worst-case scenario, progress to fibrosis. In many cases, inflammation resolves without treatment with minimal or no clinical sequelae. In this regard, regulatory T cells (Tregs) suppress granulomatous inflammation by producing mediators (IL-10, TGF-β) that suppress T cell proliferation and activation and by promoting alternative macrophage (M2) polarization. However, these same mediators can contribute to tissue fibrosis, an irreversible process resulting in the most serious disease manifestations.[9,10]

The mechanisms dictating the inflammatory (M1/Th1)/anti-inflammatory or regulatory (M2/Th2) balance are unclear in sarcoidosis. It is generally accepted that the M2/Th2 cytokine profile is proximally regulated by IL-4 and IL-13, which induces signal transducer and activator of transcription (STAT) STAT6 and Jak/STAT signaling to promote the production of IL-10 in favor of INF-γ. A more positive ratio of IL-10 relative to INF-γ typically favors disease resolution, but in some cases, it inexplicably promotes fibroblast matrix production, tissue remodeling, and fibrosis.[11,12] New disease models are needed to determine the dynamic and complex (multicellular) mechanisms dictating the fate of granulomatous inflammation and related disease manifestations in patients with diverse sarcoidosis disease phenotypes.

SARCOIDOSIS MODELS

The most fundamental environmental and host factors dictating pathological granuloma formation in sarcoidosis are yet to be fully defined and likely vary from one patient to the next, which has implications for the optimal treatment strategies. Some experts believe that sarcoidosis is a manifestation of an exaggerated immune response to common environmental exposures, whereas other experts contend that sarcoidosis represents an impaired immune response that fails to effectively clear immunogenic antigens leading to ongoing inflammation or even low-grade infection. The objective of this manuscript is to consider existing and emerging models of sarcoidosis, to consider how they could be used alone and in combination to improve our understanding of disease mechanisms, and to design more effective treatments.

In Vitro Sarcoidosis Models

In vitro models generally rely on cells derived directly or indirectly (e.g., cloned cell lines) from humans or animals, and the justifications for this approach are well founded. For the purpose of lung immunology research, as applies to sarcoidosis, in vitro models are derived primarily from three sources: (1) cell lines, (2) blood, and (3) bronchoalveolar fluid.

Sarcoidosis research involving human samples is problematic for a number of reasons. First and foremost, there is presumably a great deal of genetic variability contributing to the extreme clinical variability of sarcoidosis.[13] Secondary variables that influence in vitro immune cell research conducted on human samples include environmental factors, natural fluctuations in disease activity, and the combined effects of immunomodulating therapies, smoking, and comorbid conditions (e.g., obesity, diabetes mellitus, age, gender) which are known to influence the immune response.[14,15] Finally, maintaining a steady supply of blood or bronchoalveolar lavage (BAL) cells for the purpose of research presents a number of challenges in terms of ready access to patients, difficulty and expense (e.g., for BAL or tissue cells), and immune cell variability from one patient to the next. Despite these limitations, most of the advances in the field of sarcoidosis to date have been based on in vitro models, and in vitro models continue to evolve to match the special needs of "granuloma researchers."

Many investigators have related the clinical diversity of sarcoidosis to various T cell populations that are reflected by BAL cell analysis, and significant mechanistic discoveries continue to emerge from this approach. BAL cells are of particular interest given that they are presumed to interface with disease-promoting environmental antigens. Moreover, BAL T cell profiles of sarcoidosis are characterized by high proportions of Th1 cells,[16] which closely approximate cell patterns of diseased pulmonary tissues.[17] Thus, BAL cells may reflect the immunological features driving pathological granulomatous inflammation. For instance, Mitchell et al. recently used deep sequencing (gene expression) analysis to identify CD4+ T cell features that discriminate the relatively benign Lofgren's syndrome (LS) phenotype from more severe sarcoidosis phenotypes, leading to the discovery of specific genotype/immune phenotype characteristics that presumably respond to specific environmental, disease-causing antigens.[18] This line of research is further poised to advance the field by identifying disease-causing antigens and related immune cell receptors that promote granuloma formation in sarcoidosis, as was recently reported in berylliosis, a granulomatous model that mimics sarcoidosis.[19]

Another example of the use of BAL was recently provided by Ramstein et al., who challenged the notion that Th1 cells are the primary source of INF-γ. Using a modified flow-cytometry approach, they identified a subclass of IL-17–expressing T cells (Th17 cells) that produce large amounts of INF-γ and relatively little IL-17A, referred to as Th17.1 cells. Th17.1 cells were markedly expanded in BAL of patients with pulmonary sarcoidosis, representing up to 60% of all CD4+ T cells, suggesting that Th17.1 cells, and not Th1, are the primary source of INF-γ. This discovery has important clinical implications given that Th17.1 cells are relatively resistant to the immune-suppressing effects of glucocorticoids.[20]

Although bronchoscopy with BAL is often performed on sarcoidosis patients during initial diagnostic evaluation, studies using blood samples are more practical in terms of lower patient risk, lower cost, and patient-investigator convenience. In the context of granulomatous lung disorders, such as sarcoidosis, new evidence supports the in vitro use of peripheral blood mononuclear cells (PBMCs) for this purpose. As was long suspected, firm evidence has emerged in the last decade confirming that circulating immune cells (e.g., monocytes) intermittently cycle through the lung interstitium surveying for danger. Immune cells of animals and humans possess a number of damage-associated molecular pattern molecules (DAMPs) or pathogen-associated molecular pattern molecules (PAMPs), including aforementioned TLRs and NOD-like receptors and many others. Upon activation of these migrating immune cells by DAMPs or PAMPs, the immune cells establish residence in the lungs (or other tissues) where they initiate and propagate a local immune response. The evolution of tissue inflammation is supported by locally activated monocytes, macrophages, and T cells through the production of chemokines and cytokines to promote further cell recruitment from the circulation and to induce their local activation, respectively.[21] Under normal circumstances (e.g., pneumonia), the clearance of immunogenic antigens (e.g., bacterial) leads to resolution of inflammation through programmed cell death.[22] Thus, PBMCs are essential for the initiation and propagation of inflammatory responses in the lungs, and their altered function likely promotes sustained granuloma formation in sarcoidosis.

Indeed, PBMC populations are the primary source for monocyte and T cells that are recruited to extravascular sites of inflammation, and under appropriate circumstances, PBMCs are capable of forming multicellular granuloma-like cell aggregations. PBMC aggregates are shown to replicate many of the histological and molecular features of human granulomatous diseases, such as tuberculosis, leprosy, schistosomiasis, and sarcoidosis.[23–26] These models are unique in that they provide access to early, dynamic granuloma formation mechanisms, which are not evident from single-cell experiments or diseased tissue samples.

Some examples of in vitro granuloma-related research conducted on PBMCs are notable in the context of sarcoidosis. Many PAMPs and DAMPs have been incriminated in the pathogenesis of sarcoidosis, with particularly strong evidence supporting a role for *Mycobacterium tuberculosis* (*M.Tb.*).[27] Thus, Taflin et al. modeled sarcoidosis granuloma formation by exposing peripheral blood monocytes to immunogenic *M.Tb.* antigens derived from Bacille Calmate Guerin extract presented on sepharose beads to promote in vitro granuloma formation. They found that Treg depletion accelerated in vitro mononuclear cell aggregation in healthy controls but had no effect in those with active sarcoidosis. Taflin et al. conclude that altered responses to Tregs contribute to pathological granuloma formation in sarcoidosis.[28] Crouser et al. conducted similar experiments, wherein PBMCs were exposed to *M.Tb.*-derived purified protein derivative–coated beads. PBMCs of sarcoidosis and latent tuberculosis infection (LTBI) PBMCs showed robust in vitro multicellular granuloma formation characterized by central macrophage and peripheral T cell aggregates when compared with healthy controls. However, despite similar in vitro histology, sarcoidosis and LTBI displayed very distinctive cytokine and gene expression patterns.[23] The in vitro molecular profiles were in line with those observed in corresponding human disease. Furthermore, in keeping with the clinical diversity of the disease, significant variation in granuloma morphology (e.g., variable granulomatous responses) was observed among sarcoidosis patients. It remains to be determined if the in vitro granuloma features correspond with clinical sarcoidosis phenotypes. At the very least, the in vitro granuloma models show promise for exploration of the earliest steps during pathological granuloma formation, which are not accessible in other disease models, and for preclinical testing of potential therapeutics while minimizing research costs and risks to our patients.

In Vivo Sarcoidosis Models

There are no universally accepted animal models of sarcoidosis largely because most animals do not develop sarcoidosis spontaneously. Furthermore, genetic manipulation of animals (i.e., mice) based on human sarcoidosis gene association studies has not successfully modeled the human disease. However, generic models of granuloma formation have been used as a surrogate for the study of human granulomatous disorders, encompassing infectious and noninfectious etiologies. A few examples are highlighted in this section with special attention to one particular animal model that has serendipitously been linked to the pathogenesis of sarcoidosis.

The development of murine sarcoidosis models has been attempted using various approaches. With the exception of foreign body–mediated granuloma formation (e.g., multiwall carbon nanoparticles)[29] in which the antigen cannot be cleared and the relationship to sarcoidosis is questionable (carbon fiber–induced granuloma models), sustained granuloma formation in response to putative disease-causing infectious antigens requires prior sensitization. Unlike sarcoidosis, the granulomas so induced resolve spontaneously after several weeks.[30–32] This raises questions as to whether murine models truly represent sarcoidosis.

Chronic beryllium disease is nearly indistinguishable from sarcoidosis in its clinical, pathological, and genomic manifestations.[33,34] Transgenic mice overexpressing major histocompatibility complex class II–DP2 (HLA-DP2) when exposed to beryllium oxide via oropharyngeal aspiration develop pauci-immune mononuclear cell aggregates with peribronchovascular distribution, as is typical of sarcoidosis. In keeping with evidence from sarcoidosis patients, Treg-cell depletion in mice exacerbated lung inflammation and granuloma formation. Mack et al. linked MHC II genetic susceptibility and Treg-cell modulation of granulomatous diseases.[19] Thus, berylliosis may serve as a reasonable surrogate for sarcoidosis and has the advantage of the convenience in terms of a well-characterized and readily obtained environmental trigger.

Until very recently, gene knockout models have not offered significant insights into the pathogenesis of sarcoidosis. It was serendipity that drove investigators to link genetically altered mice with enhanced target of rapamycin complex 1 (mTORC1) activity sarcoidosis. Transgenic mice harboring deletion of an upstream inhibitor of mTORC1, tuberous sclerosis 2 (Tsc2), were noted to exhibit spontaneous sarcoidosis-like systemic nonnecrotizing granuloma formation. The compelling findings in Tsc2 −/− mice were validated in humans with progressive forms of sarcoidosis, in whom exaggerated mTORC1 activity was observed in diseased tissues. The putative mechanisms by which excessive mTORC1 activity promotes granuloma formation are not entirely clear; however, evidence suggests the involvement of a signaling pathway involving cyclin-dependent kinase four and related inhibition of nuclear factor kappa-light-chain-enhancer of activated B cells (NK-κB)–mediated apoptosis. The role of the mTOR pathway in human sarcoidosis disease progression remains to be determined; however, the pharmacological inhibition of mTORC1 in Tsc2 −/− mice was shown to effectively resolve systemic granulomas by promoting immune cell apoptosis.[35] Human studies are underway to investigate mTORC1 pathway inhibitors in patients with sarcoidosis.

The development of other transgenic animal models of sarcoidosis will be contingent upon identifying disease-causing genetic factors in humans. An alternative approach would be to "humanize" the animal models via bone marrow transplantation of animals using human sarcoidosis donors. There are inherent limitations of this approach, including impaired adaptive immunity in the humanized mice, which could prevent sarcoidosis formation in the model. That being said, a humanized model of *M.Tb.* infection which closely models human pathology has been successfully developed and shows promise as a useful experimental model.[36]

Ex Vivo Tissue Models

Human sarcoidosis tissues are the gold standard upon which all other models are compared. Explanted diseased specimens are typically preserved or stored for eventual analysis. In addition to more conventional histological and molecular platforms, the recent advent of omics and systems biology opens the door to new discoveries relating to how cells, molecules, and environmental factors (e.g., local microbiome) interact in the context of disease.[37] However, preserved tissues are representative of a snapshot in time and do not allow for experimental model manipulation.

An alternative to preserved tissue is available in the form of an organotypic explant culture, wherein partial or whole viable lung explants are maintained in vitro. Such cultures are shown to retain cellular integrity and can model in vivo functional processes and microarchitectures with high fidelity.[38] This approach has not yet been applied to the investigation of sarcoidosis.

Finally, several options exist for in vitro genesis of complex tissue cell and tissue cultures that closely approximate the human lung. One such approach uses human pluripotent stem cells that differentiate into more complex "lung bud organoids." These organoids contain a representative distribution of pulmonary cellular subtypes within a structure of branching airways. This model has been used to investigate the human airway response to respiratory syncytial virus infection and through genetic manipulation of the Hermansky-Pudlak gene (*HPS1*) to model pulmonary fibrosis.[39] The lung bud organoid model is expensive and technically difficult to manipulate, but the stems cells could theoretically be derived from sarcoidosis patients to more closely model the complex genetics of the disease. Another in vitro lung model, referred to as a lung-on-a-chip, has emerged to address some of these limitations. The lung-chip technology uses microsystems that mimic lung physiological functions and architectures by integrating cells of interest with extracellular matrix scaffold support composed of natural biological extracts or polymer materials.[40] Lung-on-a-chip has been applied in top many diseases, including asthma and chronic obstructive pulmonary disease, for preclinical drug testing.[41,42] A major advantage of this technology for sarcoidosis is being able to provide a three-dimensional lattice, including stromal cells, to support granulomas formation, and to more closely model human disease.

In Silico Models

Useful in silico models are typically based on solid mechanistic foundations. Given that the mechanisms of sarcoidosis granuloma formation are not well understood, in silico models are currently of limited use. However, with the anticipated acceleration of discovery from emerging array of sarcoidosis models discussed herein, the ultimate goal will be to develop a fully automated model that does not require human samples, laboratory equipment, or even clinical trials. As a proof of this concept, Hao et al. developed an in silico model based on available (published) disease mechanisms, including the complex interactions among cytokines, chemokines, and various immune cells that are believed to promote granuloma formation. Accordingly, each component of the model and its known interactions with other components was represented by a differential mathematical equation. The interaction among the components was shown to change over time in the model such that equilibrium was reached corresponding to the size of a "virtual" granuloma and as reflected by the predicted concentrations of various cytokines and chemokines. The mathematical model–predicted chemokine and cytokine levels were then validated against the known tissue concentrations.[43]

Mathematical models, therefore, offer the most expedient and inexpensive means to test new mechanistic hypotheses and to evaluate novel therapeutic targets by manipulating model parameters. In silico models are highly flexible and can accommodate complex molecular networks that are discovered through "omics" and "system biology" research platforms. Modern research techniques such as genomic and proteomic analyses generate an enormous amount of data. When well designed, in silico models could simulate complex biological processes of human health and diseases with high fidelity. In silico models require extensive validation from conventional experiments. Once established, however, such models could greatly accelerate the rate of scientific discovery by circumventing expensive and time-consuming conventional preclinical research conducted in animal or in vitro models. Furthermore, in silico models could rapidly explore the predicted effects of novel therapies and combined therapies or could predict the consequences of functional gene polymorphisms.

CONCLUSION

Advances in the field of sarcoidosis, such as novel therapeutics and useful biomarkers, have been greatly hindered by the lack of highly relevant and convenient research models. New laboratory models that represent the complex and dynamic intercellular interactions occurring in the context of sarcoidosis are likely to accelerate the rate of scientific discovery, including development of novel therapeutic targets and biomarkers, by attracting new talent and resources to the field.

REFERENCES

1. Tukey MH, Berman JS, Boggs DA, White LF, Rosenberg L, Cozier YC. Mortality among African American women with sarcoidosis: data from the black women's health study. *Sarcoidosis Vasc Diffuse Lung Dis*. 2013;30:128–133.
2. Judson MA, Boan AD, Lackland DT. The clinical course of sarcoidosis: presentation, diagnosis, and treatment in a large white and black cohort in the United States. *Sarcoidosis Vasc Diffuse Lung Dis*. 2012;29:119–127.
3. Erdal BS, Clymer BD, Yildiz VO, Julian MW, Crouser ED. Unexpectedly high prevalence of sarcoidosis in a representative U.S. Metropolitan population. *Respir Med*. 2012;106:893–899.
4. Maier LA, Crouser ED, Martin 2nd WJ, Eu J. Executive summary of the NHLBI workshop report: leveraging current scientific advancements to understand sarcoidosis variability and improve outcomes. *Ann Am Thorac Soc*. 2017;14:S415–S420.
5. Berger SB, Romero X, Ma C, et al. SLAM is a microbial sensor that regulates bacterial phagosome functions in macrophages. *Nat Immunol*. 2010;11:920–927.
6. Roach DR, Bean AGD, Demangel C, France MP, Briscoe H, Britton WJ. TNF regulates chemokine induction essential for cell recruitment, granuloma formation, and clearance of Mycobacterial infection. *J Immunol*. 2002;168:4620–4627.
7. Zissel G, Muller-Quernheim J. Cellular players in the immunopathogenesis of sarcoidosis. *Clin Chest Med*. 2015;36:549–560.
8. Noor A, Knox KS. Immunopathogenesis of sarcoidosis. *Clin Dermatol*. 2007;25:250–258.
9. Mortaz E, Rezayat F, Amani D, et al. The roles of T helper 1, T helper 17 and regulatory T cells in the pathogenesis of sarcoidosis. *Iran J Allergy Asthma Immunol*. 2016;15:334–339.
10. Miyara M, Amoura Z, Parizot C, et al. The immune paradox of sarcoidosis and regulatory T cells. *J Exp Med*. 2006;203:359–370.
11. Patterson KC, Hogarth K, Husain AN, Sperling AI, Niewold TB. The clinical and immunologic features of pulmonary fibrosis in sarcoidosis. *Transl Res*. 2012;160:321–331.
12. Mollers M, Aries SP, Dromann D, Mascher B, Braun J, Dalhoff K. Intracellular cytokine repertoire in different T cell subsets from patients with sarcoidosis. *Thorax*. 2001:56.
13. Moller DR, Rybicki BA, Hamzeh NY, et al. Genetic, immunologic, and environmental basis of sarcoidosis. *Ann Am Thorac Soc*. 2017;14:S429–S436.
14. Ungprasert P, Crowson CS, Matteson EL. Smoking, obesity and risk of sarcoidosis: a population-based nested case-control study. *Respir Med*. 2016;120:87–90.
15. Brito-Zeron P, Sellares J, Bosch X, et al. Epidemiologic patterns of disease expression in sarcoidosis: age, gender and ethnicity-related differences. *Clin Exp Rheumatol*. 2016;34:380–388.
16. Winterbauer RH, Lammert J, Selland M, Wu R, Corley D, Springmeyer SC. Bronchoalveolar lavage cell populations in the diagnosis of sarcoidosis. *Chest*. 1993;104:352–361.
17. D.A C, Poulter LW, du Bois RM. Immunocompetent cells in bronchoalveolar lavage reflect the cell populations in transbronchial biopsies in pulmonary sarcoidosis. *Am Rev Respir Dis*. 1985;132:1300–1306.
18. Mitchell AM, Kaiser Y, Falta MT, et al. Shared αβ TCR usage in lungs of sarcoidosis patients with Löfgren's Syndrome. *J Immunol*. 2017;199:2279–2290.
19. Mack DG, Falta MT, McKee AS, et al. Regulatory T cells modulate granulomatous inflammation in an HLA-DP2 transgenic murine model of beryllium-induced disease. *Proc Natl Acad Sci USA*. 2014;111:8553–8558.
20. Ramstein J, Broos CE, Simpson LJ, et al. IFN-gamma-producing T-helper 17.1 cells are increased in sarcoidosis and are more prevalent than T-helper type 1 cells. *Am J Respir Crit Care Med*. 2016;193:1281–1291.
21. Jakubzick C, Gautier EL, Gibbings SL, et al. Minimal differentiation of classical monocytes as they survey steady-state tissues and transport antigen to lymph nodes. *Immunity*. 2013;39:599–610.
22. Janssen WJ, Barthel L, Muldrow A, et al. Fas determines differential fates of resident and recruited macrophages during resolution of acute lung injury. *Am J Respir Crit Care Med*. 2011;184:547–560.
23. Crouser ED, White P, Caceres EG, et al. A novel in vitro human granuloma model of sarcoidosis and latent tuberculosis infection. *Am J Respir Cell Mol Biol*. 2017;57:487–498.
24. Falcao PL, Malaquias LCC, Martins-Filho OA, et al. Human schistosomiasis mansoni: IL-10 modulates the in vitro granuloma formation. *Parasite Immunol*. 1998;20:447–454.
25. Kapoor N, Pawar S, Sirakova TD, Deb C, Warren WL, Kolattukudy PE. Human granuloma in vitro model, for TB dormancy and resuscitation. *PLoS One*. 2013;8:e53657.
26. Wang H, Maeda Y, Fukutomi Y, Makino M. An in vitro model of *Mycobacterium leprae* induced granuloma formation. *BMC Infect Dis*. 2013;13:279–289.
27. Song Z, Marzilli L, Greenlee BM, et al. Mycobacterial catalase-peroxidase is a tissue antigen and target of the adaptive immune response in systemic sarcoidosis. *J Exp Med*. 2005;201:755–767.
28. Taflin C, Miyara M, Nochy D, et al. FoxP3+ regulatory T cells suppress early stages of granuloma formation but have little impact on sarcoidosis lesions. *Am J Pathol*. 2009;174:497–508.
29. Huizar I, Malur A, Midgette YA, et al. Novel murine model of chronic granulomatous lung inflammation elicited by carbon nanotubes. *Am J Respir Cell Mol Biol*. 2011;45:858–866.
30. McCaskill JG, Chason KD, Hua X, et al. Pulmonary immune responses to Propionibacterium acnes in C57BL/6 and BALB/c mice. *Am J Respir Cell Mol Biol*. 2006;35:347–356.
31. Swaisgood CM, Oswald-Richter K, Moeller SD, et al. Development of a sarcoidosis murine lung granuloma model using Mycobacterium superoxide dismutase A peptide. *Am J Respir Cell Mol Biol*. 2011;44:166–174.
32. Werner JL, Escolero SG, Hewlett JT, et al. Induction of pulmonary granuloma formation by propionibacterium acnes is regulated by MyD88 and Nox2. *Am J Respir Cell Mol Biol*. 2017;56:121–130.

33. Mayer AS, Hamzeh N, Maier LA. Sarcoidosis and chronic beryllium disease: similarities and differences. *Semin Respir Crit Care Med*. 2014;35:316–329.
34. Jonth AC, Silveira L, Fingerlin TE, et al. TGF-β1 variants in chronic beryllium disease and sarcoidosis. *J Immunol*. 2007;179:4255–4262.
35. Linke M, Pham HT, Katholnig K, et al. Chronic signaling via the metabolic checkpoint kinase mTORC1 induces macrophage granuloma formation and marks sarcoidosis progression. *Nat Immunol*. 2017;18:293–302.
36. Calderon VE, Valbuena G, Goez Y, et al. A humanized mouse model of tuberculosis. *PLoS One*. 2013;8:e63331.
37. Crouser ED, Fingerlin TE, Yang IV, et al. Application of "omics" and systems biology to sarcoidosis research. *Ann Am Thorac Soc*. 2017;14:S445–S451.
38. Konar D, Devarasetty M, Yildiz DV, Atala A, Murphy SV. Lung-on-a-chip technologies for disease modeling and drug development. *Biomed Eng Comput Biol*. 2016;7: 17–27.
39. Chen YW, Huang SX, de Carvalho A, et al. A three-dimensional model of human lung development and disease from pluripotent stem cells. *Nat Cell Biol*. 2017;19: 542–549.
40. Yang X, Li K, Zhang X, et al. Nanofiber membrane supported lung-on-a-chip microdevice for anti-cancer drug testing. *Lab Chip*. 2018;18:486–495.
41. Benam KH, Konigshoff M, Eickelberg O. Breaking the in vitro barrier in respiratory medicine: engineered microphysiological systems for COPD and beyond. *Am J Respir Crit Care Med*. 2017. https://doi.org/10.1164/rccm.201709-1795PP.
42. Benam KH, Villenave R, Lucchesi C, et al. Small airway-on-a-chip enables analysis of human lung inflammation and drug responses in vitro. *Nat Methods*. 2016;13: 151–157.
43. Hao W, Crouser ED, Friedman A. Mathematical model of sarcoidosis. *Proc Natl Acad Sci USA*. 2014;111:16065–16070.

CHAPTER 6

Pathology of Granuloma

JEAN-FRANÇOIS BERNAUDIN, MD, PHD • PHILIPPE MOGUELET, MD • FLORENCE JENY, MD • VALÉRIE BESNARD, PHD • DOMINIQUE VALEYRE, MD • MARIANNE KAMBOUCHNER, MD

Sarcoidosis is a systemic disease of unknown cause primarily involving the lung and the lymphatic system, although virtually every organ may be affected. It is characterized by the formation of immune epithelioid granulomas in affected organs.[1,2] Therefore, granuloma observation in tissue samples is not only a key step to make the diagnosis of sarcoidosis but it is also the gateway to a better understanding of the pathogenesis of the disease. Except in very special cases, detection of granulomas in at least one tissue sample is considered mandatory for diagnosis. Although granulomas may be observed in various conditions, they must display a characteristic sarcoid pattern in the setting of an evocative clinical context after exclusion of any other hypothesis to assess the diagnosis of sarcoidosis. The strategy of choice for biopsy sampling will be discussed in the diagnosis specific chapter (Diagnosis of sarcoidosis by Wim Wuyts). Briefly, the most frequent tissues biopsied are bronchial mucosa, lung parenchyma, lymph nodes, and skin, the frequency that has determined the chapter outline focused on pulmonary and skin sarcoidosis.

THE EPITHELIOID GRANULOMA IN SARCOIDOSIS

The designation of "granuloma" covers histopathologic lesions observed in diverse conditions, and it must be remembered that even in economically advanced countries, infections, mainly tuberculosis, are among the most common causes. Therefore when a pathologist observes granulomas, the first step will be to systematically exclude infectious organisms using "special stains" (Ziehl-Nielsen; Gomori-Grocott, PAS).[3,4] For more than 50 years, strict criteria were used to delineate the organized epithelioid cell granuloma, i.e., epithelioid and giant cells organized in tubercles.[5] Typical sarcoid granulomas are well-formed, compact, noncaseating granuloma that consists of epithelioid cells and multinucleated giant cells (MGCs) associated with a variable number of lymphocytes (Fig. 6.1).[6,7] The core of the granuloma consists of epithelioid cells that are highly differentiated mononuclear phagocytes with numerous interdigitated cytoplasmic projections and a nonphagocytic/secretory pattern with active metabolism feature at the ultrastructural level.[8] Epithelioid cells are in most cases in close contact with CD4+ T lymphocytes, whereas CD8+ T lymphocytes, CD4+ FOXP3+ Treg, Th17 cells, B lymphocytes, and IgA-producing plasma cells are observed in the peripheral zone.[7,9–11] Sarcoid granulomas may occasionally exhibit a focal central coagulative necrosis. Giant cells may contain cytoplasmic inclusions (asteroid or Schaumann bodies) that may be erroneously identified as exogenous contaminates. Fibrotic change is a major feature with a distinctive pattern of peripheral strapping lamellar fibrosis, ending with complete fibrosis and/or hyalinization, which may obscure the diagnostic features.

Although these features are characteristic, they are not specific for sarcoidosis, and their diagnostic value should be discussed mostly according to the affected organ. To illustrate this point, we developed, in Table 6.1, the comparison between granulomas observed in various granulomatous pulmonary diseases.

GRANULOMA IN PULMONARY SARCOIDOSIS

The lung is the most often affected organ in sarcoidosis. Table 6.1 highlights the main pulmonary granulomatous diseases involving the lung and their respective histologic patterns.[4,12] At its most basic level described previously, the nonnecrotizing sarcoid granuloma is a compact and organized aggregate of epithelioid histiocytes tightly clustered with mature macrophages, multinucleate giant cells associated to lymphocytes (Fig. 6.2A and B). This emblematic pattern of sarcoid granuloma is potentially observed in all the organs involved in the disease. However, on histological ground, pulmonary sarcoid lesions display a distinctive pattern that stands apart from some other locations (especially skin or kidney).

Sarcoidosis. https://doi.org/10.1016/B978-0-323-54429-0.00006-9

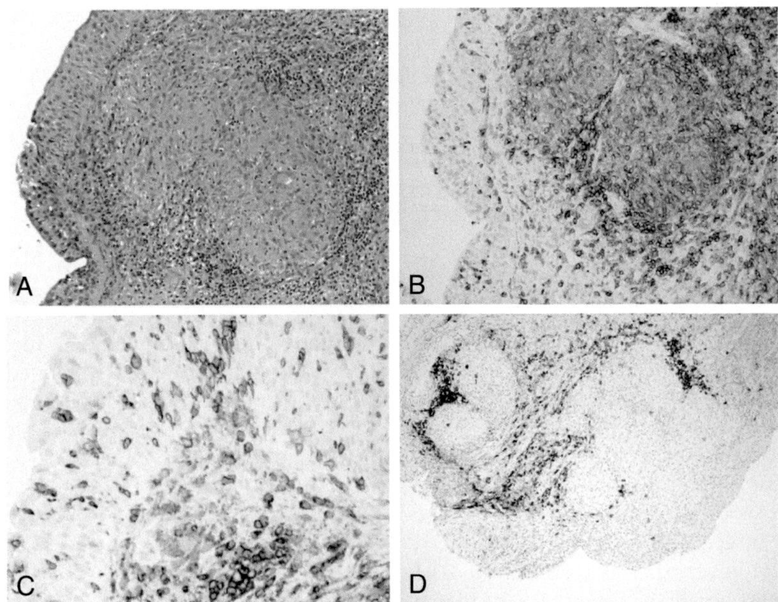

FIG. 6.1 Optic microscopy and immunohistochemistry of a bronchial mucosa biopsy in a patient with sarcoidosis. (A) Two characteristic epithelioid granulomas surrounded by lymphocytes in the connective tissue below the epithelium (hematein eosin staining). (B) The brown labeling after incubation with an anti-CD4 antibody indicates CD4+ T lymphocytes and epithelioid cells within the granuloma. (C) Higher magnification of intraepithelial CD4+ lymphocytes and periphery of the granuloma. (D) Incubation with an anti-CD19 antibody showing B lymphocytes outside of the granulomas. (final magnification: for A and B, ×100; for C, ×200; for D, ×50).

First, pulmonary sarcoid granulomas are typically distributed along lymphatic routes, sparing mediolobular areas of intervening lung parenchyma.[6,13] This topographical distribution of lesions is a crucial criterion for both radiologists and pathologists to approach the diagnosis.[14] In keeping with the lymphatic distribution, airway involvement is nearly constant. Sarcoid granulomas in the bronchial mucosa can cause airflow limitation, so called endobronchial sarcoidosis, and in the bronchiolar mucosa, a peribronchiolitis narrows the bronchiolar lumen (Fig. 6.2C).[6,15] Also, sarcoid granulomas display a peculiar tropism for the outer wall of pulmonary arteries and veins.[16,17]

Second, at the microscopic level, pulmonary granulomas are almost always surrounded by a concentric rim of lamellar collagen bundles. It is considered that the thickness of this "fibrotic coat" is correlated with the age of the granulomas.

Third, pulmonary sarcoid granulomas show a very special trend for aggregating, resulting in typical micronodules (several millimeters) and occasional macronodules (up to 5 cm). The fibrotic rim enclosing granulomas consolidates the cohesiveness of these nodules (Fig. 6.2D). Finally, nodular masses of confluent aggregates of sharply circumscribed epithelioid granulomas progressing to fibrotic hyaline nodules may replace large areas of lung parenchyma. Aspergillus infection could be occasionally observed within some excavated macronodules.

Fourth, additional changes include some degree of interstitial and alveolar inflammation in areas of intervening lung parenchyma. Although it is usually stated that alveolar and interstitial inflammatory infiltrates at distance from granulomas are quite inconspicuous,[3] evidence has been initially shown on pulmonary biopsies that alveolitis precedes granulomatous changes.[18–20] This was confirmed on data obtained by bronchoalveolar lavage.[21] In addition, gene set expression analysis on transbronchial biopsies[22] and studies of explanted lungs have demonstrated that chronic interstitial lung inflammation may be a key factor in progressive fibrotic changes in sarcoidosis.

TABLE 6.1
Histologic Patterns of Granulomatous Interstitial Pneumonias From Travis[3], Cheung[4], and Valeyre[16]

Diseases	Main Distribution of Lesions	Main Pattern of Granulomas	Associated Features
Sarcoidosis	Lymphangitic, usually located on the outer walls of pulmonary vessels, along lobular septa, visceral pleura, and airways	Well circumscribed and coalescent epithelioid and giant-cell granulomas surrounded by lymphocytes, subsequently by a ring of lamellar fibrosis; scant inflammation; extremely rare fibrinous exudate within granulomas	Frequently large polarizable crystalline structures in multinucleate giant cells. Occasionally nonspecific cytoplasmic inclusions: asteroid, Schaumann, and conchoid bodies
Berylliosis	Lymphangitic and frequently associated with scattered small lobular granulomas	Like sarcoidosis, well circumscribed coalescent +++, perigranulomatous fibrosis	Amounts of dusts depending on associated respiratory exposures
Granulomatous pneumonitis due to other inorganic agents	• Aluminum: occasional scattered sarcoid-like granulomas • Hard metal: diffuse giant-cell alveolitis	• Aluminum: pseudosarcoid granulomas • Hard metal: giant cell interstitial pneumonia	Numerous multinucleate giant cells
Infections (mycobacteria and fungi)	Early lesions: bronchiolocentric. Then, randomly distributed	Interstitial caseating and noncaseating granulomas; in late stage, palisades of epithelioid histiocytes delineating geographic-shaped necrosis; numerous inflammatory cells; few or no fibrosis. Organisms may be demonstrated by special stains	Frequently, areas of organizing pneumonia, acute inflammation, and vascular wall involvement by inflammatory cells
Hypersensitivity pneumonitis (subacute)	Airway-centered inflammation (bronchioles and alveolar ducts)	Small and loose nonnecrotizing granulomas and non fibrotizing	Interstitial infiltration by lymphocytes. Frequent areas of bronchiolitis obliterans and organizing pneumonia
Hot tub lung	Bronchiolocentric and randomly distributed within airspaces	Well-formed, nonnecrotizing granulomas	Organizing pneumonia; mild interstitial pneumonia
Sjogren's syndrome	Rare and randomly distributed over the pulmonary interstitium	Small nonnecrotizing granulomas	Peribronchial lymphoid hyperplasia, narrowing of the small airways, occasional cysts
Granulomatous pneumonitis associated with Crohn's and Whipple disease	Crohn's: rarely, randomly distributed; Whipple: patchy, around bronchioles and blood vessels	Crohn's: scattered tiny nonnecrotizing granulomas; Whipple: clusters of histiocytes	Crohn's: related to drugs used for Crohn's treatment
CVID (common variable immune deficiency)	Peribronchiolar	GL-ILD (granulomatous and lymphocytic-interstitial lung disease); clusters of alveolar and interstitial nonnecrotizing granulomas admixed with lymphocytic interstitial pneumonia	Occasional organizing pneumonia

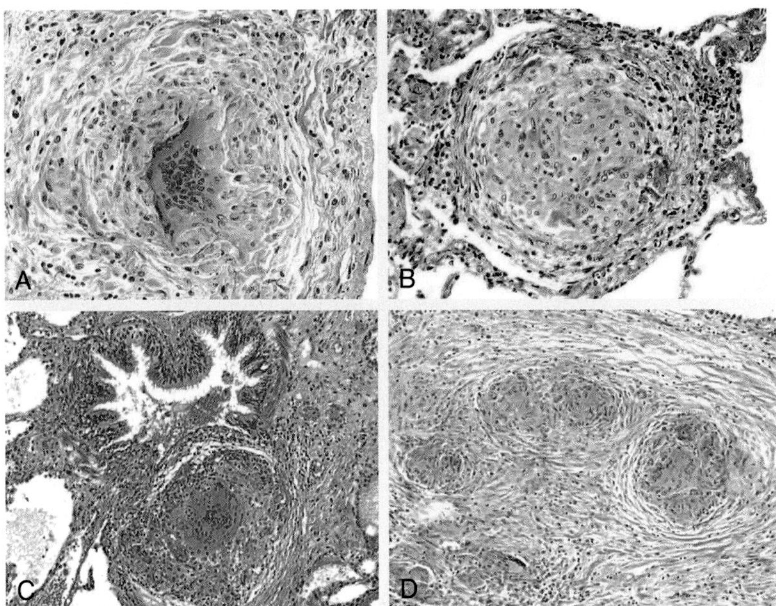

FIG. 6.2 Examples of granulomas observed in various situations in pulmonary sarcoidosis. Images obtained from paraffin-embedded surgical lung biopsies. (A) Characteristic sarcoid granuloma composed of a central multinucleated giant-cell surrounded by epithelioid cells. (B) Pulmonary sarcoid granuloma surrounded by concentric collagen bundles and lymphocytes. (C) The wall of a bronchiole is involved by a sarcoid granuloma narrowing the lumen. (D) Five coalescent old granulomas embedded in a dense fibrotic rim. (hematein-eosin-saffron staining; final magnification: for A and B, ×100; for C and D, ×50).

GRANULOMA IN SKIN SARCOIDOSIS

Skin is one of the most often affected organs in sarcoidosis.[23] Erythema nodosum and specific cutaneous lesions are in several series the more frequent extrapulmonary manifestations.[24,25] Although granulomas are not observed in erythema nodosum, easily achievable biopsies of specific lesions are particularly effective for confirming the diagnosis of sarcoidosis. Cutaneous granulomatosis is a heterogeneous group of diseases, considering the clinical presentation is the first and critical step in the process of a biopsy analysis.[26,27] Otherwise, the pathologist must keep in mind all the many skin diseases associated with a granulomatous reaction summarized in Table 6.2. Skin lesions may be the first, even the only, manifestation of sarcoidosis, and some authors prefer to talk about "sarcoid-like granulomatous diseases of unknown significance" in that situation.[28]

Granulomas observed in cutaneous sarcoidosis consist, as previously described, of well-limited grouped epithelioid and multinucleate giant cells surrounded by a merely sparse lymphocytic infiltrate, hence the name "naked" granuloma used by dermatopathologists. Depending on the clinical type of the lesion,

TABLE 6.2
Main Cutaneous Granulomatosis According to Weedon D With Modifications[33]

Sarcoidal Granulomas
SARCOIDOSIS
Foreign material granulomatous reaction (silica, silicone, tattoo pigments, beryllium, zinc, keratin scales, sea urchin, spine injury, and so forth). Blau syndrome (in children, associated with a NOD2 mutation)
TUBERCULOID GRANULOMAS
Infectious diseases (tuberculoid leprosy, mycobacteria and atypical mycobacteria, late syphilis, leishmaniasis), rosacea, perioral dermatitis, lupus miliaris faciei, Crohn's disease
NECROBIOTIC GRANULOMAS
Granuloma annulare, necrobiosis lipoidica, rheumatoid nodules, necrobiotic xanthogranuloma
SUPPURATIVE GRANULOMAS
Chromomycosis and phaeohyphomycosis, sporotrichosis, nontuberculous mycobacterial infections, blastomycosis, paracoccidioidomycosis, coccidioidomycosis, blastomycosis-like pyoderma, mycetomas, nocardiosis, and actinomycosis, Cat-scratch disease, lymphogranuloma venereum

NOD2, nucleotide-binding oligomerization domain protein 2.

granulomas are mostly observed in the dermis, superficial or throughout its depth, extending to the hypodermis (Fig. 6.3A). Granulomas may also be restricted to the subcutaneous tissue below a normal-appearing skin, classically associated with a systemic dissemination of the disease.[29] Granulomas may be isolated or more often confluent with a back-to-back distribution associated with a perigranulomatous fibrosis (Fig. 6.3B and C). Scant fibrinous material may be seen in superficial and erosive lesions, but necrosis is uncommon.[30] A transepidermal elimination of granulomas is sometimes observed.[31] By contrast with pulmonary granulomas,[13] no specific association with the lymphatic vasculature has been reported, and blood capillaries may be numerous (Fig. 6.3E).[32]

In some cases, granulomas restricted to the skin may be considered as a local sarcoid reaction to a foreign body. It should be stressed that in return, cutaneous sarcoidosis preferentially affects sites of prior injury such as scars after trauma including surgery, desensitizing injection sites, venipuncture, chronic infection, cosmetic filler injection site, and tattoo.[33–35] Polarizable foreign material consisting mainly of crystalline silica (SiO^2)[36] has been reported from 22% to 77% of biopsies, suggesting that foreign material could be a nidus for granuloma formation and a potential trigger for the disease (Fig. 6.3D).[37–39] Because foreign substances introduced in dermis may induce a sarcoid-like granulomatous disease, polarization examination of tissue sections must be systematic while bearing in mind that the presence of foreign material does not exclude the diagnosis of sarcoidosis.[37,39]

CONSTITUTION AND EVOLUTION OF GRANULOMA IN SARCOIDOSIS

The sequence of events leading to granuloma formation and evolution in sarcoidosis is for the most part still hypothetical. However, its main principle has been initially described at the time of use of the Kveim test for diagnosis, more than 60years ago: "*In developing Kveim antigen-induced granulomas, there is an accumulation of lymphocytes within a week. Giant cell may appear about the injected material, but tubercles are not seen for two or 3weeks. With time lymphocytes disappear leaving pure collection of epithelioid cell which persist unaltered for months.*"[40]

Granuloma formation is a chain of events, on site recruitment of monocytes/macrophages, their maturation and organization into a mature granuloma, and finally emergence of epithelioid cells associated in compact agglomerates.[41] Epithelioid cells are large polygonal cells derived from macrophages with pale oval nuclei and abundant cytoplasm.[5,8,40] They express CD68, a general marker of the monocyte-macrophage lineage, while no specific "epithelioid" surface marker is available.[42] By contrast to typical macrophages, no phagocytic activity has been observed. They are predominantly secretory cells, in particular for angiotensin-converting enzyme (ACE)[43] or tumor necrosis factor alpha (TNFα).[44] Other products have been detected in these cells, as cathepsin K[45,46] or osteopontin[47] both suggested to be involved in granuloma formation. In addition, epithelioid cells may play a major role in perigranuloma fibrosis because as shown in granulomas of pulmonary sarcoidosis, they contain an abundant amount of transforming growth factor (TGF-β1).[48] The significance of MGCs in granulomas of sarcoidosis is still unknown. They are classically thought to be the consequence of macrophage fusion.[49] However, it has been recently suggested that they may be polyploid macrophages related to a persistent Toll-like receptor 2 signal.[50] In other situations than in sarcoidosis, MGCs are able to sequester undegradable material (as in foreign-body granulomas) or persistent pathogens, retaining phagocytic and microbicidal activities. As they secrete interleukin (IL)-1α, TNFα, and TGF-β cytokines, they may contribute to the granuloma cellular dynamics.[51]

Granulomas are multilayered spherical structures organized around an original focal aggregate of macrophages. The mechanisms of cell cohesion are multiple: (1) intertwining of cells, thanks to numerous pseudopods;[52,53] (2) expression of E-cadherin by epithelioid cells and MGCs; and (3) even cell junctions (adherens [E-cadherin], desmosomes, and tight junctions) between macrophages[54] as in an experimental zebrafish (*Mycobacterium marinum*) model.[55] Important cell-to-cell interactions through contact between lymphocytes and macrophages rely on a large set of costimulatory and coinhibitory molecules: (1) CMH II/TCR,[56] (2) PD1/PDL-1,[57] (3) CD86/CD28,[58] (4) BTNL2,[59] and (5) ICOS/ICOSL.[60] At last, the inflammatory acute phase protein serum amyloid A is hypothesized to play a significant role in granuloma formation and cohesion.[61]

Granuloma maintenance and duration remain a mystery. In a best-case scenario, sarcoid granulomas may resolve within 2years without any treatment, whereas progressive sarcoidosis may take place for longer periods. Generally speaking, granulomas are highly dynamic structures.[62–64] Their duration depends on the balance between the rate of recruitment and local division of both macrophages and lymphocytes and their life span and death rate. Indeed, a local T-cell proliferation is observed,[65] and $CD4^+CD45RA^-FoxP3^{bright}$ Tregs lymphocytes were shown to actively proliferate and accumulate within granulomas.[66] By contrast, the

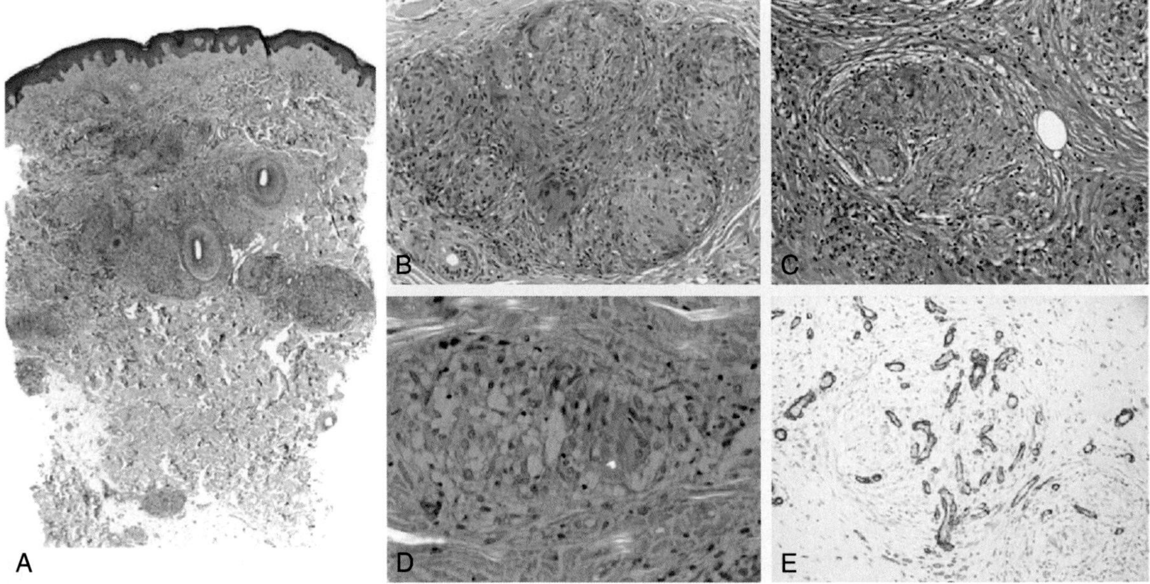

FIG. 6.3 Examples of granulomas observed in cutaneous sarcoidosis. Images obtained from paraffin-embedded skin biopsies. (A) Low magnification image showing granulomas scattered in the superficial and deep dermis. (B) The confluent back-to-back organization of granulomas. (C) A perigranulomatous fibrosis. (D) Polarized light microscopy: refringent foreign body in the cytoplasm of a giant cell. (E) Immunohistochemistry for actin showing numerous capillaries around and within granulomas. (hematein-eosin-saffron staining; final magnification: A, ×10; B and C, ×50; D and E, ×100).

apoptotic process appears to be altered within granulomas of patients with progressive sarcoidosis.[67] In that respect, interferon gamma–induced expression of the cyclin-dependant kinase inhibitor $p21^{Waf1/Cip1}$ dramatically reduces apoptosis in sarcoidosis macrophages.[68] Likewise, IL15-induction of the antiapoptotic B-cell lymphoma 2 (BCL2) protein inhibited T cells apoptosis.[69] During progressive sarcoidosis, developing fibrosis occurs around persistent granulomas. Production of Th2 cytokines, including TGF-β and IL13, is observed in fibrosing granulomas.[70] In addition, some macrophages acquire an alternative activated M2 phenotype as in granulomas in muscle or lymph node.[71,72] Notably a profibrotic M2c macrophage phenotype could potentially be induced by the chemokine CCL18 locally present in sarcoidosis tissues.[73,74]

Granulomas are metabolically active in systemic processes, for example, production of ACE of the renin angiotensin system;[75] upregulation of the extrarenal 1a–hydroxylase that converts 25–hydroxy vitamin D (25–(OH)D) to its active form: 1,25–dihydroxy vitamin D(1,25(OH)2 D);[76] and expression of parathyroid hormone–related protein (PTH–rP) both of which may result in hypercalcemia.[76] The metabolic properties of the granulomas are illustrated by the ^{18}Fluor deoxyglucose uptake, probably resulting in GLUT-1 expression (glucose transporter).[77,78]

EXPERIMENTAL MODELS OF GRANULOMAS

Attempts to identify specific exogenous components/antigens causing the granulomatous response in sarcoidosis from patients' tissue samples have been mostly inconclusive. Therefore most models of granulomatous diseases have been developed to test various potential causal agents. They have been initiated with either inorganic particles (as carbon nanotubes), mycobacterial antigens (catalase-peroxidase [mKatG], superoxide dismutase A, early secreted antigen target 6), or bacteria (*Propionibacterium acnes* in mice).[79] In most models, mainly pulmonary, formation of granulomas was observed, with presence of immune cells and production of cytokines, almost similar to what is observed in sarcoidosis patients. However, systemic disease and late clinical signs of sarcoidosis progression, including lymphadenopathy or pulmonary fibrosis, are missing in these experimental models.

Furthermore, the recent publication of a model activating the metabolic checkpoint kinase mTORC1 in macrophages by deletion of *Tsc2* opens new avenues in the understanding of the granuloma biology.[80]

CONCLUSION

Excepted in case of Lofgren's syndrome presentation or very typical other conditions such as Heerfordt syndrome or asymptomatic typical pulmonary stage 1, if an adequate monitoring is planned, diagnosis of sarcoidosis should not be made on clinical grounds alone. To assess the diagnosis of sarcoidosis, identification of typical epithelioid granulomas in an evocative clinical context after exclusion of any other hypothesis is required. Therefore, the pathologist's report describing the presence of "granulomas" in a biopsy plays a key role. Despite recent advances in the biology of macrophages, thanks to experimental models, the natural history of granulomas in sarcoidosis remains an enigma. Further developments are needed to develop more appropriate treatments in this disease.

REFERENCES

1. Valeyre D, Prasse A, Nunes H, Uzunhan Y, Brillet P-Y, Müller-Quernheim J. Sarcoidosis. *Lancet*. 2014;383(9923): 1155–1167.
2. Müller-Quernheim J, Prasse A, Zissel G. Pathogenesis of sarcoidosis. *Presse Médicale Paris Fr 1983*. 2012;41(6 Pt 2):275–287.
3. Travis W, Colby T, Koss M, Rosado-de-Christenson M, Muller N, King TE. *Non-neoplastic Disorders of the Lower Respiratory Tract. AFIP Atlas of Nontumor Pathology, First Series, Fascicle 2*; 2002.
4. Cheung OY, Muhm JR, Helmers RA, et al. Surgical pathology of granulomatous interstitial pneumonia. *Ann Diagn Pathol*. 2003;7(2):127–138.
5. Epstein WL. Granulomatous hypersensitivity. *Prog Allergy*. 1967;11:36–88.
6. Carrington CB. Structure and function in sarcoidosis. *Ann NY Acad Sci*. 1976;278:265–283.
7. Hunninghake GW, Costabel U, Ando M, et al. ATS/ERS/WASOG statement on sarcoidosis. American Thoracic Society/European respiratory Society/World association of sarcoidosis and other granulomatous disorders. *Sarcoidosis Vasc Diffuse Lung Dis Off J WASOG*. 1999;16(2):149–173.
8. Soler P, Basset F, Bernaudin J, Chretien J. Morphology and distribution of the cells of a sarcoid granuloma: ultrastructural study of serial sections. *Ann NY Acad Sci*. 1976;278:147–160.
9. Kamphuis LS, van ZMC, Lam KH, et al. Perigranuloma localization and abnormal maturation of B cells: emerging key players in sarcoidosis? *Am J Respir Crit Care Med*. 2013;187(4):406–416.
10. Miyara M, Amoura Z, Parizot C, et al. The immune paradox of sarcoidosis and regulatory T cells. *J Exp Med*. 2006;203(2):359–370.
11. Facco M, Cabrelle A, Teramo A, et al. Sarcoidosis is a Th1/Th17 multisystem disorder. *Thorax*. 2011;66(2):144–150.
12. Myers JL, Tazelaar HD. Challenges in pulmonary fibrosis: 6–Problematic granulomatous lung disease. *Thorax*. 2008;63(1):78–84.
13. Kambouchner M, Pirici D, Uhl J-F, Mogoanta L, Valeyre D, Bernaudin J-F. Lymphatic and blood microvasculature organisation in pulmonary sarcoid granulomas. *Eur Respir J*. 2011;37(4):835–840.
14. Criado E, Sánchez M, Ramírez J, et al. Pulmonary sarcoidosis: typical and atypical manifestations at high-resolution CT with pathologic correlation. *Radiogr Rev Publ Radiol Soc N Am Inc*. 2010;30(6):1567–1586.
15. Polychronopoulos VS, Prakash UBS. Airway involvement in sarcoidosis. *Chest*. 2009;136(5):1371–1380.
16. Valeyre D, Bernaudin J-F, Jeny F, et al. Pulmonary sarcoidosis. *Clin Chest Med*. 2015;36(4):631–641.
17. Takemura T, Matsui Y, Saiki S, Mikami R. Pulmonary vascular involvement in sarcoidosis: a report of 40 autopsy cases. *Hum Pathol*. 1992;23(11):1216–1223.
18. Rosen Y, Athanassiades TJ, Moon S, Lyons HA. Nongranulomatous interstitial pneumonitis in sarcoidosis. Relationship to development of epithelioid granulomas. *Chest*. 1978;74(2):122–125.
19. Keogh BA, Crystal RG. Alveolitis: the key to the interstitial lung disorders. *Thorax*. 1982;37(1):1–10.
20. Lacronique J, Bernaudin J-F, Soler P. In: Chretien J, Marsac J, Saltiel JC, eds. *Alveolitis and Granulomas: Sequential Course in Pulmonary Sarcoidosis*. Paris: Pergamon Press; 1983: 36–42.
21. Crystal RG, Bitterman PB, Rennard SI, Hance AJ, Keogh BA. Interstitial lung diseases of unknown cause. Disorders characterized by chronic inflammation of the lower respiratory tract (first of two parts). *N Engl J Med*. 1984;310(3):154–166.
22. Lockstone HE, Sanderson S, Kulakova N, et al. Gene set analysis of lung samples provides insight into pathogenesis of progressive, fibrotic pulmonary sarcoidosis. *Am J Respir Crit Care Med*. 2010;181(12):1367–1375.
23. Baughman RP, Teirstein AS, Judson MA, et al. Clinical characteristics of patients in a case control study of sarcoidosis. *Am J Respir Crit Care Med*. 2001;164(10):1885–1889.
24. Liu K-L, Tsai W-C, Lee C-H. Cutaneous sarcoidosis: a retrospective case series and a hospital-based case-control study in Taiwan. *Medicine (Baltim)*. 2017;96(40):e8158.
25. Mañá J, Rubio-Rivas M, Villalba N, et al. Multidisciplinary approach and long-term follow-up in a series of 640 consecutive patients with sarcoidosis: cohort study of a 40-year clinical experience at a tertiary referral center in Barcelona, Spain. *Medicine (Baltim)*. 2017;96(29):e7595.
26. Lodha S, Sanchez M, Prystowsky S. Sarcoidosis of the skin: a review for the pulmonologist. *Chest*. 2009;136(2):583–596.

27. Terziroli Beretta-Piccoli B, Mainetti C, Peeters M-A, Laffitte E. Cutaneous granulomatosis: a comprehensive review. *Clin Rev Allergy Immunol.* 2018;54(1):131–146.
28. Wanat KA, Rosenbach M. Cutaneous sarcoidosis. *Clin Chest Med.* 2015;36(4):685–702.
29. Marcoval J, Moreno A, Mañá J, Peyri J. Subcutaneous sarcoidosis. *Dermatol Clin.* 2008;26(4):553–556, ix.
30. Noiles K, Beleznay K, Crawford RI, Au S. Sarcoidosis can present with necrotizing granulomas histologically: two cases of ulcerated sarcoidosis and review of the literature. *J Cutan Med Surg.* 2013;17(6):377–383.
31. Ismail A, Beckum K, McKay K. Transepithelial elimination in sarcoidosis: a frequent finding. *J Cutan Pathol.* 2014;41(1):22–27.
32. Utino FL, Damiani GV, Garcia M, et al. Histomorphometric approach to differentiate skin lesions of tuberculoid leprosy from sarcoidosis. *J Cutan Pathol.* 2018;45(2):111–117.
33. Weedon D. *Weedon's Skin Pathology*. 3rd ed. Churchill Livingstone: Elsevier Masson; 2009.
34. Marcoval J, Penín RM, Mañá J. Specific skin lesions of sarcoidosis located at venipuncture points for blood sample collection. *Am J Dermatopathol.* 2018;40(5):362–366.
35. Kluger N. Sarcoidosis on tattoos: a review of the literature from 1939 to 2011. *Sarcoidosis Vasc Diffuse Lung Dis Off J WASOG.* 2013;30(2):86–102.
36. Colboc H, Bazin D, Moguelet P, et al. Detection of silica and calcium carbonate deposits in granulomatous areas of skin sarcoidosis by µFourier transform infrared spectroscopy and Field Emission Scanning Electron Microscopy coupled with Energy Dispersive X-ray Spectroscopy analysis. *Comptes Rendus Chim.* 2016;19(11):1631–1641.
37. Callen JP. The presence of foreign bodies does not exclude the diagnosis of sarcoidosis. *Arch Dermatol.* 2001;137(4):485–486.
38. Marcoval J, Moreno A, Maña J. Foreign bodies in cutaneous sarcoidosis. *J Cutan Pathol.* 2004;31(7):516.
39. Walsh NM, Hanly JG, Tremaine R, Murray S. Cutaneous sarcoidosis and foreign bodies. *Am J Dermatopathol.* 1993;15(3):203–207.
40. Rogers FJ, Haserick JR. Sarcoidosis and the Kveim reaction. *J Invest Dermatol.* 1954;23(5):389–406.
41. Broos CE, van Nimwegen M, Hoogsteden HC, Hendriks RW, Kool M, van den Blink B. Granuloma formation in pulmonary sarcoidosis. *Front Immunol.* 2013;4:437.
42. Ueda-Hayakawa I, Tanimura H, Osawa M, et al. Elevated serum BAFF levels in patients with sarcoidosis: association with disease activity. *Rheumatol Oxf Engl.* 2013;52(9):1658–1666.
43. Stanton L-A, Fenhalls G, Lucas A, et al. Immunophenotyping of macrophages in human pulmonary tuberculosis and sarcoidosis. *Int J Exp Pathol.* 2003;84(6):289–304.
44. Yanagishita T, Watanabe D, Akita Y, et al. Construction of novel in vitro epithelioid cell granuloma model from mouse macrophage cell line. *Arch Dermatol Res.* 2007;299(8):399–403.
45. Bühling F, Reisenauer A, Gerber A, et al. Cathepsin K–a marker of macrophage differentiation? *J Pathol.* 2001;195(3):375–382.
46. Samokhin AO, Gauthier JY, Percival MD, Brömme D. Lack of cathepsin activities alter or prevent the development of lung granulomas in a mouse model of sarcoidosis. *Respir Res.* 2011;12:13.
47. Carlson I, Tognazzi K, Manseau EJ, Dvorak HF, Brown LF. Osteopontin is strongly expressed by histiocytes in granulomas of diverse etiology. *Lab Investig J Tech Methods Pathol.* 1997;77(1):103–108.
48. Limper AH, Colby TV, Sanders MS, Asakura S, Roche PC, DeRemee RA. Immunohistochemical localization of transforming growth factor-beta 1 in the nonnecrotizing granulomas of pulmonary sarcoidosis. *Am J Respir Crit Care Med.* 1994;149(1):197–204.
49. TCMT van M, Vos W, van DPJ. Giant cell formation in sarcoidosis: cell fusion or proliferation with non-division? *Clin Exp Immunol.* 2009;155(3):476–486.
50. Herrtwich L, Nanda I, Evangelou K, et al. DNA damage signaling instructs polyploid macrophage fate in granulomas. *Cell.* 2016;167(5):1264–1280. e18.
51. Hernandez-Pando R, Bornstein QL, Aguilar Leon D, Orozco EH, Madrigal VK, Martinez Cordero E. Inflammatory cytokine production by immunological and foreign body multinucleated giant cells. *Immunology.* 2000;100(3):352–358.
52. Papadimitriou JM, Finlay-Jones JM, Walters MN. Surface characteristics of macrophages, epithelioid and giant cells using scanning electron microscopy. *Exp Cell Res.* 1973;76(2):353–362.
53. Adams DO. The structure of mononuclear phagocytes differentiating in vivo. I. Sequential fine and histologic studies of the effect of Bacillus Calmette-Guerin (BCG). *Am J Pathol.* 1974;76(1):17–48.
54. Wanat KA, Rosenbach M, Zoiber AF, Zhang PJ, Schaffer A. E-cadherin is expressed by mono- and multinucleated histiocytes in cutaneous sarcoidal and foreign body granulomas. *Am J Dermatopathol.* 2014;36(8):651–654.
55. Cronan MR, Beerman RW, Rosenberg AF, et al. Macrophage epithelial reprogramming underlies mycobacterial granuloma formation and promotes infection. *Immunity.* 2016;45(4):861–876.
56. Schürmann M, Reichel P, Müller-Myhsok B, Schlaak M, Müller-Quernheim J, Schwinger E. Results from a genome-wide search for predisposing genes in sarcoidosis. *Am J Respir Crit Care Med.* 2001;164(5):840–846.
57. Braun NA, Celada LJ, Herazo-Maya JD, et al. Blockade of the programmed death-1 pathway restores sarcoidosis CD4(+) T-cell proliferative capacity. *Am J Respir Crit Care Med.* 2014;190(5):560–571.
58. Agostini C, Trentin L, Perin A, et al. Regulation of alveolar macrophage-T cell interactions during Th1-type sarcoid inflammatory process. *Am J Physiol.* 1999;277(2 Pt 1):L240–L250.

59. Valentonyte R, Hampe J, Huse K, et al. Sarcoidosis is associated with a truncating splice site mutation in BTNL2. *Nat Genet.* 2005;37(4):357–364.
60. Sakthivel P, Grunewald J, Eklund A, Bruder D, Wahlström J. Pulmonary sarcoidosis is associated with high-level inducible co-stimulator (ICOS) expression on lung regulatory T cells–possible implications for the ICOS/ICOS-ligand axis in disease course and resolution. *Clin Exp Immunol.* 2016;183(2):294–306.
61. Chen ES, Song Z, Willett MH, et al. Serum amyloid A regulates granulomatous inflammation in sarcoidosis through Toll-like receptor-2. *Am J Respir Crit Care Med.* 2010;181(4):360–373.
62. Lin PL, Coleman T, Carney JPJ, et al. Radiologic responses in cynomolgus macaques for assessing tuberculosis chemotherapy regimens. *Antimicrob Agents Chemother.* 2013;57(9):4237–4244.
63. Schreiber HA, Harding JS, Hunt O, et al. Inflammatory dendritic cells migrate in and out of transplanted chronic mycobacterial granulomas in mice. *J Clin Invest.* 2011;121(10):3902–3913.
64. Schreiber HA, Harding JS, Altamirano CJ, et al. Continuous repopulation of lymphocytes subsets in transplanted mycobacterial granuloma. *Eur J Microbiol Immunol.* 2011;1(1):59–69.
65. Trentin L, Zambello R, Facco M, et al. Selection of T lymphocytes bearing limited TCR-V beta regions in the lung of hypersensitivity pneumonitis and sarcoidosis. *Am J Respir Crit Care Med.* 1997;155(2):587–596.
66. Taflin C, Miyara M, Nochy D, et al. FoxP3+ regulatory T cells suppress early stages of granuloma formation but have little impact on sarcoidosis lesions. *Am J Pathol.* 2009;174(2):497–508.
67. Agostini C, Perin A, Semenzato G. Cell apoptosis and granulomatous lung diseases. *Curr Opin Pulm Med.* 1998;4(5):261–266.
68. Xaus J, Besalduch N, Comalada M, et al. High expression of p21 Waf1 in sarcoid granulomas: a putative role for long-lasting inflammation. *J Leukoc Biol.* 2003;74(2):295–301.
69. Bulfone-Paus S, Ungureanu D, Pohl T, et al. Interleukin-15 protects from lethal apoptosis in vivo. *Nat Med.* 1997;3(10):1124–1128.
70. Marshall BG, Wangoo A, Cook HT, Shaw RJ. Increased inflammatory cytokines and new collagen formation in cutaneous tuberculosis and sarcoidosis. *Thorax.* 1996;51(12):1253–1261.
71. Shamaei M, Mortaz E, Pourabdollah M, et al. Evidence for M2 macrophages in granulomas from pulmonary sarcoidosis: a new aspect of macrophage heterogeneity. *Hum Immunol.* 2018;79(1):63–69.
72. Preusse C, Goebel H-H, Pehl D, et al. Th2-M2 immunity in lesions of muscular sarcoidosis and macrophagic myofasciitis. *Neuropathol Appl Neurobiol.* 2015;41(7):952–963.
73. Prasse A, Pechkovsky DV, Toews GB, et al. A vicious circle of alveolar macrophages and fibroblasts perpetuates pulmonary fibrosis via CCL18. *Am J Respir Crit Care Med.* 2006;173(7):781–792.
74. Chen ES. Innate immunity in sarcoidosis pathobiology. *Curr Opin Pulm Med.* 2016;22(5):469–475.
75. Silverstein E, Pertschuk LP, Friedland J. Immunofluorescent localization of angiotensin converting enzyme in epithelioid and giant cells of sarcoidosis granulomas. *Proc Natl Acad Sci USA.* 1979;76(12):6646–6648.
76. Kamphuis LS, Bonte-Mineur F, van LJA, van HPM, van DPL. Calcium and vitamin D in sarcoidosis: is supplementation safe? *J Bone Miner Res Off J Am Soc Bone Miner Res.* 2014;29(11):2498–2503.
77. Kubota R, Yamada S, Kubota K, Ishiwata K, Tamahashi N, Ido T. Intratumoral distribution of fluorine-18-fluorodeoxyglucose in vivo: high accumulation in macrophages and granulation tissues studied by microautoradiography. *J Nucl Med Off Publ Soc Nucl Med.* 1992;33(11):1972–1980.
78. Brewer S, Mc Pherson M, Fujiwara D, et al. Molecular imaging of Murine intestinal inflammation with 2-deoxy-2-[18F]Fluoro-D-glucose and positron emission tomography. *Gastroenterology.* 2008;135(3):744–755.
79. Jeny F, Pacheco Y, Besnard V, Valeyre D, Bernaudin J-F. Experimental models of sarcoidosis. *Curr Opin Pulm Med.* 2016;22(5):492–499.
80. Linke M, Pham HTT, Katholnig K, et al. Chronic signaling via the metabolic checkpoint kinase mTORC1 induces macrophage granuloma formation and marks sarcoidosis progression. *Nat Immunol.* 2017;18(3):293–302.

CHAPTER 7

Baughman's Sarcoidosis: Diagnosis

JONAS YSERBYT, MD, PHD • WIM WUYTS, MD, PHD

INTRODUCTION

Sarcoidosis is a systemic disease of unknown cause, pathophysiologically determined by granulomatous inflammation.[1] Diagnosis can be challenging as a result of variable clinical presentations both by location of the disease and by the presence of nonspecific symptomatology. In the coexistence of compatible clinical, radiological, and histopathologic features located in at least two different organs, the diagnosis can be made with high confidence. Whenever one or more of these elements are lacking, diagnostic confidence is reduced,[2] and clinical decision-making should be weighed against the potential therapeutic implications (or risk without treatment). How those four elements (clinics, radiology, histopathology, and therapeutic implications) are tiled together in the sarcoidosis jigsaw is the subject of this chapter.

GENERAL PRINCIPLES

As a potential multiorgan disease, sarcoidosis is considered to be a kaleidoscope of clinical presentations. There exists no single specific diagnostic test for sarcoidosis. A diagnosis of sarcoidosis is made in those cases in which a clinicoradiological pattern consistent with sarcoidosis is endorsed by the histopathological detection of dense, mostly noncaseating, giant cell granulomas in the absence of any evidence of another granulomatous disease.

A diagnosis of sarcoidosis is therefore a pure clinical diagnosis per *exclusionem*, and as a result, clinicians should be aware of the fact that this kind of diagnosis is potentially fallible. After all, clinical signs, radiology, or histopathology can be compatible with sarcoidosis but lack the ability to make a confident diagnosis on their own, with the exception of clear clinical presentations that are specific for sarcoidosis, such as Löfgren and Heerfordt syndromes or when multiple organs are involved in a typical manner.[3] Pathognomonic clinical characteristics or highly specific diagnostic tests are lacking, resulting in both missed diagnoses and, often unfairly less highlighted, overdiagnosis.

As a result, the clinical diagnosis of sarcoidosis is not an end point and should be put into question during the clinical evolution of the specific patient and eventually confirmed or contested. Moreover, aspecific symptoms in a patient once diagnosed with sarcoidosis should never be blindly attributed to this former diagnosis that is often made in a different time period by a different physician. Therefore the clinical firmness of such a former diagnosis should always be rechallenged.[4]

The levels of confidence in diagnosing sarcoidosis are shown in Table 7.1.

The presence of noncaseating granulomas in a single location is not specific for sarcoidosis and therefore does

TABLE 7.1
Diagnostic Levels of Confidence in Sarcoidosis

Diagnostic Level of Confidence	
Highly probable	Clinical presentation consistent with sarcoidosis, two or more organ systems involved, noncaseating granuloma on histopathological specimen obtained from presenting/symptomatic organ.
Probable	Clinical presentation consistent with sarcoidosis, noncaseating granuloma on histopathological specimen obtained from asymptomatic organ.
Possible	Clinical presentation suggestive for sarcoidosis without identification of an alternative diagnosis, histopathological specimen unobtainable/not obtained.
Unlikely	Clinical presentation suggestive for sarcoidosis, histopathological examination incompatible/absent, and/or alternative diagnosis is made.

Adapted from Govender P, Berman JS. *The Diagnosis of Sarcoidosis*. Clin Chest Med 2015;36:585–602.

Sarcoidosis. https://doi.org/10.1016/B978-0-323-54429-0.00007-0

not guarantee a firm diagnosis of sarcoidosis.[5] Moreover, cases in which only radiological or histopathological suspicion of sarcoidosis is raised without any clinical sign of the disease would be best addressed as "sarcoid-like," not only to withhold an uncertain diagnosis with little or no prognostic importance for the patient but also to clear up epidemiological data on sarcoidosis, which is now often clouded by the mix of both overt clinical sarcoidosis and case presentations that lack clinical relevance. This is not a pure semantic discussion because clinical trials of any kind addressing no matter which characteristic of the disease should also avoid this mix-up of entities with clearly distinct clinical and biological behavior.

Some argue that the term idiopathic sarcoidosis should be introduced to discriminate the textbook, classic clinical picture of sarcoidosis from sarcoid-like reactions to, for example, malignancy or pharmacological treatment of any kind (e.g., chemotherapy, antitumor necrosis factor [anti-TNF]).[6]

In general, the diagnostic process of sarcoidosis comes down to a distinct clinico-radiological pattern, the histopathological confirmation of the presence of granulomas compatible with sarcoidosis, the evaluation of the extent and organ involvement, and the evaluation of the likelihood of disease progression.

DIFFERENTIAL DIAGNOSIS

As a result of the abovementioned clinical craftsmanship that is required to correctly diagnose sarcoidosis, other potential confounding disease entities should be carefully considered throughout the diagnostic process.

Several granulomatous infectious diseases of the respiratory tract may present in a clinical and radiological pattern similar to sarcoidosis, e.g., tuberculosis, nontuberculous mycobacteriosis, and fungal granuloma (Cryptococcus, Coccidioides, Histoplasma).[7] The importance of these entities is highly dependent on the regional prevalence of these infections, and this becomes even more relevant when considering immunosuppressive treatment regimens.

Noninfectious, environmental exposure might lead to the accumulation of granulomatous disease of the respiratory tract. The most iconic example of which is berylliosis, a delayed hypersensitivity reaction as a result of sensitization to beryllium, first described in 1946 in a fluorescent lamp manufacture and in recent times related to aerospace, ceramics, and metallurgical industries.[8] There is some evidence that granulomatous lung disease might be related to (professional) exposure to other metallic agents (e.g., zirconium, aluminum, chrome, cobalt),[9] as well as to silica and inorganic dust,[10] highlighting the important role of occupational history in any patient with suspicion of sarcoidosis.

Granulomatous-lymphocytic interstitial lung disease (GLILD) can be seen in a subset of patients with common variable immunodeficiency. Among follicular bronchiolitis and lymphocytic interstitial pneumonia, sarcoid-like granulomatous lesions can be found on histopathology. GLILD is potentially multisystemic and might therefore mimic the clinical presentation of sarcoidosis.

Extrathoracic granulomatous lung disease such as Crohn's disease can rarely lead to pulmonary granulomatous lesions, which are histopathologically hard to distinguish from sarcoidosis.

Drug-induced sarcoid-like reactions have been associated with the use of anti-TNF treatment (class effect seen with infliximab, etanercept, adalimumab), methotrexate, leflunomide, 5-aminosalicylate derivates, interferon, and sirolimus.[7] More recently, immune checkpoint inhibitor therapy has been associated with both the apparition of sarcoid-like lesions and the aggravation of preexistent sarcoidosis. Although these adverse events have originally been described with ipilimumab and nivolumab in the treatment of metastatic melanoma, reports in other solid tumors and hematologic malignancies as well as similar observations with pembrolizumab suggest a class effect.[11]

SYMPTOMATOLOGY

When considering a clinical diagnosis of sarcoidosis in general, large epidemiological surveys have shown that almost half of the cases refer to asymptomatic patients in whom granulomatous inflammation has been detected in an incidental manner. Most often, these cases result from the fortuitous finding of enlarged hilar/mediastinal lymph nodes in the workup of a different medical problem or the biopsy of a solitary localized asymptomatic skin lesion (e.g., scar granulomatosis).

When symptomatic, common signs include fever, dyspnea, cough, arthralgia, eye symptoms, and skin eruptions. In up to 70% of patients fatigue is prominent and might even be the most decapacitating symptom in many patients.[12]

Two distinct clinical presentations are Löfgren syndrome (ankle arthritis, erythema nodosum, and bilateral hilar lymphadenopathy) and Heerfordt syndrome (protracted fever, parotitis, uveitis, and facial nerve palsy).

Beside the classic clinical signs, patients with sarcoidosis often present with more nonspecific symptoms. These signs are often referred to as autonomous dysfunction and are related to small fiber neuropathy,[13,14] a pathophysiological pathway that has gained recent interest among both researchers and clinicians. Another pathway to evaluate whenever aspecific symptoms are increasing in a patient with sarcoidosis is the calcium metabolism. Hypercalcemia is estimated to occur in about 4% of all cases[15] and might result in fatigue, asthenia, depression, digestive upset, nausea and vomiting, and diffuse pain.

The modern clinical approach to systemic diseases is multidisciplinary. The assessment of patients with sarcoidosis therefore combines the expertise of pulmonary physicians, cardiologists, dermatologists, ophthalmologists, rheumatologists, and neurologists. The organ systems that are most often affected include the respiratory tract (95% of cases), skin (16%), lymph nodes (15%), eye (12%), and liver.[15] Although arthralgia and myalgia are frequent symptoms, granulomatous inflammation of bones, joints, or muscles is estimated to occur in less than 1% of patients. Although potentially life-threatening, neurosarcoidosis and cardiac sarcoidosis are rare, with estimates ranging 3%–5% and 2%–15%, respectively. The considerable variation in the prevalence of cardiac sarcoidosis is related to the methodology of epidemiological evidence (case-control vs. autopsy studies) and the specific population (high interest in cardiac sarcoidosis and higher prevalence in Japan). A practically useful overview of organ systems with their respective symptomatology is provided by the World Association of Sarcoidosis and Other Granulomatous diseases.[16]

As in every diagnostic process, pretest probability should be taken into account when assessing the overall diagnostic yield of a diagnostic approach to sarcoidosis. Several epidemiological factors may increase or decrease the likelihood of a clinical diagnosis of sarcoidosis in a specific context, for example, age, ethnicity, smoking status, familial precedents, and occupational exposure. For example, the clinical likelihood of sarcoidosis is decreased in patients aged under 18 years or in male patients older than 50 years,[17] as well as in current smokers.[18] The diagnostic likelihood is increased in Afro-Americans[19] and northern Europeans,[20] as well as in first- and second-degree members of patients.[21] A confounder in the diagnostic process is the exposure to silica[22] and beryllium[23] because this may lead to clinical presentations that mimic sarcoidosis; exposure to antigens causing hypersensitivity pneumonitis should encourage to look for an alternative diagnosis.

SEROLOGY

No stand-alone biomarker exists to date that is clinically validated to offer sufficient diagnostic accuracy in the diagnosis of sarcoidosis. Inflammatory changes can evidently be seen in the serum of the patient, although serologic inflammation is often absent or only marginally present in patients with sarcoidosis. Hypergammaglobulinemia can be seen; a decrease in gammaglobulin dosage is atypical for sarcoidosis.

The use of serum angiotensin-converting enzyme (SACE) has been propagated for three decennia as a marker of total body granuloma activity,[24] but it has no value as a stand-alone diagnostic tool or as a marker for disease activity in sarcoidosis.[25] The lack of diagnostic power of SACE is in part attributable to the existence of polymorphisms of the angiotensin-converting enzyme gene, not only influencing SACE titers but also leading to important differences between ethnicities, theoretically necessitating corrected reference values.[26] Nevertheless, an SACE increase of greater than 2 times the upper limit of normal is rarely seen in other diseases.[27] The largest survey on the diagnostic value of SACE included nearly 2000 patients with sarcoidosis, a control group of healthy subjects, and a large group of patients with other diseases. The sensitivity of SACE for the diagnosis of sarcoidosis was 57%, the specificity was 90%, positive predictive value was 90%, and negative predictive value was 60%.[28]

A case-control study on 430 sarcoidosis patients and 264 healthy controls calculated sensitivity and specificity of SACE (upper limit of normal 32.0 U/L) at 66% and 54%, respectively.[29] The authors reported no correlation between SACE and fludeoxyglucose (FDG) avidity in a subset of patients. The same paper propagates the use of serum chitotriosidase, a serum marker of macrophage activation,[30,31] as a diagnostic marker of sarcoidosis with a sensitivity of 83% and a specificity of 74% (upper limit of normal 100 nmol/mL/h) and with the advantage over SACE that it is correlated with chest X-ray (CXR) abnormalities and FDG uptake on positron emission tomography (PET) scan, as well as with disease duration.

Other biomarkers have shown promising results, but currently available data are not yet robust enough to suggest their use routinely. Serum soluble interleukin two receptor (sIL-2R) and sIL-2R in bronchoalveolar lavage (BAL) fluid, both originating from activated T-lymphocytes, have been shown to correlate with various indices of disease severity and might be a marker for extrapulmonary disease activity.[32,33] A recent cross-sectional study in cases of uveitis showed that using a cutoff value of 4000 pg/mL, sIL-2R had a sensitivity of 81% and a specificity of 64%. There was no significant correlation between sIL-2R and activity of the uveitis.[34] Neopterin, a marker for the activation of the monocyte/

macrophage system, has been shown to be increased in serum and in breath condensate of patients with sarcoidosis.[35,36] Serum adenosine deaminase and serum amyloid A protein both showed promising diagnostic accuracy in a case-control setting.[37]

Recently, omics and system biology have been applied in the field of sarcoidosis to characterize a disease-specific and/or phenotype-specific "fingerprint." The aim of such approach is not to identify a single specific biomarker for sarcoidosis but to characterize groups of proteins/nucleotides/mediators as potential targets for further research. Micro-RNAs, proteins related to transdermal growth factor beta pathway, tumor necrosis factor (TNF) alpha, and vitamin D might be able to work out different clinical phenotypes in sarcoidosis.[38,39] The potential use of miRNA as a fingerprint for the diagnosis of sarcoidosis has been highlighted in a recent paper from the a case control etiologic study of sarcoidosis (ACCESS) research group. In addition, the authors stress the future use of miRNA subtyping in the prediction of clinical outcome.[40]

IMAGING

From a historical point of view, the diagnostic use of plain CXR for the diagnosis and radiological staging of sarcoidosis is well established since the introduction of the Scadding stages in 1961. Bilateral hilar lymphadenopathy on CXR in the appropriate clinical setting is highly specific for the diagnosis of sarcoidosis.[41] The radiological staging based on CXR has even prognostic implications although with considerable variability.[42] Although the radiographic stages of sarcoidosis have their merit and are often referred to in a clinical context, the change in disease extent over time scored on CXR is more sensitive than change in stage and is the most appropriate way for the radiological assessment of the evolution in pulmonary sarcoidosis.[43]

The most commonly observed abnormalities on high-resolution computerized tomography (HRCT) consist of enlarged mediastinal lymph nodes and nodular abnormalities at the level of the lung parenchyma. The latter reflecting the histopathological characteristics of pulmonary sarcoidosis, granular inflammatory lesions with a bronchovascular/perilymphatic, and interstitial distribution. These nodules might be dispersed in early phases of the disease but can coalesce over time to form larger lesions, at which moment peribronchial fibrosis may occur.

The additional value of chest computed tomography (CT) scan is undeniable from a morphologic point of view—increased detection rate of more subtle parenchymal and mediastinal abnormalities. CT features in combination with composite physiological index have been successfully used to indicate prognosis.[44] Nevertheless, the prognostic and therapeutic guidance provided by chest CT is still questionable, making sarcoidosis one of few pulmonary diseases in which CXR still has a considerable clinical value.

Several papers report on the correlation between CT findings and other clinical factors used to mirror disease activity.[45] In general, pulmonary function data and radiological patterns might be surprisingly discordant in a substantial number of cases. A recent report found that force vital capacity (FVC) and total lung capacity (TLC) were inversely correlated with consolidation and ground-glass opacity CT scores (two radiological patterns that are less often seen in sarcoidosis), but not with semiquantitative scores for micronodules and macronodules.[46] The same authors state that a relative decrease in lymphocyte count on BAL together with an increase in BAL neutrophil number is associated with an increased radiographic stage of sarcoidosis.

The value of serial HRCT in the follow-up of patients and the assessment of disease progression has been studied.[47] This report in 73 cases of sarcoidosis shows that there is moderate agreement between change in FVC and TLC and change in disease extent on HRCT. The same agreement was not found for change in diffusion capacity of carbon monoxide (DLCO) and HRCT, concluding that a morphological correlate of change in gas transfer cannot be reproduced on HRCT. As a result of these findings, the use of HRCT abnormalities and current scoring methodology is unlikely to add any clinical value in the long-term follow-up of disease activity in pulmonary sarcoidosis and is therefore not proposed as a routine clinical procedure. This being said, HRCT does have a pivotal role in the diagnosis of alternative causes of progressive pulmonary symptoms in a patient in whom the diagnosis of sarcoidosis has been previously established.

Another emerging imaging modality in daily clinical practice is FDG-PET. FDG-PET has shown to have a high sensitivity for the detection of inflammation in sarcoidosis both inside and outside the chest cavity.[48] FDG-PET is able to highlight sites of inflammation that are concealed from so-called best-practice clinical assessment.[49] However, the true added value of FDG-PET in a clinical setting, beyond the world of scientific reports and clinical trials, seems to be disappointing. First of all, the indication of FDG-PET in sarcoidosis is unclear. As shown by a retrospective cohort study, the additional value of PET is negligible in those cases in which the clinical probability of active inflammation is high, e.g., based on clinical, radiological, and serological markers.[50] There could be a potential role for PET in those patients with persistent nonorganic disabling symptoms but without clinical, serological, or radiological abnormalities suggestive for active inflammation within the clinical routine. Unlike the "binary" outcome of PET in oncology (presence/absence of FDG uptake) with the primary tumor as point of reference, FDG uptake in inflammatory conditions should preferably be assessed on a scale, ideally reflecting inflammation activity. Unfortunately, FDG uptake quantification is hard to standardize and to reproduce. In addition, robust data are lacking to advocate the use of PET in the clinical assessment of treatment response. The change in FDG uptake as a marker for treatment response has been evaluated in several papers, but findings are inconsistent. A retrospective cohort, in which only a minority of patients had repeated FDG-PET during treatment, showed a potential role of FDG-PET in monitoring treatment response.[49] Another trial used FGD-PET to assess the effect of anti-TNF treatment[51] and found that the increased mediastinal standardized uptake value (SUV) at initiation of therapy predicted response but also that PET was not able to produce consistent findings during the course of treatment. The same authors used FDG-PET for the selection of patients for a trial with infliximab and showed that maximum SUV levels of pulmonary parenchyma decreased during treatment.[52] Somewhat contradictory to the clinical observation that steroid treatment lacks efficacy in stage IV sarcoidosis, patients with fibrotic lung disease show increased FDG uptake in a majority of cases.[53] Moreover, cost and radiation exposure in case of repeated scanning should be taken into consideration. The CT scan provided in combined PET/CT procedures lacks resolution and is often obtained in incomplete inspiration. As a result, HRCTs are often performed in addition to PET/CT scans to obtain qualitative morphological data, often considered to provide additional clinical information in comparison to PET/CT.[54]

In conclusion, no clinically relevant conclusions about the use of FDG-PET can be drawn from the evidence that is provided in small selected cohorts of patients with an often retrospective data collection. Although several papers tried to demonstrate the value of PET in the evaluation of disease extent and activity in sarcoidosis,[52,53,55] PET remains in the domain of preclinical study and adds no fundamental benefit in patient management.[56]

ENDOSCOPIC DIAGNOSTICS

Bronchoalveolar Lavage

From a global perspective, the diagnostic usefulness of BAL in the diagnosis of ILD is not generally accepted and uniformity concerning its application within different guidelines is lacking.[57] Nevertheless, from a local point of view, BAL is an indispensable piece of the diagnostic workup, not as a result of its explicit accuracy in detecting single specific pathologies, but as a guidance within the differential diagnosis. In sarcoidosis, the use of BAL is able to significantly increase the diagnostic likelihood (from 34% to 68%) when lymphocyte counts are between 30% and 50% and granulocyte counts are low. On the other hand, the likelihood for usual interstitial pneumonia increases from 16% to 33% when lymphocyte counts are below 30%, and the number of BAL granulocytes is increased.[58] To a lesser extent, these findings have recently been corroborated.[59] There might be a diagnostic value of CD4/CD8 in the diagnosis of sarcoidosis, although sensitivity and specificity are depending on the proposed cutoff values.[57,60] It is generally accepted that a CD4/CD8 ratio > 3.5 is highly specific for sarcoidosis in the absence of an increased proportion of other inflammatory cell types. In other words, BAL lymphocytosis is sensitive for sarcoidosis, whereas CD4/CD8 ratio, although highly variable,[61] has a high specificity for sarcoidosis.[58,62,63]

Because BAL lymphocytosis reflects the intensity of the Th1 response in sarcoidosis, the BAL profile may vary with time and corresponding inflammatory activity. Unfortunately, lymphocyte counts show a considerable degree of variability and are therefore not validated to assess disease activity or monitor treatment response in clinical practice.[64]

Although the specificity of BAL cellular analysis is insufficient to diagnose sarcoidosis as a stand-alone tool, it is a piece of the sarcoidosis jigsaw and may well support the diagnosis when considered in the clinical and radiographic context.[65] The BAL pattern that is most often described as compatible with sarcoidosis shows a normal/mildly elevated total cell count with a predominance of lymphocytes, a normal percentage of eosinophils and neutrophils, and the lack of plasma cells and "foamy" alveolar macrophages.[62,64]

Several papers have described the use of BAL analysis to discriminate sarcoidosis from sarcoid-like pathologies such as pulmonary lymphoma[66] and environmental exposure (foreign bodies, bi-refringent material, inclusion bodies in alveolar macrophages).[10,67]

Needless to say that these recommendations are valid in case the BAL was obtained through high-quality sampling. The latter includes the thorough selection of

TABLE 7.2
Diagnostic Yield of Endoscopic Techniques in Detecting Granulomatous Inflammation

	DIAGNOSTIC YIELD OF ENDOSCOPIC TECHNIQUES				
			DIAGNOSTIC YIELD (%)		
Technique	**Number of Studies**	**Total Number of Patients Included**	**Median**	**Minimal**	**Maximal**
EBB	10	1378	30	5	80
TBLB	12	1256	45	30	78
EBB + TBLB	6	673	54	33	81
TBNA	7	275	61	22	83
EBUS-TBNA	16	1823	80	57	96
EBB + TBLBL + TBNA	2	123	87	86	93
EBB + TBLB + EBUS + EBUS-TBNA	5	475	92	86	100

Median, minimal, and maximal values for a mix of randomized and nonrandomized, retro and prospective trials are provided in the table. *EBB*, endobronchial biopsy; *EBUS*, endobronchial ultrasound; *TBLB*, transbronchial lung biopsy; *TBNA*, conventional transbronchial needle aspiration.

Data from Hu L, Chen R, Huang H, Shao C, Wang P, Liu Y, et al. Endobronchial ultrasound-guided transbronchial needle aspiration versus standard bronchoscopic modalities for diagnosis of sarcoidosis: a meta-analysis. Chin Med J 2016;129(13):1607–1615.

the target area based on a recent chest CT,[68,69] a wedged position of the bronchoscope, the use of 100–300 mL of saline solution divided into three to five aliquots,[65] and the recovery of at least 30% of the instilled volume with an optimal volume exceeding 20 mL. Cell analysis itself is best performed after cytocentrifugation (filtration might underestimate the proportion of neutrophils), staining, and manual enumeration. Manual counting or flow cytometry are preferred over automated cell counting/cell sorting (cytospin) in case of inflammatory conditions[70] because automated cell counting might overestimate the proportion of neutrophils.[71] It is established that active smoking status blurs BAL analysis.[72]

Diagnostic Yield of Bronchoscopic Techniques

Several endoscopic procedures can be indicated, separately or in combination, to obtain cytology and/or histopathology and detect granulomas, each with their individual diagnostic yield. Several papers have been published, either retrospective, prospective, and/or randomized, reporting a wide range in diagnostic yields. A recent meta-analysis on a total of 1823 cases from different reports with a variety in methodology[73] reports a median diagnostic yield of 30% for endobronchial biopsy (EBB) (range 5%–80%), 45% for transbronchial lung biopsy (TBLB) (range 30%–78%), 61% for conventional transbronchial needle aspiration (TBNA) (range 22%–83%), and 80% for endobronchial ultrasound (EBUS)-guided TBNA (EBUS-TBNA) (range 57%–96%) (Table 7.2).

The wide spread diagnostic yield among reports is attributable to a certain degree of selection in both enrolled patients and different technical aspects of the procedure. Previous data have shown that the diagnostic yield of TBLB increases when four to five biopsies are taken.[74] EBB obtained from macroscopically normal mucosa has a lower likelihood of showing granulomas than a biopsy of nodular or inflamed mucosa.[75] The same is true for TBLB in regard to the presence/absence of parenchymal abnormalities on HRCT and their specific location.

Combined endoscopic procedures result in higher diagnostic yield than the procedures performed separately, with a reported median diagnostic yield of TBLB combined to EBB of 54% (range, 33%–81%), reaching 92% (range, 86%–100%) for the combination of TBLB, EBB, and EBUS-TBNA.

The to-date largest randomized trial on endosonography in 304 cases of sarcoidosis[70] reports a diagnostic yield to detect granulomas of 80% (95% confidence interval [CI], 73%–86%) when EBUS or endoscopic ultrasound fine needle aspiration (EUS-FNA) is performed and of 53% (95% CI, 45%–61%) for standard bronchoscopy (EBB, TBLB, or EBB and TBLB in the same procedure).

Nevertheless, Hu et al.[73] reported an odds ratio for the combination of EBB, TBLB, and EBUS-TBNA of 0.55 (95% CI, 0.39–0.78) in favor of the combination of these endoscopic modalities, indicating that even in the EBUS-TBNA era, conventional forceps biopsies still have an additional value in the bronchoscopic diagnosis of sarcoidosis. A report on 36 patients with sarcoidosis, selected from a retrospective cohort, shows that transbronchial lung cryobiopsy may also have an additional benefit over EBUS-TBNA at the expense of a pneumothorax rate of 11%.[76]

A recent randomized trial from Poland[77] focused more in extent on the combined approach of bronchoscopic forceps biopsies and endosonography. The study design included randomization to EBUS or EUS in a cross-over design whenever the first endosonographic procedure (EBUS or EUS) did not detect lymph node granulomas. Only if both EBUS and/or EUS were negative, mediastinoscopy was performed (4% of cases). This survey shows that the sensitivity of EUS is better than that of EBUS for detecting nodal granulomas. Moreover, the combination of both EUS and EBUS reaches highest diagnostic yield, opening the way for a combined bronchoscopic approach of forceps biopsies, EBUS and EUS-b (performing nodal sampling through the airways and down the esophagus with one and the same echo-endoscope).

Based on the aforementioned findings, the scope of endoscopic diagnostics in sarcoidosis had broadened, and therefore, mediastinoscopy should be avoided as a first-line diagnostic tool for the detection of mediastinal granulomatous lymphadenitis in sarcoidosis because of its invasive nature with a substantial risk of (post-)operative complications.

HISTOPATHOLOGY

The histologic or cytological detection of granulomatous disease as such is not specific for sarcoidosis. Undoubtedly, histopathology is able to enhance the likelihood of a diagnosis of sarcoidosis in a suggestive clinical and radiological presentation. But when granulomatous inflammation is detected, the possibility of alternative causes of granulomatosis should at least be considered. Nevertheless, microscopic examination might be able to discriminate between distinct types of granulomas that may be highly suspicious of sarcoidosis and other types of granulomas that are more specific for other respiratory conditions, e.g., hypersensitivity pneumonitis and granulomatosis with polyangiitis. Although the scope of histopathological findings in sarcoidosis is broad, sarcoid granulomas are multiple, well formed, and, in essence, nonnecrotizing. Therefore, it is commonly stated that the presence of caseating granulomas is incompatible with a diagnosis of sarcoidosis and as such necessitates the need to exclude infectious disease. Nevertheless, one should be aware of the exceptional existence of focal central coagulative necrosis in sarcoid granulomas (see Chapter "Pathology of granuloma"). Sarcoid granulomas show compact clusters of epitheloid and multinucleated histiocytes with frequent inclusion bodies, and they are surrounded by a crown of lymphocytes. In sarcoidosis these granulomas show a bronchovascular distribution.[78]

The above scribed endoscopic procedures will often be applied in cases of suspected sarcoidosis to obtain cytological or histological material for histopathological diagnosis. Evidently, more easily accessible location such as skin lesions or peripheral lymph nodes can provide a histopathological diagnosis in a less invasive manner, when applicable.[79] For isolated parenchymal lung lesions or subpleural lesions, CT guided needle biopsy can be a well-tolerated technique with low procedural risk. When biopsies cannot be obtained with a minimally invasive procedure at easily accessible sites, surgical biopsies such as video-assisted thoracic surgery (VATS) lung biopsy or mediastinoscopy may be unavoidable. In general, it is not recommended to obtain liver biopsy for the diagnosis of sarcoidosis because of the lack of specificity since there is a wide array of histological findings potentially compatible with other primary liver diseases on the one hand,[80] and hepatic granulomas may be an incidental finding on the other hand.[81] It makes no sense to biopsy clearly defined erythema nodosum because these lesions do not contain granulomatous inflammation.

Histopathological confirmation of a clinicoradiological suspicion of sarcoidosis is warranted in most cases with the exception of clearly defined clinical presentations (Heerfordt and Löfgren syndromes, asymptomatic bilateral hilar adenopathy on CXR, Lamda-Panda sign).[4] In cases in which sarcoidosis is clinically suspected and it is clear that therapeutic consequences are completely lacking, histopathological sampling can be renounced. However, this implies that a thorough search has been performed to identify potential systemic disease, and this does not dismiss the clinician from a certain degree of follow-up because cases judged to be limited at diagnosis might progress over time and might evolve toward more severe disease in which treatment strategies become necessary and at which point histopathology is yet relevant. In clinical practice, these limited presentations of sarcoidosis almost always concern cases of asymptomatic patients in whom the radiological discovery enlarged bilateral hilar with or without and/or mediastinal lymph nodes is mere incidental.[82] On the other hand, in case any atypical lesion is observed either clinically (e.g., skin) or on imaging (e.g., irregular or spicular lung nodules), a guided biopsy should be considered to rule out synchronous oncological diseases.

A mere clinical diagnosis of sarcoidosis in cases in which histopathology is unable to provide confirmation should be avoided in patients whose clinical picture is predominantly characterized by fatigue or nonspecific symptoms of generalized pain. To avoid a downward spiral of self-confirming fatigue and physical deconditioning, alternative reasons for patient symptoms should be excluded. In such cases, in which no consistent medical diagnosis can be made and clinical, radiological, and histopathological elements offer no or only a limited confidence for a diagnosis of sarcoidosis, the focus should be on reconditioning and psychosocial rehabilitation, more than on an incomplete or even mystifying diagnosis of alleged sarcoidosis. Such a low confidence diagnosis offers patients insecurity and may propagate an endless diagnostic process to prove a diagnosis that cannot be proven. The energy of patients and medical staff will be absorbed by such a futile diagnostic process, evading the defying challenge of taking the future in hand and working hard on physical and psychosocial rehabilitation, the latter often being a winding road of trial and error.

GLOBAL PATIENT ASSESSMENT

Once a diagnosis of sarcoidosis is established with significant confidence, a systemic diagnostic workup should be performed aiming at a screening for asymptomatic systemic disease and assessing functionality.

The extent to which asymptomatic systemic disease has to be investigated is unknown. In general, peripheral blood counts and blood chemistry (calcium, liver enzymes, creatinine, BUN), urine analysis, spirometry, electrocardiography, and ophthalmologic examination are the essential diagnostic tests for any case of sarcoidosis. The indication of any additional testing should be guided by clinical assessment, e.g., transthoracic ultrasonography of the heart can be helpful in many cases because it can assess the presence of pulmonary hypertension or cardiac dysfunction, both important prognostic parameters. Whenever neurological symptoms appear, thorough clinical neurological assessment with or without brain imaging and cerebrospinal fluid analysis should be performed. The cost-effectiveness of a broader and more thorough screening for asymptomatic multiorgan disease is questionable, and scientific data are lacking. This kind of deeper search is prone to result in fortuitous findings, most often without any therapeutic implication.

Pulmonary function testing is the cornerstone of the functional assessment in pulmonary sarcoidosis. The typical finding is a restrictive pattern, whereas an obstructive pattern is seen in up to 30% of patients, and bronchial hyperreactivity is present in 25%. Pulmonary function testing should be performed in any case of sarcoidosis at the initiation of follow-up. When respiratory symptoms develop or increase during follow-up, the decline in FVC and/or DLCO can guide therapeutic decisions. Changes in gas exchange with exercise are more sensitive than lung function tests at rest and should be performed whenever there is an incongruity between increased respiratory symptoms and decline in exercise tolerance on the one hand and radiological and lung functional abnormalities on the other hand. Exercise testing may also be performed to assess the global fitness of the patient, to address the problem of chronic fatigue, and to guide functional rehabilitation.

REFERENCES

1. Judson MA, Thompson BW, Rabin DL, et al. The diagnostic pathway to sarcoidosis. *Chest.* 2003;123:406–412.
2. Judson MA, Baughman RP, Teirstein AS, Terrin ML, Yeager Jr H. Defining organ involvement in sarcoidosis: the ACCESS proposed instrument. ACCESS Research Group. A case control etiologic study of sarcoidosis. *Sarcoidosis Vasc Diffuse Lung Dis.* 1999;16:75–86.
3. Baughman RP, Culver DA, Judson MA. A concise review of pulmonary sarcoidosis. *Am J Respir Crit Care Med.* 2011;183:573–581.
4. Govender P, Berman JS. The diagnosis of sarcoidosis. *Clin Chest Med.* 2015;36:585–602.
5. Costabel U, Guzman J, Drent M. Diagnostic approach to sarcoidosis. *Eur Respir Monogr.* 2005;32:259–264.
6. Leqouy M. Sarcoidosis lung nodules in colorectal cancer follow-up: sarcoidosis or not? *Am J Med.* 2013;126:642–645.
7. Ohshimo S, Guzman J, Costabel U, Fl B. Differential diagnosis of granulomatous lung disease: clues and pitfalls. *Eur Respir Rev.* 2017;26:170012.
8. Newman KL, Newman LS. Occupational causes of sarcoidosis. *Curr Opin Allergy Clin Immunol.* 2012;12(2):145–150.
9. Fireman E, Shai AB, Alcalay Y, Ophir N, Kivity S, Stejskal V. Identification of metal sensitization in sarcoid-like metal-exposed patients by the MELISA® lymphocyte proliferation test - a pilot study. *J Occup Med Toxicol.* 2016;11:18.
10. Drent M, Bomans PH, Van Suylen RJ, Lamers RJ, Bast A, Wouters EF. Association of man-made mineral fibre exposure and sarcoid like granulomas. *Respir Med.* 2000;94(8):815–820.

11. Chopra A, Nautiyal A, Kalkanis A, Judson MA. Drug-induced sarcoidosis-like reactions. *Chest*. 2018. https://doi.org/10.1016/j.chest.2018.03.056. [Epub ahead of print].
12. Valeyre D, Prasse A, Nunes H, Uzunhan Y, Brillet PY, Müller-Quernheim J. Sarcoidosis. *Lancet*. 2014;383:1155-1167.
13. Parambil JG, Tavee JO, Zhou L, Pearson K, Culver DA. Efficacy of intravenous immunoglobulin for small fiber neuropathy associated with sarcoidosis. *Respir Med*. 2010;105:101-105.
14. Tavee J, Culver D. Sarcoidosis and small-fiber neuropathy. *Curr Pain Headache Rep*. 2011;15(3):201-206.
15. Baughman RP, Teirstein AS, Judson MA, et al. Clinical characteristics of patients in a case control study of sarcoidosis. *Am J Respir Crit Care Med*. 2001;164(10):1886.
16. Judson MA, Costabel U, Drent M, et al. The WASOG sarcoidosis organ assessment instrument: an update of a previous clinical tool. *Sarcoidosis Vasc Diffuse Lung Dis*. 2014;31(1):19-27.
17. Iannuzzi MC, Rybicki BA, Teirstein AS. Sarcoidosis. *N Engl J Med*. 2007;357:2153-2165.
18. Valeyre D, Soler P, Clerici C, et al. Smoking and pulmonary sarcoidosis: effect of cigarette smoking on prevalence, clinical manifestations, alveolitis, and evolution of the disease. *Thorax*. 1988;43:516-524.
19. Cozier YC, Berman JS, Palmer JR, Boggs DA, Serlin DM, Rosenberg L. Sarcoidosis in black women in the United States: data from the black Women's health study. *Chest*. 2011;139:144-150.
20. O'Regan A, Berman JS. Sarcoidosis. *Ann Intern Med*. 2012;156:1-15.
21. Rybicki BA, Iannuzzi MC, Frederick MM, et al. Familial aggregation of sarcoidosis. A case-control etiologic study of sarcoidosis (ACCESS). *Am J Respir Crit Care Med*. 2001;164:2085-2091.
22. Solà R, Boj M, Hernandez-Flix S, Camprubí M. Silica in oral drugs as a possible sarcoidosis-inducing antigen. *Lancet*. 2009;373(9679):1943-1944.
23. Kreiss K, Day GA, Schuler CR. Beryllium: a modern industrial hazard. *Annu Rev Public Health*. 2007;28:259-277.
24. Muthuswamy PP, Lopez-Majano V, Panginwala M, Trainor WD. Serum angiotensin-converting enzyme as an indicator of total body granuloma load and prognosis in sarcoidosis. *Sarcoidosis*. 1987;4:142-148.
25. Turner-Warwick M, McAllister W, Lawrence R, Britten A, Ha slam PL. Corticosteroid treatment in pulmonary sarcoidosis: do serial lavage lymphocyte counts, serum angiotensin-converting enzyme measurements and gallium-67 scans help management? *Thorax*. 1986;41:903-913.
26. Kruit A, Grutters JC, Gerritsen WB, et al. ACE I/D-corrected Z-scores to identify normal and elevated ACE activity in sarcoidosis. *Respir Med*. 2007;101(3):510-515.
27. Stouten K, van de Werken M, Tchetverikov I, et al. Extreme elevation of serum angiotensin-converting enzyme (ACE) activity: always consider familial ACE hyperactivity. *Ann Clin Biochem*. 2014;51:289-293.
28. Studdy PR, James DG. The specificity and sensitivity of serum angiotensin-converting enzyme in sarcoidosis and other diseases. In: Chretien J, Marsac J, Saltiel JC, eds. *Sarcoidosis*. Paris, France: Pergamon Press; 1983:332-344.
29. Popević S, Šumarac Z, Jovanović D, et al. Verifying sarcoidosis activity: chitotriosidase versus ACE in sarcoidosis - a case-control study. *J Med Biochem*. 2016;35:390-400.
30. Brunner J, Scholl-Bürgi S, Zimmerhackl LB. Chitotriosidase as a marker of disease activity in sarcoidosis. *Rheumatol Int*. 2007;27:1171-1172.
31. Bargaglia E, Margollicci M, Luddi A, et al. Chitotriosidase activity in patients with interstitial lung diseases. *Respir Med*. 2007;101:2176-2181.
32. Grutters JC, Fellrath JM, Mulder L, Janssen R, van den Bosch JM, van Velzen-Blad H. Serum soluble interleukin-2 receptor measurement in patients with sarcoidosis: a clinical evaluation. *Chest*. 2003;124(1):186-195.
33. Gundlach E, Hoffmann MM, Prasse A, Heinzelmann S, Ness T. Interleukin-2 receptor and angiotensin-converting enzyme as markers for ocular sarcoidosis. *PLoS One*. 2016;11(1):e0147258.
34. Groen-Hakan F, Eurelings L, Ten Berge JC, et al. Diagnostic value of serum-soluble interleukin 2 receptor levels vs angiotensin-converting enzyme in patients with sarcoidosis-associated uveitis. *JAMA Ophthalmol*. 2017;135(12):1352-1358.
35. Ahmadzai H, Cameron B, Chui J, Lloyd A, Wakefield D, Thomas PS. Measurement of neopterin, TGF-β1 and ACE in the exhaled breath condensate of patients with sarcoidosis. *J Breath Res*. 2013;7(4):046003.
36. Ziegenhagen MW, Rothe ME, Schlaak M, Muller-Quernheim J. Bronchoalveolar and serological parameters reflecting the severity of sarcoidosis. *Eur Respir J*. 2003;21:407-413.
37. Gungor S, Ozseker F, Yalcinsoy M, et al. Conventional markers in determination of activity of sarcoidosis. *Int Immunopharmacol*. 2015;25(1):174-179.
38. Carleo A, Bennett D, Rottoli P. Biomarkers in sarcoidosis: the contribution of system biology. *Curr Opin Pulm Med*. 2016;22(5):509-514.
39. Crouser ED, Fingerlin TE, Yang IV, et al. Application of 'omics' and systems biology to sarcoidosis research. *Ann Am Thorac Soc*. 2017;14(supplement 6):S445-S451.
40. Ascoli C, Huang Y, Schott C, et al. A circulating micro-RNA signature serves as a diagnostic and prognostic indicator in sarcoidosis. *Am J Respir Cell Mol Biol*. August 16, 2017. https://doi.org/10.1165/rcmb.2017-0207OC. [Epub ahead of print].
41. Calandriello L, Walsh SLF. Imaging for sarcoidosis. *Semin Respir Crit Care Med*. 2017;38(4):417-436.
42. Zappala CJ, Desai SR, Copley SJ, et al. Optimal scoring of serial change on chest radiography in sarcoidosis. *Sarcoidosis Vasc Diffuse Lung Dis*. 2011;28(2):130-138.
43. Baughman RP, Shipley R, Desai S, et al. Sarcoidosis Investigators. Changes in chest roentgenogram of sarcoidosis patients during a clinical trial of infliximab therapy: comparison of different methods of evaluation. *Chest*. 2009;136(2):526-535.

44. Walsh SL, Wells AU, Sverzellati N, et al. An integrated clinicoradiological staging system for pulmonary sarcoidosis: a case-cohort study. *Lancet Respir Med.* 2014;2(2):123–130.
45. Nunes H, Uzunhan Y, Gille T, Lamberto C, Valeyre D, Brillet PY. Imaging of sarcoidosis of the airways and lung parenchyma and correlation with lung function. *Eur Respir J.* 2012;40:750–765.
46. Aleksonienė R, Zeleckienė I, Matačiūnas M, et al. Relationship between radiologic patterns, pulmonary function values and bronchoalveolar lavage fluid cells in newly diagnosed sarcoidosis. *J Thorac Dis.* 2017;9(1):88–95.
47. Zappala CJ, Desai SR, Copley SJ, et al. Accuracy of individual variables in the monitoring of long-term change in pulmonary sarcoidosis as judged by serial high resolution CT scan data. *Chest.* 2014;145:101–107.
48. Keijsers RG, Grutters JC, Thomeer M, et al. Imaging the inflammatory activity of sarcoidosis: sensitivity and inter observer agreement of (67)Ga imaging and (18)F-FDG PET. *Q J Nucl Med Mol Imaging.* 2011;55:66–71.
49. Teirstein AS, Machac J, Almeida O, Lu P, Padilla ML, Iannuzzi MC. Results of 188 whole-body fluorodeoxyglucose positron emission tomography scans in 137 patients with sarcoidosis. *Chest.* 2007;132:1949–1953.
50. Mostard RL, Van Kuijk SM, Verschakelen JA, et al. A predictive tool for an effective use of (18)F-FDG PET in assessing activity of sarcoidosis. *BMC Pulm Med.* 2012;12:57.
51. Vorselaars AD, Verwoerd A, van Moorsel CH, Keijsers RG, Rijkers GT, Grutters JC. Prediction of relapse after discontinuation of infliximab therapy in severe sarcoidosis. *Eur Respir J.* 2014;43(2):602–609.
52. Vorselaars AD, Crommelin HA, Deneer VH, et al. Effectiveness of infliximab in refractory FDG PET-positive sarcoidosis. *Eur Respir J.* 2015;46(1):175–185.
53. Mostard RL, Verschakelen JA, van Kroonenburgh MJ, et al. Severity of pulmonary involvement and (18)F-FDG PET activity in sarcoidosis. *Respir Med.* 2013;107(3):439–447.
54. Ambrosini V, Zompatori M, Fasano L, et al. (18)F-FDG PET/CT for the assessment of disease extension and activity in patients with sarcoidosis: results of a preliminary prospective study. *Clin Nucl Med.* 2013;38:e171–e177.
55. Rubini G, Cappabianca S, Altini C, et al. Current clinical use of 18FDG-PET/CT in patients with thoracic and systemic sarcoidosis. *Radiol Med.* 2014;119:64–74.
56. Mohapatra PR, Vivek KU, Panigrahi MK, Bhuniya S. Managing FDG PET-positive sarcoidosis: "a riddle wrapped in a mystery inside an enigma". *Eur Respir J.* 2016;47:346–347.
57. Lee W, Chung WS, Hong KS, Huh J. Clinical usefulness of bronchoalveolar lavage cellular analysis and lymphocyte subsets in diffuse interstitial lung diseases. *Ann Lab Med.* 2015;35:220–225.
58. Welker L, Jorres RA, Costabel U, Magnussen H. Predictive value of BAL cell differentials in the diagnosis of interstitial lung diseases. *Eur Respir J.* 2004;24:1000–1006.
59. Efared B, Ebang-Atsame G, Rabiou S, et al. The diagnostic value of the bronchoalveolar lavage in interstitial lung diseases. *J Negat Results Biomed.* 2017;16(1):4.
60. Tanrıverdi H, Uygur F, Örnek T, et al. Comparison of the diagnostic value of different lymphocyte subpopulations in bronchoalveolar lavage fluid in patients with biopsy proven sarcoidosis. *Sarcoidosis Vasc Diffuse Lung Dis.* 2016;32(4):305–312.
61. Costabel U. CD4/CD8 ratios in bronchoalveolar lavage fluid: of value for diagnosing sarcoidosis? *Eur Respir J.* 1997;10:2699–2700.
62. Winterbauer RH, Lammert J, Selland M, Wu R, Corley D, Springmeyer SC. Bronchoalveolar lavage cell populations in the diagnosis of sarcoidosis. *Chest.* 1993;104:352–361.
63. Shen Y, Pang C, Wu Y, et al. Diagnostic performance of bronchoalveolar lavage fluid CD4/CD8 ratio for sarcoidosis: a meta-analysis. *EBioMedicine.* 2016;8:302–308.
64. Drent M, Mansour K, Linssen C. Bronchoalveolar lavage in sarcoidosis. *Semin Respir Crit Care Med.* 2007;28(5):486–495.
65. Meyer KC, Raghu G, Baughman RP, et al. An official American Thoracic Society clinical practice guideline: the clinical utility of bronchoalveolar lavage cellular analysis in interstitial lung disease. *Am J Respir Crit Care Med.* 2012;185:1004–1014.
66. Drent M, Wagenaar SS, Mulder PH, van Velzen-Blad H, Diamant M, van den Bosch JM. Bronchoalveolar lavage fluid profiles in sarcoidosis, tuberculosis, and non-Hodgkin's and Hodgkin's disease: an evaluation of differences. *Chest.* 1994;105:514–519.
67. Muller-Quernheim J, Gaede KI, Fireman E, Zissel G. Diagnoses of chronic beryllium disease within cohorts of sarcoidosis patients. *Eur Respir J.* 2006;27:1190–1195.
68. Sterclova M, Vasakova M, Dutka J, Kalanin J. Extrinsic allergic alveolitis: comparative study of the bronchoalveolar lavage profiles and radiological presentation. *Postgrad Med J.* 2006;82:598–601.
69. Ziora D, Grzanka P, Mazur B, Niepsuj G, Oklek K. BAL from two different lung segments indicated by high resolution computed tomography (HRCT) in patients with sarcoidosis. I. Evaluation of alveolitis homogeneity and estimation of HRCT usefulness in selection of lung region for BAL. *Pneumonol Alergol Pol.* 1999;67:422–434.
70. von Bartheld MB, Dekkers OM, Szlubowski A, et al. Endosonography vs conventional bronchoscopy for the diagnosis of sarcoidosis: the GRANULOMA randomized clinical trial. *JAMA.* 2013;309(23):2457–2464.
71. Comparison of cell counting methods in rodent pulmonary toxicity studies: automated and manual protocols and considerations for experimental design. *Inhal Toxicol.* 2016;28(9):410–420.
72. Drent M, van Velzen Blad H, Diamant M, Hoogsteden HC, van den Bosch JM. Relationship between presentation of sarcoidosis and T lymphocyte profile: a study in bronchoalveolar lavage fluid. *Chest.* 1993;104:795–800.
73. Hu L, Chen R, Huang H, et al. Endobronchial ultrasound-guided transbronchial needle aspiration versus standard bronchoscopic modalities for diagnosis of sarcoidosis: a meta-analysis. *Chin Med J.* 2016;129(13):1607–1615.

74. Gilman MJ, Wang KP. Transbronchial lung biopsy in sarcoidosis: an approach to determine the optimal number of biopsies. *Am Rev Respir Dis*. 1980;122:721–724.
75. Armstrong JR, Radke JR, Kvale PA, Eichenhorn MS, Popovich Jr J. Endoscopic findings in sarcoidosis. Characteristics and correlations with radiographic staging and bronchial mucosal biopsy yield. *Ann Otol*. 1981;90:339–434.
76. Aragaki-Nakahodo AA, Baughman RP, Shipley RT, Benzaquen S. The complimentary role of transbronchial lung cryobiopsy and endobronchial ultrasound fine needle aspiration in the diagnosis of sarcoidosis. *Respir Med*. 2017;131:65–69.
77. Kocoń P, Szlubowski A, Kużdżał J, et al. Endosonography-guided fine-needle aspiration in the diagnosis of sarcoidosis: a randomized study. *Pol Arch Intern Med*. 2017;127(3):154–162.
78. Rossi G, Cavazza A, Colby TV. Pathology of sarcoidosis. *Clin Rev Allergy Immunol*. 2015;49(1):36–44.
79. Baughman RP, Lower EE, du Bois RM. Sarcoidosis. *Lancet*. 2003;361:1111–1118.
80. Devaney K, Goodman Z, Epstein M, Zimmerman H, Ishak K. Hepatic sarcoidosis. Clinicopathologic features in 100 patients. *Am J Surg Pathol*. 1993;17(12):1272–1280.
81. Hussain N, Feld JJ, Kleiner DE, et al. Hepatic abnormalities in patients with chronic granulomatous disease. *Hepatology*. 2007;45(3):675–683.
82. Reich JM. Tissue confirmation of presumptive stage I sarcoidosis. *J Bronchol Interv Pulmonol*. 2013;20:103–105.

CHAPTER 8

Bronchoscopic Modalities to Diagnose Sarcoidosis

SADIA BENZAQUEN, MD • ALEJANDRO ARAGAKI, MD

INTRODUCTION

Sarcoidosis is a multisystemic granulomatous disease of unknown cause. It commonly affects young and middle-aged adults and frequently presents with bilateral hilar lymphadenopathy, pulmonary infiltration, and ocular and skin lesions. A diagnosis of the disorder usually requires the demonstration of typical lesions (noncaseating epithelioid cell granulomas) in more than one organ system and exclusion of other disorders known to cause granulomatous disease.[1]

Because lung involvement in sarcoidosis is highly prevalent, a biopsy of the intrathoracic lymph nodes and/or the lung parenchyma is usually considered if tissue diagnosis is desired when a presumptive diagnosis cannot be based on clinicoradiographic findings alone.[2,3] The gold standard approach to sampling the lung and mediastinal/hilar lymph nodes is surgical lung biopsy and cervical mediastinoscopy. However, the diagnostic yield from bronchoscopic procedures has decreased the need for invasive surgical procedures in the majority of cases.

We recently reviewed different bronchoscopic modalities available to procure tissue samples from the lung and/or mediastinum: bronchoalveolar lavage (BAL), endobronchial biopsy (EBB), conventional transbronchial needle aspiration (cTBNA), endobronchial ultrasound-guided transbronchial needle aspiration (EBUS-TBNA), esophageal ultrasound-guided fine needle aspiration (EUS-FNA), transbronchial lung biopsy (TBLB), and transbronchial lung cryobiopsy (TBLC). We updated our literature search to include an unexplored additional bronchoscopic modality: endobronchial ultrasound miniforceps biopsies (EBUS-MFB) from hilar/mediastinal lymph nodes.

METHODS

A computerized search of the literature was performed using the search terms "sarcoidosis," "tissue diagnosis," and "bronchoscopy." A total of 223 references were identified in PubMed. Reference lists of relevant studies were checked to identify additional references not found in PubMed: CINAHL, Scopus, and Embase. Studies included in this review met the following criteria: the study objective was to describe single or multiple diagnostic modalities in bronchoscopy to diagnose sarcoidosis; the study population consisted of only sarcoidosis patients or included a subgroup of sarcoidosis patients; the reference was published in English and in a peer-reviewed journal.

After full inspection, 16 references met the selection criteria from the initial 223; an additional 48 were included in this review. See Fig. 8.1.

BRONCHOALVEOLAR LAVAGE

BAL is the simplest and least invasive bronchoscopic procedure. Currently, there are two well-known techniques to obtain a bronchoalveolar lavage: low-pressure wall suction through a trap versus low pressure generated by a handheld syringe. In our institution we prefer to perform BAL with a trap connected to wall suction. For further details, refer to this BAL review paper by Baughman.[4]

It is well known that activated pulmonary CD4+ T lymphocytes of the Th-1 type are essential for the inflammatory process in sarcoidosis. For this reason a BAL CD4/CD8 ratio is usually ordered (a cutoff value of 3.5 usually suggests sarcoidosis). However, this CD4/CD8 ratio is highly variable.[5–11] Some authors postulate that the CD4/CD8 ratio needs to be adjusted for symptomatic/asymptomatic disease and with increased Scadding stage.[12] Additional testing in BAL such as CD103 + CD4+/CD4+ ratio[13] or chitotriosidase activity[14] has not proven to be of additional benefit for the diagnosis of sarcoidosis. The actual value of a BAL is to rule out granulomatous infections such as fungal or mycobacterial infection. The BAL should be performed before any biopsy attempt to avoid blood contamination.

ENDOBRONCHIAL BIOPSY

EBB is performed under direct visualization with a biopsy forceps instrument. We keep the biopsy forceps as close

Sarcoidosis. https://doi.org/10.1016/B978-0-323-54429-0.00008-2

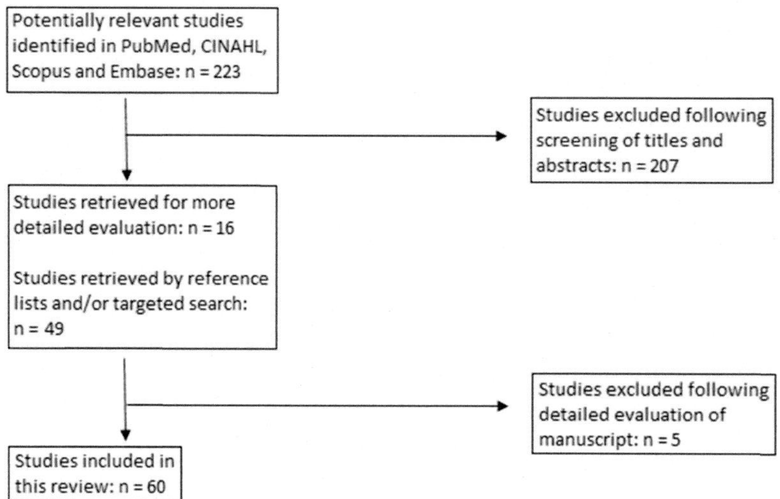

FIG. 8.1 Study selection process.

to the edge of the bronchoscope as possible to avoid the "parallel effect" (loss of anatomical planes and depth due to visualization of a three-dimensional structure in a two-dimensional screen). Once an EBB is taken (biopsy forceps is closed), rather than pulling the biopsy forceps through the working channel, we "lock" the biopsy forceps at the level of the working channel valve and pull the bronchoscope "en-bloc." This maneuver provides bigger samples.

EBB is particularly useful in patients with endobronchial sarcoidosis who experience cough, wheezing, stridor, or signs of obstruction of the main airway.[15,16] In this clinical scenario it is common to find cobblestone mucosa and, in some cases, nodules in the anterior wall of the trachea and bronchi as well as tracheal and/or bronchial stenosis. We obtain EBBs if any of the above is noted. Available literature describes the diagnostic yield ranging from 20% to 61%. Diagnostic yield appears to increase with additional biopsies[17] and is markedly higher when endobronchial sarcoidosis features are present.[18] In patients with normal-appearing endobronchial mucosa, the diagnostic yield is around 30%.[19] If narrow band image is available, consider its use to direct endobronchial tissue sampling.[20] Because the EBB technique has a very low risk even in the absence of endobronchial sarcoidosis features, we strongly suggest to obtain at least three to four different samples from the main carina and subsegmental carinas (right upper, right middle, and right lower).

CONVENTIONAL TRANSBRONCHIAL NEEDLE ASPIRATION

cTBNA, as any other bronchoscopic technique, depends on operator experience. For further details in this particular technique, we recommend this review paper by Wang.[21]

With the advent of endobronchial ultrasonography to guide transbronchial needle aspiration in the early 1990s and availability of real-time convex probe EBUS-TBNA, the use of cTBNA is decreased during the last decade. Nevertheless, cTBNA diagnostic yield is described to be between 6% and 90%.[18,22–26] In one study the diagnostic yield was 48.4% when sampling the right paratracheal or subcarinal station that measured >10 mm in largest dimension.[23] A recent publication established that rapid on-site evaluation (ROSE) can increase cTBNA diagnostic yield, being comparable with EBUS-TBNA.[24] In the absence of EBUS-TBNA, cTBNA should be considered in patients with Scadding stages 1 and 2 with ROSE (if available).

ENDOBRONCHIAL ULTRASOUND-GUIDED TRANSBRONCHIAL NEEDLE ASPIRATION

EBUS-TBNA emerged as a new tool to biopsy and stage the mediastinum in patients with lung cancer. With the advent of personalized medicine (mutation markers for lung cancer), there is a growing need for more tissue sampling. We alternate between the Olympus 19- and

21-gauge needles in each lymph node station to procure adequate tissue samples. For further details in this particular technique, we recommend the review paper by Herth et al.[25]

Its use in patients with suspected sarcoidosis has increased dramatically because of the easy accessibility of the lymph nodes in the mediastinal/hilar locations. The diagnostic yield ranges between 80% and 94%.[23–35] There is no difference between EBUS-TBNA samples obtained with a 21- or 22-gauge needle.[36] Additionally, there is no difference in diagnostic yield whether ROSE is available or not for EBUS-TBNA;[24,29] however, an EBUS-TBNA aspirate can obviate further lung biopsies if the typical noncaseating epithelioid cell granulomas are identified via ROSE.[37] The current literature suggests 3 to 5 passes in the largest mediastinal/hilar lymph node station to achieve a higher diagnostic yield.[38] Careful examination during the EBUS-TBNA procedure could increase the diagnostic yield, based on specific ultrasound findings while evaluating the hilar/mediastinal lymph nodes: granular appearance and distinct margins.[39] Our current approach is to perform 5 passes per station (If the lymph node is enlarged more than 5 mm in largest dimension). One of the passes from each station should be sent for flow cytometry to rule out lymphoproliferative disorders that sometimes are difficult to differentiate from sarcoidosis. As with BAL, EBUS-TBNA CD4/CD8 ratio is highly variable.[40] Some authors have described different BAL and EBUS-TBNA CD4/CD8 ratios in patients with sarcoidosis.[41] EBUS-TBNA should be used routinely in patients who undergo bronchoscopy for the diagnosis of sarcoidosis, especially in patients with Scadding stage 1 or 2 (with enlarged mediastinal and/or hilar adenopathy).

ESOPHAGEAL ULTRASOUND-GUIDED FINE NEEDLE ASPIRATION

EUS-FNA is able to access the mediastinal lymph node stations: 2 (higher paratracheal), 4 (lower paratracheal), 7 (subcarinal), 8 (paraesophageal), and 9 (pulmonary ligament). It is better tolerated than EBUS-TBNA and usually can be performed with moderate sedation. Its use was initially described back in 2010: it was indicated after a negative conventional bronchoscopy.[42,43] Its diagnostic yield ranges between 77% and 94%. EUS-FNA probably is indicated in patients with poor lung function and/or intractable cough. If there is mediastinal adenopathy that has been sampled without success (ROSE negative) via EBUS-TBNA, we typically extubate the patient and intubate the esophagus with the EBUS bronchoscope.

The technique is essentially the same as for EBUS-TBNA, although visualization of the needle sheath is particularly difficult once in the esophagus. Our recommendation is to push out the needle sheath as long as the EBUS image of the lymph node is visible enough before deploying the needle into the lymph node. Once the esophagus is accessed and samples obtained, the procedure is terminated (to avoid introducing gastric acid content into the tracheobronchial tree).

TRANSBRONCHIAL LUNG BIOPSY

The TBLB technique has been previously described by Kvale.[44] Although there is no difference between TBLB with or without fluoroscopic guidance in terms of post-procedural complications, we prefer to perform TBLB with fluoroscopic guidance in our institution.

The TBLB diagnostic yield for suspected sarcoidosis ranges from 37% to 90% (when at least four samples are obtained). Intuitively the diagnostic yield increases in patients with Scadding stages 2 and 3 (cases with parenchymal involvement) when compared with Scadding stage 1 (66% in stage 1, 80% in stage 2, and 83% in stage 3).[16,22,30,36–38] However, this technique has fallen behind during the last decade, favoring EBUS-TBNA for tissue diagnosis of sarcoidosis. Our recommendation is that at least four samples through TBLB should be obtained in all patients with suspected sarcoidosis, regardless of their Scadding stage.

TRANSBRONCHIAL LUNG CRYOBIOPSY

Surgical lung biopsy achieves 100% diagnostic yield in patients with suspected stage 1 sarcoidosis, with less extent of granulomatous inflammation and fibrosis than patients with group two or three sarcoidosis.[45] Variable "granuloma density" may explain differences in diagnostic yield by lung biopsy and disease stage, highlighting the need for bigger specimens in patients with less "granuloma density": Scadding stages 0 and 1.[46] An alternative to surgical lung biopsy is TBLC. For undifferentiated interstitial lung disease, TBLC diagnostic yield ranges from 74% to 98% when interpreted in isolation, with a pooled estimate around 80%,[47–49] with lower complication and mortality rates than surgical lung biopsy. The interest in TBLC, when compared to TBLB, is the ability to retrieve bigger biopsies with preserved architecture (avoiding the crush effect of TBLB). See Picture 1. In the era of "personalized medicine," time will only tell if TBLC could facilitate genetic profiling for sarcoidosis.[50]

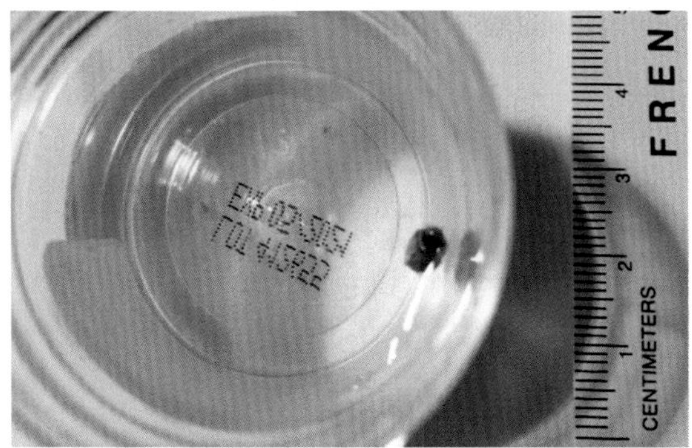

PICTURE 1 Macroscopic difference between TBLB and TBLC. *TBLB*, transbronchial lung biopsy; *TBLC*, transbronchial lung cryobiopsy.

There are significant variations in technique for TBLC[47–49] with criticism toward patient safety. Our two-scope technique has been described elsewhere.[51] We also described our institutional experience with an unselected cohort with a clinical suspicion for sarcoidosis.[52] Out of 36 patients, 18 of them had tissue diagnosis compatible with sarcoidosis: 12 of 18 had positive EBUS-TBNA biopsies, whereas 12 of /18 had positive TBLC biopsies. The combined diagnostic yield (EBUS-TBNA + TBLC) achieved 100%. The pneumothorax rate for the whole cohort was 11.1%, easily managed with a small bore chest tube placement and a short stay in the hospital. We believe this increased pneumothorax rate was due to the low number of patients. In our first publication with TBLC for diffuse parenchymal lung disease, the pneumothorax rate was 6.7% (74 patients in total). No significant bleeding and mortality were observed in our cohort.

To decrease the risk of possible complications, we use general anesthesia with an airway (laryngeal mask airway or endotracheal tube) during the procedure, with the patient spontaneously breathing. To further decrease the risk of pneumothorax, we perform TBLC under fluoroscopy guidance (allows us to determine the best airway to be biopsied, i.e., ideally the one that follows a straight line to the lung periphery). Once the cryobiopsy is retrieved, a second bronchoscope is introduced and wedged immediately in the segment where the TBLC was retrieved for bleeding control. A postprocedural thoracic ultrasound and portable chest x-ray are performed to rule out iatrogenic pneumothorax. Prospective randomized trials are needed to establish the value of TBLC in the diagnosis of suspected sarcoidosis.

ENDOBRONCHIAL ULTRASOUND LYMPH NODE MINIFORCEPS BIOPSY

EBUS-MFB biopsies of mediastinal and/or hilar lymph nodes have been recently described with different miniforceps tools.[53–55] Although its use is not widespread as EBUS-TBNA, this technique, along with TBLC, could be helpful in the bronchoscopic diagnosis of sarcoidosis. Two of the miniforceps tools (Olympus FB-56D-1; Boston Scientific M00546270) require a previous puncture in the bronchial wall by the EBUS-TBNA needle (preferably the 19 gauge) as the cusps are ellipsoid and would not pierce the bronchial mucosa. Similar to the EBUS-TBNA technique, under direct EBUS guidance, the miniforceps are pushed into the lymph node to obtain a core biopsy. It is important to remember the puncture site area from the EBUS-TBNA sampling through the EBUS images so the miniforceps can be pushed in the same area. Once in the same area, the miniforceps tool is advanced into the lymph node under direct visualization, "negotiating" (push and pull) until the lymph node is accessed. See Picture 2.

Herth et al.[53] compared the diagnostic yield of EBUS-TBNA with the 22- and 19-gauge needle with the EBUS-MFB in subcarinal masses (with low likelihood to be malignancy). The EBUS-TBNA diagnostic yield was 36% versus 88% of EBUS-MFB. Although the size of EBUS-MFB are small when compared with that of TBLB or TBLC, the "core" biopsy is definitely bigger than the cytology specimens of the EBUS-TBNA. Again, the "granuloma density" and the ability to retrieve bigger biopsies through EBUS-MFB probably explain the difference in diagnostic yield. Prospective randomized trials are needed to establish the value of EBUS-MFB in the diagnosis of suspected sarcoidosis when mediastinal/hilar adenopathy is sampled (Scadding stages 1 and 2).

DISCUSSION

We recently reviewed the different bronchoscopic techniques to biopsy the lung parenchyma and/or mediastinal/hilar adenopathy in patients with suspected sarcoidosis.[56]

The combination of different bronchoscopic techniques maximizes the chance of achieving tissue diagnosis[18,23,29,57] through conscientious and careful procedural planning. Goyal et al.,[18] for example, described the diagnostic yield of the following: EBB (49.6%), cTBNA (22.4%), TBLB (68.7%), and EBUS-TBNA (57.1%). When combined in two different groups, the diagnostic yield increased: cTBNA + EBB + TBLB (86.9%) versus EBUS-TBNA + EBB + TBLB (86.4%). See Table 8.1.

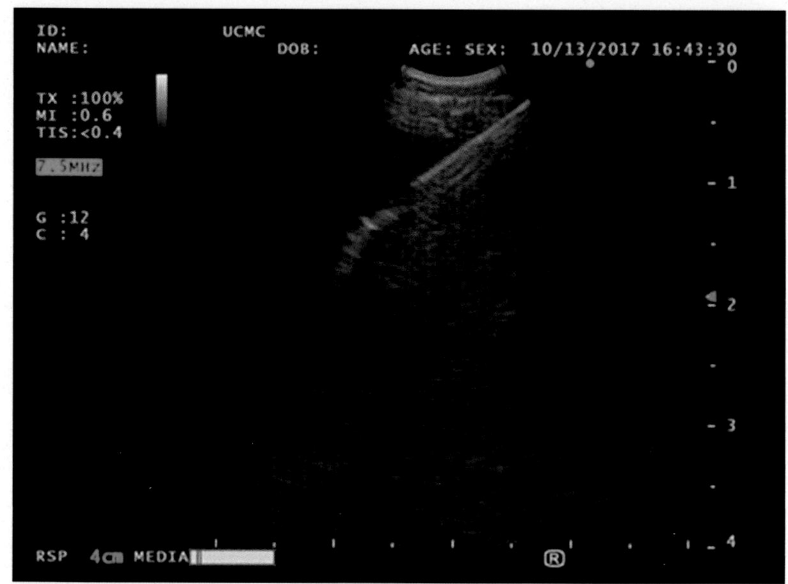

PICTURE 2 EBUS-MFB of subcarinal lymph node station. *EBUS-MFB*, endobronchial ultrasound-guided miniforceps biopsies.

TABLE 8.1
Summary of Studies Adding Different Bronchoscopic Techniques in Diagnosis Sarcoidosis

Author/Year	Study Design	Scadding Stage	No. of Patients	Study Protocol	Diagnostic Yield
Goyal[18] 2014	PCS	1, 2, 3, and 4	151	cTBNA + TBLB + EBB vs. EBUS-TBNA + TBLB + EBB	cTBNA + TBLB + EBB 86.9%; EBUS-TBNA + TBLB + EBB 86.4%
Shorr[19] 2001	PCS	1, 2, and 3	34	EBB, TBLB, and EBB + TBLB	EBB 61.8%; TBLB 58.5%; EBB + TBLB 79.4%
Agarwal[22] 2013	MA	1 and 2	915	cTBNA and cTBNA + TBLB	cTBNA 61.6%; cT-BNA + TBLB 83%
Gupta[23] 2014	RCT	1 and 2	117	cTBNA + TBLB + EBB; EBUS-TBNA + TBLB + EBB	cTBNA + TBLB + EBB 85.5%; EBUS-TBNA + TBLB + EBB 92.7%
Dziedzic[29] 2017	RCS	1,2	653	EBB; TBLB; EBUS-TBNA; and EBB + TBLB + EBUS-TBNA	EBB 29.7%; TBLB 43.9%; EBUS-TBNA 84%; EBB + TBLB + EBUS-FNA 89%
Plit[58] 2012	PCS	1,2	40	EBB; TBLB; EBUS-TBNA; and EBB + TBLB + EBUS-TBNA	EBB 27%; TBLB 78%; EBUS-TBNA 84%; EBB + TBLB + EBUS-TBNA 100%
Aragaki[52] 2017	RCS	0,1,2,3,4	36	EBUS-TBNA; TBLC; and EBUS-TBNA + TBLC	EBUS-TBNA 66.7%; TBLC 66.7%; EBUS-TBNA + TBLC 100%

cTBNA, conventional transbronchial needle aspiration; *EBB*, endobronchial biopsy; *EBUS-TBNA*, endobronchial ultrasound-guided transbronchial needle aspiration; *MA*, meta-analysis; *PCS*, prospective case series; *RCS*, retrospective case series; *RCT*, randomized controlled trial; *TBLB*, transbronchial lung biopsy; *TBLC*, transbronchial lung cryobiopsy.

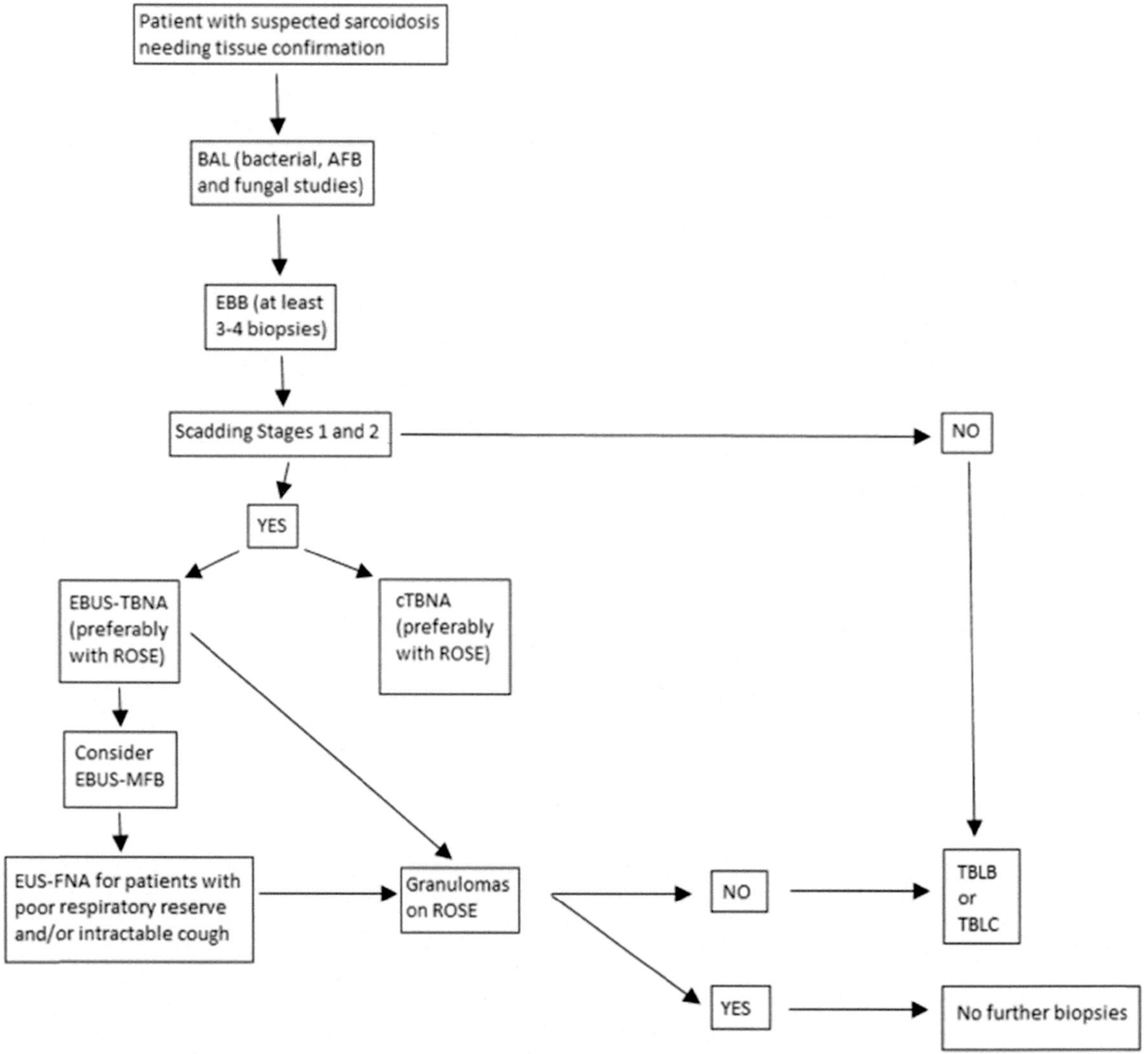

FIG. 8.2 A proposed flowchart to diagnose sarcoidosis via flexible bronchoscopy. *BAL*, bronchoalveolar lavage; *cTBNA*, conventional transbronchial needle aspiration; *EBB*, endobronchial biopsy; *EBUS-TBNA*, endobronchial ultrasound-guided transbronchial needle aspiration; *ROSE*, rapid on-site evaluation; *TBLB*, transbronchial lung biopsy; *TBLC*, transbronchial lung cryobiopsy.

A significant amount of references in this review come from India, a country with a high prevalence of tuberculosis (TB). Because TB and sarcoidosis can both cause mediastinal/hilar adenopathy, the decision to pursue tissue diagnosis might be different in countries with a lower prevalence of TB or if malignancy is suspected (lymphoma). The aggressiveness of diagnostic testing depends on the level of confidence the clinician has for his/her patient. The bronchoscopic approach will depend on the patient's preference, clinician expertise, and local capabilities.

CONCLUSION

For bronchoscopic tissue diagnosis of sarcoidosis, we propose the following diagnostic flowchart (see Fig. 8.2):

1. For all patients (with and without hilar/mediastinal adenopathy), a BAL should be obtained at the beginning of the bronchoscopic procedure.
2. With or without bronchoscopic evidence of endobronchial sarcoidosis, EBB should be taken (at least three samples from different sites; for example, main carina and subsegmental carinal areas and/or endobronchial nodules).

3. For patients with hilar/mediastinal adenopathy, EBUS-TBNA or cTBNA should be obtained. Consider EBUS-MFB.
4. In patients with poor respiratory reserve and/or intractable cough, EUS-FNA can be considered.
5. For patients with/without parenchymal disease, either TBLB or TBLC should be obtained.
6. A combination of different techniques maximizes the chance of achieving tissue diagnosis in patients with suspected sarcoidosis.

REFERENCES

1. Hunninghake GW, Costabel U, Ando M, et al. ATS/ERS/WASOG statement on sarcoidosis. American thoracic society/European Respiratory Society/World Association of sarcoidosis and other granulomatous disorders. *Am J Respir Crit Care Med*. 1999;160:736–755.
2. Govender P, Berman JS. The diagnosis of sarcoidosis. *Clin Chest Med*. 2015;36(4):585–602.
3. Baughman RP, Culver DA, Judson MA. A concise review of pulmonary sarcoidosis. *Am J Respir Crit Care Med*. 2011;183:583–581.
4. Baughman RP. Technical aspects of bronchoalveolar lavage: recommendations for a standard procedure. *Semin Respir Crit Care Med*. 2007;28:475–485.
5. Valeyre D, Bernaudin JF, Uzunhan Y, et al. Clinical presentation of sarcoidosis and diagnostic work-up. *Semin Respir Crit Care Med*. 2014;35(3):336–351.
6. Drent M, Mansour K, Linssen C. Bronchoalveolar lavage in sarcoidosis. *Semin Respir Crit Care Med*. 2007;28(5):486–495.
7. Grunewald J, Eklund A. Role of CD4+ T cells in sarcoidosis. *Proc Am Thorac Soc*. 2007;4(5). 416–4.
8. Kantrow SP, Meyer KC, Kidd P, et al. The CD4/CD8 ratio in BAL fluid is highly variable in sarcoidosis. *Eur Respir J*. 1997;10(2):2716–2721.
9. Costabel U, Bonella F, Ohshimo S, et al. Diagnostic modalities in sarcoidosis: BAL, EBUS, and PET. *Semin Respir Crit Care Med*. 2010;31(4):404–408.
10. Tanriverdi H, Uygur F, Ornek T, et al. Comparison of the diagnostic value of different lymphocyte subpopulations in bronchoalveolar lavage fluid in patients with biopsy proven sarcoidosis. *Sarcoidosis Vasc Diffuse Lung Dis*. 2015;32:305–312.
11. Aleksoniene R, Zeleckiene I, Mataciunas M, et al. Relationship between radiologic patterns, pulmonary function values and bronchoalveolar lavage fluid cells in newly diagnosed sarcoidosis. *J Thorac Dis*. 2017;9(1):88–95.
12. Danila E, Norkuniene J, Jurgauskiene L, et al. Diagnostic role of BAL fluid CD4/CD8 ratio in different radiographic and clinical forms of pulmonary sarcoidosis. *Clin Respir J*. 2009;4:214–221.
13. Bretagne L, Diatta ID, Faouzi M, et al. Diagnostic value of the CD103+CD4+/CD4+ ratio to differentiate sarcoidosis from other causes of lymphocytic alveolitis. *Respiration*. 2016;91(6):486–496.
14. Harlander M, Salobir B, Zupancic M, et al. Bronchoalveolar lavage chitotriosidase activity as a biomarker of sarcoidosis. *Sarcoidosis Vasc Diffuse Lung Dis*. 2016;32(4):313–317.
15. Hadfield JW, Page RL, Flower CD, et al. Localised airway narrowing in sarcoidosis. *Thorax*. 1982;37(6):443–447.
16. Polychronopoulos VS, Prakash UB. Airway involvement in sarcoidosis. *Chest*. 2009;136(5):1371–1380.
17. Bybee JD, Bahar D, Greenberg SD, et al. Bronchoscopy and bronchial mucosal biopsy in the diagnosis of sarcoidosis. *Am Rev Respir Dis*. 1968;97(2):232–239.
18. Goyal A, Gupta D, Agarwal R, et al. Value of different bronchoscopic sampling techniques in diagnosis of sarcoidosis: a prospective study of 151 patients. *J Bronchology Interv Pulmonol*. 2014;21(3):220–226.
19. Shorr AF, Torrington KG, Hnatiuk OW. Endobronchial biopsy for sarcoidosis: a prospective study. *Chest*. 2001;120(1):109–114.
20. Hakim R, Sabath B, Kaplan T, et al. Use of narrow band imaging in the diagnosis of hypovascular endobronchial sarcoidosis. *J Bronchol Interv Pulmonol*. 2017;24(4):315–318.
21. Wang KP. How I do it. Transbronchial needle aspiration. *J Bronchol*. 1994;1:63–68.
22. Agarwal R, Aggarwal AN, Gupta D. Efficacy and safety of conventional transbronchial needle aspiration in sarcoidosis: a systematic review and meta-analysis. *Respir Care*. 2013;58:683–693.
23. Gupta D, Dadhwal DS, Agarwal R, et al. Endobronchial ultrasound-guided transbronchial needle aspiration vs conventional transbronchial needle aspiration in the diagnosis of sarcoidosis. *Chest*. 2014;146(3):547–556.
24. Madan K, Dhungana A, Mohan A, et al. Conventional transbronchial needle aspiration versus endobronchial ultrasound-guided transbronchial needle aspiration, with or without rapid on-site evaluation, for the diagnosis of sarcoidosis: a randomized controlled trial. *J Bronchol Intervent Pulmonol*. 2017;24:48–58.
25. Herth FJF, Krasnik M, Yasufuku K, et al. How I do it. Endobronchial ultrasound-guided transbronchial needle aspiration. *J Bronchol*. 2006;13:84–91.
26. Li K, Jiang SA. Randomized controlled study of conventional TBNA versus EBUS-TBNA for diagnosis of suspected stage I and II sarcoidosis. *Sarcoid Vasc Diffuse Lung Dis*. 2014;31(3):211–218.
27. Tremblay A, Stather DR, MacEachern P, et al. A randomized controlled trial of standard vs endobronchial ultrasonography-guided transbronchial needle aspiration in patients with suspected sarcoidosis. *Chest*. 2009;136(2):340–346.
28. Von Bartheld MB, Dekkers OM, Szlubowski A, et al. Endosonography vs conventional bronchoscopy for the diagnosis of sarcoidosis. The GRANULOMA randomized controlled trial. *J Am Med Assoc*. 2013;309(23):2457–2464.
29. Dziedzic DA, Peryt A, Orlowski T. The role of EBUS-TBNA and standard bronchoscopic modalities in the diagnosis of sarcoidosis. *Clin Respir J*. 2017;11:58–63.
30. Nakajima T, Yasufuku K, Kurosu K, et al. The role of EBUS-TBNA for the diagnosis of sarcoidosis – comparisons with other bronchoscopic diagnostic modalities. *Respir Med*. 2009;103:1796–1800.

31. Oki M, Saka H, Kitagawa C, et al. Prospective study of endobronchial ultrasound-guided transbronchial needle aspiration of lymph nodes versus transbronchial lung biopsy of lung tissue for diagnosis of sarcoidosis. *J Thorac Cardiovasc Surg*. 2012;143:1324–1329.
32. Agarwal R, Srinivasan A, Aggarwal AN, et al. Efficacy and safety of convex probe EBUS-TBNA in sarcoidosis: a systematic review and meta-analysis. *Respir Med*. 2012;106(6):883–892.
33. Trisolini R, Agli LL, Tinelli C, et al. Endobronchial ultrasound-guided transbronchial needle aspiration for diagnosis of sarcoidosis in clinically unselected study populations. *Respirology*. 2015;20(2):226–234.
34. Eckardt J, Olsen KE, Jorgensen OD, et al. Minimally invasive diagnosis of sarcoidosis by EBUS when conventional diagnostics fail. *Sarcoidosis Vasc Diffuse Lung Dis*. 2010;27:43–48.
35. Wong M, Yasufuku K, Nakajima T, et al. Endobronchial ultrasound: new insight for the diagnosis of sarcoidosis. *Eur Respir J*. 2007;29:1182–1186.
36. Muthu V, Gupta N, Dhooria S, et al. A prospective, randomized, double-blind trial comparing the diagnostic yield of 21- and 22- gauge aspiration needles for performing endobronchial ultrasound-guided transbronchial needle aspiration in sarcoidosis. *Chest*. 2016;149(4):1111–1112.
37. Plit ML, Havryk AP, Hodgson A, et al. Rapid cytological analysis of endobronchial ultrasound-guided aspirates in sarcoidosis. *Eur Respir J*. 2013;42:1302–1308.
38. Sun J, Yang H, Teng J, et al. Determining factors in diagnosing pulmonary sarcoidosis by endobronchial ultrasound-guided transbronchial needle aspiration. *Ann Thorac Surg*. 2015;99:441–446.
39. Ozgul MA, Centikaya E, Kirkil G, et al. Lymph node characteristics of sarcoidosis with endobronchial ultrasound. *Endosc Ultrasound*. 2014;3(4):232–237.
40. Ruiz SJ, Zhang Y, Mukhopadhyay S. CD4/CD8 ratio in mediastinal lymph nodes involved by sarcoidosis. Analysis of flow cytometry data obtained by endobronchial ultrasound-guided transbronchial needle aspiration. *J Bronchol Intervent Pulmonol*. 2016;23:288–297.
41. Oda K, Ishimoto H, Yatera K, et al. Relationship between the ratios of CD4/CD8 T-lymphocytes in the bronchoalveolar lavage fluid and lymph nodes in patients with sarcoidosis. *Res Inv*. 2014:179–183.
42. Tournoy KG, Bolly A, Aerts JG, et al. The value of endoscopic ultrasound after bronchoscopy to diagnose thoracic sarcoidosis. *Eur Respir J*. 2010;35:1329–1335.
43. von Bartheld MB, Veselic-Charvat M, Rabe KF, et al. Endoscopic ultrasound-guided fine-needle aspiration for the diagnosis of sarcoidosis. *Endoscopy*. 2010;42(3):213–217.
44. Kvale PA. How I do it. Bronchoscopic lung biopsy. *J Bronchol*. 1994;1:321–326.
45. Rosen Y, Amorosa JK, Moon S, Cohen J, Lyons HA. Occurrence of lung granulomas in patients with stage I sarcoidosis. *AJR*. 1977;129:1083–1085.
46. Burke RR, Stone CH, Havstad S, et al. Racial differences in sarcoidosis granuloma density. *Lung*. 2009;187(1):1–7.
47. Johannson KA, Marcoux VS, Ronksley PE, et al. Diagnostic yield and complications of transbronchial lung cryobiopsy for interstitial lung disease. A systematic review and metaanalysis. *Ann Am Thorac Soc*. 2016;13(10):1828–1838.
48. Hagmeyer L, Theegarten D, Wohlschlager J, et al. The role of transbronchial lung cryobiopsy and surgical lung biopsy in the diagnostic algorithm of interstitial lung disease. *Clin Respir J*. 2016;10(5):589–595.
49. Ravaglia C, Bonifazi M, Wells AU, et al. Safety and diagnostic yield of transbronchial lung cryobiopsy in diffuse parenchymal lung diseases: a comparative study versus video-assisted thoracoscopic lung biopsy and a systematic review of the literature. *Respiration*. 2016;91(3):215–227.
50. Christophi GP, Caza T, Curtiss C, et al. Gene expression profiles in granuloma tissue reveal novel diagnostic markers in sarcoidosis. *Exp Mol Pathol*. 2014;96(3):393–399.
51. Sriprasart T, Aragaki A, Baughman R, et al. A single US center experience of transbronchial lung cryobiopsy for diagnosing interstitial lung disease with a two-scope technique. *J Bronchol Interv Pulmonol*. 2017;24(2):131–135.
52. Aragaki-Nakahodo AA, Baughman RP, Shipley RT, et al. The complimentary role of transbronchial lung cryobiopsy and endobronchial ultrasound fine needle aspiration in the diagnosis of sarcoidosis. *Respir Med*. 2017;131:65–69.
53. Herth FJF, Morgan RK, Eberhardt R, et al. Endobronchial ultrasound-guided miniforceps biopsy in the biopsy of subcarinal masses in patients with low likelihood of non-small cell lung cancer. *Ann Thorac Surg*. 2008;85:1874–1879.
54. Chrissian A, Misselhorn D, Chen A. Endobronchial-ultrasound guided miniforceps biopsy of mediastinal and hilar lesions. *Ann Thorac Surg*. 2011;92:284–289.
55. Darwiche K, Freitag L, Nair A, et al. Evaluation of a novel endobronchial ultrasound-guided lymph node forceps in enlarged mediastinal lymph nodes. *Respiration*. 2013;86:229–236.
56. Benzaquen S, Aragaki-Nakahodo AA. Bronchoscopic modalities to diagnose sarcoidosis. *Curr Opin Pulm Med*. 2017;23(5):433–438.
57. Gilman MJ, Wang KP. Transbronchial lung biopsy in sarcoidosis. An approach to determine the optimal number of biopsies. *Am Rev Respir Dis*. 1980;122(5):721–724.
58. Plit M, Pearson R, Havryk A, et al. The diagnostic utility of endobronchial ultrasound-guided transbronchial needle aspiration compared with transbronchial and endobronchial biopsy for suspected sarcoidosis. *Intern Med J*. 2012;42:434–438.

FURTHER READING

1. Roethe RA, Byrd RB, Hafermann DR. Transbronchoscopic lung biopsy in sarcoidosis. Optimal number and sites for diagnosis. *Chest*. 1980;77(3):400–402.

CHAPTER 9

Cardiac Sarcoidosis: Questions for the Clinician

MERILYN VARGHESE, MD • ZARTASHIA SHAHAB, MD • EDWARD J. MILLER, MD, PHD

INTRODUCTION

Sarcoidosis can affect the heart by causing conduction system disease, arrhythmias, and ventricular remodeling. In some patients the adverse remodeling leads to left ventricular dysfunction and/or aneurysm formation. However, it is difficult for clinicians to know with certainty which patients are at the highest risk for poor outcomes from CS. In patients with sarcoidosis, cardiac involvement may account for up to a quarter of deaths. The true prevalence for CS is unknown, but studies have demonstrated a range from 25% to 40% of patients with systemic sarcoidosis have some evidence of CS. Patients may report dyspnea, orthopnea, palpitations, syncope, or near-syncope which should prompt further evaluation. Sudden cardiac death is unfortunately a common presentation of CS, predominantly secondary to ventricular arrhythmias or conduction disturbances. Therefore it is important to help prevent mortality secondary to CS by empowering clinicians to screen, diagnose, risk-stratify, and treat patients to potentially improve outcomes.

Despite the importance of understanding the risk of CS, there are many current clinical controversies in its care stemming from a lack of large-scale randomized or observational trials. However, there is some emerging consensus on aspects of CS care generated by expert opinion, and a summary of recent expert consensus documents will be the focus of this chapter by putting the data in these guidelines into a broader clinical context.[1–3] Aspects of CS management will be addressed by framing the discussion in the form of commonly posed questions in CS, including appropriate screening, methods for diagnosis, and consideration of the different imaging modalities.

Who Do You Screen for CS?

There are multiple cohorts of patients who should be screened for CS based on consensus guidelines (Table 9.1).[1–3] These include patients with known extracardiac sarcoidosis and the particular cardiac presentations described in the following.

TABLE 9.1
Indications for Screening

Who?	How?
Patients with extracardiac sarcoidosis	Symptom review, echocardiogram, ECG
Patients with extracardiac sarcoidosis with: symptoms (palpitations, new-onset heart failure, syncope), abnormal findings on echocardiogram or abnormal findings on ECG	FDG-PET and CMR
Less than 60 years old with advanced AV block	FDG-PET and CMR
Idiopathic VT	FDG-PET and CMR

Data from the study by Birnie DH, Sauer WH, Bogun F, et al. HRS expert consensus statement on the diagnosis and management of arrhythmias associated with cardiac sarcoidosis. *Heart Rhythm*. 2014;11(7):1304–1323. https://doi.org/10.1016/j.hrthm.2014.03.043; Slart RHJA, Glaudemans AWJM, Lancellotti P, et al. A joint procedural position statement on imaging in cardiac sarcoidosis: from the cardiovascular and inflammation & infection committees of the European association of nuclear medicine, the European association of cardiovascular imaging, and the American Society of Nuclear Cardiology. *J Nuclear Cardiol*. February 2018:298–319.

Sarcoidosis. https://doi.org/10.1016/B978-0-323-54429-0.00009-4

Patients with extracardiac sarcoidosis should be evaluated at the time of initial diagnosis and then yearly for symptoms or signs of possible CS. These screening visits can be performed by the patient's primary sarcoidosis clinician, depending on the clinician's expertise and comfort with CS, or by a cardiologist or cardiac sarcoid expert. Symptoms that may prompt concern include palpitations, pre-syncope, syncope, and/or heart failure symptoms (orthopnea, paroxysmal nocturnal dyspnea, and lower extremity edema). Signs of CS can include ECG abnormalities and/or structural heart changes on imaging. The ECG should be reviewed for signs of conduction system disease (>240 ms first degree atrioventricular (AV) block, second-/third-degree atrioventricular nodal block (AVB), left anterior fascicular block (LAFB), right bundle branch block (RBBB), and left bundle branch block (LBBB)), abnormal Q waves, and/or premature ventricular contractions (PVCs).[1] Although not useful or needed in all patients, an echocardiogram can look for structural changes, recognizing that it is insensitive for many aspects of CS. Nonetheless, abnormal echo findings may include regional wall motion abnormalities, focal aneurysms, basal septal thinning, or a depressed systolic function. Any patient with extracardiac sarcoidosis and an abnormal ECG or echocardiogram should prompt further discussion about testing with cardiac MRI (cardiac magnetic resonance imaging (CMR)) and/or FDG-PET imaging, which can demonstrate the pathological features of CS (inflammation/scar) with greater sensitivity/specificity than ECG or echo.[1]

Two other specific groups of patients who should prompt further evaluation for CS are (1) patients aged less than 60 years with new evidence of second- or third-degree AV block of unknown cause and (2) patients with idiopathic ventricular tachycardia (VT) not attributable to a known ischemic or nonischemic cardiomyopathy. Even if extracardiac sarcoidosis was not previously identified in these patients, the possibility of occult sarcoidosis as the cause of their new conduction system dysfunction or arrhythmias should prompt further evaluation for CS. While ECGs and echocardiography can be used in these patients, in most cases a combination of both CMR and FDG-PET should be considered as the testing strategy for diagnosis. In particular, CMR late gadolinium enhancement (LGE) in classic patterns for CS provides powerful diagnostic and risk stratification. FDG-PET imaging can identify not only cardiac inflammation but also extracardiac sites of sarcoidosis that were previously unrecognized.

How Do You Diagnose CS?

The diagnosis of cardiac sarcoidosis can be challenging. The historical gold standard for cardiac sarcoidosis diagnosis is endomyocardial biopsy (EMBx). However, EMBx is insensitive compared with clinical and imaging diagnostic strategies. EMBx yields a diagnosis in only 20%–30% of samples because it relies on accurately acquiring a sample with evidence of granulomatous inflammation which may be missed due to the patchy nature of inflammation.[3] As a result, even if the biopsied sample does not have evidence of inflammation, it does not rule out cardiac sarcoidosis as it could be present elsewhere in the heart. In many cases it is difficult to justify EMBx as the initial diagnostic strategy because it requires subjecting patients to an invasive procedure that is not likely to be of diagnostic yield. Thus finding alternative methods by which to diagnose CS becomes paramount.

There are three major imaging modalities that can be used to assist in the diagnosis of CS: echocardiogram, cardiac MRI, and FDG-PET (Table 9.2). No finding in any of these modalities is pathognomonic or possesses absolute specificity. Echocardiography may be useful in assessing features suggestive of CS, such as focal aneurysm formation or left ventricular dysfunction. However, no single echo feature is sensitive or specific for cardiac sarcoidosis. In contrast to echocardiography, both CMR and FDG-PET provide insight into the pathophysiologic processes of CS. FDG uptake on PET and T2/T1 mapping on CMR can identify inflammation, while perfusion imaging on PET and late gadolinium enhancement (LGE) along with postcontrast T1 on CMR may image fibrosis. However, neither of these techniques is specific to sarcoidosis, and their use is challenging in many CS patients. For example, FDG-PET imaging requires a complicated and prolonged dietary preparation to alter cardiac metabolism to highlight inflammation. The optimal FDG-PET patient preparation has not been defined, varies by site, and fails in 10%–25% of patients. CMR may be contraindicated in patients with ICDs or pacemakers that are not MRI compatible. Fig. 9.1 demonstrates the different findings on MRI and FDG-PET that correlate with the likelihood of CS. Table 9.2 presents a comparison of common findings seen in CS in each imaging modality. The choice of CMR versus FDG-PET is based on imaging availability, clinician expertise, and individual patient characteristics.

Clinical criteria have been proposed as methods to standardize the diagnostic approach to CS. Three commonly used criteria are compared in Table 9.3. The Heart Rhythm Society (HRS) and Japanese Ministry of Health and Welfare (JMHW; 2006 version) guidelines separate their diagnostic criteria into histological criteria, which relies on endomyocardial biopsy, and clinical criteria.[1,4] The JMHW, HRS, and World Association of Sarcoidosis and Other Granulomatous Diseases Organ Assessment

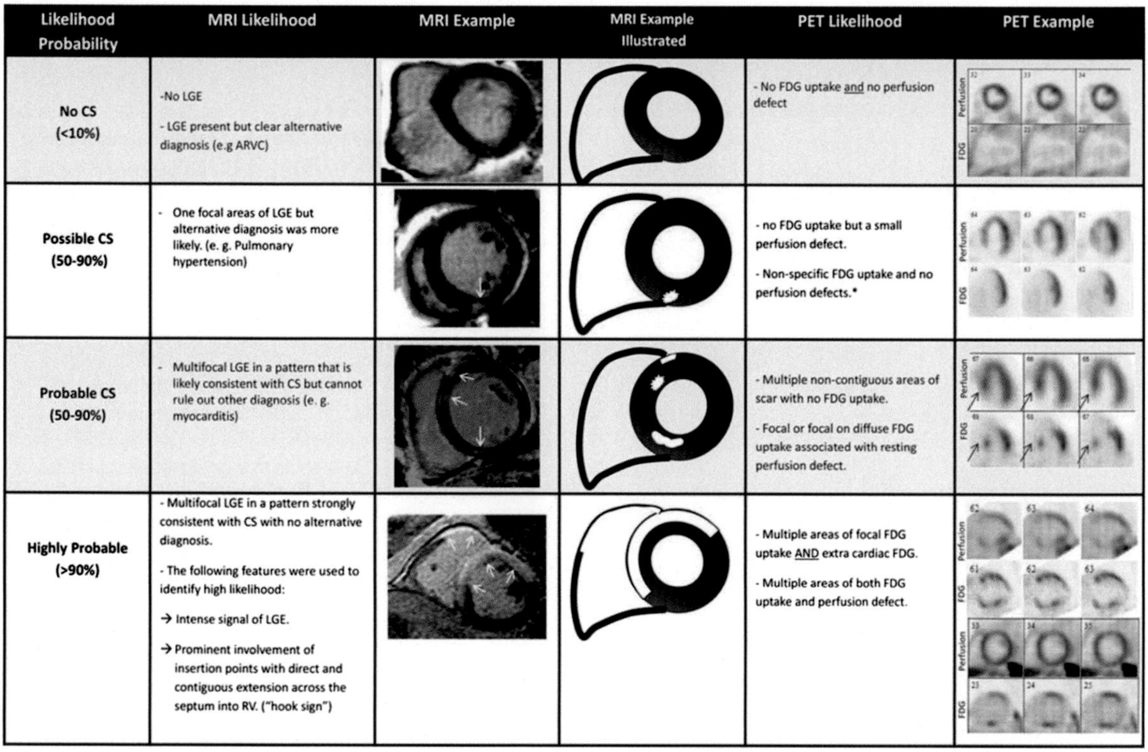

Likelihood Probability	MRI Likelihood	MRI Example	MRI Example Illustrated	PET Likelihood	PET Example
No CS (<10%)	-No LGE - LGE present but clear alternative diagnosis (e.g ARVC)			- No FDG uptake and no perfusion defect	
Possible CS (50-90%)	- One focal areas of LGE but alternative diagnosis was more likely. (e. g. Pulmonary hypertension)			- no FDG uptake but a small perfusion defect. - Non-specific FDG uptake and no perfusion defects.*	
Probable CS (50-90%)	- Multifocal LGE in a pattern that is likely consistent with CS but cannot rule out other diagnosis (e. g. myocarditis)			- Multiple non-contiguous areas of scar with no FDG uptake. - Focal or focal on diffuse FDG uptake associated with resting perfusion defect.	
Highly Probable (>90%)	- Multifocal LGE in a pattern strongly consistent with CS with no alternative diagnosis. - The following features were used to identify high likelihood: → Intense signal of LGE. → Prominent involvement of insertion points with direct and contiguous extension across the septum into RV. ("hook sign")			- Multiple areas of focal FDG uptake AND extra cardiac FDG. - Multiple areas of both FDG uptake and perfusion defect.	

FIG. 9.1 This figure correlates the probability of CS with MRI and FDG-PET findings. *CS*, cardiac sarcoidosis. (Adapted from the study by Vita T, Okada DR, Veillet-Chowdhury M, et al. Complementary value of cardiac magnetic resonance imaging and positron emission tomography/computed tomography in the assessment of cardiac sarcoidosis. *Circ Cardiovasc Imaging*. 2018;11(1):e007030. https://doi.org/10.1161/CIRCIMAGING.117.007030.)

TABLE 9.2
Features of CS on Each Imaging Modality (Echo, CMR, and FDG-PET)

Echocardiogram	Cardiac MRI	FDG-PET-CT
Atria • atrial wall hypertrophy Ventricles: • Focal Aneurysms • Regional wall motion abnormalities without corresponding coronary anatomy • Mild wall thickening or thinning • Increased wall echogenicity, "speckled/snowstorm" patterns • Localized thinning/akinesia of basal septum • Early on, decreased longitudinal myocardial function • End-stage RV dilation and dysfunction with basal septal findings	Focal or multifocal hyperenhancement on LGE (most specific) Midwall/subepicardial enhancement in basal ventricular/lateral walls or septum Subendocardial/transmural enhancement Edema-sensitive images with high-signal regions	Focal or multifocal FDG uptake in the left or right ventricle (high risk) Focal on diffuse pattern (less specific) Perfusion defects on myocardial perfusion imaging

Data From the study by Birnie DH, Sauer WH, Bogun F, et al. HRS expert consensus statement on the diagnosis and management of arrhythmias associated with cardiac sarcoidosis. *Heart Rhythm*. 2014;11(7):1304–1323. https://doi.org/10.1016/j.hrthm.2014.03.043; Chareonthaitawee P, Beanlands RS, Chen W, et al. Joint SNMMI–ASNC expert consensus document on the role of 18F-FDG PET/CT in cardiac sarcoid detection and therapy monitoring. *J Nuclear Med*. 2017;58(8):1341–1353. https://doi.org/10.2967/jnumed.117.196287.
CS, cardiac sarcoidosis; *LGE*, late gadolinium enhancement.

TABLE 9.3
Comparison of Guidelines—HRS/JMHW/WASOG

Japanese Ministry of Health and Welfare Criteria (2006)	Heart Rhythm Society Expert Consensus Statement (2014)	World Association of Sarcoidosis and Other Granulomatous Diseases Organ Assessment Instrument (2014)
Histological: Endomyocardial biopsy with noncaseating granulomas with histological or clinical diagnosis of extracardiac sarcoidosis	Histological: Endomyocardial biopsy with noncaseating granuloma	At least probable diagnosis of CS: Treatment responsive CM or AVNB Reduced LVEF in the absence of other clinical risk factors Spontaneous or inducible sustained VT with no other risk factor Mobitz type II or 3rd degree heart block Patchy uptake on dedicated cardiac PET Delayed enhancement on CMR Positive gallium uptake Defect on perfusion scintigraphy or SPECT scan T2 prolongation on CMR
Clinical diagnosis (Extracardiac sarcoidosis is diagnosed clinically or histologically AND 2 or more of 4 major criteria OR 1 in 4 of major criteria and 2 or more of 5 minor criteria are satisfied) Major criteria: Advanced AV block Basal thinning of interventricular septum Positive ^{67}gallium uptake in the heart Depressed EF of the left ventricle (<50%) Minor criteria: Abnormal ECG findings Abnormal Echo Nuclear medicine-perfusion defect Gadolinium enhanced CMR imaging- delayed enhancement of myocardium Endomyocardial biopsy with interstitial or monocyte infiltration	Clinical diagnosis: Probable if Histological diagnosis of extra-CS AND one or more of following is present Steroid/Immunosuppressant responsive cardiomyopathy or heart block Unexplained reduced LVEF (<40%) Unexplained sustained (spontaneous or induced) VT Mobitz type II 2nd degree or 3rd degree heart block Patchy uptake on dedicated cardiac PET (in a pattern consistent with CS) Late gadolinium enhancement on CMR (in a pattern consistent with CS) Positive gallium uptake (in a pattern consistent with CS) AND other causes for cardiac manifestations have been reasonably excluded	Possible diagnosis of CS: Reduced LVEF in the presence of other risk factors Atrial dysrhythmias

Data from the study by Birnie DH, Sauer WH, Bogun F, et al. HRS expert consensus statement on the diagnosis and management of arrhythmias associated with cardiac sarcoidosis. *Heart Rhythm*. 2014;11(7):1304–1323. https://doi.org/10.1016/j.hrthm.2014.03.043; Diagnostic standard and guidelines for sarcoidosis. *Jpn J Sarcoidosis Granulomatous Disord*. 2007;27:89–102; Judson MA, Costabel U, Drent M, et al. The WASOG Sarcoidosis organ assessment instrument: an update of a previous clinical tool. *Sarcoidosis Vasc Diffuse Lung Dis*. 2014;31(1):19–27.

AVNB, Atrioventricular nodal block; *CM*, Cardiomyopathy; *CS*, Cardiac Sarcoidosis; *EF*, Ejection fraction; *HRS*, Heart Rhythm Society; *JMHW*, Japanese Ministry of Health and Welfare; *LVEF*, Left ventricular ejection fraction; *SPECT*, Single photon emission computed tomography; *VT*, Ventricular tachycardia; *WASOG*, World Association of Sarcoidosis and Other Granulomatous Diseases Organ Assessment Instrument.

Instrument (WASOG) clinical criteria[5] share some similarities; however, all of these criteria suffer significant limitations that limit their utility. First, none of these criteria were experimentally derived. Rather, they arose from expert consensus opinion from limited panels of specialists. Second, they all require the presence of extracardiac sarcoidosis to make the diagnosis. This is in conflict with data that suggest a certain minority of patients who have sarcoidosis isolated to the heart and not present in any other organs. In a recent study, more than 60% (33 of 52) of patients with known CS had CS isolated to the heart.[6] Third, these criteria are inferior to FDG-PET and CMR in determining prognosis. Thus the lack of inclusion of imaging modalities is a significant problem for the JMHW criteria as it does not include FDG-PET imaging as a criterion. Lastly, neither the HRS nor the WASOG criteria provide diagnostic certainty. The HRS criteria, if met, provide a "greater than 50% likelihood" of CS being present, whereas the WASOG instrument provides only a "possible diagnosis of CS." This lack of diagnostic certainty can be frustrating to clinicians and patients who are searching for a clinically useful diagnostic framework.

The advent of advanced imaging modalities, the existence of multiple conflicting clinical guidelines for CS, and the limitations of endomyocardial biopsy argue for a new approach to CS diagnosis. One potentially useful method is the use of a probabilistic approach that integrates cardiac imaging and clinical data. This framework attempts to determine a specific patient's likelihood of a CS diagnosis, analogous to a commonly used multidisciplinary diagnostic strategy used for diseases such as idiopathic pulmonary fibrosis.[7] Recent data using this approach provide a framework that integrates clinical data with CMR and FDG-PET findings to create a probabilistic framework of CS as follows (**refer also to** Fig. 9.1):

No Cardiac Sarcoidosis (<10%)—No evidence of CS or an alternative diagnosis established.

Possible Cardiac Sarcoidosis (10%–50%)—When imaging findings are not specific for CS, CS could not be excluded but an alternative diagnosis is more likely.

Probable Cardiac Sarcoidosis (50%–90%)—When imaging findings are suggestive but not definitive for CS.

Highly Probable Cardiac Sarcoidosis (>90%)—When imaging findings are highly specific for CS.

While experimental validation of this approach is needed, this concept of a probabilistic diagnostic approach to CS holds great promise.

Who Should Be Treated for CS and How Should Treatment Be Monitored?

There are challenging aspects in the management of cardiac sarcoidosis, including deciding whether to treat with immunosuppressive medications, which medications to use, and the duration of treatment. Clinicians should recognize that there are no randomized controlled trials, or even large observational studies, to provide evidence to answer these questions. Therefore patients and clinicians should have discussions about the risks and side effects of immunosuppression, as well as the goals of treatment. Patients should be carefully monitored for complications during treatment. In addition to immunosuppression, many questions frequently arise regarding the utility and indications for implantable cardiac defibrillators (ICDs).

Immunosuppression

The concept behind the use of immunosuppressive agents in CS is to reduce active sarcoidosis inflammation to slow the progression of the disease and/or prevent complications. These goals include the preservation of left ventricular function and prevention of myocardial remodeling. Corticosteroids are historically considered first line for patients requiring immunosuppressive therapy with evidence of active myocardial inflammation either on imaging studies or myocardial biopsy. There is a lack of consensus about timing of treatment, optimal dosage, duration of steroid use, and addition of alternate steroid sparing immunosuppressive agents.

Based on these data and our experience, we advocate for demonstration of the presence of active cardiac inflammation on FDG-PET imaging as a gate keeper for discussion of immunosuppression. Once inflammation on FDG-PET is defined, the clinical scenario can assist with deciding on the appropriateness of immunosuppression. Based on HRS consensus statement guidelines, steroid use is recommended in Mobitz type II second-degree or third-degree AV block, frequent ventricular ectopy/nonsustained and sustained ventricular arrhythmias with evidence of myocardial inflammation. There is some literature to suggest that steroids are more useful for AV block than for treatment of arrhythmias.[8] In patients who have a reduction of inflammation on FDG-PET in response to steroids, some studies suggest left ventricular function is preserved or improved with treatment.[9,10] Treatment for asymptomatic or minimally symptomatic patients with preserved ejection fraction is controversial and needs individualized assessment for risks and benefits of this approach.

Generally the initial dose of prednisone is 20–40 mg/day (based on patient size). We recommend an empiric 3–4-month course at this dose, followed by repeat FDG-PET imaging to define therapeutic efficacy.

TABLE 9.4A
Dietary Instructions and Yale Diet Prep for FDG-PET for Cardiac Sarcoidosis

The 24 h before Examination	High-fat and low-carbohydrate diet. Finish evening meal no later than 12 h before examination.
	Eat fatty unsweetened, nonbreaded foods including chicken, turkey, fish, meats, fried eggs, bacon, scrambled eggs prepared without milk, fried eggs, bacon, and hamburgers (plain, without the bun or vegetables).
	Do not eat any food containing carbohydrates and sugars including milk, cheese, bread, bagels, cereal, cookies, grits, oatmeal, toast, pasta, crackers, muffins, peanut butter, peanuts, fruit juice, potatoes, candy, fruit, rice, chewing gum, mints, cough drops, beans, alcohol, or any natural or artificial sweeteners
	Drink clear liquids without milk or sugars or artificial sweeteners: coffee without milk or sugar, no drinks with natural or artificial sweeteners (ex. Diet Pepsi, Diet Coke, Nutra-sweet), tea without milk or sugar, water.
After evening meal (~ 6 p.m.)	Fast until the test is finished the next day (water is allowed).
The morning of exam	Do not eat any food Drink water, coffee, or tea (no sugar or milk). Do not drink any sugary drinks, sodas, or juice

At that point, we wean prednisone slowly over the course of several months and repeat a third FDG-PET scan while on the lowest tolerated prednisone dose (usually 5–10 mg/day prednisone) to ensure there is no rebound of cardiac inflammation.

Owing to side effects associated with the use of steroids, alternative agents such as methotrexate (up 20 mg oral weekly), azathioprine (100 mg oral daily), infliximab (3–5 mg/kg initially then every 4–8 weeks), or mycophenolate are considered in addition to or as a replacement for steroids. They are more widely used in systemic sarcoidosis—data in CS are limited.

TABLE 9.4B
Patient Food Diary

Day Before Exam	Time	Food/Drinks	Comments
Breakfast			
Lunch			
Dinner			
Snacks			
Day of Exam			

Treatment monitoring with FDG-PET

FDG-PET imaging can be used for monitoring of treatment response in cardiac sarcoidosis. Increased FDG uptake in metabolically active macrophages, which rely on glucose as substrate for metabolism, are assumed to represent active ongoing inflammation and CS disease activity. Patient preparation for FDG-PET requires specific dietary mechanisms to reduce physiological FDG uptake in myocardial cells and shift myocardial metabolism to fatty acids. Although the ideal patient preparation is an area of controversy, our approach combines prolonged fasting (12–18 h) with dietary modification of high fat and low carbohydrates. Specifically, we recommend a high-fat/low-carbohydrate diet beginning at breakfast the day before the scan, followed by a strict fast (except clear water) after 6 p.m. the night before the study. Imaging laboratory personnel should contact all patients several days before the scan and provide specific written dietary instructions (Table 9.4a) and ask them to maintain a food diary (Table 9.4b) to help ensure compliance and consistency in preparation for serial FDG-PET scans. Common pitfalls for patients include the inclusion of cream in coffee, breath mints, antacids, and so on. These can all lead to incomplete suppression of myocardial glucose uptake, and if the patient admits to consuming any glucose-containing foods after 6 p.m. the night prior to the examination, then the examination should be canceled and rescheduled. In addition to FDG images, we recommend all patients receive resting perfusion imaging with either SPECT (Tc-99m sestamibi or tetrofosmin) or PET (Rb-82 or N-13 ammonia) to evaluate for perfusion defects assumed to be from myocardial scar. Myocardial perfusion images are acquired followed by injection of FDG and acquiring images after an uptake period of 90 min. FDG images are interpreted qualitatively by visual

TABLE 9.5
Quantitative Metrics for FDG-PET

SUV max	Maximal SUV Intensity Pixel in Myocardium Corrected by Injected Dose and Patients Weight
SUV mean	Mean of segmental, ROI, or LV SUVs
Coefficient of Variance	Standard deviation of uptake divided by mean uptake in 17 segments
CMV	Volume of abnormal myocardial FDG-positive voxels above a predetermined threshold (ex. 1.5× left ventricular blood pool SUV)
CMA	Volume of abnormal myocardial FDG-positive voxels (CMV) multiplied by the mean activity in that region. Expressed in "grams of glucose"

CMA, Cardiac metabolic activity; *CMV*, Cardiac metabolic volume; *ROI*, Region of interest; *SUV*, standardized uptake value.

TABLE 9.6
Recommendations for ICD Placement in Patients With Cardiac Sarcoidosis (HRS Expert Consensus Statement Guidelines)[1]

Class I	Spontaneous sustained ventricular arrhythmias, including prior cardiac arrest
	Left ventricular ejection fraction 35% or less despite optimal medical/immunosuppressive therapy
Class IIa	An indication for permanent pacemaker placement independent of ejection fraction Symptomatic Mobitz type II second-degree and third-degree heart block even if there is transient reversibility Cardiogenic syncope Inducible sustained ventricular tachycardi
	Postablation treatment for ventricular tachycardia
Class IIb	LVEF 36%–49% or Right ventricular ejection fraction less than 40% despite optimal medical/immunosuppressive treatment

assessment of FDG uptake and quantitatively by using standardized uptake value (SUV)–based parameters for cardiac sarcoidosis (Table 9.5). Quantitative interpretation of FDG uptake is critical to increase the specificity of the reads and determine response to therapy on serial scans.

ICD placement

There is a high rate of ventricular arrhythmias, conduction abnormalities, and sudden cardiac deaths in patients with cardiac sarcoidosis. The HRS consensus statement includes general primary and secondary prevention guidelines for ICD placement in cardiac sarcoidosis patients (Table 9.6). Secondary prevention ICD implantation (Class I) is recommended in patients with a history of VT/VF or sudden cardiac death. For primary prevention, patients who meet other ICD criteria (e.g., LVEF<35%) warrant ICDs. In CS patients with a need for a pacemaker due to conduction system disease, simultaneous ICD implantation can be considered (Class IIa). In asymptomatic CS patients with preserved LVEF, primary prevention ICD placement is an area of some controversy. Holter monitoring and/or programmed electrical stimulation can be used to assess arrhythmic risk, as can LGE volume on CMR or focal FDG uptake on PET. An individualized decision-making approach involving the patient, cardiologist, electrophysiologist, and sarcoid physician is often needed in cases of uncertainty.

What Constitutes "Complicated CS" and Who/When Do You Refer to a CS Specialist?

As described previously, cardiac sarcoidosis is not a singular diagnosis. There is a spectrum of disease that can range from a patient with extracardiac sarcoidosis who has mild LGE on CMR and infrequent PVCs to a patient with persistent inflammation on FDG-PET, large myocardial scars, congestive heart failure, pacemaker dependency, and need for heart transplantation evaluation. Obviously, these two patients

TABLE 9.7
Complicated CS

Clinical Features	Advanced Imaging
Sustained ventricular tachycardia	Multifocal FDG uptake and resting perfusion defects
Acute AV block	FDG uptake in right ventricle
Transplant evaluation	Left ventricular dysfunction. Late gadolinium enhancement on CMR including focal LGE and the extent of LGE (LGE mass ≥20% of LV mass). Perfusion defects on perfusion imaging
Symptomatic CS with coexisting pulmonary involvement	Depressed left ventricular ejection fraction, large left ventricle end diastolic diameter on echocardiography

CS, cardiac sarcoidosis; *LGE*, late gadolinium enhancement.

require much different capabilities and expertise involved in their care. This suggests the concept of "complicated" cardiac sarcoidosis, in which certain high-risk features should prompt consideration of referral to a center with multidisciplinary expertise in sarcoidosis care.

Recently, WASOG in partnership with the Foundation for Sarcoidosis Research has established "WASOG Sarcoidosis Centers of Excellence" that include a "multidisciplinary team of specialized medical and paramedical professionals with a shared specialized facility that has proven sustainability over years and provides leadership, best practices, research, support, and/or training for sarcoidosis patients and professionals." In the case of cardiac sarcoidosis, the multidisciplinary team can include experts in heart failure/transplantation, immunosuppression, arrhythmias, cardiac MRI, and cardiac FDG-PET imaging, in collaboration with pulmonary, rheumatology, neurology, and other multispecialty colleagues. Given the crucial nature of cardiac imaging to the diagnosis and management of CS patients, the inclusion of expert cardiac imagers is very important.

Some high-risk features that should warrant consideration of Cardiac Sarcoidosis Center referrals (Table 9.7) can include advanced left ventricular dysfunction, need for transplantation evaluation, need for immunosuppression for cardiac inflammation, need for adjunctive immunosuppression (either persistent or progressing inflammation on FDG-PET), complex arrhythmias, and/or diagnostic uncertainty. In particular, a lack of experience with or access to FDG-PET imaging or a lack of knowledge of its use in CS patients should prompt referral to CS centers of excellence.

SUMMARY AND CONCLUSIONS

In summary, cardiac sarcoidosis remains a diagnosis with life-changing implications for patients. Appropriate screening can range from an ECG to FDG-PET or CMR imaging depending on the clinical condition of the patient. JMHW, HRS, and WASOG guidelines include important criteria to be aware of when assessing patients. Combining these criteria with advanced imaging modalities for CS diagnosis is nuanced and optimally requires the input of an experienced clinician. Treatment of patients with immunosuppression or ICD placement, particularly in a complicated CS population, requires consideration of the risks and benefits tailored to the individual patient. CS centers with multidisciplinary teams are ideally trained to provide specialized services to this unique patient population.

REFERENCES

1. Birnie DH, Sauer WH, Bogun F, et al. HRS expert consensus statement on the diagnosis and management of arrhythmias associated with cardiac sarcoidosis. *Heart Rhythm*. 2014;11(7):1304–1323. https://doi.org/10.1016/j.hrthm.2014.03.043.
2. Chareonthaitawee P, Beanlands RS, Chen W, et al. Joint SNMMI–ASNC expert consensus document on the role of 18F-FDG PET/CT in cardiac sarcoid detection and therapy monitoring. *J Nuclear Med*. 2017;58(8):1341–1353. https://doi.org/10.2967/jnumed.117.196287.
3. Slart RHJA, Glaudemans AWJM, Lancellotti P, et al. A joint procedural position statement on imaging in cardiac sarcoidosis: from the cardiovascular and inflammation & infection committees of the European association of nuclear medicine, the European association of cardiovascular imaging, and the American Society of Nuclear Cardiology. *J Nuclear Cardiol*. 2018:298–319.

4. Diagnostic standard and guidelines for sarcoidosis. *Jpn J Sarcoidosis Granulomatous Disord.* 2007;27:89–102.
5. Judson MA, Costabel U, Drent M, et al. The WASOG Sarcoidosis organ assessment instrument: an update of a previous clinical tool. *Sarcoidosis Vasc Diffuse Lung Dis.* 2014;31(1):19–27.
6. Kandolin R, Lehtonen J, Graner M, et al. Diagnosing isolated cardiac sarcoidosis. *J Intern Med.* 2011;270(5):461–468. https://doi.org/10.1111/j.1365-2796.2011.02396.x.
7. Vita T, Okada DR, Veillet-Chowdhury M, et al. Complementary value of cardiac magnetic resonance imaging and positron emission tomography/computed tomography in the assessment of cardiac sarcoidosis. *Circ Cardiovasc Imaging.* 2018;11(1):e007030. https://doi.org/10.1161/CIRCIMAGING.117.007030.
8. Sadek MM, Yung D, Birnie DH, Beanlands RS, Nery PB. Corticosteroid therapy for cardiac sarcoidosis: a systematic review. *Can J Cardiol.* 2013;29(9):1034–1041. https://doi.org/10.1016/j.cjca.2013.02.004.
9. Osborne MT, Hulten EA, Singh A, et al. Reduction in ^{18}F-fluorodeoxyglucose uptake on serial cardiac positron emission tomography is associated with improved left ventricular ejection fraction in patients with cardiac sarcoidosis. *J Nuclear Cardiol.* 2014;21(1):166–174. https://doi.org/10.1007/s12350-013-9828-6.
10. Ahmadian A, Pawar S, Govender P, Berman J, Ruberg FL, Miller EJ. The response of FDG uptake to immunosuppressive treatment on FDG PET/CT imaging for cardiac sarcoidosis. *J Nuclear Cardiol.* 2017;24(2):413–424. https://doi.org/10.1007/s12350-016-0490-7.

CHAPTER 10

Neurosarcoidosis

FLEUR COHEN AUBART, MD, PHD • THIBAUD CHAZAL, MD • RAPHAËL LHOTE, MD • ZAHIR AMOURA, MD, MSC

Sarcoidosis is a multisystemic granulomatous disease of unknown cause characterized by the presence of noncaseating granuloma in various organs.[1,2] Affected organs are mainly the lung, eyes, skin, lymph nodes, spleen, and liver. The neurological localizations of sarcoidosis, so-called neurosarcoidosis, are rare (5%–40% depending on criteria, arising from clinical or autopsy studies). Any part of the central nervous system (CNS) or peripheral nervous system (PNS) may be affected, leading to protean manifestations. Among sarcoidosis manifestations, neurological involvement is characterized by diagnosis and therapeutic difficulties. First, neurosarcoidosis may be the first manifestation of the disease, and the other localizations may be clinically silent. Then, nervous system tissue is difficult to access for histological documentation. Finally, neurosarcoidosis has a protracted course, and the treatment management is affected by the blood-brain barrier. In this chapter, we will describe clinical, biological, and imaging presentations of neurosarcoidosis, as well as treatments and general management. From 1985 to 2017, 20 series of more than 10 patients with CNS sarcoidosis have been described in the English literature. The percentages given in this chapter are summarized from these series.

CLINICAL PRESENTATIONS OF NEUROSARCOIDOSIS

Clinical involvement of nervous system is rare during sarcoidosis (5%–10% of cases).[3] Neurological manifestations often reveal sarcoidosis (50%–70% of patients) and may constitute the unique localization of the disease (20% of cases).[4–9] Although all parts of the nervous system can be affected, some presentations are more common. The CNS is more frequently affected (85% of cases), whereas the PNS, including muscle, is affected in 10%–15% of cases.[10,11]

CENTRAL NERVOUS SYSTEM LOCALIZATIONS OF SARCOIDOSIS

The CNS localizations of sarcoidosis have been described in several series, all of them being retrospective. The localizations in the CNS may be divided into meningeal (50%), cerebral intraparenchymal (50%), cranial nerves (11%–80%) including optic nerves (3%–38%), medullary (3%–43%), and pituitary (20%) localizations.[4,6–9,12–24] The clinical signs of CNS sarcoidosis depend on the localization of granulomas and are detailed in Table 10.1; headache, motor or sensory deficits, sphincter disturbances, psychiatric manifestations, cognitive disturbances, and epilepsy are the most frequently seen signs.[25–28]

The most frequently affected cranial nerves are the optic, trigeminal, and facial nerves,[21] followed by cochleovestibular and oculomotor nerves. Cranial nerves palsy may be transient or lead to persistent deficit. Optical neuropathy is usually associated with classical signs of optic nerve involvement (progressive or subacute visual loss, retro-orbital pain, color vision changes).[29]

Diffuse meningeal involvement may lead to cognitive disturbances, depression (10% of cases), or other types of psychiatric disorders.[30] Seizures may also be observed in case of diffuse meningeal involvement. Intracranial hypertension may be associated with meningeal granuloma and is associated with a worse prognosis.[31] Intracranial hypertension may present with headache resistant to level one analgesics, nausea or vomiting, and/or papilledema. A high cerebrospinal fluid (CSF) protein level is an indirect sign of elevated intracranial hypertension and may prompt urgent treatment. In the most severe cases, intracranial hypertension requires urgent neurosurgical management with implantation of ventriculoperitoneal, ventriculoatrial, or external shunt valves, which may be transient or more often definitive.[32]

Sarcoidosis. https://doi.org/10.1016/B978-0-323-54429-0.00010-0

TABLE 10.1
Presentations of Neurosarcoidosis

Localizations	Clinical Presentation	Frequency*	Main Differential Diagnoses	Notes
CNS		85%–90%		
Meningeal	Heterogeneous presentation: headache, cognitive impairment, psychiatric manifestations, epilepsy, intracranial hypertension; may be asymptomatic	10%–50%	• Infectious diseases (tuberculosis, Lyme disease, Whipple disease, HIV infection, PML, other bacteria, viruses, and fungi) • Solid or hematological malignancies • Autoimmune disorders: systemic lupus erythematosus, Behcet's disease, granulomatosis with polyangiitis • IgG4-associated disease, histiocytoses	May be defined by meningeal gadolinium enhancement on MRI or pleocytosis in CSF analyses
Parenchymal	Various presentations: motor or sensory deficits, epilepsy, ataxia, cerebellar impairment; may be asymptomatic	20%–40%	• Demyelinating disorders: MS, NMO spectrum disorder • Infectious and autoimmune diseases Solid or hematological malignancies	May be supratentorial or infratentorial
Medullar	Motor and/or sensory deficits; Sphincter disorders; Conus medullaris syndrome	3%–43%	• MS • NMO spectrum disorders • Neoplasia • Behcet's disease • Vitamin B12 deficiency Cervical arthrosis	Inflammatory lesions may be located next to compression area
Pituitary	Anterior pituitary insufficiency; Diabetes Insipidus	≈20%		Associated with sinonasal localizations
Optic nerves	Optical neuritis; may be associated with posterior or anterior uveitis	3%–38%		

Cranial nerves (optic nerves excluded)	Most frequently involved: V, VII More rarely: VIII, III, IV, VI May be bilateral or alternating right/left	11%–80%	May recover spontaneously; frequently relapsing
Others	Brain parenchymal involvement of variable localization Pseudotumoral presentations Temporal localization with pseudodementia presentation Stroke-like presentations Central venous thrombosis	NA	Rarely intracranial hemorrhage
PNS		10%–15%	
Radiculopathies	Monoradicular or pluriradicular presentations; Cauda equina syndrome; thoracic nerves involvement	NA	
Muscle	Nodular form; myopathic form; mixed neuropathic and myopathic form; smoldering form	5%	The myopathic form has a less good prognosis
Others	Axonal motor and/or sensory neuropathy; pseudo-demyelinating neuropathy; multiplex mononeuritis; small fibers neuropathy	Rare	

*Relative frequency.
CNS, central nervous system; *MS,* multiple sclerosis; *NA,* not applicable; *NMO,* neuromyelitis optica; *PML,* progressive multifocal leukoencephalopathy; *PNS*, peripheral nervous system.

Pituitary involvement may lead to diabetes insipidus, hyperphagia, and abnormalities of the thermal regulation.[20,33] Owing to the diffusion of granuloma in adjacent structures, pituitary involvement is often associated with optic nerves involvement and sometimes with lupus pernio.

Myelopathies occur in 3%–43% of patients with neurosarcoidosis and lead to significant morbidity.[25] Differential diagnoses include clinical isolated syndromes; multiple sclerosis; vascular myelopathy; optical neuromyelitis spectrum disorder; compressive, infectious, or nutritional myelitis.[34] Back or radicular pain is more frequent in spinal cord sarcoidosis than in other myelopathies and may guide the diagnosis.

PNS LOCALIZATIONS OF SARCOIDOSIS

PNS involvement may be responsible for a broad spectrum of PNS manifestations, including radiculopathy, axonal, or pseudo-demyelinating neuropathy.[11,35] Pure motor neuropathy may mimic anterior horn disease.[36] A classical presentation is multiradicular, proximal, symmetrical, or nonacute or chronic onset neuropathy mimicking inflammatory demyelinating polyneuropathy. These patterns are readily associated with lymphocytic meningitis on CSF analysis (so-called "meningoradiculopathy"). Small intraepidermal fiber involvement has been described[37] and may be suspected ahead of painful presentation, with or without large fibers neuropathy.

Muscular localization may present with distinct clinical presentations: (1) a nodular pattern with palpable nodules, (2) an acute form, also rare and occurring at the beginning of the evolution of the disease, and (3) a pseudo-myopathic form, of later occurrence especially in women, which is the most frequent presentation of the muscular lesions of sarcoidosis.[10,38] Muscular localization may also be typically associated with neuropathy. The nodular pattern is associated with cutaneous involvement.[39]

EXTRANEUROLOGICAL INVOLVEMENT DURING NEUROSARCOIDOSIS

The extraneurological lesions associated with neurosarcoidosis may be clinically silent.[22] Mediastino-pulmonary involvement can be found in 30%–94% of cases with or without thoracic symptoms; ocular involvement in 25%–56% of cases; skin in 7%–30% of cases; peripheral lymph nodes in 10% of cases; and eye, nose, and throat involvement histologically proven in 10%–15% of cases. Sinonasal involvement is readily associated with hypothalamic-pituitary localization.[33] Cardiac involvement is found in 30% of cases.[14] An analysis of clinical phenotypes of sarcoidosis demonstrated the association of ocular, cardiac, cutaneous, and central nervous system disease involvements.[40]

BIOLOGICAL CHARACTERISTICS OF NEUROSARCOIDOSIS

As in sarcoidosis without neurological involvement, the serum angiotensin-conversion enzyme (ACE) is elevated in only 25%–50% of cases and is not a diagnostic test. Other blood laboratory abnormalities may be found such as lymphopenia, moderately increased C-reactive protein, elevated liver or muscle enzymes, polyclonal hypergammaglobulinemia. Hypercalcemia and hypercalciuria are more specific and should be evaluated in case of suspicion of neurosarcoidosis.

Phenotyping of regulatory T cells may show an expansion of activated regulatory T cells and a decrease in quiescent regulatory T cells but is not routinely performed.[41]

The CSF analysis obtained by lumbar puncture usually displays pleocytosis (50% of cases) with elevated lymphocyte count, sometimes associated with hypoglycorachia (up to 50% of cases when there is hypercellularity). In 20%–50% of cases, the presence of CSF-specific oligoclonal bands may be observed. Pleiocytosis and hypoglycorachia are biological signs of activity during neurosarcoidosis.[42] ACE dosage in CSF is not useful as it may be elevated in sarcoidosis and also in other inflammatory neurological disorders.[25,43] The interest of CSF lymphocytes phenotype and cytokines (such as interleukin 6 and 10) dosages has to be studied.[16,44,45]

IMAGING IN NEUROSARCOIDOIS

Brain and spinal magnetic resonance imaging (MRI) are useful for detecting CNS neurosarcoidosis. Brain MRI shows T2 or Fluid-Attenuated Inversion Recovery (FLAIR) parenchymal hyperintensities that have a nonspecific appearance (Fig. 10.1). T2 hyperintensities sometimes meet the Barkhof criteria.[46] Hyperintensities may be found in supratentorial white matter, brainstem, gray nuclei, and/or cerebellum.[19,32] However, some localizations are particularly suggestive of neurosarcoidosis: (1) involvement of the optic nerves, brainstem, and cerebellar peduncles and (2) involvement of the pituitary axis.[33] Leptomeningeal gadolinium enhancement is frequently observed in brain or spinal MRI. It is highly suggestive of neurosarcoidosis when

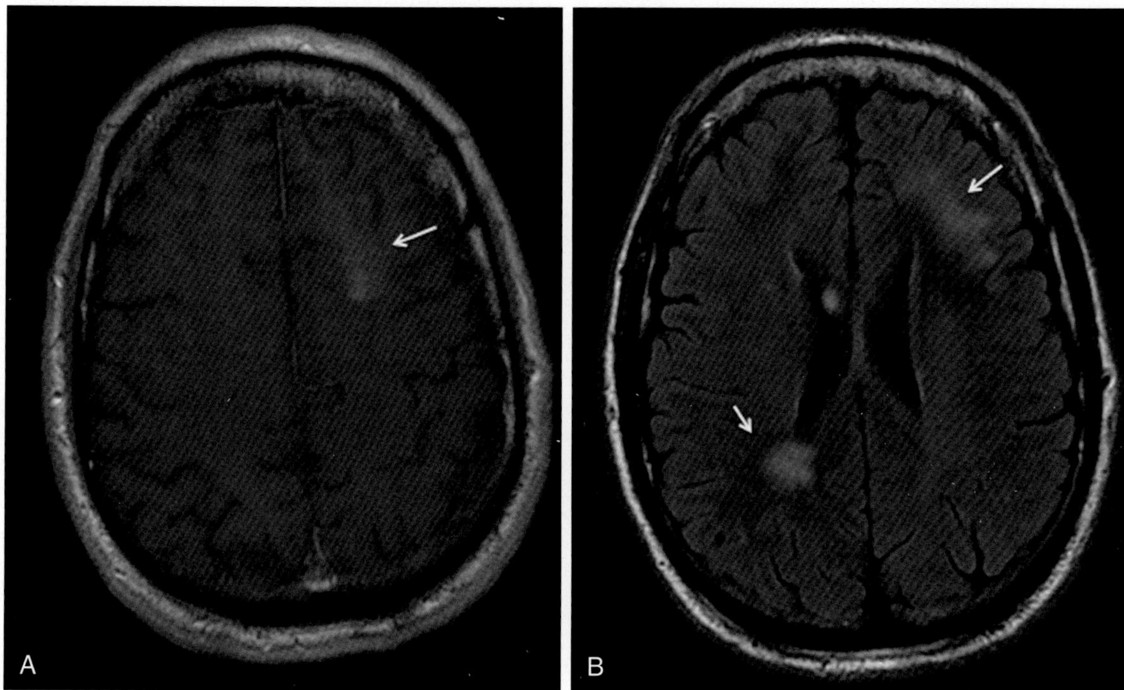

FIG. 10.1 Brain magnetic resonance imaging of central nervous system sarcoidosis. **(A)** Gadolinium enhancement of the parenchymal lesion (*arrows*) (brain magnetic resonance imaging, T1 weighted). **(B)** Parenchymal lesions in T2-weighted FLAIR imaging (same patient seen in **A**).

it has a confluent micronodular appearance (Fig. 10.1). The cranial nerves can be thickened or enhanced on gadolinium T1-weighted images. In the same way, the optic nerves can be enlarged and hyperintense in FLAIR images and may be enhanced in gadolinium T1 images. As in diffuse meningeal involvement, gadolinium enhancement is typically around the nerves and has a micronodular appearance. Ventricular dilation can be observed and should prompt the diagnosis of intracranial hypertension that requires urgent treatment (as mentioned previously). There are exceptional "stroke-like" ischemic or hemorrhagic forms.[47,48] However, it is essential to differentiate these rare presentations of neurosarcoidosis, in which granulomas are present in the wall of the vessels or around it, from other conditions, which can also lead to stroke episodes during sarcoidosis (e.g., atheroma, atrial fibrillation). Stroke-like presentations should not be confused from cerebral granulomatous vasculitis, a rare condition mostly occurring during the course of hematologic or infectious diseases such as tuberculosis (Figs. S1 and S2).

Spinal cord MRI may also show meningeal enhancement and/or intramedullary hypersignal. Gadolinium enhancement and T2 hyperintensities are generally extensive (more than three vertebral bodies).[25,26] This can help to differentiate sarcoidosis myelopathy from other demyelinating affections where the T2 hyperintense image is less than one vertebral body height. The spinal cord often presents with edema. When sarcoidosis myelopathy is seen next to a herniated disk ("Kubner" phenomenon in spinal cord), it may be confused with compressive myelopathy.[49] The extension of images beyond the area of compression should evoke sarcoidosis myelopathy. At a late stage of sarcoidomyelopathy, MRI shows bone marrow atrophy. The main differential diagnosis of extensive spinal cord injury is optic neuromyelitis spectrum disorders,[50] and the determination of the antiaquaporin four antibodies is essential. Other differential diagnoses include lupus and primary Sjogren syndrome myelopathies, Behcet's disease, infectious or tumoral myelopathies, and B12 deficiency.

DIAGNOSIS CRITERIA

Examples of differential diagnoses of neurosarcoidosis are listed in Table 10.1 and depend of the clinical presentation. Definite neurosarcoidosis is defined

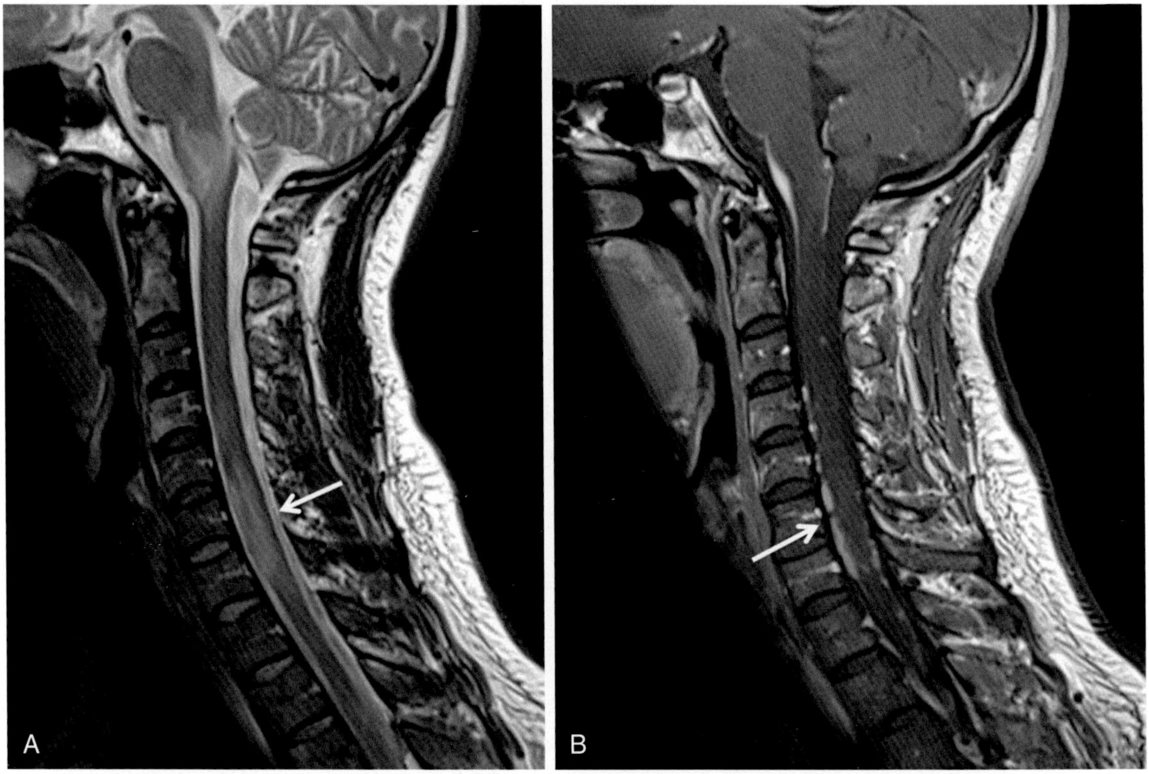

FIG. S1 Sarcoidosis myelitis. Sagittal cervical spine MRI. **(A)** T2-weighted images showing longitudinally extensive myelitis with T2-hyperintensity (*arrow*). **(B)** T1-weighted images showing leptomeningeal gadolinium enhancement (*arrow*). *MRI*, magnetic resonance imaging.

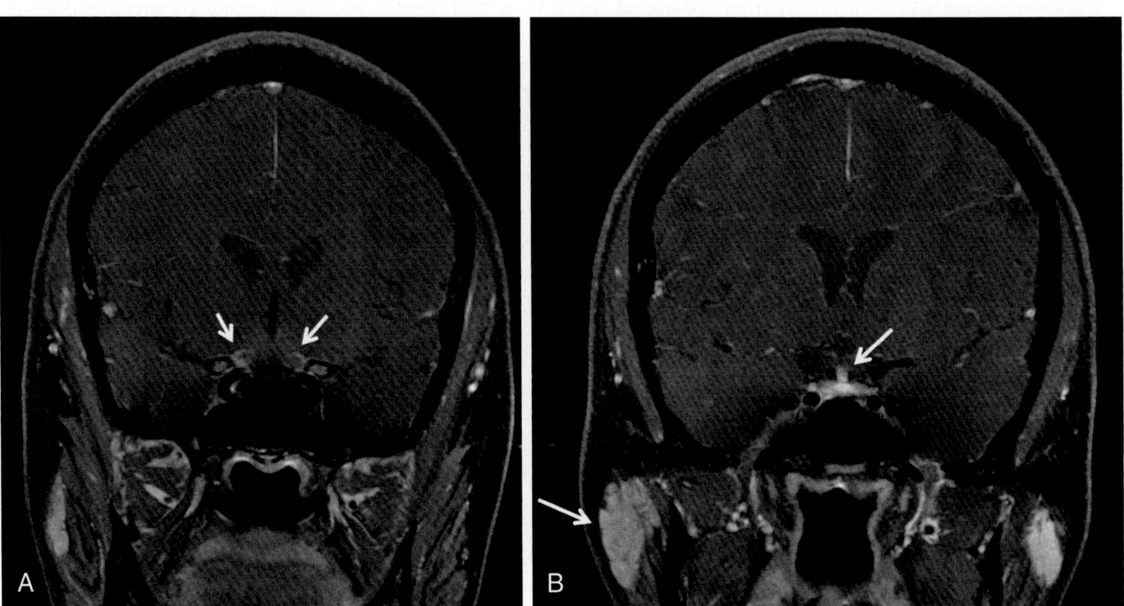

FIG. S2 Sarcoidosis optic nerves and pituitary involvements. Coronal brain MRI, T1-weighted images. **(A)** Leptomeningeal enhancement with granulomatous appearance surrounding the optic nerves (*arrows*). **(B)** Pituitary thickening and parotidomegaly (*arrows*).

TABLE 10.2
Diagnosis Criteria of Neurosarcoidosis

Definite neurosarcoidosis	• Clinical presentation compatible with neurosarcoidosis • Exclusion of differential diagnoses • Documentation of noncaseating granuloma in CNS or PNS tissue
Probable	• Clinical presentation compatible with neurosarcoidosis • Presence of indirect signs of neurological inflammation (elevated CSF level, CSF pleocytosis) and/or brain or spine MRI or electrophysiological studies compatible with neurosarcoidosis • Exclusion of differential diagnoses • Documentation of noncaseating granuloma in a tissue other than CNS or PNS
Possible	• Clinical presentation compatible with neurosarcoidosis • Exclusion of differential diagnoses • Criteria for definite or probable neurosarcoidosis are not fulfilled

CNS, central nervous system; *CSF*, cerebrospinal fluid; *MRI*, magnetic resonance imaging; *PNS*, peripheral nervous system.
Adapted from Zajicek et al.

as neurological involvement with documentation of granuloma in the nervous system. The diagnosis of sarcoidosis is based on the combination of[1] compatible clinical and radiological features[2] of histological documentation of noncaseating epithelioid granuloma[3] and exclusion of other causes of granulomatosis.[51] Probable neurosarcoidosis is considered if the neurological involvement is associated with the presence of granuloma in an extraneurological organ. Finally, possible neurosarcoidosis may be considered if the aforementioned conditions are not met[18] (Table 10.2, adapted from Zajicek[18]), considering that an extensive workout has been realized.

Compared to other localizations of sarcoidosis, neurosarcoidosis is characterized with the difficulty of obtaining histological evidence of granulomas in the CNS.[31] The response to treatment is a major additional argument for neurosarcoidosis diagnosis. Whether sarcoidosis is documented or not, resistance to treatment should question the diagnosis. The diagnosis of neurosarcoidosis without histological evidence ("possible neurosarcoidosis" according to Zajicek criteria) leads to diagnosis errors in a number of cases. A specialized advice is recommended in these cases.

The most easily accessible organs for obtaining histological evidence in case of neurological presentation suggestive of neurosarcoidosis are minor salivary glands (20%–40% positivity), bronchial biopsies (20%–35% positivity), peripheral or mediastinal lymph nodes, skin, liver, and bones. Skin localization is an easy site for obtaining histological evidence when present (consider recent modification of scars). Liver biopsy may be considered in case of blood liver tests abnormalities. Muscle biopsy should be performed only in case of clinical or laboratory signs of muscle involvement. The choice of biopsy sites can be guided by 18 fludeoxyglucose (FDG)–positron emission tomography (PET) scanner.[52]

MANAGEMENT OF NEUROLOGICAL SIGNS OCCURRING AT ONSET OR DURING THE COURSE OF SARCOIDOSIS

In 1 of 3 cases, the neurological signs occur during the course of sarcoidosis. In this case, the challenge is to be sure that neurological manifestations are related to sarcoidosis. Other diagnoses, such as infections, tumors, and multiple sclerosis may be ruled out.

When the diagnosis of sarcoidosis has not been previously made, the challenge is to discuss the diagnosis of sarcoidosis and to obtain histological evidence.

The 18FDG-PET scanner can help finding hypermetabolic areas, which can be biopsied, if the first-line examinations are not suggestive of sarcoidosis localizations.[52,53] Its added value when previous examinations are normal or negative has not been evaluated.[52,54] If finally the neurosarcoidosis diagnosis could not be confirmed, a nervous system biopsy will have to be discussed if the lesions are reachable.

When histological evidence of epithelioid granulomas is found outside the CNS (probable neurosarcoidosis), physicians must be ensured that the biological presentation (especially CSF) and imaging are at least compatible, if not typical, with neurosarcoidosis because other conditions may be responsible for a neurological involvement associated with the presence of granulomas (lymphomas, neoplasia, and Rosai-Dorfman's disease in particular).[55]

Differential diagnoses must also be ruled out, in particular, tuberculosis or other infections (Lyme disease, infection with the human immunodeficiency virus, progressive multifocal leukoencephalopathy), vasculitis associated with antineutrophil cytoplasmic antibodies, such as granulomatosis with polyangiitis, Sjögren syndrome, systemic lupus erythematosus, histiocytosis, IgG4-related disease, and also multiple sclerosis, optic neuromyelitis spectrum disorders, lymphomas, and cancers (Table 10.1). Neurosarcoidosis presentation is usually different from multiple sclerosis, which is characterized by the presence of extraneurological signs, hypercellularity and elevated CSF protein level, and low CSF glucose level. CSF-specific oligoclonal bands may be found in sarcoidosis (as mentioned previously) and is not helpful to differentiate these two entities.

The diagnostic approach ahead of PNS manifestation is easier because a nerve or muscle sample can be more easily performed. For radicular lesions, the same diagnosis approach as for the CNS may apply.

TREATMENTS OF NEUROSARCOIDOSIS

There is currently no randomized clinical trial that specifically addressed the question of the treatment of neurosarcoidosis. The treatment propositions that are detailed below are based on retrospective studies. In all cases, it is recommended to get an advice from a tertiary care center because of the rarity of this condition.

Corticosteroids are the cornerstone of the treatment of neurosarcoidosis. Steroids have a rapid anti-inflammatory action, which is usually necessary when neurological manifestation occur. Prednisone should be preferred to prednisolone because of a better bioavailability. In life-threatening situations, methylprednisolone should be given intravenously. The steroid dosage is not well established, usually higher (1 mg/kg/day) in case of motor or visual deficit, intracranial hypertension, or sphincter disturbances. In other cases, steroids dosage may be reduced (0.5 mg/kg/day), e.g., in pure and moderate sensory impairment.[31]

The need for an immunosuppressive drug is not proven in neurosarcoidosis.[13,15] However, CNS or PNS localizations usually indicate that the disease will have a chronic course and that the treatment will have to be prolonged for several years.[2] Immunosuppressive drugs may help to limit the total cumulative dose of steroids and may help to reduce the doses without relapse to reach a daily dosage of prednisone less than 0.1 mg/kg/day. The immunosuppressive drugs that are the most used in neurosarcoidosis are methotrexate, azathioprine, and mycophenolate mofetil.[56–58] Methotrexate was shown to be more efficacious to prevent relapses than mycophenolate mofetil in a retrospective study of neurosarcoidosis.[59] Hydroxychloroquine has also been used in some moderate forms.[60] Cyclosporine, cladribine, and rituximab have also been successfully used but always in combination with corticosteroids.[61–63] In case of incomplete response to corticosteroid therapy, or in severe cases, particularly in myelopathies, immunosuppressive drugs may also help the action of steroids; infliximab, an anti–TNF-alpha, and cyclophosphamide may be chosen.[64–66] Anti–TNF-alpha drugs, in particular infliximab, a chimeric monoclonal antibody directed against TNF-alpha, have shown an efficacy for the treatment of neurosarcoidosis reported in several series.[65,67–70] Infliximab is usually used at a dose of 3–5 mg/kg (D1-D15 then every 4–8 weeks).[71] A high incidence of infectious adverse events during infliximab therapy has been reported, probably related to the multiple lines of previous immunosuppressive therapy received by these patients. Anti–TNF-alpha drugs, as other drugs, do not cure sarcoidosis, and relapses are frequent when discontinued.[72] A biosimilar agent of infliximab has also been used in a small series and seems efficacious.[73] Radiotherapy had been described for neurosarcoidosis treatment but should not be used nowadays given the efficacy of anti–TNF-alpha. The neurosurgical indications are limited to refractory intracranial hypertension or for obtaining a histological documentation if not possible outside the nervous system.

In all cases, the treatment must be prolonged because relapse rate is high in neurosarcoidosis. There is no consensual duration, but usually a minimal period of 2 years is recommended. During follow-up, opportunistic infections may occur, some of which may mimic neurological involvement of sarcoidosis.[74,75]

Finally, there is an increased thromboembolic risk in case of neurosarcoidosis; this should be particularly remembered in case of symptoms such as dyspnea or chest pain, particularly in patients whose mobility is impaired.[76]

OUTCOMES

The neurological locations of sarcoidosis are serious; 2 of 3 patients have clinical, motor, sensory, sphincter or cognitive sequelae. Some localizations have a severe prognosis and have increased morbidity, including spinal cord injury and axonal motor neuropathy. Conversely, meningeal or cranial nerves' involvements have typically a better prognosis.

Treatments are often prolonged and lead to complications, such as opportunistic infections.[77]

CONCLUSIONS

The neurological localizations of sarcoidosis are rare although severe. The diagnosis may be difficult when neurological signs are inaugural. The spectrum of differential diagnoses is broad, and this adds to diagnosis difficulties. When neurological signs occur during the course of sarcoidosis, infectious diseases may be ruled out. Specialized advice may be useful for diagnosis and treatment.

REFERENCES

1. Iannuzzi MC, Rybicki BA, Teirstein AS. Sarcoidosis. *N Engl J Med.* 2007;357(21):2153–2165.
2. Valeyre D, Prasse A, Nunes H, Uzunhan Y, Brillet PY, Muller-Quernheim J. Sarcoidosis. *Lancet.* 2014;383(9923): 1155–1167.
3. Fritz D, van de Beek D, Brouwer MC. Clinical features, treatment and outcome in neurosarcoidosis: systematic review and meta-analysis. *BMC Neurol.* 2016;16(1):220.
4. Ferriby D, de Seze J, Stojkovic T, et al. Long-term follow-up of neurosarcoidosis. *Neurology.* 2001;57(5):927–929.
5. Hoitsma E, Faber CG, Drent M, Sharma OP. Neurosarcoidosis: a clinical dilemma. *Lancet Neurol.* 2004;3(7):397–407.
6. Joseph FG, Scolding NJ. Neurosarcoidosis: a study of 30 new cases. *J Neurol Neurosurg Psychiatry.* 2009;80(3):297–304.
7. Lower EE, Broderick JP, Brott TG, Baughman RP. Diagnosis and management of neurological sarcoidosis. *Arch Intern Med.* 1997;157(16):1864–1868.
8. Luke RA, Stern BJ, Krumholz A, Johns CJ. Neurosarcoidosis: the long-term clinical course. *Neurology.* 1987;37(3):461–463.
9. Pawate S, Moses H, Sriram S. Presentations and outcomes of neurosarcoidosis: a study of 54 cases. *QJM Mon J Assoc Phys.* 2009;102(7):449–460.
10. Le Roux K, Streichenberger N, Vial C, et al. Granulomatous myositis: a clinical study of thirteen cases. *Muscle Nerve.* 2007;35(2):171–177.
11. Burns TM, Dyck PJ, Aksamit AJ, Dyck PJ. The natural history and long-term outcome of 57 limb sarcoidosis neuropathy cases. *J Neurol Sci.* 2006;244(1–2):77–87.
12. Spencer TS, Campellone JV, Maldonado I, Huang N, Usmani Q, Reginato AJ. Clinical and magnetic resonance imaging manifestations of neurosarcoidosis. *Semin Arthritis Rheum.* 2005;34(4):649–661.
13. Scott TF, Yandora K, Valeri A, Chieffe C, Schramke C. Aggressive therapy for neurosarcoidosis: long-term follow-up of 48 treated patients. *Arch Neurol.* 2007;64(5):691–696.
14. Chapelon C, Ziza JM, Piette JC, et al. Neurosarcoidosis: signs, course and treatment in 35 confirmed cases. *Medicine.* 1990;69(5):261–276.
15. Agbogu BN, Stern BJ, Sewell C, Yang G. Therapeutic considerations in patients with refractory neurosarcoidosis. *Arch Neurol.* 1995;52(9):875–879.
16. Stern BJ, Griffin DE, Luke RA, Krumholz A, Johns CJ. Neurosarcoidosis: cerebrospinal fluid lymphocyte subpopulations. *Neurology.* 1987;37(5):878–881.
17. Sharma OP. Neurosarcoidosis: a personal perspective based on the study of 37 patients. *Chest.* 1997;112(1):220–228.
18. Zajicek JP, Scolding NJ, Foster O, et al. Central nervous system sarcoidosis–diagnosis and management. *QJM Mon J Assoc Phys.* 1999;92(2):103–117.
19. Dumas JL, Valeyre D, Chapelon-Abric C, et al. Central nervous system sarcoidosis: follow-up at MR imaging during steroid therapy. *Radiology.* 2000;214(2):411–420.
20. Bihan H, Christozova V, Dumas JL, et al. Sarcoidosis: clinical, hormonal, and magnetic resonance imaging (MRI) manifestations of hypothalamic-pituitary disease in 9 patients and review of the literature. *Medicine.* 2007;86(5):259–268.
21. Carlson ML, White Jr JR, Espahbodi M, et al. Cranial base manifestations of neurosarcoidosis: a review of 305 patients. *Otol Neurotol.* 2015;36(1):156–166.
22. Nozaki K, Scott TF, Sohn M, Judson MA. Isolated neurosarcoidosis: case series in 2 sarcoidosis centers. *Neurol.* 2012;18(6):373–377.
23. Gascon-Bayarri J, Mana J, Martinez-Yelamos S, Murillo O, Rene R, Rubio F. Neurosarcoidosis: report of 30 cases and a literature survey. *Eur J Intern Med.* 2011;22(6):e125–e132.
24. Leonhard SE, Fritz D, Eftimov F, van der Kooi AJ, van de Beek D, Brouwer MC. Neurosarcoidosis in a tertiary referral center: a cross-sectional cohort study. *Medicine.* 2016;95(14):e3277.
25. Cohen-Aubart F, Galanaud D, Grabli D, et al. Spinal cord sarcoidosis: clinical and laboratory profile and outcome of 31 patients in a case-control study. *Medicine.* 2010;89(2):133–140.
26. Durel CA, Marignier R, Maucort-Boulch D, et al. Clinical features and prognostic factors of spinal cord sarcoidosis: a multicenter observational study of 20 BIOPSY-PROVEN patients. *J Neurol.* 2016;263(5):981–990.
27. Sohn M, Culver DA, Judson MA, Scott TF, Tavee J, Nozaki K. Spinal cord neurosarcoidosis. *Am J Med Sci.* 2014;347(3):195–198.
28. Sakushima K, Yabe I, Nakano F, et al. Clinical features of spinal cord sarcoidosis: analysis of 17 neurosarcoidosis patients. *J Neurol.* 2011;258(12):2163–2167.
29. Kefella H, Luther D, Hainline C. Ophthalmic and neuro-ophthalmic manifestations of sarcoidosis. *Curr Opin Ophthalmol.* 2017;28(6):587–594.
30. Westhout FD, Linskey ME. Obstructive hydrocephalus and progressive psychosis: rare presentations of neurosarcoidosis. *Surg Neurol.* 2008;69(3):288–292; discussion 92.
31. Nozaki K, Judson MA. Neurosarcoidosis. *Curr Treat Options Neurol.* 2013;15(4):492–504.
32. Nozaki K, Judson MA. Neurosarcoidosis: clinical manifestations, diagnosis and treatment. *Presse Med.* 2012;41(6 Pt 2):e331–e348.

33. Langrand C, Bihan H, Raverot G, et al. Hypothalamo-pituitary sarcoidosis: a multicenter study of 24 patients. *QJM Mon J Assoc Phys*. 2012;105(10):981–995.
34. Zalewski NL, Flanagan EP, Keegan BM. Evaluation of idiopathic transverse myelitis revealing specific myelopathy diagnoses. *Neurology*. 2018;90(2):e96–e102.
35. Kerasnoudis A, Woitalla D, Gold R, Pitarokoili K, Yoon MS. Sarcoid neuropathy: correlation of nerve ultrasound, electrophysiological and clinical findings. *J Neurol Sci*. 2014;347(1–2):129–136.
36. Souayah N, Hassan AE, Krivitskaya N, et al. Neurosarcoidosis presenting as an anterior horn syndrome. *J Neuroimmunol*. 2010;225(1–2):132–136.
37. Bakkers M, Merkies IS, Lauria G, et al. Intraepidermal nerve fiber density and its application in sarcoidosis. *Neurology*. 2009;73(14):1142–1148.
38. Maeshima S, Koike H, Noda S, et al. Clinicopathological features of sarcoidosis manifesting as generalized chronic myopathy. *J Neurol*. 2015;262(4):1035–1045.
39. Cohen Aubart F, Abbara S, Maisonobe T, et al. Symptomatic muscular sarcoidosis. *Neurol Neuroimmunol Neuroinflammation*. 2018;5(3):e452.
40. Schupp JC, Freitag-Wolf S, Bargagli E, et al. Phenotypes of organ involvement in sarcoidosis. *Eur Respir J*. 2018;51(1).
41. Miyara M, Amoura Z, Parizot C, et al. The immune paradox of sarcoidosis and regulatory T cells. *J Exp Med*. 2006;203(2):359–370.
42. Wengert O, Rothenfusser-Korber E, Vollrath B, et al. Neurosarcoidosis: correlation of cerebrospinal fluid findings with diffuse leptomeningeal gadolinium enhancement on MRI and clinical disease activity. *J Neurol Sci*. 2013;335(1–2):124–130.
43. Bridel C, Courvoisier DS, Vuilleumier N, Lalive PH. Cerebrospinal fluid angiotensin-converting enzyme for diagnosis of neurosarcoidosis. *J Neuroimmunol*. 2015;285:1–3.
44. Hashiguchi S, Momoo T, Murohashi Y, et al. Interleukin 10 level in the cerebrospinal fluid as a possible biomarker for Lymphomatosis cerebri. *Intern Med*. 2015;54(12):1547–1552.
45. Alvermann S, Hennig C, Stuve O, Wiendl H, Stangel M. Immunophenotyping of cerebrospinal fluid cells in multiple sclerosis: in search of biomarkers. *JAMA Neurol*. 2014;71(7):905–912.
46. Filippi M, Rocca MA, Ciccarelli O, et al. MRI criteria for the diagnosis of multiple sclerosis: MAGNIMS consensus guidelines. *Lancet Neurol*. 2016;15(3):292–303.
47. O'Dwyer JP, Al-Moyeed BA, Farrell MA, et al. Neurosarcoidosis-related intracranial haemorrhage: three new cases and a systematic review of the literature. *Eur J Neurol*. 2013;20(1):71–78.
48. Macedo PJ, da Silveira VC, Ramos LT, Nobrega FR, Vasconcellos LF. Isolated central nervous system vasculitis as a manifestation of neurosarcoidosis. *J Stroke Cerebrovasc Dis*. 2016;25(6):e89–92.
49. Isabel C, Cohen Aubart F, Dodet P, Galanaud D, Amoura Z, Maillart E. Spinal Koebner phenomenon: medullar sarcoidosis facing a discal hernia. *Joint Bone Spine*. 2017;84(4):497–498.
50. Flanagan EP, Kaufmann TJ, Krecke KN, et al. Discriminating long myelitis of neuromyelitis optica from sarcoidosis. *Ann Neurol*. 2016;79(3):437–447.
51. Statement on sarcoidosis. Joint Statement of the American thoracic Society (ATS), the European Respiratory Society (ERS) and the World association of sarcoidosis and other granulomatous disorders (WASOG) adopted by the ATS board of Directors and by the ERS Executive Committee, February 1999. *Am J Respir Crit Care Med*. 1999;160(2):736–755.
52. Bartels S, Kyavar L, Blumstein N, et al. FDG PET findings leading to diagnosis of neurosarcoidosis. *Clin Neurol Neurosurg*. 2013;115(1):85–88.
53. Soussan M, Augier A, Brillet PY, Weinmann P, Valeyre D. Functional imaging in extrapulmonary sarcoidosis: FDG-PET/CT and MR features. *Clin Nucl Med*. 2014;39(2):e146–e159.
54. Bolat S, Berding G, Dengler R, Stangel M, Trebst C. Fluorodeoxyglucose positron emission tomography (FDG-PET) is useful in the diagnosis of neurosarcoidosis. *J Neurol Sci*. 2009;287(1–2):257–259.
55. Judson MA, Costabel U, Drent M, et al. The WASOG Sarcoidosis Organ Assessment Instrument: an update of a previous clinical tool. *Sarcoidosis Vasc Diffuse Lung Dis*. 2014;31(1):19–27.
56. Androdias G, Maillet D, Marignier R, et al. Mycophenolate mofetil may be effective in CNS sarcoidosis but not in sarcoid myopathy. *Neurology*. 2011;76(13):1168–1172.
57. Baughman RP, Winget DB, Lower EE. Methotrexate is steroid sparing in acute sarcoidosis: results of a double blind, randomized trial. *Sarcoidosis Vasc Diffuse Lung Dis*. 2000;17(1):60–66.
58. Vorselaars AD, Wuyts WA, Vorselaars VM, et al. Methotrexate vs azathioprine in second-line therapy of sarcoidosis. *Chest*. 2013;144(3):805–812.
59. Bitoun S, Bouvry D, Borie R, et al. Treatment of neurosarcoidosis: a comparative study of methotrexate and mycophenolate mofetil. *Neurology*. 2016;87(24):2517–2521.
60. Sharma OP. Effectiveness of chloroquine and hydroxychloroquine in treating selected patients with sarcoidosis with neurological involvement. *Arch Neurol*. 1998;55(9):1248–1254.
61. Stern BJ, Schonfeld SA, Sewell C, Krumholz A, Scott P, Belendiuk G. The treatment of neurosarcoidosis with cyclosporine. *Arch Neurol*. 1992;49(10):1065–1072.
62. Bhagwan S, Bhagwan B, Bhigjee AI. The use of cladribine in neurosarcoidosis: a report of two cases. *Clin Neurol Neurosurg*. 2015;136:79–81.
63. Bomprezzi R, Pati S, Chansakul C, Vollmer T. A case of neurosarcoidosis successfully treated with rituximab. *Neurology*. 2010;75(6):568–570.
64. Vorselaars AD, Crommelin HA, Deneer VH, et al. Effectiveness of infliximab in refractory FDG PET-positive sarcoidosis. *Eur Respir J*. 2015;46(1):175–185.
65. Moravan M, Segal BM. Treatment of CNS sarcoidosis with infliximab and mycophenolate mofetil. *Neurology*. 2009;72(4):337–340.

66. Lorentzen AO, Sveberg L, Midtvedt O, Kerty E, Heuser K. Overnight response to infliximab in neurosarcoidosis: a case report and review of infliximab treatment practice. *Clin Neuropharmacol*. 2014;37(5):142–148.
67. Judson MA, Baughman RP, Costabel U, et al. Efficacy of infliximab in extrapulmonary sarcoidosis: results from a randomised trial. *Eur Respir J*. 2008;31(6):1189–1196.
68. Santos E, Shaunak S, Renowden S, Scolding NJ. Treatment of refractory neurosarcoidosis with Infliximab. *J Neurol Neurosurg Psychiatry*. 2010;81(3):241–246.
69. Gelfand JM, Bradshaw MJ, Stern BJ, et al. Infliximab for the treatment of CNS sarcoidosis: a multi-institutional series. *Neurology*. 2017;89(20):2092–2100.
70. Cohen Aubart F, Bouvry D, Galanaud D, et al. Long-term outcomes of refractory neurosarcoidosis treated with infliximab. *J Neurol*. 2017;264(5):891–897.
71. Drent M, Cremers JP, Jansen TL, Baughman RP. Practical eminence and experience-based recommendations for use of TNF-alpha inhibitors in sarcoidosis. *Sarcoidosis Vasc Diffuse Lung Dis*. 2014;31(2):91–107.
72. Vorselaars AD, Verwoerd A, van Moorsel CH, Keijsers RG, Rijkers GT, Grutters JC. Prediction of relapse after discontinuation of infliximab therapy in severe sarcoidosis. *Eur Respir J*. 2014;43(2):602–609.
73. Schimmelpennink MC, Vorselaars ADM, van Beek FT, et al. Efficacy and safety of infliximab biosimilar Inflectra((R)) in severe sarcoidosis. *Respir Med*. 2018;138S:S7–S13.
74. Jamilloux Y, Neel A, Lecouffe-Desprets M, et al. Progressive multifocal leukoencephalopathy in patients with sarcoidosis. *Neurology*. 2014;82(15):1307–1313.
75. Bernard C, Maucort-Boulch D, Varron L, et al. Cryptococcosis in sarcoidosis: cryptOsarc, a comparative study of 18 cases. *QJM Mon J Assoc Phys*. 2013;106(6):523–539.
76. Ungprasert P, Srivali N, Wijarnpreecha K, Thongprayoon C. Sarcoidosis and risk of venous thromboembolism: a systematic review and meta-analysis. *Sarcoidosis Vasc Diffuse Lung Dis*. 2015;32(3):182–187.
77. Girard N, Cottin V, Hot A, Etienne-Mastroianni B, Chidiac C, Cordier JF. Opportunistic infections and sarcoidosis. *Rev Mal Respir*. 2004;21(6 Pt 1):1083–1090.

CHAPTER 11

Cutaneous Sarcoidosis

SOTONYE IMADOJEMU, MD, MBE • KAROLYN A. WANAT, MD • MEGAN NOE, MD, MPH, MSCE • JOSEPH C. ENGLISH III, MD • MISHA ROSENBACH, MD

Sarcoidosis is a systemic granulomatous disease that can affect any organ. Skin is second only to the lungs as most frequently affected organ in this disease. Cutaneous manifestations of sarcoidosis are highly variable. Skin findings in patients with sarcoidosis can be specific, representing direct involvement of the skin with sarcoidal granulomas, or they can represent a reactive nonspecific inflammatory reaction, as is seen in erythema nodosum. Skin sarcoid can be the initial presenting sign or develop later in the course of the disease. In some patients the skin will be the most involved and impactful organ system and will drive therapy. In other cases the skin will be an incidental finding but may be easily accessible for biopsy to confirm the diagnosis or to track response to therapy. While sarcoidosis is a multiorgan disease, this chapter will discuss cutaneous involvement in detail.

HISTORY

Sarcoidosis is a systemic disorder with a prominent cutaneous component. In fact, the elucidation of the clinical manifestations and pathology of sarcoidosis was predominantly discovered by dermatologists. Sarcoidosis was first described by a British dermatologist named Jonathan Hutchinson in 1869.[1,2] Hutchinson's most famous sarcoidosis patient is Mrs. Mortimer. She was a 64-year-old woman who presented with raised, dusky red skin lesions on the face and forearm. These later progressed, affecting the bridge of the nose—making it swollen, red, and indurated.[3] Later in 1889 a French dermatologist named Ernest Besnier coined the term "lupus pernio" to describe purplish swelling of the nose, ears, and fingers. Then around 1900, a Norwegian dermatologist, Caesar Boeck coined the term "sarkoid" as the lesions resembled benign sarcoma-like disease and described the histologic findings. Boeck was also the first person to describe sarcoidosis as a systemic, rather than a cutaneous, disease, noting the disease's ability to involve of the lungs, conjunctiva, bones, and lymph nodes.[1]

EPIDEMIOLOGY

In the United States, large and generalizable epidemiologic studies are needed to accurately comment on incidence and prevalence of cutaneous manifestations of sarcoidosis. While overall the annual incidence of sarcoidosis is 35.5 per 100,000 black Americans and 10.9 per 100,000 white Americans, and skin involvement is more common in African American patients, the overall incidence of cutaneous sarcoidosis is uncertain. An epidemiologic study performed in a predominantly Caucasian population in Minnesota from 1976 to 2013 found an annual age- and sex-adjusted incidence of sarcoidosis-specific skin lesions to be 1.9 per 100,000 population.[4] Skin is the second most common organ affected in sarcoidosis, occurring in 25%–30% of reported cases.[5–7] Cutaneous sarcoidosis is commonly the presenting sign of systemic disease.[8] Although sarcoidosis can affect people of all races, at any age, the clinical presentation may vary by ethnic background. Of note, African Americans have the highest rates of sarcoidosis in the United States and appear more likely to have chronic cutaneous sarcoidosis than Caucasians.[6] Females appear more likely to have skin involvement than men.[7] Recently an increasing number of medications have been reported to induce cutaneous sarcoidosis and sarcoid-like granulomatous eruptions, including interferon, immune checkpoint inhibitors, targeted kinase inhibitors and, paradoxically, tumor necrosis factor (TNF) inhibitors.[9–15]

PATHOPHYSIOLOGY

Sarcoidosis is a granulomatous disease characterized by dysregulation of the cell-mediated portion of the immune system.[16] It may be that exposure to an antigen (environmental, infectious. or autoimmune) coupled with a genetic predisposition leads to activation of macrophages and T cells, with subsequent granuloma formation.[17] Sarcoidosis is a polygenic disease. Specific HLA alleles appear to be associated with increased risk of developing sarcoidosis, particularly HLA-DRB1

Sarcoidosis. https://doi.org/10.1016/B978-0-323-54429-0.00011-2

variants.[18,19] HLA-B8/DR3 may be associated with the development of Lofgren syndrome (discussed in the following). In African Americans, HLA-DQB1 alleles may play a role.[20] ANXA11, BTNL2, and CCR5 gene polymorphisms have also been identified in specific populations. A variant in the promoter for tumor necrosis factor (lymphotoxin alpha/TNF gene cluster) was found to be associated with erythema nodosum in female Caucasian sarcoidosis patients.[21]

As part of the immune response to defend from a foreign antigen that cannot be easily cleared, but for which cell-mediated immunity is intact, tissue macrophages and T lymphocytes form granulomas with a fibrous capsule to surround the pathogen. The granuloma walls off the pathogen from the rest of the tissue, while the immune system slowly destroys it. The antigen responsible for the granuloma formation in sarcoidosis is yet to be identified. It may be that any number of triggers, such as mycobacteria, *Propionobacterium acnes*, a misfolded self-antigen, or organic or inorganic molecules from the environment, precipitate disease.[22–28] It is possible that different antigens trigger a similar sarcoidal phenotype in different groups of patients or that different antigens lead to the variety of observed clinical phenotypes. The increased incidence of involvement of organs that interact with the outside world, such as the skin, lungs, and eyes, supports a possible environmental trigger. No matter the etiologic agent, a predominantly Th1 immune response with contributions of the innate and Th17 arms of the immune system occurs in sarcoidosis. Important cytokines in the pathophysiology of sarcoidosis includes IL-1, IL-2, IL-12, IL-17, IL-18, interferon gamma (IFN-γ), and tumor necrosis factor alpha (TNF-α), with TNF-α and IFN-γ consistently shown to play key roles.[29]

CLINICAL MANIFESTATIONS

Skin findings of systemic sarcoidosis develop before or at the time of diagnosis in 80% of patients.[30] There are 'specific' and 'nonspecific' findings of cutaneous sarcoidosis, based on the presence or absence of characteristic sarcoidal granulomas on biopsy. Some patterns of cutaneous involvement may be associated with specific extracutaneous manifestations of sarcoidosis, whereas other patterns of cutaneous involvement may predict response to treatment. There are secondary skin findings that are iatrogenic and may be associated with treatments of sarcoidosis. Cutaneous sarcoidosis is one of the great mimickers in dermatology, and the differential diagnosis is broad (see Table 11.1).

Cutaneous lesions can aid in the diagnosis of sarcoidosis and is easily accessible tissue for pathology. There should be a low threshold to refer to dermatology for evaluation and potential biopsy of patients in whom a diagnosis of sarcoidosis is considered.

Additionally, skin involvement has been shown to be a reliable, reproducible measure of disease activity and can be evaluated to monitor response to treatment. Clinical assessment tools such as the Cutaneous Sarcoidosis Activity and Morphology Instrument (CSAMI) and the Sarcoidosis Activity and Severity Index (SASI) can be used to trend clinical response to treatment in both the clinical and research settings.[31,32]

Specific Cutaneous Sarcoidosis Findings

Specific cutaneous findings of sarcoidosis have granulomas on histology (discussed in the following). There are a wide variety of sarcoidosis-specific skin lesions, including common and less common (Table 11.1). The clinical appearance may vary based on both the lesion morphologic type and the patients' skin type.

Bedside diagnostic tools such as diascopy and dermoscopy may be helpful in identifying these lesions, particularly in lighter skinned patients. Diascopy involves applying pressure to skin lesions with a clear glass slide to blanch the erythema. Behind the erythema, yellow-brown "apple jelly" color can be visualized. This finding is suggestive but not specific for cutaneous sarcoidosis.

Dermoscopy is a noninvasive tool allowing for the visualization of pigmented and vascular structures in the skin that are not visible to the unaided eye. Although traditionally used for the diagnosis of pigmented skin tumors, recently dermoscopy has gained increasing interest as an aid in the clinical diagnosis of inflammatory and infectious skin manifestations in general dermatology.[33] In a small 2010 Italian retrospective study, linear vessels overlying translucent orange ovoid structures or within scar-like areas were seen in all 7 cases of cutaneous sarcoidosis and may represent dermatoscopic findings suggestive of cutaneous sarcoidosis. More research is needed in this area.[33]

Papules and papulonodules

Papules are small, raised cutaneous lesions, whereas papulonodules are small raised lesions with a concomitant deeper, dermal component. Papules are the most common morphology of the specific cutaneous manifestations of sarcoidosis (Fig. 11.1). This morphology often presents with numerous, firm, typically nonscaly, papules usually smaller than 1 cm in

TABLE 11.1
Differential Diagnosis for Common and Uncommon Cutaneous Sarcoidosis Morphologies

	Cutaneous Sarcoid Morphology	Differential Diagnosis
Common	Papules and papulonodules	Acne, rosacea, granuloma annulare, cutaneous tuberculosis, warts, prurigo, and secondary syphilis
	Plaques	Rosacea, psoriasis, lichen planus, discoid lupus, granuloma annulare, cutaneous T-cell lymphoma, secondary syphilis, keloids, and Kaposi sarcoma
	Lupus pernio	Rhinophymatous rosacea, granulomatosis with polyangiitis, cutaneous tuberculosis, deep fungal infection, and leprosy
	Subcutaneous nodules	Lipomas, cysts, panniculitis, cellulitis, rheumatoid nodule, medium vessel vasculitis, epithelioid sarcoma, lymphoma, subcutaneous granuloma annulare, foreign body reaction, erythema nodosum, and sarcoidosis of the muscle
Uncommon	Ichthyosiform	Ichthyosis vulgaris, inherited ichthyoses and acquired ichthyosis from lymphoma, HIV, or other causes
	Atrophic and ulcerative	Lues maligna, morphea, lichen sclerosis, trauma, malignancy, infection, and necrobiosis lipoidica
	Genital	Cutaneous Crohn's disease, foreign body reaction, tuberculosis, syphilis, granuloma inguinale, and lymphogranuloma venereum
	Mucosal	Squamous cell carcinoma, drug-induced gingivitis, and vasculitis
	Erythroderma	Drug hypersensitivity, psoriasis, atopic dermatitis, cutaneous T-cell lymphoma, and other inflammatory dermatoses
	Alopecic	Alopecia areata, seborrheic dermatitis, lichen planopilaris, necrobiosis lipoidica, central centrifugal alopecia, and discoid lupus erythematosus
	Nail sarcoidosis	Nail lichen planus, nail sarcoid, and trachyonychia
	Macules and patches	Leprosy

size. The papules can be the same color as the normal surrounding skin (i.e., flesh-colored), yellow-brown, red-brown, or purple-brown, often based on the patient's underlying skin color.[34] Papules of sarcoidosis can also be hypopigmented. Additionally, they can have prominent hyperkeratosis, which can be described as verrucous or can resemble perforating disorders.[34] Papules typically present on the face, often on the eyelids or alar rim, but also on the trunk and extremities. The papules and papulonodules of cutaneous sarcoidosis can present in a miliary pattern in rare cases, with wide dissemination of a hundreds of 1–5 mm papules. "Papular sarcoidosis of the knee" has been reported in Caucasians in association with Lofgren syndrome and is suggested to portend a good prognosis. Foreign bodies are often seen on histology of papules in this location. Notably this is a common location for trauma, and patients with sarcoidosis can develop cutaneous lesions at sites of remote foreign body exposure, such as from superficial trauma to the knees during childhood.

Plaques

Plaques are broad, flat-surfaced, slightly elevated lesions. Plaque sarcoidosis can be oval or annular in shape, often well demarcated, typically firm to the touch, and they can sometimes have scales (Figs. 11.1–11.3). They range in color from red-brown to flesh-colored to purple brown and sometimes yellow-brown. Plaques can be found on the trunk, buttocks, shoulders, and arms.[35] Variants of plaque sarcoidosis include psoriasiform sarcoidosis that is characterized by thick scales; verrucous sarcoidosis that is characterized by hyperkeratosis (Fig. 11.4); hypopigmented sarcoidosis with light-colored thin plaques (Figs. 11.5 and 11.6); as well as angiolupoid sarcoidosis that is characterized by prominent telangiectasias and may be at particularly high risk for being mistaken for rosacea.

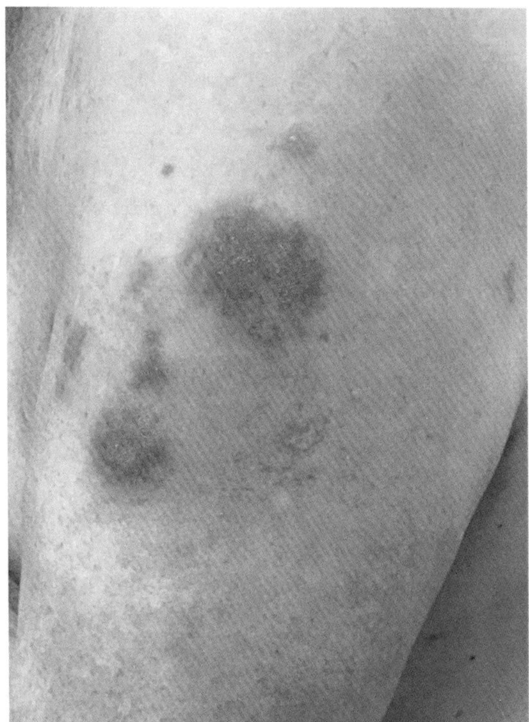

FIG. 11.1 Papular and plaque sarcoidosis. Pink-red, slightly scaly papules and plaques of cutaneous sarcoidosis. Note the apple-jelly, yellow-orange color in the center of the larger plaques.

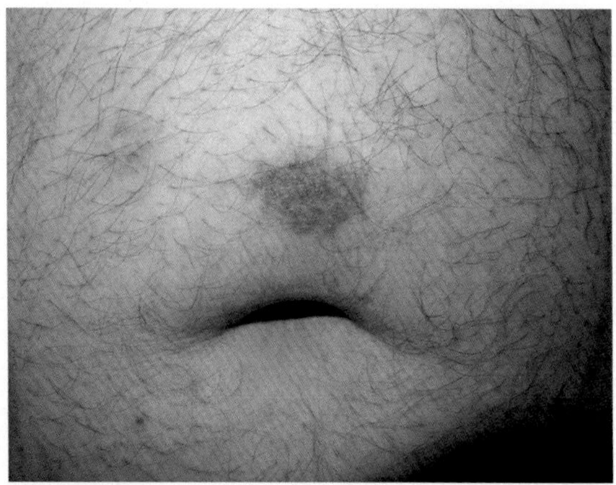

FIG. 11.2 Plaque sarcoidosis. Red-brown thin plaques on the abdomen.

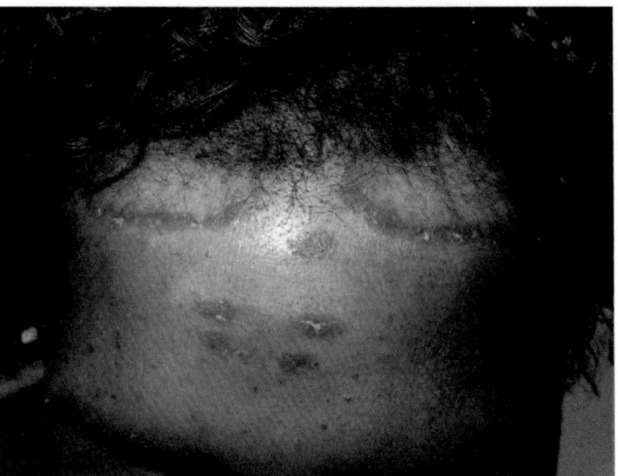

FIG. 11.3 Annular sarcoidosis. Ring-like red-brown plaques with hypopigmented centers on the forehead.

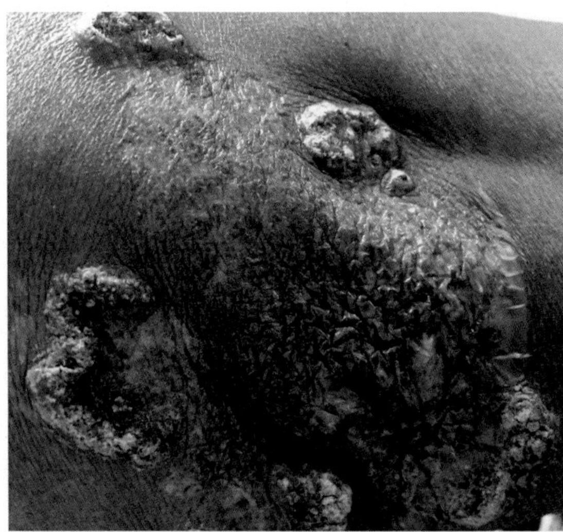

FIG. 11.4 Verrucous sarcoidosis. Dark, deep purple-gray and hyperpigmented plaques with thick keratotic scale on the elbows. Some are scar associated as the lesion was initially mistaken for a squamous cell carcinoma and excised.

Psoriasiform lesions of sarcoidosis are an established, but rare, cutaneous manifestation of sarcoidosis. Only 0.9% of sarcoidosis patients develop this form of the disease, and the majority of these cases have been reported in dark-skinned patients.[36] Psoriasis may occur in patients with sarcoidosis as a comorbid condition as both are Th1/Th17-mediated diseases, and biopsy may be necessary to determine which entity a particular skin lesion represents.[36,37]

Scar sarcoidosis

Cutaneous sarcoidosis may occur in scar tissue, at traumatized sites, and around imbedded foreign material, such as tattoos.[38] Scar sarcoidosis is a common pattern

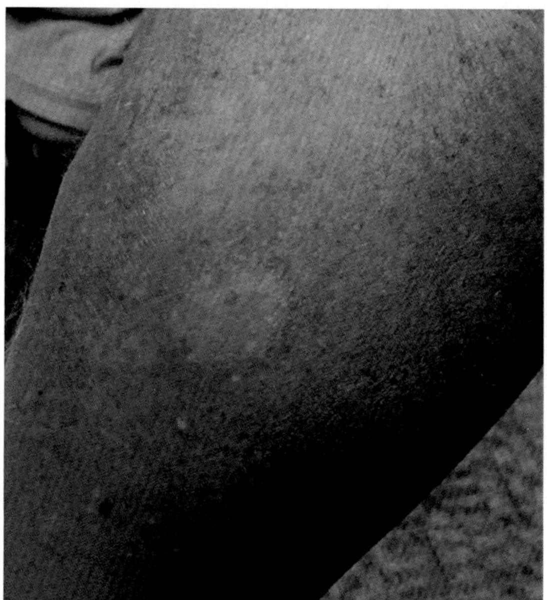

FIG. 11.5 Hypopigmented sarcoidosis. Hypopigmented thin plaque with an erythematous annular rim on the leg of a darker skinned patient.

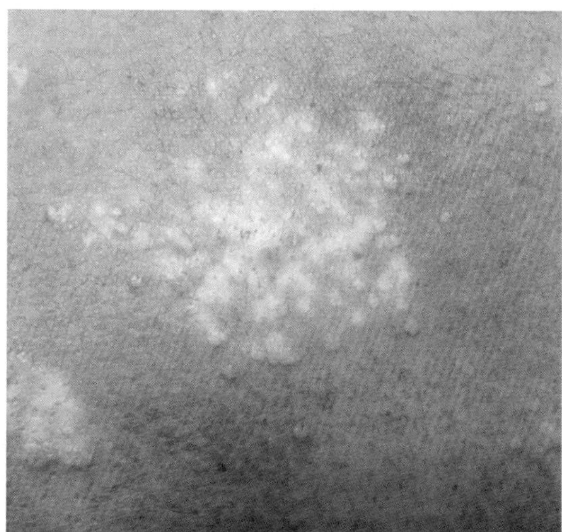

FIG. 11.6 Hypopigmented sarcoidosis. Hypopigmented macules, coalescing into patches in some areas, with pink, slightly scaly papules, in a lighter skinned patient.

and an important variant of papular and plaque sarcoidosis. Scars from surgical incisions, venipuncture, acne, herpes zoster virus, and other forms of skin trauma that were previously flat can become raised and erythematous to violaceous. These lesions may be

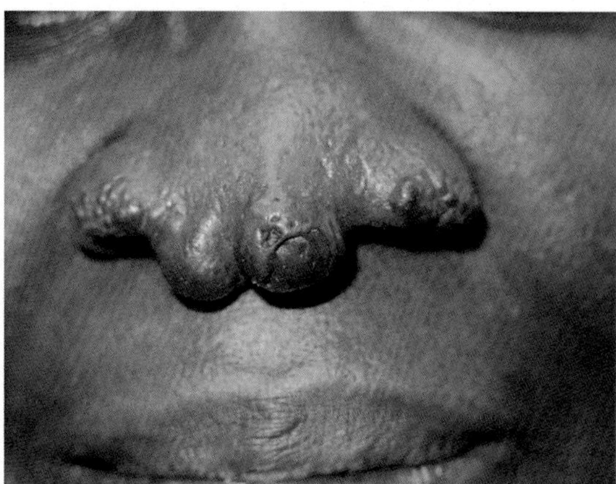

FIG. 11.7 Lupus pernio. Extensive subcutaneous nodules and plaques with destruction of the nasal cartilage and resultant deformity.

confused with hypertrophic scars or keloids. Involvement of tattoos may be an early sign of sarcoidosis and is often confused with granulomatous hypersensitivity reactions to tattoo pigment. The appearance of disease in previously inactive scars is thought to herald signs of increased disease activity.[38] Notably in patients in whom sarcoidosis is not recognized, lesions may develop in response to treatment such as laser-induced sarcoidosis in patients who were mistakenly thought to have rosacea.

This pattern of cutaneous involvement highlights the Koebner isomorphic response, the appearance of skin lesions at sites of injury that are morphologically similar to the existing skin disease,[38,39] which may be seen in cutaneous sarcoidosis. It is unclear if this pattern of organ involvement occurs in extracutaneous sarcoidosis.

The relationship between systemic sarcoidosis and scar sarcoidosis is unclear.

Lupus pernio

This clinical variant of plaque sarcoidosis is characterized by brown to violaceous or erythematous smooth shiny plaques, which may develop scales and often located on the central face, specifically the nose, cheeks, lips, forehead, and ears (Figs. 11.7 and 11.8). These lesions are at times infiltrating and can be very disfiguring. Lupus pernio tends to affect African Americans and women disproportionately.[40]

Lupus pernio has prognostic implications. This clinical variant is associated with a prolonged, chronic, and refractory course, often requiring aggressive systemic therapy, particularly with TNF inhibitors.[7,30,41]

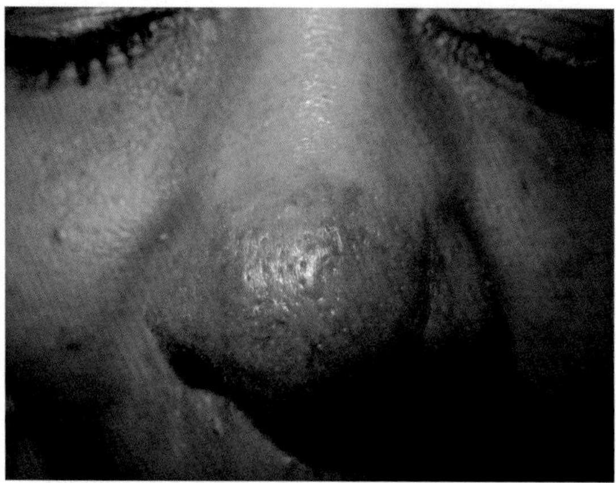

FIG. 11.8 Lupus pernio. Pink-red indurated plaque with some telangiectasias on the nasal tip.

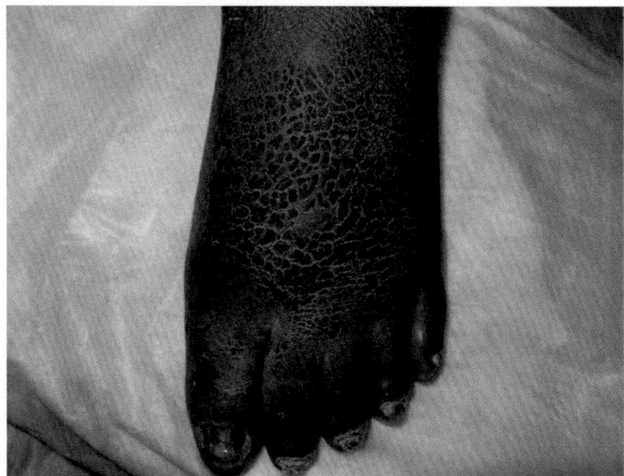

FIG. 11.9 Ichthyosiform sarcoidosis. Fish scale–like hyperkeratotic, dark-brown plate-like scaly plaque on the dorsal foot.

Involvement of the upper aerodigestive tract is also quite common, and lesions wrapping from the external nose to obliterate the internal nasal mucosa can be seen on clinical examination. The evaluation of a patient with lupus pernio clinical variant should prompt otorhinolaryngology evaluation as sinus disease can be severe in patients with lupus pernio.

The frequency of bone involvement, most commonly of the fingers and toes,[40] has been reported as higher in patients with lupus pernio in comparison with other types of skin sarcoidosis.[42] Severe treatment-refractory arthritis has also been reported in association with lupus pernio.[43]

Subcutaneous nodules

Subcutaneous nodules are deep-seated lesions in the skin, located in the deep dermis and subcutis, often with minimal changes appreciated on the surface of the skin. They are often easier to feel than see. Subcutaneous nodules of sarcoidosis are sometimes referred to as Darier-Roussy sarcoidosis. [44] The skin overlying the nodules can appear normal, erythematous, flesh colored, violaceous, or hyperpigmented. The nodules of subcutaneous sarcoidosis typically involve the trunk and extremities, mainly upper extremities.[45] They can be distributed in a linear fashion on an extremity, which is termed lymphangiectic or sporotrichoid pattern. The lesions are typically firm to touch, mobile, round to oval, and asymptomatic. There is also a lipodermatosclerosis-like variant of subcutaneous sarcoidosis, which is characterized by subcutaneous nodules and progress to indurated, circumferential, progressively fibrotic plaques on the lower extremities.[46]

While published reports have noted that subcutaneous sarcoidosis tends to be associated with systemic involvement, it is important to note that as sarcoidosis is a multiorgan disease in almost all cases, almost every form of sarcoid-specific skin lesion is also associated with systemic involvement. It has been thought that subcutaneous sarcoid is associated with benign internal disease, but that assertion is debated of late.[44,45]

Less Common Morphological Variants

Ichthyosiform

Ichthyosiform sarcoidosis resembles fish scales, with adherent, polygonal, brown or white-gray scales (Fig. 11.9). This variant commonly involves the lower extremities of dark-skinned patients of African descent.[47] The differential diagnosis includes ichthyosis vulgaris, inherited ichthyoses and acquired ichthyosis from lymphoma, HIV, or other causes. Biopsy revealing noncaseating diagnosis will distinguish ichthyosiform sarcoidosis from other ichthyotic dermatoses.

Atrophic and ulcerative

Atrophic sarcoidosis is characterized by depressed plaques that have a tendency to ulcerate. The atrophic plaques can be firm and sclerotic, as in the morpheaform variant, or yellow-pink to violaceous plaques on the shins, as in the necrobiosis lipoidica variant.[48] Ulcers in sarcoidosis can be primary, or they can secondarily affect other primary lesions of sarcoidosis. This is a relatively rare variant of cutaneous sarcoidosis.

Genital

Sarcoidosis of the vulva is a very rare condition. Sarcoidosis has also been reported in fallopian tubes, ovaries, and uterus. The uterine involvement usually presents as menometrorrhagia, and the diagnosis is based on the result of endometrial curettage.[49] Biopsies of vulvar sarcoidosis may be atypical and can show transepidermal elimination of the granulomas.[50] Sarcoidosis of the penis and scrotum is not uncommon and can present with genital edema.[51–53] Crohn's disease may clinically and histologically resemble sarcoidosis, and involvement at this site should prompt consideration of inflammatory bowel disease.

Mucosal

Involvement of the mucosa by sarcoidosis is uncommon but has been reported to involve the buccal mucosa, hard palate, tongue, posterior pharynx, and salivary glands as papules, plaques, nodules, and localized edema; gingiva as papules or infiltrative thickening, sometimes presenting as strawberry gingiva; nasal mucosa, particularly in lupus pernio, in the form of papules and nodules, or the urethra as infiltrative thickening.[54–57]

Erythroderma

Erythroderma is a cutaneous state characterized by erythematous involvement of an eruption involving greater than 80% of body surface area. In erythrodermic sarcoidosis, an extremely rare variant, indurated, yellow-brown, red-brown, or purple-brown scaly plaques coalesce to involve large areas of skin, often with fine superficial scale or mild exfoliative dermatitis. Such extensive cutaneous disease is often accompanied by systemic signs and symptoms such as fever, arthralgias, dehydration, weight loss, and dyspnea.[58] This variant has been reported to be precipitated by TNF inhibitor therapy.[59]

Alopecic

Involvement of the scalp with sarcoidosis can lead to scarring or nonscarring alopecia (hair loss) (Figs. 11.10 and 11.11). This finding can sometimes be confused with alopecia areata, seborrheic dermatitis, lichen planopilaris, necrobiosis lipoidica, central centrifugal alopecia, or discoid lupus erythematosus.[60,61]

Nail sarcoidosis

Granulomatous infiltration of the nail matrix, where the nail plate is made, can lead to a wide variety of nail dystrophy morphologies, is often coincident with phalangeal bone disease, and can be painful (Fig. 11.12). As such, nail sarcoidosis can present as thinning, brittle nails, thickened nails, pitting, ridging, trachyonychia (rough nails), hyperpigmentation, clubbing or pseudoclubbing, or destruction of the nail plate and scarring (ptyerigum).[62] Nail sarcoidosis can rarely be the

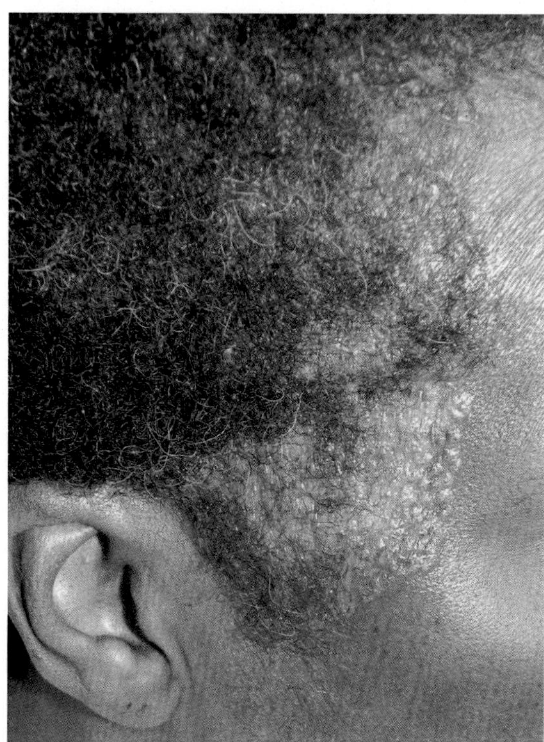

FIG. 11.10 Alopecic sarcoidosis. Annular red-brown thin, scaly plaque with hypopigmented sclerosis on the scalp. Note the decreased hair growth within the affected scalp.

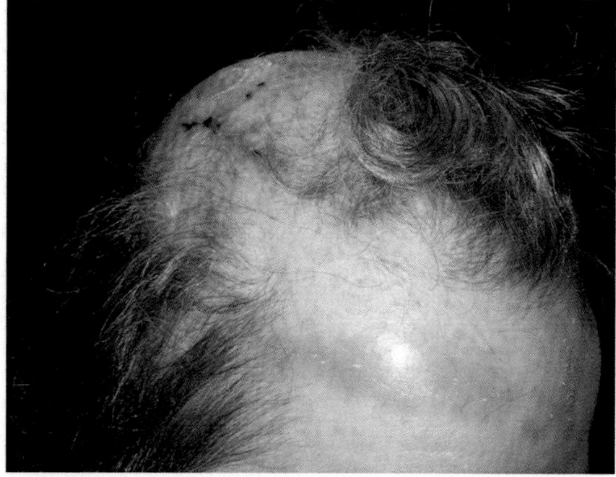

FIG. 11.11 Alopecic sarcoidosis. Brown-yellow plaque studded with flesh-colored to hyperpigmented papules. Note the hair is thin or absent within the plaque.

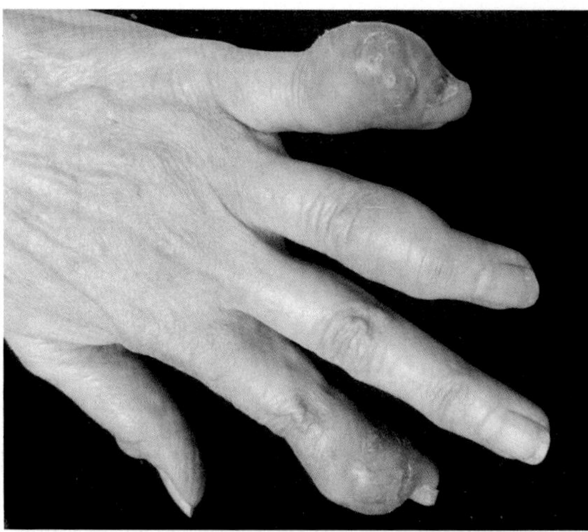

FIG. 11.12 Nail sarcoidosis. Thin, ridged, and brittle fingernails with destruction of the nail plate associated with extensive, large pink nodules on the distal second and fifth digits. Note the fusiform swelling of the fourth digit.

initial or sole manifestation of cutaneous sarcoidosis but more often is associated with systemic sarcoidosis involvement, particularly pulmonary involvement and lymphadenopathy. [62] Sarcoidal dactylitis, characterized by fusiform swelling of a digit is associated with lupus pernio.[62,63]

Macules and patches

Macules are small, flat cutaneous lesions, whereas patches are large, flat cutaneous lesions. Macules are an uncommon presentation of sarcoidosis. This is because cutaneous sarcoidosis is due to infiltration of macrophages and granulomatous inflammation into the skin which typically leads to induration. However, macules and patches can be present, especially as cutaneous disease is resolving, either spontaneously or as a result of treatment. The hypopigmented variant of sarcoidosis is often a patch or a thin plaque. These lesions can resemble some forms of leprosy, and depending on the geographic location of the patient, differentiating the two entities may be challenging. Sarcoidal granulomas do not tend to be neurotrophic, whereas those in leprosy are frequently near or around cutaneous nerve bundles.

Nonspecific Cutaneous Findings Associated With Sarcoidosis

Erythema nodosum

Erythema nodosum is a reactive inflammatory panniculitis that develops in up to 25% of patients with sarcoidosis. Erythema nodosum is characterized by erythematous to violaceous to brown, tender, warm subcutaneous nodules, classically located on the pretibial leg (Fig. 11.13). It is often associated with arthralgias and periarthritis, lower extremity edema, and fever. In patients with sarcoidosis, erythema nodosum has been associated with a favorable prognosis, a pattern that has been seen in patients of Scandinavian European descent.[64,65]

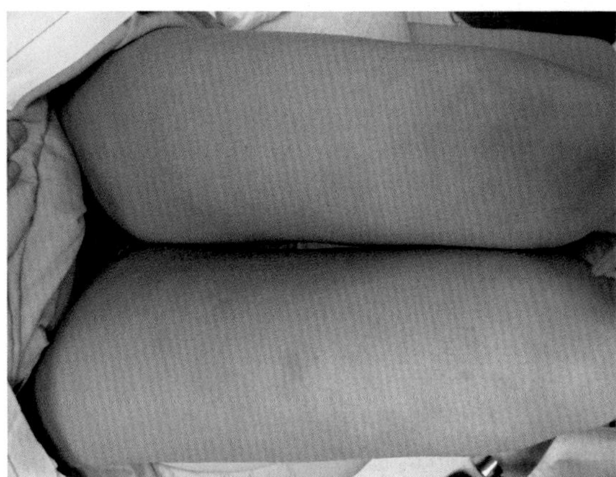

FIG. 11.13 Erythema nodosum. Erythematous subcutaneous nodules on the thighs.

Specifically, Lofgren's syndrome is characterized by the tetrad of erythema nodosum, hilar adenopathy, migratory polyarthralgia, and fever. In Caucasians, Lofgren syndrome is associated with a good prognosis and spontaneous resolution, although in the acute phase can be very symptomatic.[60,66,67] It is typically managed with nonsteroidal antiinflammatory drugs, although severe cases often require systemic corticosteroids.

Other nonspecific cutaneous findings of sarcoidosis include calcinosis cutis, clubbing, and prurigo. Importantly, medications used to treat sarcoidosis can lead to skin findings. For example, corticosteroid therapy can lead to steroid acne, and TNF inhibitors have been associated with the development to psoriasiform eruptions. It is important to recognize these as drug-related eruptions and not representative of treatment failure in the form of recurrent or recalcitrant cutaneous sarcoidosis.

DIAGNOSIS AND EVALUATION

The diagnosis of cutaneous sarcoidosis requires skin biopsy and histopathological analysis. When cutaneous sarcoidosis is suspected, a systemic evaluation is necessary. Thorough systemic evaluation is discussed elsewhere in this book, but it is important for physicians diagnosing cutaneous sarcoidosis to recognize how to evaluate patients for systemic internal involvement.

Workup should include a detailed history (including birth and travel history as well as occupational exposures) and physical examination along with chest radiograph, pulmonary function tests with diffusion capacity, and ophthalmologic evaluation. Laboratory testing should include complete blood count, comprehensive serum chemistries, electrocardiogram and transthoracic echocardiogram (with additional testing if any abnormalities are detected or if patients report palpitations on review of systems), tuberculin skin test or IFN-γ release assay, vitamin D25 and vitamin D1,25, as well as thyroid testing. Laboratory testing in advance of immunosuppression may be needed including HIV screen and hepatitis serologies, in addition to tuberculosis screening, depending on the therapeutic agent being considered. Consultants, such as pulmonologists, ophthalmologists, otorhinolaryngologists, cardiologists, or rheumatologists, may be necessary to manage extracutaneous manifestations.

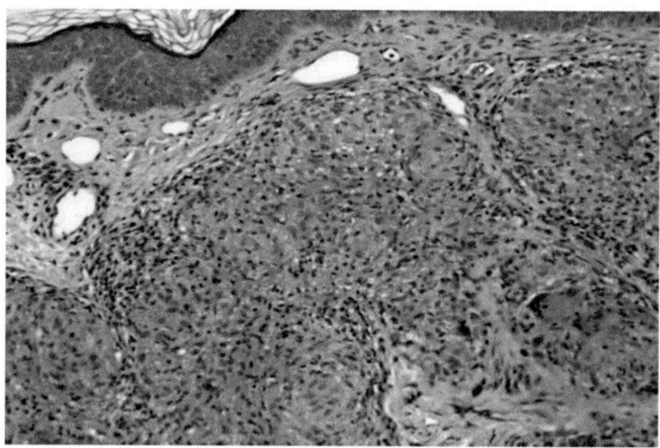

FIG. 11.14 Histopathology of cutaneous sarcoidosis. There are collections of histiocytes and giant cells organized into granulomas with few surrounding lymphocytes in the dermis.

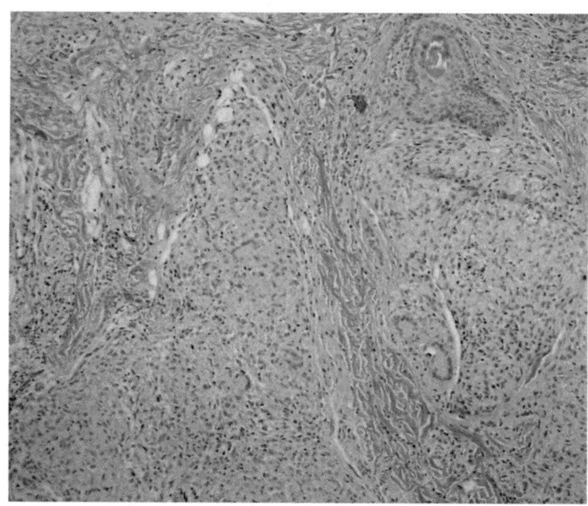

FIG. 11.15 Histopathology of cutaneous sarcoidosis. There are collections of histiocytes and giant cells organized into granulomas with few surrounding lymphocytes in the mid-dermis.

HISTOPATHOLOGY

The skin is easily accessible and represents a high-yield location of involvement to confirm the diagnosis of sarcoidosis. Skin biopsy, using the punch or incisional technique, should be pursued over biopsy of other organs if skin involvement in suspected cases, given the ease and safety of the procedure. Given the protean nature of the disease and the potential for subtle cutaneous involvement, physicians should have a low threshold to refer patients with suspected sarcoidosis to an experienced medical dermatologist for a full skin examination and evaluation for possible accessible cutaneous lesions amenable to biopsy.

The formation of the noncaseating granuloma is the hallmark of cutaneous sarcoidosis. This pattern is recapitulated in all affected organs. Histopathology of cutaneous sarcoidosis classically reveals superficial, deep dermal, and, occasionally, subcutaneous epithelioid granulomas, organized into tubercles, without a prominent surrounding lymphoplasmacytic infiltrate (Figs. 11.14 and 11.15). Central necrosis or caseation is typically absent.[68] Giant cells are typically present and may contain asteroid bodies (stellate eosinophilic inclusion bodies) or Schaumann bodies (round, laminated basophilic inclusion bodies).[69] Of note, up to 20% of biopsies of cutaneous sarcoidosis contain polarizable material.[69] As such, the presence of a foreign body does not exclude the diagnosis of sarcoidosis.

Histologic differential diagnosis includes infections such as leprosy and other mycobacterial infections as well as deep fungal infections such as histoplasmosis or coccidioidomycosis. Tissue culture and microbial stains should be performed to exclude infections, when clinically appropriate. Other entities with granulomatous inflammation include the epithelioid granulomas of Crohn's disease, granulomatous rosacea, and Melkersson-Rosenthal syndrome; palisading patterns of necrobiosis lipoidica, granuloma annulare, annular elastolytic giant cell granuloma, interstitial granulomatous dermatitis, and rheumatoid nodule; and xanthomatous granulomatous entities such as necrobiotic xanthogranuloma, and juvenile xanthogranuloma. Other granulomatous processes include foreign body reactions, granulomatous vasculitis, and granulomatous mycosis fungoides.[68]

TREATMENT

Because sarcoidosis is a multisystem disease, a therapeutic regimen should be constructed to address the most severely affected organ. Additionally, whenever possible, a regimen should be selected that can help all affected organs as some agents have relatively stronger or weaker organ-specific activity. Although the cutaneous manifestations of sarcoidosis are not life-threatening, their psychosocial impact may be devastating and may warrant treatment. This section will focus on the treatment for cutaneous sarcoidosis, whereas the treatment of extracutaneous disease is outside the scope of this chapter. It is important to note that there is overlap in the treatment of cutaneous and extracutaneous sarcoidosis, and treatment for extracutaneous sarcoidosis may control skin disease. However, control of cutaneous disease does not always correlate with control of extracutaneous disease. A skin-directed therapeutic ladder is recommended for patients with primary cutaneous disease or cutaneous disease that is not controlled by treatments for extracutaneous disease (Figs. 11.16 and 11.17). Treatment of stable, limited, asymptomatic cutaneous sarcoidosis can be deferred. As sarcoidosis involves chronic inflammatory cells, patience is essential when initiating a treatment, and patient counseling is important. Cutaneous sarcoidosis response to treatment is typically seen after 2–3 months of therapy and rarely sooner.

There are no Food and Drug Administration (FDA)–approved therapies for cutaneous sarcoidosis. Treatment recommendations are based on small case series, retrospective studies, and expert opinion.

Topical and Local Therapy

First line

Topical steroids. High-potency topical steroids such as clobetasol, halobetasol and betamethasone applied twice daily can lead to resolution of cutaneous disease.[70,71] This effect is enhanced with occlusion. High-potency topical steroids can induce skin thinning and should not be used for long periods of time on sensitive sites, such as the face.

Intralesional corticosteroids. Intralesional injections of triamcinolone acetonide in concentrations ranging from 5 to 40 mg/mL, administered every 3–6 weeks, deliver the corticosteroid to the dermis and is thought to be more effective than topical preparation. Injections can be painful and difficult for patients to tolerate. Importantly, topical and, even more so, intralesional corticosteroids are impractical in cases of generalized or widespread lesions.[72] The risks of topical and intralesional steroids include skin atrophy, dyspigmentation, telangiectasias, striae, purpura, and acne.

Topical calcineurin inhibitors. Twice daily application of topical calcineurin inhibitors has been shown to be efficacious in small case series and does not come with the risk of cutaneous side effects of corticosteroids.[73,74] If used on mucosal sites or ulcerated lesions, there is the potential for systemic absorption.

Second line

Topical retinoids. In the authors' opinion, topical retinoids can be used as an adjuvant therapy to mitigate dyspigmentation and scaling due to both antigranulomatous effects and their effects on keratinocyte biology and dyspigmentation.

Phototherapy and photodynamic therapy. Phototherapy is an umbrella term for the treatment of skin disorders with the application of light. Treatment modalities differ based on the wavelength of light used and the use of a photosensitizer. Ultraviolet A phototherapy has been reported to be helpful after 30–50 sessions or 10–16 weeks of treatment but may not penetrate to sufficient depth to help some types of sarcoidosis.[75]

Photodynamic therapy is a type of phototherapy treatment in which a photosensitizing chemical is applied to the skin or given systemically followed by irradiation with visible light to elicit cell death. It has been used in the treatment of cutaneous sarcoidosis with beneficial, although transient, results.[76–78] Skin disease tends to recur after discontinuation of therapy.

Laser therapy. Laser therapy has been reported to be helpful in the treatment of limited cutaneous sarcoidosis, with intense pulsed light alone[79] and with nonablative fractional resurfacing,[80] pulsed dye,[81,82] CO_2,[83] and ruby[84] being reported. Notably, laser therapy has also been reported to worsen sarcoidosis, including induction of ulcerative lesions in previously stable disease, and should be used with caution and only by experienced providers.

Surgical excision. Surgical excision can be used in certain situation, particularly when lesions are inactive. However, it is important to note the importance of using laser and surgery with caution given the predilection for cutaneous sarcoidosis to affect areas of trauma or prior scars.

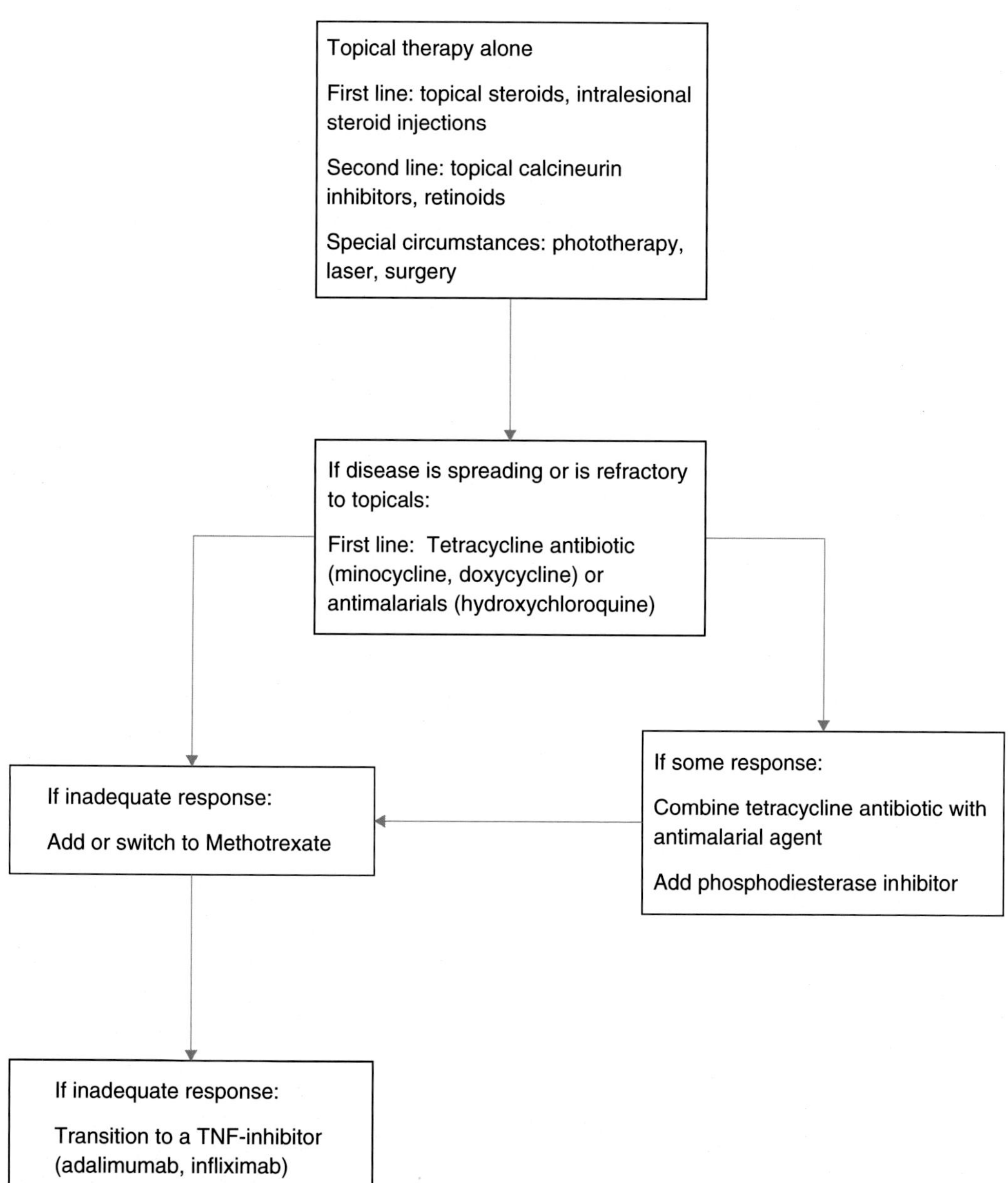

FIG. 11.16 Treatment algorithm: localized cutaneous disease or minimal cosmetic or psychosocial impact. *TNF*, tumor necrosis factor.

Immunomodulatory Systemic Therapy

Oral tetracycline antibiotics

Minocycline, doxycycline, and tetracycline are used in the treatment of cutaneous sarcoidosis because of their antiinflammatory properties, rather than an antimicrobial effect.[85,86] Response to treatment is slow, and partial-to-complete response can be seen in up to 70%–75% of patients.[86] Doxycycline is recommended given its efficacy and side effect profile. Potential side effects of tetracyclines include photosensitivity and gastrointestinal (GI) distress, as well as a lupus-like syndrome with minocycline. Minocycline is known to induce pigmentation in ~5% of patients in general; in sarcoidosis

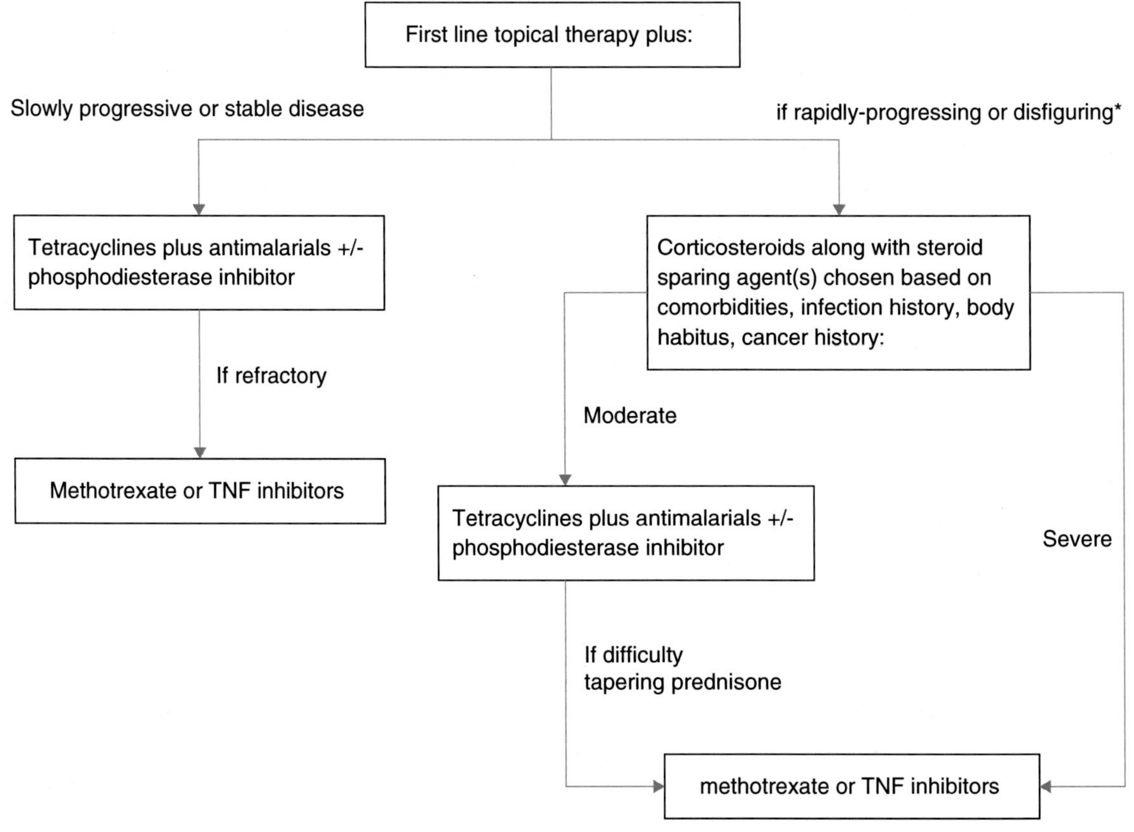

FIG. 11.17 Treatment algorithm: widespread cutaneous disease or significant cosmetic or psychosocial impact*. *TNF*, tumor necrosis factor.

patients this pigmentation may deposit within the lesions of sarcoidosis or in the gingiva, which can lead to suboptimal cosmetic results in some cases.

Antimalarials

Antimalarials, such as hydroxychloroquine and chloroquine, are the first-line systemic treatment for widespread skin sarcoidosis or next line of treatment in patients who fail skin-directed topical therapy. The mechanism of action of antimalarials is thought to involve blockade of presentation of antigen to CD4+ T-helper cells and a decrease in the activity of cytokines, such as IL-1 and TNFα, which lead to the formation of granulomas. The medications can take up to 3 months to see improvement but is helpful in two-thirds to three-quarters of cases.[87,88] The most common side effects include GI distress, risk for skin dyspigmentation, and potential for ocular toxicity, generally seen in patients on long-term use.

Phosphodiesterase inhibitors

Pentoxifylline inhibits the synthesis of TNF in vitro and in vivo by inhibiting phosphodiesterase type

4 activity.[71,89,90] Although there is a theoretical and anecdotal benefit to pentoxifylline in cutaneous sarcoidosis, studies evaluating for cutaneous efficacy are limited. There is, however, some evidence to suggest that pentoxifylline may have some efficacy in pulmonary sarcoidosis.[91] It has a very benign side effect profile with the most common side effect being GI upset. Dosed at 400 mg three times daily, it is often best used in combination with other therapies such as corticosteroids, antimalarials, and tetracyclines, rather than as monotherapy.

Apremilast, a new PDE-4 inhibitor dosed at 20 mg twice daily, was added to the regimen of patients with stable systemic therapy for persistent cutaneous sarcoidosis and was associated with improvement in skin lesions.[92]

Isotretinoin. Isotretinoin is a synthetic retinoid with immunomodulatory effects, suppressing antigen-directed T-cell activation and proliferation.[71] The evidence to support the use of isotretinoin in sarcoidosis is limited to case reports, which demonstrated at least partial control of disease with doses ranging from 0.5 to 1.3 mg/kg/day over six or more months.[93–95]

Immunosuppressive Systemic Therapy

Corticosteroids

Corticosteroids are the traditional, systemic immunosuppressive medication for systemic and cutaneous sarcoidosis. Corticosteroids work quickly but have side effects and toxicities that require close follow-up and monitoring. Prednisone can be used for rapidly progressing cutaneous disease. Starting doses ranging from prednisone 20–40 mg per day and are tapered slowly to the minimal dose which maintains control in an effort to minimize side effects.[96] The risks of corticosteroids are well established and include glucose intolerance, hypertension, mood instability, insomnia, osteoporosis, gastroesophageal reflux disease, stomach ulcers, weight gain, fluid retention, and opportunistic infections. As such, other therapies described in this section are used to aid in tapering systemic steroids or avoiding steroids altogether.

Acthar

Acthar, also known as corticotropin, was the first medication approved by the FDA for sarcoidosis in the 1950s, albeit based on only a handful of cases.[97] The proposed mechanism of action is via stimulation of alternative melanocortin receptors leading to a decrease in inflammation. Acthar gel therapy consists of a twice weekly intramuscular or subcutaneous administration of 80 IU. Reports have detailed improvement in advanced systemic sarcoidosis and in lupus pernio.[98,99] Common side effects include agitation and peripheral edema secondary to the mineralocorticoid effect of Acthar gel. This can be mitigated with spironolactone.[99] Acthar can be helpful in advanced, refractory cutaneous, and extracutaneous sarcoidosis and can aid in lowering glucocorticoid dose.

Methotrexate

Methotrexate is the first-line systemic medication for extensive or treatment-refractory cutaneous sarcoidosis.[100,101] It may be effective in up to 80% of patients.[102] Dosing is 7.5–25 mg/kg per week. Methotrexate can take up to 3 months for clinical improvement. Laboratory monitoring is important. Side effects include hepatotoxicity, GI upset, stomatitis, leukopenia, and pulmonary fibrosis. The risk of GI upset, hepatotoxicity, and stomatitis is reduced with supplementation with folic acid; severe adverse effects are more common in patients with preexisting renal disease or elderly patients. Patients with severe GI side effects may be treated with subcutaneous methotrexate.

Thalidomide and its derivatives

Thalidomide is thought to be effective in sarcoidosis due to its anti-TNF properties and has been found to be effective in the management of cutaneous sarcoidosis.[103–105] The majority of patients respond to 100–200 mg/day within 2 months of starting treatment.[105] A recent randomized trial failed to demonstrate benefits with thalidomide, and with the emergency of newer, stronger anti-TNF agents (biologics; see below), thalidomide is used less frequently.[106] Lenalidomide, a thalidomide derivative, appears to be safer with greater anti-TNF activity. Pomalidomide is a newer, more potent thalidomide-derivative. Given the side effect profile, some limit therapy with thalidomide to 3 months. Adverse events with thalidomide and its derivatives include nonreversible peripheral neuropathy, sedation, and venous thromboembolism. More studies are needed to evaluate lenalidomide and pomalidomide for cutaneous sarcoidosis.

TNF inhibitors

Adalimumab and infliximab have been shown to clear chronic, treatment-refractory, and severe cutaneous disease such as lupus pernio and ulcerative sarcoidosis.[107,108] Infliximab, dosed at 3–7 mg/kg at 0, 2, and 6 weeks, with maintenance every 4–8 weeks, has been shown to lead to rapid improvement of refractory cutaneous sarcoidosis.[109–113] Adalimumab, dosed at 40 mg weekly, has been shown to be efficacious in refractory cutaneous sarcoidosis in both a randomized controlled trial and numerous case reports.[114–119] Etanercept was studied for pulmonary sarcoidosis, and the trial was halted due to increased adverse events and lack of efficacy and generally is not used for cutaneous sarcoidosis.[120] TNF inhibitors, etanercept more frequently than adalimumab and infliximab, have been associated with paradoxical development of sarcoidosis when used for treatment of psoriasis, Crohn's disease, or rheumatoid arthritis.[59,121–123] Clinicians should consider discontinuation of TNF inhibitors if worsening disease is noted. Evaluation for latent tuberculosis and hepatitis, laboratory monitoring, and consideration of other comorbidities such as malignancy, congestive heart failure, or demyelinating disease need to be considered in all patients before the initiation of TNF inhibitors.

Mycophenolate mofetil and azathioprine

Less frequently used steroid-sparing agents used to treat cutaneous sarcoidosis include mycophenolate mofetil and azathioprine. Mycophenolate mofetil inhibits lymphocyte proliferation and function. At a dose of 500–1500 mg twice a day, it can be used to aid in steroid tapering although its efficacy as monotherapy is not known.[124] Azathioprine is an antimetabolite that has been used in extracutaneous sarcoidosis, but its efficacy in cutaneous sarcoidosis appears low.[125] Typical dosing is 50–200 mg once a day. Given the limited data, these medications should be considered in those patients who are unable to tolerate or have contraindications to other steroid-sparing agents.

Future Therapies

It has been shown that chronic nicotine exposure reduces the incidence of granulomatous diseases.[126] There are very early data to suggest that nicotine's immunomodulatory effects may be beneficial in patients with pulmonary sarcoidosis.[127] The implication for cutaneous sarcoidosis is yet unknown. Cytokine modulators such as ustekinumab via IL12/23 inhibition or secukinumab via IL17 inhibition may prove useful in the treatment of cutaneous sarcoidosis. A randomized, double-blind safety and efficacy study of ustekinumab with corticosteroid taper did not show efficacy in pulmonary or cutaneous sarcoidosis.[128] Knowing the role the Th17 arm of the immune system plays in granuloma formation and in the pathophysiology of sarcoidosis, targeted IL17 inhibitors may be a future target of investigation in the treatment of sarcoidosis, although there have been reports of induction of Crohn's disease, another granulomatous inflammatory condition, with some IL-17 inhibitors. More randomized trials to evaluate safety and efficacy of cytokine modulators, ideally using cutaneous sarcoidosis-specific severity indices such as the CSAMI or the SASI, in sarcoidosis are needed.

REFERENCES

1. Spagnolo P. Sarcoidosis: a critical review of history and milestones. *Clin Rev Allergy Immunol*. 2015;49(1):1–5.
2. Caesar Peter Moeller Boeck (1845–1917). Boeck's sarcoidosis. *JAMA*. 1970;211(9):1537–1538.
3. Sharma OP. Sarcoidosis: a historical perspective. *Clin Dermatol*. 2007;25(3):232–241.
4. Ungprasert PWD, Crowson CS, Matteson EL. Epidemiology of cutaneous sarcoidosis, 1976–2013: a population-based study from Olmsted County, Minnesota. *J Eur Acad Dermatol Venereol*. 2016;3:1799–1804.
5. Brito-Zerón PSJ, Bosch X, Hernández F, et al. Epidemiologic patterns of disease expression in sarcoidosis: age, gender and ethnicity-related differences. *Clin Exp Rheumatol*. 2016;34(3):380–388.
6. Baughman RP, Teirstein AS, Judson MA, et al. Clinical characteristics of patients in a case control study of sarcoidosis. *Am J Respir Crit Care Med*. 2001;164(10 Pt 1):1885–1889.
7. Yanardag H, Pamuk ON, Karayel T. Cutaneous involvement in sarcoidosis: analysis of the features in 170 patients. *Respir Med*. 2003;97(8):978–982.
8. Esteves TC, Aparicio G, Ferrer B, Garcia-Patos V. Prognostic value of skin lesions in sarcoidosis: clinical and histopathological clues. *Eur J Dermatol : EJD*. 2015;25(6):556–562.
9. Amber KT, Bloom R, Mrowietz U, Hertl M. TNF-alpha: a treatment target or cause of sarcoidosis? *J Eur Acad Dermatol Venereol*. 2015;29(11):2104–2111.
10. Leclerc S, Myers RP, Moussalli J, Herson S, Poynard T, Benveniste O. Sarcoidosis and interferon therapy: report of five cases and review of the literature. *Eur J Intern Med*. 2003;14(4):237–243.
11. Gaughan EM. Sarcoidosis, malignancy and immune checkpoint blockade. *Immunotherapy*. 2017;9(13):1051–1053.
12. Reddy SB, Possick JD, Kluger HM, Galan A, Han D. Sarcoidosis following anti-PD-1 and anti-CTLA-4 therapy for metastatic melanoma. *J Immunother*. 2017;40(8):307–311.
13. Collins LK, Chapman MS, Carter JB, Samie FH. Cutaneous adverse effects of the immune checkpoint inhibitors. *Current Problems Cancer*. 2017;41(2):125–128.
14. Lheure C, Kramkimel N, Franck N, et al. Sarcoidosis in patients treated with vemurafenib for metastatic melanoma: a paradoxical autoimmune activation. *Dermatology*. 2015;231(4):378–384.
15. Adam A, Thomas L, Bories N, et al. Sarcoidosis associated with vemurafenib. *Br J Dermatol*. 2013;169(1):206–208.

16. Goldstein RA, Janicki BW, Mirro J, Foellmer JW. Cell-mediated immune responses in sarcoidosis. *Am Rev Respirat Dis*. 1978;117(1):55–62.
17. Bindoli S, Dagan A, Torres-Ruiz JJ, et al. Sarcoidosis and autoimmunity: from genetic background to environmental factors. *Isr Med Assoc J*. 2016;18(3–4):197–202.
18. Rybicki BA, Maliarik MJ, Poisson LM, Iannuzzi MC. Sarcoidosis and granuloma genes: a family-based study in African-Americans. *Eur Respir J*. 2004;24(2):251–257.
19. Rybicki BA, Maliarik MJ, Poisson LM, et al. The major histocompatibility complex gene region and sarcoidosis susceptibility in African Americans. *Am J Respir Crit Care Med*. 2003;167(3):444–449.
20. Fischer A, Grunewald J, Spagnolo P, Nebel A, Schreiber S, Muller-Quernheim J. Genetics of sarcoidosis. *Semin Respir Crit Care Med*. 2014;35(3):296–306.
21. McDougal KE, Fallin MD, Moller DR, et al. Variation in the lymphotoxin-alpha/tumor necrosis factor locus modifies risk of erythema nodosum in sarcoidosis. *J Invest Dermatol*. 2009;129(8):1921–1926.
22. Oswald-Richter KA, Beachboard DC, Seeley EH, et al. Dual analysis for mycobacteria and propionibacteria in sarcoidosis BAL. *J Clin Immunol*. 2012;32(5):1129–1140.
23. Eishi Y. Etiologic aspect of sarcoidosis as an allergic endogenous infection caused by Propionibacterium acnes. *BioMed Res Int*. 2013;2013:935289.
24. Dubaniewicz A, Kampfer S, Singh M. Serum anti-mycobacterial heat shock proteins antibodies in sarcoidosis and tuberculosis. *Tuberculosis*. 2006;86(1):60–67.
25. Iannuzzi MCRB, Teirstein AS. Sarcoidosis. *N Engl J Med*. 2007;357:268–281.
26. Izbicki G, Chavko R, Banauch GI, et al. World Trade Center "sarcoid-like" granulomatous pulmonary disease in New York City Fire Department rescue workers. *Chest*. 2007;131(5):1414–1423.
27. Sola R, Boj M, Hernandez-Flix S, Camprubi M. Silica in oral drugs as a possible sarcoidosis-inducing antigen. *Lancet*. 2009;373(9679):1943–1944.
28. Chen ES, Moller DR. Sarcoidosis–scientific progress and clinical challenges. *Nat Rev Rheumatol*. 2011;7(8):457–467.
29. Sakthivel P, Bruder D. Mechanism of granuloma formation in sarcoidosis. *Curr Opin Hematol*. 2017;24(1):59–65.
30. Marcoval J, Mana J, Rubio M. Specific cutaneous lesions in patients with systemic sarcoidosis: relationship to severity and chronicity of disease. *Clin Exp Dermatol*. 2011;36(7):739–744.
31. Rosenbach M, Yeung H, Chu EY, et al. Reliability and convergent validity of the cutaneous sarcoidosis activity and morphology instrument for assessing cutaneous sarcoidosis. *JAMA Dermatol*. 2013;149(5):550–556.
32. Yeung H, Farber S, Birnbaum BK, et al. Reliability and validity of cutaneous sarcoidosis outcome instruments among dermatologists, pulmonologists, and rheumatologists. *JAMA Dermatol*. 2015;151(12):1317–1322.
33. Pellicano R, Tiodorovic-Zivkovic D, Gourhant JY, et al. Dermoscopy of cutaneous sarcoidosis. *Dermatology*. 2010;221(1):51–54.
34. Elgart ML. Cutaneous sarcoidosis: definitions and types of lesions. *Clin Dermatol*. 1986;4(4):35–45.
35. Lodha S, Sanchez M, Prystowsky S. Sarcoidosis of the skin: a review for the pulmonologist. *Chest*. 2009;136(2):583–596.
36. Vega ML, Abrahams J, Keller M. Psoriasiform sarcoidosis: collision of two entities or expression of one common pathogenesis? *J Clin Aesthetic Dermatol*. 2016;9(4):55–57.
37. Khalid U, Gislason GH, Hansen PR. Sarcoidosis in patients with psoriasis: a population-based cohort study. *PLoS One*. 2014;9(10):e109632.
38. Martires K, Shvartsbeyn M, Brinster N, Ramachandran S, Franks Jr AG. Sarcoidosis. *Dermatol Online J*. 2015;21(12).
39. Buss G, Cattin V, Spring P, Malinverni R, Gilliet M. Two cases of interferon-alpha-induced sarcoidosis Koebnerized along venous drainage lines: new pathogenic insights and review of the literature of interferon-induced sarcoidosis. *Dermatology*. 2013;226(4):289–297.
40. Spiteri MA, Matthey F, Gordon T, Carstairs LS, James DG. Lupus pernio: a clinico-radiological study of thirty-five cases. *Br J Dermatol*. 1985;112(3):315–322.
41. Mana JMJ, Rubio M, et al. Granulomatous cutaneous sarcoidosis: diagnosis, relationship to systemic disease, prognosis and treatment. *Sarcoidosis Vasc Diffuse Lung Dis*. 2013;30:268–281.
42. Nagai Y, Igarashi N, Ishikawa O. Lupus pernio with multiple bone cysts in the fingers. *J Dermatol*. 2010;37(9):812–814.
43. Efthimiou P, Kukar M. Lupus pernio: sarcoid-specific cutaneous manifestation associated with chronic sarcoid arthropathy. *J Clin Rheumatol*. 2011;17(6):343.
44. Ando MME, Hatano Y, Nishio S, et al. Subcutaneous sarcoidosis: a clinical analysis of nine patients. *Clin Rheumatol*. 2016;35(9):2277–2281.
45. O'Neill JL, Moustafa F, Teague D, Huang WW. Subcutaneous sarcoidosis without systemic involvement. *Dermatol Online J*. 2014;20(8).
46. Huang CL, Mutasim DF. Sarcoidosis mimicking lipodermatosclerosis. *Cutis*. 2005;75(6):322–324.
47. Cather JC, Cohen PR. Ichthyosiform sarcoidosis. *J Am Acad Dermatol*. 1999;40(5 Pt 2):862–865.
48. Chiba T, Takahara M, Nakahara T, et al. Cutaneous sarcoidosis clinically mimicking necrobiosis lipoidica in a patient with systemic sarcoidosis. *Ann Dermatol*. 2012;24(1):74–76.
49. Decavalas G, Adonakis G, Androutsopoulos G, Gkermpesi M, Kourounis G. Sarcoidosis of the vulva: a case report. *Arch Gynecol Obstet*. 2007;275(3):203–205.
50. Ismail ABK, McKay K. Transepithelial elimination in sarcoidosis: a frequent finding. *J Cutan Pathol*. 2014;41(1):22–27.

51. Weinberger LN, Zirwas MJ, English 3rd JC. A diagnostic algorithm for male genital oedema. *J Eur Acad Dermatol Venereol*. 2007;21(2):156–162.
52. Mahmood N, Afzal N, Joyce A. Sarcoidosis of the penis. *Br J Urol*. 1997;80(1):155.
53. Vahid B, Weibel S, Nguyen C. Scrotal swelling and sarcoidosis. *Am J Med*. 2006;119(11):e3.
54. Ho KC, Blair FM. Sarcoidosis of the gingiva–a case report. *Dent Update*. 2003;30(5):264–268.
55. Ho KL, Hayden MT. Sarcoidosis of urethra simulating carcinoma. *Urol*. 1979;13(2):197–199.
56. Suresh L, Radfar L. Oral sarcoidosis: a review of literature. *Oral Dis*. 2005;11(3):138–145.
57. Kowalczyk JP, Ricotti CA, de Araujo T, Drosou A, Nousari CH. "Strawberry gums" in sarcoidosis. *J Am Acad Dermatol*. 2008;59(suppl 5):S118–S120.
58. Wirth FA, Gould WM, Kauffman CL. Erythroderma in a patient with arthralgias, uveitis, and dyspnea. *Arch Dermatol*. 1999;135(11):1411, 4.
59. Park SK, Hwang PH, Yun SK, Kim HU, Park J. Tumor necrosis factor alpha blocker-induced erythrodermic sarcoidosis in with juvenile rheumatoid arthritis: a case report and review of the literature. *Ann Dermatol*. 2017;29(1):74–78.
60. Wanat KA, Rosenbach M. Cutaneous sarcoidosis. *Clin Chest Med*. 2015;36(4):685–702.
61. Katta R, Nelson B, Chen D, Roenigk H. Sarcoidosis of the scalp: a case series and review of the literature. *J Am Acad Dermatol*. 2000;42(4):690–692.
62. Momen SE, Al-Niaimi F. Sarcoid and the nail: review of the literature. *Clin Exp Dermatol*. 2013;38(2):119–124; quiz 25.
63. Cohen PD, Lester RS. Sarcoidosis presenting as nail dystrophy. *J Cutan Med Surg*. 1999;3(6):302–305.
64. Neville E, Walker AN, James DG. Prognostic factors predicting the outcome of sarcoidosis: an analysis of 818 patients. *Q J Med*. 1983 Autumn;52(208):525–533.
65. Milman N, Selroos O. Pulmonary sarcoidosis in the Nordic countries 1950-1982. II. Course and prognosis. *Sarcoidosis*. 1990;7(2):113–118.
66. Ponhold W. The Lofgren syndrome: acute sarcoidosis (author's transl). *Rontgen-Blatter; Zeitschrift fur Rontgen-Technik und medizinisch-wissenschaftliche Photographie*. 1977;30(6):325–327.
67. James DG, Thomson AD, Willcox A. Erythema nodosum as a manifestation of sarcoidosis. *Lancet*. 1956;271(6936):218–221.
68. Ball NJ, Kho GT, Martinka M. The histologic spectrum of cutaneous sarcoidosis: a study of twenty-eight cases. *J Cutan Pathol*. 2004;31(2):160–168.
69. Mangas C, Fernandez-Figueras MT, Fite E, Fernandez-Chico N, Sabat M, Ferrandiz C. Clinical spectrum and histological analysis of 32 cases of specific cutaneous sarcoidosis. *J Cutan Pathol*. 2006;33(12):772–777.
70. Khatri KA, Chotzen VA, Burrall BA. Lupus pernio: successful treatment with a potent topical corticosteroid. *Arch Dermatol*. 1995;131(5):617–618.
71. Doherty CB, Rosen T. Evidence-based therapy for cutaneous sarcoidosis. *Drugs*. 2008;68(10):1361–1383.
72. Singh SK, Singh S, Pandey SS. Cutaneous sarcoidosis without systemic involvement: response to intralesional corticosteroid. *Indian J Dermatol Venereol Leprol*. 1996;62(4):273–274.
73. Katoh N, Mihara H, Yasuno H. Cutaneous sarcoidosis successfully treated with topical tacrolimus. *Br J Dermatol*. 2002;147(1):154–156.
74. Green CM. Topical tacrolimus for the treatment of cutaneous sarcoidosis. *Clin Exp Dermatol*. 2007;32(4):457–458.
75. Mahnke N, Medve-Koenigs K, Berneburg M, Ruzicka T, Neumann NJ. Cutaneous sarcoidosis treated with medium-dose UVA1. *J Am Acad Dermatol*. 2004;50(6):978–979.
76. Penrose C, Mercer SE, Shim-Chang H. Photodynamic therapy for the treatment of cutaneous sarcoidosis. *J Am Acad Dermatol*. 2011;65(1):e12–e14.
77. Karrer S, Abels C, Wimmershoff MB, Landthaler M, Szeimies RM. Successful treatment of cutaneous sarcoidosis using topical photodynamic therapy. *Arch Dermatol*. 2002;138(5):581–584.
78. Wilsmann-Theis D, Bieber T, Novak N. Photodynamic therapy as an alternative treatment for cutaneous sarcoidosis. *Dermatology*. 2008;217(4):343–346.
79. Rosende L, del Pozo J, de Andres A, Perez Varela L. Intense pulsed light therapy for lupus pernio. *Actas Dermosifiliograficas*. 2012;103(1):71–73.
80. Emer J, Uslu U, Waldorf H. Improvement in lupus pernio with the successive use of pulsed dye laser and nonablative fractional resurfacing. *Dermatol Surg*. 2014;40(2):201–202.
81. Holzmann RD, Astner S, Forschner T, Sterry G. Scar sarcoidosis in a child: case report of successful treatment with the pulsed dye laser. *Dermatol Surg*. 2008;34(3):393–396.
82. Roos S, Raulin C, Ockenfels HM, Karsai S. Successful treatment of cutaneous sarcoidosis lesions with the flashlamp pumped pulsed dye laser: a case report. *Dermatol Surg*. 2009;35(7):1139–1140.
83. Zaouak A, Koubaa W, Hammami H, Fenniche S. Unconventional use of fractional ablative CO_2 laser in facial cutaneous sarcoidosis. *Dermatol Ther*. 2017.
84. Grema H, Greve B, Raulin C. Scar sarcoidosis–treatment with the Q-switched ruby laser. *Laser Surg Med*. 2002;30(5):398–400.
85. Miyazaki E, Ando M, Fukami T, Nureki S, Eishi Y, Kumamoto T. Minocycline for the treatment of sarcoidosis: is the mechanism of action immunomodulating or antimicrobial effect? *Clin Rheumatol*. 2008;27(9):1195–1197.
86. Steen T, English JC. Oral minocycline in treatment of cutaneous sarcoidosis. *JAMA Dermatol*. 2013;149(6):758–760.

87. Jones E, Callen JP. Hydroxychloroquine is effective therapy for control of cutaneous sarcoidal granulomas. *J Am Acad Dermatol.* 1990;23(3 Pt 1):487–489.
88. Zic JA, Horowitz DH, Arzubiaga C, King Jr LE. Treatment of cutaneous sarcoidosis with chloroquine. Review of the literature. *Arch Dermatol.* 1991;127(7):1034–1040.
89. Zabel P, Entzian P, Dalhoff K, Schlaak M. Pentoxifylline in treatment of sarcoidosis. *Am J Respir Crit Care Med.* 1997;155(5):1665–1669.
90. Badgwell C, Rosen T. Cutaneous sarcoidosis therapy updated. *J Am Acad Dermatol.* 2007;56(1):69–83.
91. Park MK, Fontana Jr , Babaali H, et al. Steroid-sparing effects of pentoxifylline in pulmonary sarcoidosis. *Sarcoidosis Vasc Diffuse Lung Dis.* 2009;26(2):121–131.
92. Baughman RP, Judson MA, Ingledue R, Craft NL, Lower EE. Efficacy and safety of apremilast in chronic cutaneous sarcoidosis. *Arch Dermatol.* 2012;148(2): 262–264.
93. Waldinger TP, Ellis CN, Quint K, Voorhees JJ. Treatment of cutaneous sarcoidosis with isotretinoin. *Arch Dermatol.* 1983;119(12):1003–1005.
94. Georgiou S, Monastirli A, Pasmatzi E, Tsambaos D. Cutaneous sarcoidosis: complete remission after oral isotretinoin therapy. *Acta Dermato-venereologica.* 1998;78(6):457–459.
95. Chong WS, Tan HH, Tan SH. Cutaneous sarcoidosis in Asians: a report of 25 patients from Singapore. *Clin Exp Dermatol.* 2005;30(2):120–124.
96. Baughman RP, Lower EE. Evidence-based therapy for cutaneous sarcoidosis. *Clin Dermatol.* 2007;25(3):334–340.
97. Philbin M, Niewoehner J, Wan GJ. Clinical and economic evaluation of repository corticotropin injection: a narrative literature review of treatment efficacy and healthcare resource utilization for seven key indications. *Adv Ther.* 2017;34(8):1775–1790.
98. Zhou Y, Lower EE, Li H, Baughman RP. Sarcoidosis patient with lupus pernio and infliximab-induced myositis: response to Acthar gel. *Respirat Med Case Rep.* 2016;17:5–7.
99. Baughman RP, Barney JB, O'Hare L, Lower EE. A retrospective pilot study examining the use of Acthar gel in sarcoidosis patients. *Respir Med.* 2016;110:66–72.
100. Lower EE, Baughman RP. Prolonged use of methotrexate for sarcoidosis. *Arch Intern Med.* 1995;155(8):846–851.
101. Webster GF, Razsi LK, Sanchez M, Shupack JL. Weekly low-dose methotrexate therapy for cutaneous sarcoidosis. *J Am Acad Dermatol.* 1991;24(3):451–454.
102. Mosam A, Morar N. Recalcitrant cutaneous sarcoidosis: an evidence-based sequential approach. *J Dermatol Treat.* 2004;15(6):353–359.
103. Carlesimo M, Giustini S, Rossi A, Bonaccorsi P, Calvieri S. Treatment of cutaneous and pulmonary sarcoidosis with thalidomide. *J Am Acad Dermatol.* 1995;32(5 Pt 2):866–869.
104. Lee JB, Koblenzer PS. Disfiguring cutaneous manifestation of sarcoidosis treated with thalidomide: a case report. *J Am Acad Dermatol.* 1998;39(5 Pt 2):835–838.
105. Baughman RP, Lower EE. Newer therapies for cutaneous sarcoidosis: the role of thalidomide and other agents. *Am J Clin Dermatol.* 2004;5(6):385–394.
106. Droitcourt C, Rybojad M, Porcher R, et al. A randomized, investigator-masked, double-blind, placebo-controlled trial on thalidomide in severe cutaneous sarcoidosis. *Chest.* 2014;146(4):1046–1054.
107. Wanat KA, Rosenbach M. Case series demonstrating improvement in chronic cutaneous sarcoidosis following treatment with TNF inhibitors. *Arch Dermatol.* 2012;148(9):1097–1100.
108. Heidelberger V, Ingen-Housz-Oro S, Marquet A, et al. Efficacy and tolerance of anti-tumor necrosis factor alpha agents in cutaneous sarcoidosis: a French study of 46 cases. *JAMA Dermatol.* 2017;153(7):681–685.
109. Rosen T, Doherty C. Successful long-term management of refractory cutaneous and upper airway sarcoidosis with periodic infliximab infusion. *Dermatol Online J.* 2007;13(3):14.
110. Tu J, Chan J. Cutaneous sarcoidosis and infliximab: evidence for efficacy in refractory disease. *Australas J Dermatol.* 2014;55(4):279–281.
111. Tuchinda P, Bremmer M, Gaspari AA. A case series of refractory cutaneous sarcoidosis successfully treated with infliximab. *Dermatol Ther.* 2012;2(1):11.
112. Sene T, Juillard C, Rybojad M, et al. Infliximab as a steroid-sparing agent in refractory cutaneous sarcoidosis: single-center retrospective study of 9 patients. *J Am Acad Dermatol.* 2012;66(2):328–332.
113. Baughman RP, Judson MA, Lower EE, et al. Infliximab for chronic cutaneous sarcoidosis: a subset analysis from a double-blind randomized clinical trial. *Sarcoidosis Vasc Diffuse Lung Dis.* 2016;32(4):289–295.
114. Pariser RJ, Paul J, Hirano S, Torosky C, Smith M. A double-blind, randomized, placebo-controlled trial of adalimumab in the treatment of cutaneous sarcoidosis. *J Am Acad Dermatol.* 2013;68(5):765–773.
115. Kaiser CA, Cozzio A, Hofbauer GF, Kamarashev J, French LE, Navarini AA. Disfiguring annular sarcoidosis improved by adalimumab. *Case Rep Dermatol.* 2011;3(2):103–106.
116. Field S, Regan AO, Sheahan K, Collins P. Recalcitrant cutaneous sarcoidosis responding to adalimumab but not to etanercept. *Clin Exp Dermatol.* 2010;35(7):795–796.
117. Thielen AM, Barde C, Saurat JH, Laffitte E. Refractory chronic cutaneous sarcoidosis responsive to dose escalation of TNF-alpha antagonists. *Dermatology.* 2009;219(1):59–62.
118. Heffernan MP, Smith DI. Adalimumab for treatment of cutaneous sarcoidosis. *Arch Dermatol.* 2006;142(1):17–19.
119. Philips MA, Lynch J, Azmi FH. Ulcerative cutaneous sarcoidosis responding to adalimumab. *J Am Acad Dermatol.* 2005;53(5):917.

120. Utz JP, Limper AH, Kalra S, et al. Etanercept for the treatment of stage II and III progressive pulmonary sarcoidosis. *Chest*. 2003;124(1):177–185.
121. Santos G, Sousa LE, Joao AM. Exacerbation of recalcitrant cutaneous sarcoidosis with adalimumab–a paradoxical effect? A case report. *Anais Brasileiros de Dermatologia*. 2013;88(6 suppl 1):26–28.
122. Numakura T, Tamada T, Nara M, et al. Simultaneous development of sarcoidosis and cutaneous vasculitis in a patient with refractory Crohn's disease during infliximab therapy. *BMC Pulm Med*. 2016;16:30.
123. Lamrock E, Brown P. Development of cutaneous sarcoidosis during treatment with tumour necrosis alpha factor antagonists. *Australas J Dermatol*. 2012;53(4):e87–e90.
124. Kouba DJ, Mimouni D, Rencic A, Nousari HC. Mycophenolate mofetil may serve as a steroid-sparing agent for sarcoidosis. *Br J Dermatol*. 2003;148(1):147–148.
125. Baughman RP, Lower EE. Treatment of sarcoidosis. *Clin Rev Allergy Immunol*. 2015;49(1):79–92.
126. Newman LS, Rose CS, Bresnitz EA, et al. A case control etiologic study of sarcoidosis: environmental and occupational risk factors. *Am J Respir Crit Care Med*. 2004;170(12):1324–1330.
127. Julian MW, Shao G, Schlesinger LS, et al. Nicotine treatment improves Toll-like receptor 2 and Toll-like receptor 9 responsiveness in active pulmonary sarcoidosis. *Chest*. 2013;143(2):461–470.
128. Judson MA, Baughman RP, Costabel U, et al. Safety and efficacy of ustekinumab or golimumab in patients with chronic sarcoidosis. *Eur Respir J*. 2014;44(5):1296–1307.

CHAPTER 12

Ocular Sarcoidosis

KAREEM GENENA, MBBCH • SUMIT SHARMA, MD • DANIEL A. CULVER, DO

INTRODUCTION

Sarcoidosis is a disease characterized by the formation of noncaseating granulomas in affected organs. The lungs are the most commonly affected organs, followed by the skin and the eyes. About a quarter of patients with sarcoidosis in the United States have ocular disease,[1] which often presents early in the disease course.[2] Uveitis is the most common manifestation of ocular sarcoidosis, but any part of the eye can be affected. The terms ocular and ophthalmic sarcoidosis are often used interchangeably in the literature and refer to any eye involvement. The term intraocular sarcoidosis, however, strictly refers to sarcoidosis uveitis.[3] For the purpose of this review, the term ocular sarcoidosis will be used to indicate eye involvement in general, and the term intraocular sarcoidosis will be used to refer to sarcoidosis uveitis. The term ocular sarcoidosis should be used to refer to both isolated ocular sarcoidosis and ocular involvement in systemic disease.

Pathogenesis

Sarcoidosis is a disease characterized by the formation of noncaseating granulomas in affected organs. The name was coined by the Norwegian dermatologist Caesar Boeck who examined skin lesions of sarcoidosis thinking they resembled sarcomas.[4] Although the etiology and pathogenesis of sarcoidosis have not been fully elucidated, there is evidence that it is an antigen-driven response, based on several observations. Studies of T-lymphocytes from bronchoalveolar lavage (BAL) fluid from patients with sarcoidosis exhibit downregulation of surface αβ T-cell receptor expression and increased β-chain mRNA transcript numbers, consistent with antigen-stimulated T-cell activation.[5] Transcripts of the β chain of the T-cell receptors from BAL fluid show evidence of oligoclonal expansion of T cells.[6] Cytokine gene expression patterns from lung parenchymal sarcoidosis granulomas and from BAL cells demonstrate a predilection toward secretion of cytokines (interleukin-2, interferon-gamma) conventionally associated with a Th-1 immunophenotype.[7] More recently, several authors have identified that most of the response is actually produced by cells with features also exhibiting Th-17 lineage, so-called Th17.1 cells.[8] Sarcoidosis patients tend to display cutaneous anergy to tuberculin skin testing. Blood and BAL fluid lymphocytes from patients with sarcoidosis have been shown to "under-react" to stimulation by purified protein derivative compared with normal controls.[9] This phenomenon is yet to be fully explained, but suppression of naïve T-cell proliferation by T regulatory cells has been demonstrated by some investigators.[10] Hypercalcemia associated with sarcoidosis occurs in about 6%–8% of patients and is thought to be secondary to elevated 1-α hydroxylase enzyme levels by sarcoid granulomas.[11,12] Based on current knowledge, the immunology of sarcoidosis uveitis is similar to that of sarcoidosis in general.[13,14]

Family members of patients with sarcoidosis are at increased risk for the disease, pointing to a genetic predisposition.[15] A higher incidence of the disease has also been observed in people sharing the same occupation or the same residence, suggesting environmental and communicable roles in sarcoidosis.[16–18] Associations have been observed between certain gene alleles, such as HLA-DRB1, and disease phenotypes and also between certain gene alleles and prognosis.[19] Genetic variants in human leukocyte antigen genes, RAB23 and ANXA11, have all been associated with risk of sarcoidosis uveitis, although the associations are often dependent on what population is studied.[20,21]

Epidemiology

According to a recent cross-sectional study in the United States, incidence and prevalence rates of sarcoidosis are higher for African Americans (17.8 and 141.4 per 100,000, respectively) than for Caucasian individuals (8.1 and 49.8), Hispanics (4.3 and 21.7), or Asians (3.2 and 18.9). Women are approximately two times more likely to have sarcoidosis, with the highest prevalence noted in African-American women (178.5 per 100,000).[22] The onset of sarcoidosis is earlier in African Americans than in Caucasians, with more organs involved and more advanced Scadding radiographic changes.[1]

Sarcoidosis. https://doi.org/10.1016/B978-0-323-54429-0.00012-4

Ocular manifestations are the initial presenting symptoms in about 20%–54% of patients[23,24] and can precede nonocular manifestations.[25] Contrary to the common belief that sarcoidosis is a disease of younger people, more than half of the patients develop manifestations of the disease after the age of 55 years.[22] The median age of patients in A Case Control Study of Sarcoidosis (ACCESS) was 42.1 years, with a range of 18–83 years.[26] In the ACCESS population, ocular involvement was more common in women and African-American subjects.[27]

Worldwide, ocular sarcoidosis is most common in Japan, affecting up to 79% of all sarcoidosis patients.[24] In the United States, ocular involvement was reported in 23% of a cohort of 1774 patients in a sarcoidosis clinic in South Carolina.[1] A similar prevalence of 26% was reported in a retrospective review of 183 patients with chronic sarcoidosis in Maryland in 1986.[2] Uveitis was present at the time of diagnosis of sarcoidosis in 32 of 35 (91%) patients. Lacrimal gland, conjunctival, and eyelid involvement was present in 85%, 75%, and 50% of patients at the time of diagnosis, respectively, indicating that those who have ocular involvement often experience it earlier in their disease course. In a large US epidemiologic study of incident sarcoidosis, 12% of patients had ocular disease at the outset, but only 2% of the cohort without ocular sarcoidosis at presentation went on to develop it within the 2-year follow-up period.[27,28]

A French study, which followed up patients for >7 years, showed that when ocular sarcoidosis was the presenting manifestation of sarcoidosis, isolated uveitis remained a strictly ocular condition in most patients.[29]

Reports of the prevalence of ocular sarcoidosis in other countries have varied. A Turkish cross-sectional study of 139 patients with sarcoidosis identified ocular sarcoidosis in 12.9%.[30] In contrast, the reported prevalence of ocular sarcoidosis in the Netherlands is as high as 41%–44%.[25] In the formerly mentioned Japanese series,[24] 54% (87/159) of the patients had initially presented with ocular manifestations. However, even in the 56% (72/159) who had initially presented with chest symptoms, intraocular involvement was identified in 54% (39/71).

When considering the entire spectrum of uveitis, sarcoidosis accounts for less than 5% of cases in most series.[31–33] However, in areas such as the Southeast United States, it may be seen in up to 11% of uveitis patients.[34] This observation may be due to higher prevalence in African-American patients (25%) who constituted a large proportion of the patients.

TABLE 12.1
Uveitis Nomenclature

Type	Primary Site of Inflammation	Includes
Anterior uveitis	Anterior chamber	Iritis Iridocyclitis Anterior cyclitis
Intermediate uveitis	Vitreous	Pars planitis Posterior cyclitis Hyalitis
Posterior uveitis	Retina or choroid	Focal, multifocal, or diffuse choroiditis Chorioretinitis Retinochoroiditis Retinitis Neuroretinitis
Panuveitis	Anterior chamber, vitreous and retina or choroid	

Data from the Standardization of Uveitis Nomenclature Working Group.

CLINICAL PRESENTATION

Constitutional symptoms such as fatigue, anorexia, weight loss, and night sweats are common.[4,35] Uveitis is the most common manifestation of ocular sarcoidosis, occurring in about 40%–70% of cases.[2,25,36] However, sarcoidosis can affect any part of the eye.[37] The lacrimal glands and conjunctivae are the next most common parts of the eye affected by sarcoidosis.[2,38]

Sarcoidosis uveitis is bilateral[39] in more than 70% of patients.[29,40,41] Although 60%–90% of patients have a chronic persistent course, some individuals have recurrent flares or only a single acute episode.[29,41] Recurrence of sarcoidosis after complete remission is unusual, but when it does happen, it is more common in females.[42] In a Spanish population, an initial presentation with Lofgren's syndrome carried a higher risk for recurrence.[42]

Uveitis can be classified according to the anatomy of the affected structure. Intermediate uveitis involves the middle layer of the eye, which includes the vitreous, peripheral retina, and pars plana portion of the ciliary body; anterior uveitis involves the iris and ciliary body, and posterior uveitis involves any of the choroid or central retina. An effort toward the standardization of the nomenclature of uveitis was made by the Standardization of Uveitis Nomenclature working group in 2005.[43] Definitions are summarized in Table 12.1.

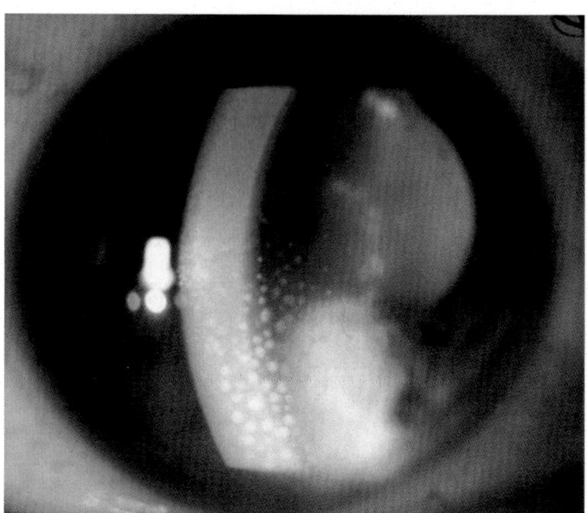

FIG. 12.1 Keratic precipitates. Clusters of leukocytes on the corneal endothelium, the innermost layer of the cornea. Acute precipitates tend to be rounded and whitish, as in this example.

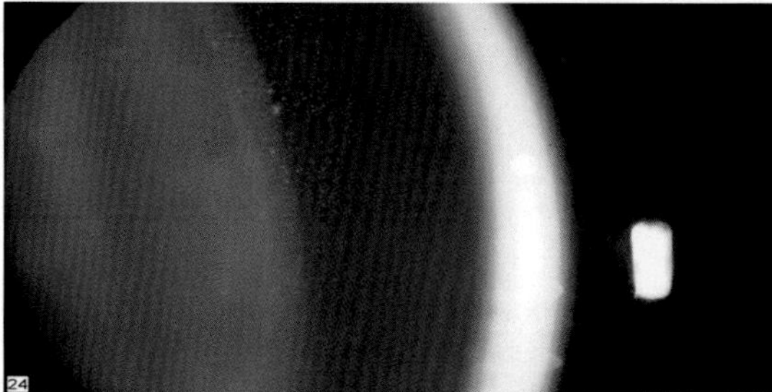

FIG. 12.2 Anterior chamber cells visualized by slit-lamp examination.

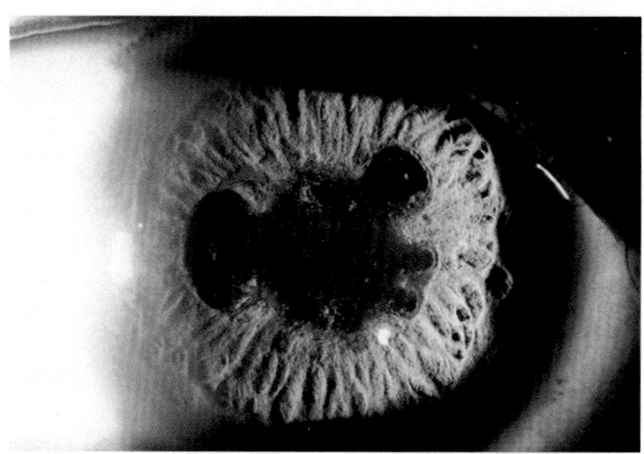

FIG. 12.3 Anterior synechiae exhibiting misshapen iris. Synechiae occur as a consequence of inflammation that leads to adherence of the iris to the cornea (anterior synechiae) or the lens (posterior synechiae).

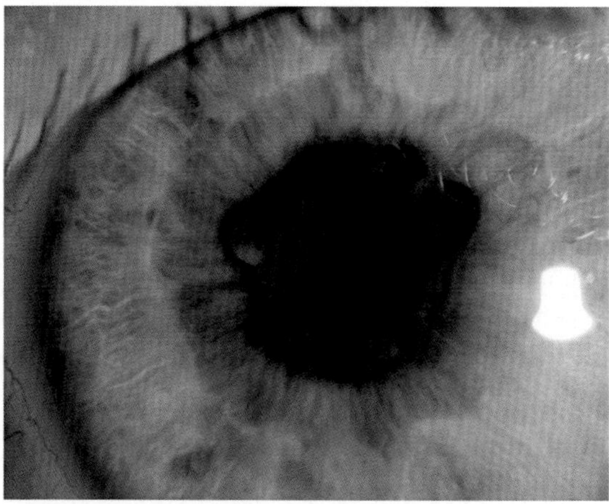

FIG. 12.4 Iris granulomas. The granulomas are visible as yellowish deposits around the periphery of the iris.

The term granulomatous uveitis is used when at least one of the following clinical signs is observed: (1) large mutton-fat keratic precipitates (KPs) (accumulation of inflammatory leukocytes that deposit on the corneal endothelium; Fig. 12.1); (2) iris or trabecular meshwork (TM) nodules; or (3) choroidal granulomas. Not all cases of sarcoidosis uveitis present with these signs though, especially early in the disease. When the term nongranulomatous uveitis is used by some authors, it simply means that the former signs were not observed.[37]

Anterior uveitis is the most common form of sarcoidosis uveitis, occurring in about 70%–84% of patients with sarcoid uveitis, including isolated anterior uveitis and that associated with inflammation of other segments of the uvea.[2,44]

Patients with anterior uveitis often present with red eyes, eye pain, photophobia, and decreased visual acuity.[37] Clinical findings on examination include anterior chamber cells/flare (Fig. 12.2), TM nodules, posterior synechiae, peripheral anterior synechiae (Fig. 12.3), and iris nodules (Fig. 12.4). Accumulation of inflammatory cells in the anterior chamber can raise intraocular pressure by obstructing the aqueous humor outflow tract. Peripheral anterior synechiae can similarly obstruct aqueous outflow.

TM nodules and tent-shaped peripheral anterior synechiae are believed to be two points on the same spectrum of disease. One hypothesis is that tent-shaped peripheral anterior synechiae are formed during the

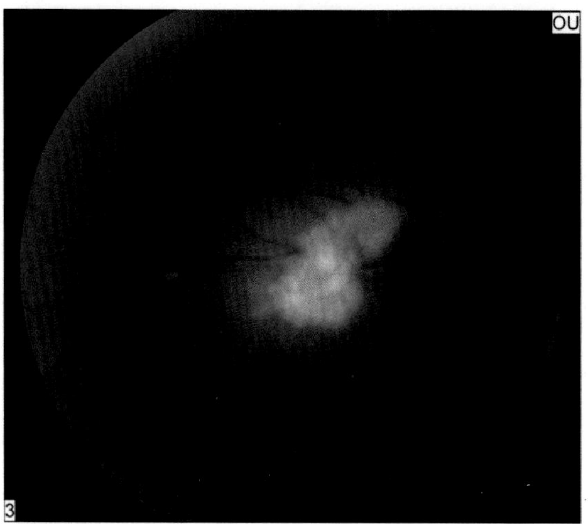

FIG. 12.5 Retinal granulomas.

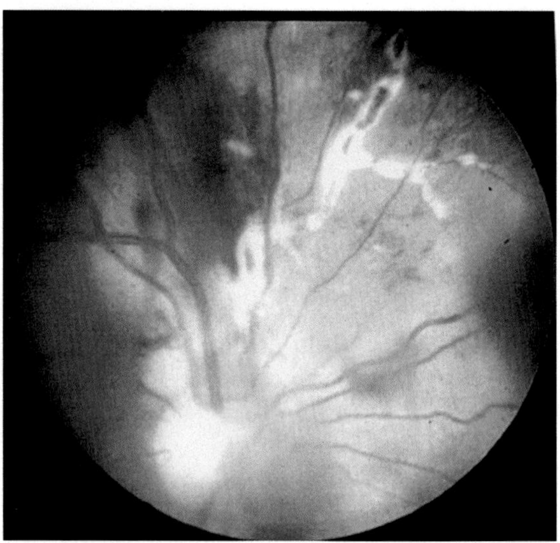

FIG. 12.6 Retinal periphlebitis with sheathing and exudates, known as "candle wax drippings".

healing process of the trabecular nodules.[24] The latter two signs had the highest sensitivity, specificity, and positive and negative predictive values for sarcoidosis in a Japanese study.[39]

Intermediate uveitis occurs in about 21% of patients with ocular sarcoidosis.[40] Findings on clinical examination include vitreous cells, haze, and snowballs, as well as peripheral snowbanks. Snowballs are yellow-white inflammatory aggregates typically seen in the mid-vitreous and inferior periphery, whereas snowbanks are exudates on the pars plana and are typically found inferiorly. Snowballs can form aggregates which are seen as a string of pearls. Snow banking is usually associated with more severe disease and can warrant aggressive therapy.

Posterior uveitis refers to the inflammation of the choroid and displays a distinct epidemiologic pattern where the incidence has been reported to be higher in Caucasian populations, especially females.[25] It is often associated with retinal inflammation (chorioretinitis), though retinal lesions can occur independently from choroidal ones (Fig. 12.5). Choroidal lesions are typically bilateral but can be asymmetric. Lesions can be tiny, or very large, simulating choroidal tumors. Choroidal neovascularization and exudative retinal detachment can develop in severe cases. Severe posterior segment involvement can lead to permanent visual disability.

Retinal vasculitis can manifest as perivascular sheathing, which is typically mid-peripheral, with or without perivascular exudates known as candle wax drippings (Fig. 12.6). Retinal macroaneurysms can be seen as well. In severe cases, hemorrhages and retinal/optic disc neovascularization can occur, as well as retinal artery and vein occlusions.

Cystoid macular edema (Fig. 12.7) is a consequence of inflammation in any part of the eye, including uveitis isolated to the anterior chamber; it is thought to result from vascular incompetence due an increase in inflammatory mediators in the eye. It does not always represent direct inflammation of the macula; however, it needs to be treated promptly as it can lead to irreversible vision loss from damage to the macula.

In a Japanese study,[24] iritis, trabecular nodules, and perivasculitis (mostly periphlebitis) were the most common intraocular findings, seen in 74%, 61%, and 67%, respectively. Tent-like peripheral anterior synechiae were seen in 54%.

Prognostic factors for poor visual outcome include intermediate and posterior uveitis, chronic uveitis, multifocal choroiditis, the presence of secondary glaucoma, delay in presentation to a subspecialist, and an age of >55 years.[2,29,40,41] In a British study,[40] poor visual outcome, defined as best corrected visual acuity (BCVA) of 20/40 or less, was found in 71% of patients with multifocal choroiditis and 46% of patients with panuveitis without multifocal choroiditis versus 12% of patients with anterior uveitis, after the completion of the treatment. On the other hand, a French study[29] showed that cystoid macular edema was found in 89% of patients with BCVA ≤ 20/50 versus 39% of patients with BCVA > 20/50. Age and multifocal choroiditis were not associated with poor visual outcome in that study.

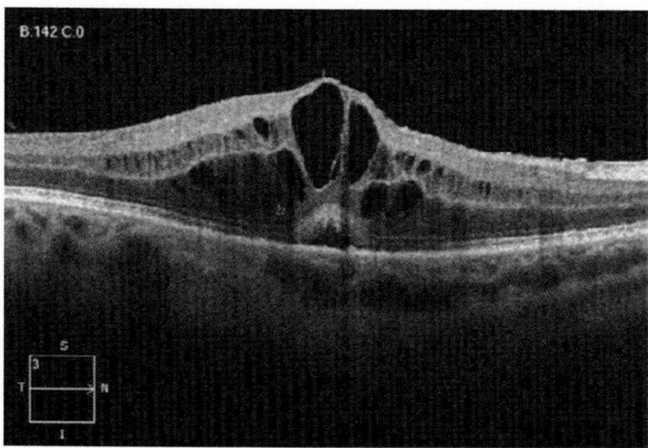

FIG. 12.7 Cystoid macular edema visualized by optical coherence tomography. Note the hyperlucent cysts in the central retina in this cross-sectional image.

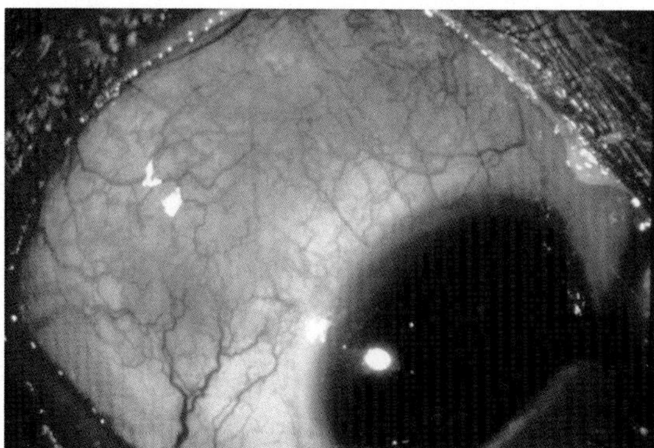

FIG. 12.8 Scleritis.

Nonuveitis Ocular Manifestations

Lacrimal gland involvement can present with a palpable mass, eyelid swelling, or dry eyes, secondary to decreased tear production.[45,46] Keratoconjunctivitis sicca has been reported in up to 70% of patients with ocular sarcoidosis.[44] Concurrent inflammation of the uvea and the parotid gland, accompanied by fever and facial nerve palsy, is known as Heerfordt's syndrome or uveoparotid fever. However, not all cases will manifest all four components of the syndrome. Facial nerve palsy might be unilateral or bilateral.[47,48] The uncommon simultaneous involvement of lacrimal and parotid glands gives the unique "panda sign" on gallium scintigraphy.[49]

Conjunctival involvement has been reported in 14%–46% of patients with ocular sarcoidosis[2,25,44]; it may occur more often in females.[25] Conjunctival involvement is typically discovered on examination of asymptomatic patients.[37,50] Manifestations include conjunctival follicles or nodules that can even be large enough to cause diplopia.[25,51] Conjunctival nodules can be found on the palpebral or bulbar conjunctivae, as well as on the fornix.[37,44,52] Conjunctival sarcoidosis has been reported to present as follicular conjunctivitis,[50,53] a condition with a main differential diagnosis of infection, making the diagnosis challenging.

Eyelid manifestations of sarcoidosis include "millet seed" nodules, ulcerated nodules, plaques, and swollen eyelids. Inflammation of the eyelid can result in loss of the Meibomian glands, trichiasis, eyelid notching, entropion, or symblepharon. Dry eyes can result from the destruction of the Meibomian glands. Trichiasis or entropion can lead to keratitis.[54,55]

Corneal involvement is usually secondary to other orbital structure involvement. As mentioned earlier, keratitis could be the sequela of keratoconjunctivitis sicca or trichiasis and entropion. Corneal calcium deposits have been described in sarcoidosis, with an association with hypercalcemia and a response to a low-calcium diet.[44] Peripheral corneal deposits of calcium may form a band-like opacity, known as band keratopathy.[37,44] Interstitial keratitis and ulcerative keratitis have been reported to occur in patients with sarcoidosis.[56,57] Scleritis may be in the form of scleral nodules or diffuse scleral inflammation (Fig. 12.8).[58–60]

Neuro-Ophthalmic Sarcoidosis

Neurosarcoidosis affects about 5%–10% of patients with sarcoidosis.[1,61,62] Neuro-ophthalmic sarcoidosis is a term that encompasses involvement of the optic nerve, chiasm, or tracts; the three cranial nerves controlling extraocular motion (oculomotor, trochlear, and abducens); as well as facial nerve involvement due to its effects of the eyelid and cornea.[63] The disease affects about one-third of patients with neurosarcoidosis[61] and occurs more frequently in women.[62,64] Cranial neuropathy is the most common manifestation of neuro-ophthalmic sarcoidosis. The facial and optic nerves are the two most commonly affected nerves.[37] Optic neuropathy has been reported in up to 70% of patients.[64] Evidence of intraocular inflammation concurrent with neuro-ophthalmic disease is common,[62] and there is a higher association of optic neuritis with uveitis.[65]

Common symptoms of neuro-ophthalmic sarcoidosis are vision loss, double vision, and pain. Extraocular muscle palsy may be apparent on examination. Ptosis and miosis might occur in Horner syndrome. The optic disk commonly appears swollen in optic neuritis but could appear normal in cases of retrobulbar neuritis. Occasionally, inflammation of the optic nerve results in retinal exudates, a condition known as neuroretinitis.[61]

Neuro-ophthalmic sarcoidosis, including involvement of the optic nerve, is typically considered within the spectrum of neurosarcoidosis and will not be discussed in detail in this chapter.

DIAGNOSTIC APPROACH

The diagnosis of ocular sarcoidosis often requires the joint efforts of ophthalmologists and pulmonologists. Up to 50% of patients who initially present to ophthalmologists with ocular symptoms receive the diagnosis of sarcoidosis after referral to a pulmonologist when sarcoidosis is suspected.[25] Enough diagnostic test results to confirm a diagnosis of sarcoidosis are not necessarily present at the time of referral, and the time interval between initial referral and the final diagnosis could exceed 1 year.[25] On the other hand, screening ocular examination by ophthalmologists for patients who carry the diagnosis of sarcoidosis can reveal signs of ocular sarcoidosis in the absence of symptoms.[41]

Concurrent involvement of multiple ocular structures should raise concern for sarcoidosis.[37] Sarcoidosis should be considered in any patient who presents with uveitis, whether it be granulomatous or nongranulomatous.[3]

Diagnostic Criteria

The most widely referenced diagnostic criteria were proposed by an international consensus conference, International Workshop on Ocular Sarcoidosis (IWOS).[3] The World Association of Sarcoidosis and Other Granulomatous Disorders (WASOG) has developed an alternate set of criteria.[66] Both sets of criteria are based on clinical signs, laboratory and imaging findings, and biopsy results, but the IWOS criteria provide a pathway to diagnose sarcoidosis even when extraocular sarcoidosis has not been confirmed by biopsy (presumed ocular sarcoidosis). Unfortunately, the IWOS criteria do not include several other widely used biomarkers that can improve diagnostic suspicion of sarcoidosis, such as the soluble interleukin-2 receptor level and indices of excess vitamin D bioconversion. Neither set of criteria has been validated.

Seven intraocular signs were identified by IWOS to be compatible with a diagnosis of intraocular sarcoidosis:

1. mutton-fat KPs/small granulomatous KPs and/or iris nodules at the pupillary margin (Koeppe) or in stroma (Busacca);
2. TM nodules and/or tent-shaped peripheral anterior synechiae;
3. vitreous opacities displaying snowballs/strings of pearls;
4. multiple chorioretinal peripheral lesions (active and/or atrophic);
5. nodular and/or segmental periphlebitis (with or without candle wax drippings) and/or retinal macroaneurysm in an inflamed eye;
6. optic disk nodule(s)/granuloma(s) and/or solitary choroidal nodule;
7. bilaterality.

TABLE 12.2
Diagnostic Levels of Certainty

Definite ocular sarcoidosis	Biopsy-supported diagnosis with a compatible uveitis.
Presumed ocular sarcoidosis	Compatible uveitis in the setting of a chest X-ray showing bilateral hilar lymphadenopathy with no biopsy.
Probable ocular sarcoidosis	3 intraocular signs and 2 positive laboratory tests when no biopsy was performed, and chest X-ray did not show bilateral hilar lymphadenopathy.
Possible ocular sarcoidosis	At least 4 intraocular signs and 2 positive laboratory tests when a biopsy was performed and showed no evidence of sarcoidosis.

Data from the International Workshop on Ocular Sarcoidosis.

Five laboratory and imaging investigations were identified as valuable in the diagnosis of ocular sarcoidosis in patients who had intraocular signs of uveitis:

1. Negative tuberculin skin test in a Bacille Calmette-Guerin–vaccinated patient or in a patient having had a positive tuberculin skin test previously.
2. Elevated serum angiotensin-converting enzyme (ACE) levels and/or elevated serum lysozyme.
3. Chest X-ray revealing bilateral hilar lymphadenopathy.
4. Abnormal liver enzyme tests.
5. Chest computed tomography (CT) scan in patients with a negative chest X-ray result.

Based on these clinical, laboratory, and imaging findings, sarcoidosis can be diagnosed with four levels of certainty, as demonstrated in Table 12.2. The IWOS criteria are useful for the diagnosis of sarcoidosis uveitis but not for other orbital involvement.

Diagnostic Evaluation

Gonioscopy should be performed on all patients with sarcoidosis looking for TM nodules and peripheral anterior synechiae. The presence of TM nodules is not always associated with other clinical signs of anterior uveitis but is often associated with a higher intraocular pressure.[24]

Conjunctival examination may be useful in patients with suspected sarcoidosis. The presence of conjunctival follicles or nodules represents a readily accessible source for possible tissue diagnosis. The diagnostic yield of conjunctival biopsies is higher in the presence of conjunctival follicles, but blind conjunctival biopsies are occasionally performed, typically from the inferior fornix.[67] In patients with suspected sarcoidosis, the diagnostic yield varies in different reports between 25% and 40%.[53,68,69] It should be noted that this procedure could lead to conjunctival scarring and is not very commonly used in clinical practice.

Accessory salivary gland biopsy is another available diagnostic tool, with highly variable reported diagnostic yields.[70,71] Vitreous, choroidal or retinal biopsies are uncommonly performed in cases of uveitis and are a last resort when the diagnosis cannot be reached by other diagnostic methods, since they carry the risk of visual loss and generally have low diagnostic yields.[72]

Histologic confirmation is the gold standard for the diagnosis of sarcoidosis, except for a few specific situations such as Löfgren's or Heerfordt's syndrome. Biopsies of involved organs should be performed when feasible. In the absence of an obvious ocular source for a biopsy, blind conjunctival or accessory salivary gland biopsies represent useful diagnostic tools, with yields that are generally higher in the presence of a compatible clinical picture or a proven diagnosis of sarcoidosis in other sites.

Operator experience often dictates which diagnostic tool is used. When the lungs are involved, evidence of non-caseating granulomas obtained from intrathoracic lymph nodes or pulmonary parenchyma, together with a clinically compatible ocular involvement, is sufficient to confirm the diagnosis of sarcoidosis. Many authors also consider the diagnosis of ocular sarcoidosis secure when BAL findings (elevated percent lymphocytes, elevated CD4/CD8 ratio) are demonstrated in a patient with ocular findings typical of sarcoidosis. In the future, it is possible that a confident diagnosis of sarcoidosis might be reached in certain scenarios without the requirement for a biopsy.[73] Obviously, the diagnosis of ocular sarcoidosis also requires expert ophthalmologic evaluation to exclude conditions that could mimic it.

Chest CT is more sensitive than X-ray for detection of mediastinal and parenchymal involvement,[74] and is useful in guiding biopsies. The presence of typical imaging features of sarcoidosis is associated with a higher yield of bronchial biopsies.[75] Endobronchial ultrasound-guided biopsy has largely replaced mediastinoscopy for the evaluation of mediastinal lymph nodes.[76]

In the absence of chest radiographic involvement or readily ascertainable non-thoracic organ involvement, fluorodeoxyglucose positron emission tomography (FDG-PET scan) may be useful for identifying alternative biopsy sites. FDG-PET can reveal foci of uptake in up to 50% of patients with a negative CT,[77] and is preferred to gallium scintigraphy. FDG-PET involves less radiation exposure; image acquisition can be done within 2h of injection, compared to 48–72h in the case of gallium scintigraphy; and is more sensitive than gallium scintigraphy in the detection of extrapulmonary involvement.[78,79] A suggested diagnostic approach is summarized in Fig. 12.9.

Differentiating neuro-ophthalmic sarcoidosis from demyelinating disorders such as multiple sclerosis or neuromyelitis optica (Devic's diease) can be daunting, especially for patients without other overt manifestations of sarcoidosis. Multiorgan involvement supports the diagnosis of sarcoidosis. Brain/orbital magnetic resonance imaging (MRI) with and without contrast can often help differentiate multiple sclerosis from neurosarcoidosis based on the sometimes-characteristic distribution and appearance of white matter lesions in the former; and more importantly, the potential presence of non-myelin related masses, leptomeningeal, or dural involvement in the latter.[61] Seen in approximately 40% of patients with neurosarcoidosis, leptomeningeal involvement with diffuse or focal/multi-focal enhancement is the most commonly reported imaging abnormality. Enlargement and enhancement of cranial nerves on T1-weighted images is suggestive of neurosarcoidosis. An elevated ACE level on cerebrospinal fluid analysis, or an elevated CD4:CD8 ratio could support the diagnosis but is not very sensitive or specific.[80] Neuromyelitis optica usually also causes transverse myelitis but not intracranial inflammation; most patients have elevated aquaporin four antibodies.[81]

Treatment

Anterior uveitis often responds to topical corticosteroids. Intermediate, posterior and panuveitis usually require regional therapy with periocular corticosteroid injections or systemic immunosuppressive treatment.

Prednisolone acetate is the most commonly used topical corticosteroid for anterior uveitis.[37] Treatment is often initiated as frequently as hourly; a regimen which compromises compliance. Difluprednate is a newer topical steroid that has shown at least equal efficacy in endogenous anterior uveitis with half as often application.[82] Side effects of topical steroids include glaucoma and cataract. Topical mydriatics/cycloplegics, such as cyclopentolate and atropine, are used to relieve pain from ciliary spasm, and to break or prevent anterior synechiae.[37]

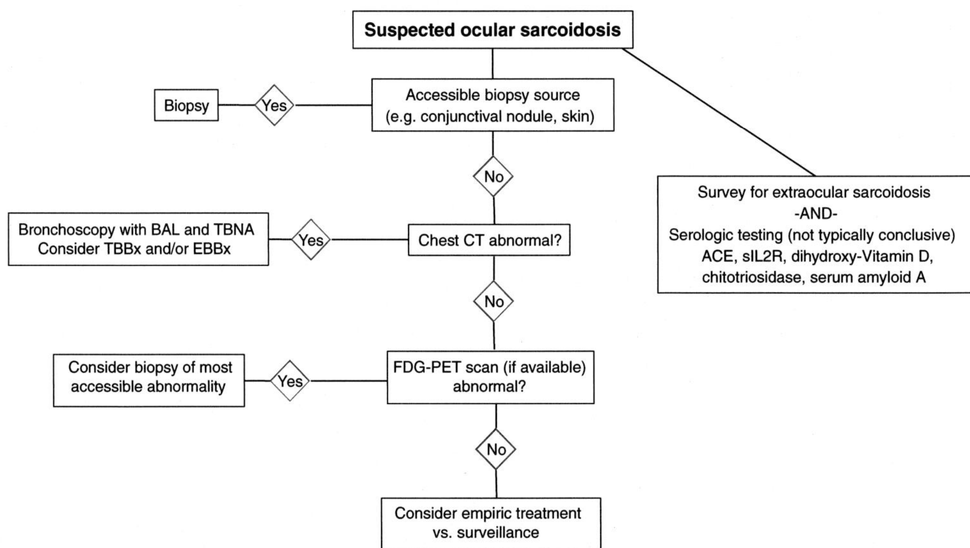

FIG. 12.9 Proposed diagnostic strategy in patients with suspected ocular sarcoidosis. When the ophthalmologic findings are highly suggestive of sarcoidosis (see text), the biopsy proof of granulomas in any organ is sufficient to confidently diagnose sarcoidosis. In situations where there is no biopsy proof of sarcoidosis, serologic markers and other evidence of extraocular abnormalities consistent with sarcoidosis may enhance diagnostic confidence. When bronchoscopy is performed, bronchoalveolar lavage with cell count and CD4/CD8 ratio assessed by flow cytometry is useful; even in technically nonenlarged lymph nodes, granulomatous inflammation may be found by endobronchial ultrasound-guided TBNA, supporting the diagnosis. *BAL*, bronchoalveolar lavage; *TBNA*, transbronchial needle aspiration; *TBBx*, transbronchial forceps biopsy; *EBBx*, endobronchial forceps biopsy; *CT*, computed tomography; *FDG-PET*, fluorodeoxyglucose positron emission tomography; *ACE*, angiotensin-converting enzyme; *sIL2R*, soluble interleukin-2 receptor

Regional steroid therapy options include subconjunctival, periocular/subtenons, and intravitreal injections.[83] Periocular injections can be repeated every 4–6 weeks. Intravitreal injections suppress inflammation for 3–6 months.[37] Steroid-releasing intravitreal implants are newer treatment modalities that avoid some of the procedural risks of repeated intraocular injections. They have been shown to reduce the recurrence rate of non-infectious uveitis by about 70% at 24 months,[84] but at the cost of a higher frequency of side effects; most notably cataract and glaucoma. Implants in wide use at present include an injectable biodegradable dexamethasone implant which releases steroids for 3 months; and a surgically-implanted fluocinolone acetonide implant which releases steroids for 3 years. Patients who received the fluocinolone acetonide implant were shown, in a recent systematic review, to have a threefold elevated risk of cataract formation or progression; a threefold risk of having cataract surgery; and a sevenfold risk of requiring intraocular pressure-lowering surgery, compared to standard of care therapy.[85] However, patients with the fluocinolone acetonide implant were able to have their uveitis controlled without systemic medications while maintaining the same visual acuity as the systemic therapy group. In our experience, the fluocinolone acetonide implant is a good option for patients with severe uveitis without systemic manifestations and those with difficult to control uveitis. Benefits and risks should be explained as these treatment modalities are being offered to patients.

Systemic steroids are indicated in patients not responding to topical therapy when regional therapy is not preferred, such as in cases of severe bilateral uveitis, and when therapy is indicated for other systemic disease.[37,86] Oral prednisone doses as high as 1–1.5 mg/kg/day are commonly used initially with tapers to avoid relapses and minimize complications. However, there are no dose-ranging data that demonstrate the superiority of this practice compared to lower induction doses. In our clinic, we typically initiate prednisone at 40–80 mg daily depending on the severity of ocular involvement. Intravenous methylprednisolone can occasionally be used in cases of acute vision-threatening inflammation.

Systemic immunosuppressive agents should be started in most patients in order to minimize both intraocular and extraocular steroid complications. In patients with threatened vision loss, avoiding additional complications from therapy should be a priority. Some useful agents include methotrexate, leflunomide, azathioprine, mycophenolate mofetil, and the calcineurin inhibitors cyclosporine and tacrolimus.[87–91] The expected onset of action for the these agents ranges from 2 to 12 weeks,[37] so they should generally be initiated early in the treatment course in order to facilitate steroid tapering. The practical use of these agents is beyond the scope of this chapter, but it is covered elsewhere in this publication.

Tumor necrosis factor-alpha inhibitors are useful for sarcoidosis uveitis. Adalimumab has been shown to reduce the rate of recurrence in patients who had been uncontrolled on prednisone for at least 2 weeks.[92] In a trial of adalimumab versus placebo in patients with non-infectious uveitis, the median time to treatment failure was 24 weeks, compared to 13 weeks, in patients treated with adalimumab, compared to placebo. Studies evaluating infliximab have shown mixed results.[93,94] Compared to placebo, etanercept was associated with no significant improvement.[95] Rare cases of granulomatous uveitis have been reported as side effects of TNF-alpha inhibitors.[37,96]

Oral nonsteroidal anti-inflammatory agents are usually used as first-line agents to control scleritis,[37] but more than half the patients with scleritis, regardless of etiology, will need systemic corticosteroids or immunosuppressive therapy.[97] A low-calcium diet could lead to successful resolution of corneal and conjunctival calcifications.[44] Topical cyclosporin and intralesional steroid injections have been used for conjunctival nodules as well.[51,98] Cutaneous eyelid lesions often respond to intralesional steroid injections.

Treatment of keratoconjunctivits sicca, also known as dysfunctional tear syndrome or dry eye disease, depends on severity of symptoms. Lifestyle modification and tear supplementation might be sufficient for mild symptoms. Short courses of topical steroids or cyclosporine could be used for patients with moderate to severe symptoms, but they are often ineffective since the poor tear production tends to be a result of lacrimal gland fibrosis. Physical measures such as punctum plugs, and moisture-retaining eye wear are sometimes useful.[99–101]

Treatment of neuro-ophthalmic sarcoidosis is analogous to that of neurosarcoidosis, warranting aggressive therapy at the outset to optimize outcomes. Further information about the management of neurosarcoidosis is available in this publication as well as elsewhere.[65]

CONCLUSION

Sarcoidosis is a disease that continues to challenge physicians in terms of pathogenesis, diagnosis and treatment. A compatible clinical picture of intraocular inflammation is key to the diagnosis of intraocular sarcoidosis, requiring a close collaboration between ophthalmologists and physicians who diagnose and manage systemic sarcoidosis. The presence of concomitant lung involvement facilitates the diagnosis since findings from lung imaging and bronchoscopy could, in all practicality, secure the diagnosis of intraocular sarcoidosis. Based on our current understanding of the disease, treatment is largely directed at modulating the immune response to suppress ocular inflammation. Steroids remain the first-line treatment for rapid control of severe disease, but steroid-sparing agents are typically the primary agents used for long-term disease control.

REFERENCES

1. Judson MA, Boan AD, Lackland DT. The clinical course of sarcoidosis: presentation, diagnosis, and treatment in a large white and black cohort in the United States. *Sarcoidosis Vasc Diffuse Lung Dis.* 2012;29(2):119–127.
2. Jabs DA, Johns CJ. Ocular involvement in chronic sarcoidosis. *Am J Ophthalmol.* 1986;102(3):297–301.
3. Herbort CP, Rao NA, Mochizuki M. International criteria for the diagnosis of ocular sarcoidosis: results of the first International Workshop on Ocular Sarcoidosis (IWOS). *Ocul Immunol Inflamm.* 2009;17(3):160–169.
4. Iannuzzi MC, Rybicki BA, Teirstein AS. Sarcoidosis. *N Engl J Med.* 2007;357(21):2153–2165.
5. Du Bois RM, Kirby M, Balbi B, Saltini C, Crystal RG. T-lymphocytes that accumulate in the lung in sarcoidosis have evidence of recent stimulation of the T-cell antigen receptor. *Am Rev Respir Dis.* 1992;145(5):1205–1211.
6. Bellocq A, Lecossier D, Pierre-Audigier C, Tazi A, Valeyre D, Hance AJ. T cell receptor repertoire of T lymphocytes recovered from the lung and blood of patients with sarcoidosis. *Am J Respir Crit Care Med.* 1994;149(3 Pt 1):646–654.

7. Baumer I, Zissel G, Schlaak M, Muller-Quernheim J. Th1/Th2 cell distribution in pulmonary sarcoidosis. *Am J Respir Cell Mol Biol*. 1997;16(2):171–177.
8. Ramstein J, Broos CE, Simpson LJ, et al. IFN-gamma-Producing T-helper 17.1 cells are increased in sarcoidosis and are more prevalent than T-helper type 1 cells. *Am J Respir Crit Care Med*. 2016;193(11):1281–1291.
9. Lecossier D, Valeyre D, Loiseau A, et al. Antigen-induced proliferative response of lavage and blood T lymphocytes. Comparison of cells from normal subjects and patients with sarcoidosis. *Am Rev Respir Dis*. 1991;144(4):861–868.
10. Miyara M, Amoura Z, Parizot C, et al. The immune paradox of sarcoidosis and regulatory T cells. *J Exp Med*. 2006;203(2):359–370.
11. Kamphuis LS, Bonte-Mineur F, van Laar JA, van Hagen PM, van Daele PL. Calcium and vitamin D in sarcoidosis: is supplementation safe? *J Bone Miner Res*. 2014;29(11): 2498–2503.
12. Baughman RP, Janovcik J, Ray M, Sweiss N, Lower EE. Calcium and vitamin D metabolism in sarcoidosis. *Sarcoidosis Vasc Diffuse Lung Dis*. 2013;30(2):113–120.
13. Chan AS, Sharma OP, Rao NA. Review for disease of the year: immunopathogenesis of ocular sarcoidosis. *Ocul Immunol Inflamm*. 2010;18(3):143–151.
14. Nagata K, Maruyama K, Uno K, et al. Simultaneous analysis of multiple cytokines in the vitreous of patients with sarcoid uveitis. *Invest Ophthalmol Vis Sci*. 2012;53(7):3827–3833.
15. Grunewald J. Review: role of genetics in susceptibility and outcome of sarcoidosis. *Semin Respir Crit Care Med*. 2010;31(4):380–389.
16. Hills SE, Parkes SA, Baker SB. Epidemiology of sarcoidosis in the Isle of Man–2: evidence for space-time clustering. *Thorax*. 1987;42(6):427–430.
17. Edmondstone WM. Sarcoidosis in nurses: is there an association? *Thorax*. 1988;43(4):342–343.
18. Kern DG, Neill MA, Wrenn DS, Varone JC. Investigation of a unique time-space cluster of sarcoidosis in firefighters. *Am Rev Respir Dis*. 1993;148(4 Pt 1):974–980.
19. Grunewald J, Eklund A, Olerup O. Human leukocyte antigen class I alleles and the disease course in sarcoidosis patients. *Am J Respir Crit Care Med*. 2004;169(6):696–702.
20. Sato H, Woodhead FA, Ahmad T, et al. Sarcoidosis HLA class II genotyping distinguishes differences of clinical phenotype across ethnic groups. *Hum Mol Genet*. 2010;19(20):4100–4111.
21. Davoudi S, Chang VS, Navarro-Gomez D, et al. Association of genetic variants in RAB23 and ANXA11 with uveitis in sarcoidosis. *Mol Vis*. 2018;24:59–74.
22. Baughman RP, Field S, Costabel U, et al. Sarcoidosis in America. Analysis based on health care use. *Ann Am Thorac Soc*. 2016;13(8):1244–1252.
23. Heiligenhaus A, Wefelmeyer D, Wefelmeyer E, Rosel M, Schrenk M. The eye as a common site for the early clinical manifestation of sarcoidosis. *Ophthalmic Res*. 2011;46(1):9–12.
24. Ohara K, Okubo A, Sasaki H, Kamata K. Intraocular manifestations of systemic sarcoidosis. *Jpn J Ophthalmol*. 1992;36(4):452–457.
25. Rothova A, Alberts C, Glasius E, Kijlstra A, Buitenhuis HJ, Breebaart AC. Risk factors for ocular sarcoidosis. *Doc Ophthalmol*. 1989;72(3–4):287–296.
26. Newman LS, Rose CS, Bresnitz EA, et al. A case control etiologic study of sarcoidosis: environmental and occupational risk factors. *Am J Respir Crit Care Med*. 2004;170(12):1324–1330.
27. Baughman RP, Teirstein AS, Judson MA, et al. Clinical characteristics of patients in a case control study of sarcoidosis. *Am J Respir Crit Care Med*. 2001;164(10 Pt 1):1885–1889.
28. Judson MA, Baughman RP, Thompson BW, et al. Two year prognosis of sarcoidosis: the ACCESS experience. *Sarcoidosis Vasc Diffuse Lung Dis*. 2003;20(3):204–211.
29. Rochepeau C, Jamilloux Y, Kerever S, et al. Long-term visual and systemic prognoses of 83 cases of biopsy-proven sarcoid uveitis. *Br J Ophthalmol*. 2017;101(7):856–861.
30. Atmaca LS, Atmaca-Sonmez P, Idil A, Kumbasar OO, Celik G. Ocular involvement in sarcoidosis. *Ocul Immunol Inflamm*. 2009;17(2):91–94.
31. Islam SM, Tabbara KF. Causes of uveitis at the Eye Center in Saudi Arabia: a retrospective review. *Ophthalmic Epidemiol*. 2002;9(4):239–249.
32. Rathinam SR, Namperumalsamy P. Global variation and pattern changes in epidemiology of uveitis. *Indian J Ophthalmol*. 2007;55(3):173–183.
33. Paivonsalo-Hietanen T, Tuominen J, Vaahtoranta-Lehtonen H, Saari KM. Incidence and prevalence of different uveitis entities in Finland. *Acta Ophthalmol Scand*. 1997;75(1):76–81.
34. Merrill PT, Kim J, Cox TA, Betor CC, McCallum RM, Jaffe GJ. Uveitis in the southeastern United States. *Curr Eye Res*. 1997;16(9):865–874.
35. Newman LS, Rose CS, Maier LA. Sarcoidosis. *N Engl J Med*. 1997;336(17):1224–1234.
36. Evans M, Sharma O, LaBree L, Smith RE, Rao NA. Differences in clinical findings between Caucasians and African Americans with biopsy-proven sarcoidosis. *Ophthalmology*. 2007;114(2):325–333.
37. Pasadhika S, Rosenbaum JT. Ocular sarcoidosis. *Clin Chest Med*. 2015;36(4):669–683.
38. Rothova A. Ocular involvement in sarcoidosis. *Br J Ophthalmol*. 2000;84(1):110–116.
39. Kawaguchi T, Hanada A, Horie S, Sugamoto Y, Sugita S, Mochizuki M. Evaluation of characteristic ocular signs and systemic investigations in ocular sarcoidosis patients. *Jpn J Ophthalmol*. 2007;51(2):121–126.
40. Lobo A, Barton K, Minassian D, du Bois RM, Lightman S. Visual loss in sarcoid-related uveitis. *Clin Exp Ophthalmol*. 2003;31(4):310–316.
41. Dana MR, Merayo-Lloves J, Schaumberg DA, Foster CS. Prognosticators for visual outcome in sarcoid uveitis. *Ophthalmology*. 1996;103(11):1846–1853.

42. Mana J, Montero A, Vidal M, Marcoval J, Pujol R. Recurrent sarcoidosis: a study of 17 patients with 24 episodes of recurrence. *Sarcoidosis Vasc Diffuse Lung Dis*. 2003;20(3):212–221.
43. Jabs DA, Nussenblatt RB, Rosenbaum JT. Standardization of uveitis nomenclature for reporting clinical data. Results of the First International Workshop. *Am J Ophthalmol*. 2005;140(3):509–516.
44. Crick RP, Hoyle C, Smellie H. The eyes in sarcoidosis. *Br J Ophthalmol*. 1961;45(7):461–481.
45. Mavrikakis I, Rootman J. Diverse clinical presentations of orbital sarcoid. *Am J Ophthalmol*. 2007;144(5):769–775.
46. Prabhakaran VC, Saeed P, Esmaeli B, et al. Orbital and adnexal sarcoidosis. *Arch Ophthalmol*. 2007;125(12):1657–1662.
47. Petropoulos IK, Zuber JP, Guex-Crosier Y. Heerfordt syndrome with unilateral facial nerve palsy: a rare presentation of sarcoidosis. *Klin Monbl Augenheilkd*. 2008;225(5):453–456.
48. Chappity P, Kumar R, Sahoo AK. Heerfordt's syndrome presenting with recurrent facial nerve palsy: case report and 10-year literature review. *Sultan Qaboos Univ Med J*. 2015;15(1):e124–e128.
49. Cakmak SK, Gonul M, Gul U, Gunduz H, Han O, Kulacoglu S. Sarcoidosis involving the lacrimal, submandibular, and parotid glands with panda sign. *Dermatol Online J*. 2009;15(3):8.
50. Manrique Lipa RK, de los Bueis AB, De los Rios JJ, Manrique Lipa RD. Sarcoidosis presenting as acute bulbar follicular conjunctivitis. *Clin Exp Optom*. 2010;93(5):363–365.
51. Schilgen G, Sundmacher R, Pomjanski N, Bocking A, Reinecke P, Gabbert HE. Bilateral large conjunctival tumours as primary manifestation of sarcoidosis–successful treatment with steroid-depot-injections. *Klin Monbl Augenheilkd*. 2006;223(4):326–329.
52. Dithmar S, Waring 3rd GO, Goldblum TA, Grossniklaus HE. Conjunctival deposits as an initial manifestation of sarcoidosis. *Am J Ophthalmol*. 1999;128(3):361–362.
53. Bastiaensen LA, Verpalen MC, Pijpers PM, Sprong AC. Conjunctival sarcoidosis. *Doc Ophthalmol*. 1985;59(1):5–9.
54. Collins ME, Petronic-Rosic V, Sweiss NJ, Marcet MM. Full-thickness eyelid lesions in sarcoidosis. *Case Rep Ophthalmol Med*. 2013;2013:579121.
55. Moin M, Kersten RC, Bernardini F, Kulwin DR. Destructive eyelid lesions in sarcoidosis. *Ophthal Plast Reconstr Surg*. 2001;17(2):123–125.
56. Lennarson P, Barney NP. Interstitial keratitis as presenting ophthalmic sign of sarcoidosis in a child. *J Pediatr Ophthalmol Strabismus*. 1995;32(3):194–196.
57. Siracuse-Lee D, Saffra N. Peripheral ulcerative keratitis in sarcoidosis: a case report. *Cornea*. 2006;25(5):618–620.
58. Babu K, Kini R, Mehta R. Scleral nodule and bilateral disc edema as a presenting manifestation of systemic sarcoidosis. *Ocul Immunol Inflamm*. 2010;18(3):158–161.
59. Heiligenhaus A, Michel D, Koch JM. Nodular scleritis in a patient with sarcoidosis. *Br J Ophthalmol*. 2003;87(4):507–508.
60. Dursun D, Akova YA, Bilezikci B. Scleritis associated with sarcoidosis. *Ocul Immunol Inflamm*. 2004;12(2):143–148.
61. Baughman RP, Weiss KL, Golnik KC. Neuro-ophthalmic sarcoidosis. *Eye Brain*. 2012;4:13–25.
62. Kidd DP, Burton BJ, Graham EM, Plant GT. Optic neuropathy associated with systemic sarcoidosis. *Neurol Neuroimmunol Neuroinflamm*. 2016;3(5):e270.
63. Kefella H, Luther D, Hainline C. Ophthalmic and neuro-ophthalmic manifestations of sarcoidosis. *Curr Opin Ophthalmol*. 2017;28(6):587–594.
64. Koczman JJ, Rouleau J, Gaunt M, Kardon RH, Wall M, Lee AG. Neuro-ophthalmic sarcoidosis: the University of Iowa experience. *Semin Ophthalmol*. 2008;23(3):157–168.
65. Culver DA, Ribeiro Neto ML, Moss BP, Willis MA. Neurosarcoidosis. *Semin Respir Crit Care Med*. 2017;38(4):499–513.
66. Judson MA, Costabel U, Drent M, et al. The WASOG Sarcoidosis Organ Assessment Instrument: an update of a previous clinical tool. *Sarcoidosis Vasc Diffuse Lung Dis*. 2014;31(1):19–27.
67. Gambrelle J, Jacob M, Le Breton F, et al. Conjunctival biopsy: a useful procedure for the diagnosis of sarcoidosis. *J Fr Ophtalmol*. 2006;29(5):579–582.
68. Karcioglu ZA, Brear R. Conjunctival biopsy in sarcoidosis. *Am J Ophthalmol*. 1985;99(1):68–73.
69. Spaide RF, Ward DL. Conjunctival biopsy in the diagnosis of sarcoidosis. *Br J Ophthalmol*. 1990;74(8):469–471.
70. Chevalet P, Clement R, Rodat O, Moreau A, Brisseau JM, Clarke JP. Sarcoidosis diagnosed in elderly subjects: retrospective study of 30 cases. *Chest*. 2004;126(5):1423–1430.
71. Blaise P, Fardeau C, Chapelon C, Bodaghi B, Le Hoang P. Minor salivary gland biopsy in diagnosing ocular sarcoidosis. *Br J Ophthalmol*. 2011;95(12):1731–1734.
72. Lim LL, Suhler EB, Rosenbaum JT, Wilson DJ. The role of choroidal and retinal biopsies in the diagnosis and management of atypical presentations of uveitis. *Trans Am Ophthalmol Soc*. 2005;103:84–91; discussion 91–82.
73. Bickett AN, Lower EE, Baughman RP. Sarcoidosis diagnostic score (SDS): a systematic evaluation to enhance the diagnosis of sarcoidosis. *Chest*. 2018.
74. Kaiser PK, Lowder CY, Sullivan P, et al. Chest computerized tomography in the evaluation of uveitis in elderly women. *Am J Ophthalmol*. 2002;133(4):499–505.
75. Takahashi T, Azuma A, Abe S, Kawanami O, Ohara K, Kudoh S. Significance of lymphocytosis in bronchoalveolar lavage in suspected ocular sarcoidosis. *Eur Respir J*. 2001;18(3):515–521.
76. Wessendorf TE, Bonella F, Costabel U. Diagnosis of sarcoidosis. *Clin Rev Allergy Immunol*. 2015;49(1):54–62.
77. Seve P, Billotey C, Janier M, Grange JD, Broussolle C, Kodjikian L. Fluorodeoxyglucose positron emission tomography for the diagnosis of sarcoidosis in patients with unexplained chronic uveitis. *Ocul Immunol Inflamm*. 2009;17(3):179–184.

78. Nishiyama Y, Yamamoto Y, Fukunaga K, et al. Comparative evaluation of 18F-FDG PET and 67Ga scintigraphy in patients with sarcoidosis. *J Nucl Med.* 2006;47(10):1571–1576.
79. Schuster DM, Alazraki N. Gallium and other agents in diseases of the lung. *Semin Nucl Med.* 2002;32(3):193–211.
80. Lower EE, Weiss KL. Neurosarcoidosis. *Clin Chest Med.* 2008;29(3):475–492.
81. Sato DK, Callegaro D, de Haidar Jorge FM, et al. Cerebrospinal fluid aquaporin-4 antibody levels in neuromyelitis optica attacks. *Ann Neurol.* 2014;76(2):305–309.
82. Sheppard JD, Toyos MM, Kempen JH, Kaur P, Foster CS. Difluprednate 0.05% versus prednisolone acetate 1% for endogenous anterior uveitis: a phase III, multicenter, randomized study. *Invest Ophthalmol Vis Sci.* 2014;55(5):2993–3002.
83. Yang SJ, Salek S, Rosenbaum JT. Ocular sarcoidosis: new diagnostic modalities and treatment. *Curr Opin Pulm Med.* 2017;23(5):458–467.
84. Pavesio C, Zierhut M, Bairi K, Comstock TL, Usner DW. Evaluation of an intravitreal fluocinolone acetonide implant versus standard systemic therapy in noninfectious posterior uveitis. *Ophthalmology.* 2010;117(3): 567–575.e561.
85. Brady CJ, Villanti AC, Law HA, et al. Corticosteroid implants for chronic non-infectious uveitis. *Cochrane Database Syst Rev.* 2016;2:Cd010469.
86. Varron L, Abad S, Kodjikian L, Seve P. Sarcoid uveitis: diagnostic and therapeutic update. *Rev Med Interne.* 2011;32(2):86–92.
87. Dev S, McCallum RM, Jaffe GJ. Methotrexate treatment for sarcoid-associated panuveitis. *Ophthalmology.* 1999;106(1):111–118.
88. Baughman RP, Winget DB, Lower EE. Methotrexate is steroid sparing in acute sarcoidosis: results of a double blind, randomized trial. *Sarcoidosis Vasc Diffuse Lung Dis.* 2000;17(1):60–66.
89. Bhat P, Cervantes-Castaneda RA, Doctor PP, Anzaar F, Foster CS. Mycophenolate mofetil therapy for sarcoidosis-associated uveitis. *Ocul Immunol Inflamm.* 2009;17(3):185–190.
90. Galor A, Jabs DA, Leder HA, et al. Comparison of antimetabolite drugs as corticosteroid-sparing therapy for noninfectious ocular inflammation. *Ophthalmology.* 2008;115(10):1826–1832.
91. Kacmaz RO, Kempen JH, Newcomb C, et al. Cyclosporine for ocular inflammatory diseases. *Ophthalmology.* 2010;117(3):576–584.
92. Jaffe GJ, Dick AD, Brezin AP, et al. Adalimumab in patients with active noninfectious uveitis. *N Engl J Med.* 2016;375(10):932–943.
93. Judson MA, Baughman RP, Costabel U, et al. Efficacy of infliximab in extrapulmonary sarcoidosis: results from a randomised trial. *Eur Respir J.* 2008;31(6):1189–1196.
94. Doty JD, Mazur JE, Judson MA. Treatment of sarcoidosis with infliximab. *Chest.* 2005;127(3):1064–1071.
95. Baughman RP, Lower EE, Bradley DA, Raymond LA, Kaufman A. Etanercept for refractory ocular sarcoidosis: results of a double-blind randomized trial. *Chest.* 2005;128(2):1062–1047.
96. Seve P, Kodjikian L, Jamilloux Y. Ocular sarcoidosis: what the internist should know? *Rev Med Interne.* 2017.
97. Jabs DA, Mudun A, Dunn JP, Marsh MJ. Episcleritis and scleritis: clinical features and treatment results. *Am J Ophthalmol.* 2000;130(4):469–476.
98. Akpek EK, Ilhan-Sarac O, Green WR. Topical cyclosporin in the treatment of chronic sarcoidosis of the conjunctiva. *Arch Ophthalmol.* 2003;121(9):1333–1335.
99. Jackson WB. Management of dysfunctional tear syndrome: a Canadian consensus. *Can J Ophthalmol.* 2009;44(4):385–394.
100. Dogru M, Nakamura M, Shimazaki J, Tsubota K. Changing trends in the treatment of dry-eye disease. *Expert Opin Investig Drugs.* 2013;22(12):1581–1601.
101. Behrens A, Doyle JJ, Stern L, et al. Dysfunctional tear syndrome: a Delphi approach to treatment recommendations. *Cornea.* 2006;25(8):900–907.

FURTHER READING

1. Scadding JG. *Mycobacterium tuberculosis* in the aetiology of sarcoidosis. *Br Med J.* 1960;2(5213):1617–1623.
2. Almenoff PL, Johnson A, Lesser M, Mattman LH. Growth of acid fast L forms from the blood of patients with sarcoidosis. *Thorax.* 1996;51(5):530–533.
3. Brown ST, Brett I, Almenoff PL, Lesser M, Terrin M, Teirstein AS. Recovery of cell wall-deficient organisms from blood does not distinguish between patients with sarcoidosis and control subjects. *Chest.* 2003;123(2):413–417.
4. Fidler HM, Rook GA, Johnson NM, McFadden J. *Mycobacterium tuberculosis* DNA in tissue affected by sarcoidosis. *Bmj.* 1993;306(6877):546–549.
5. Wilsher ML, Menzies RE, Croxson MC. *Mycobacterium tuberculosis* DNA in tissues affected by sarcoidosis. *Thorax.* 1998;53(10):871–874.
6. Drake WP, Pei Z, Pride DT, Collins RD, Cover TL, Blaser MJ. Molecular analysis of sarcoidosis tissues for mycobacterium species DNA. *Emerg Infect Dis.* 2002;8(11):1334–1341.
7. Gazouli M, Ikonomopoulos J, Trigidou R, Foteinou M, Kittas C, Gorgoulis V. Assessment of mycobacterial, propionibacterial, and human herpesvirus 8 DNA in tissues of Greek patients with sarcoidosis. *J Clin Microbiol.* 2002;40(8):3060–3063.
8. Oswald-Richter KA, Beachboard DC, Zhan X, et al. Multiple mycobacterial antigens are targets of the adaptive immune response in pulmonary sarcoidosis. *Respir Res.* 2010;11:161.

CHAPTER 13

Other Extra-pulmonary Visceral Involvement

HUIPING LI, MD • ROBERT PHILLIP BAUGHMAN, MD

HEPATIC AND SPLENIC SARCOIDOSIS

After the lung and lymph nodes, the liver is the third most frequently affected organ in sarcoidosis according to pathology. Histologic features of hepatic sarcoidosis can mimic other liver diseases (infections, drugs, metabolites, autoimmune disease) which have to be excluded.[1] Even when sarcoidosis is confirmed, any associated liver disease needs to be considered before liver manifestations are relied to sarcoidosis. Hepatic sarcoidosis can present with a wide variety of manifestations (Table 13.1).[1,3] The clinical manifestations of liver sarcoidosis are usually not specific. Only 5%–30% of patients with liver sarcoidosis show clinical symptoms,[4] which include fever of unknown origin; occasional increases in serum transaminases, alkaline phosphatase, γ-glutamyltranspeptidase, and/or bilirubin; rare chronic cholestasis resulting from intrahepatic biliary granuloma; and very rare (1% patients) portal hypertension and cirrhosis.[3,5] In one series, a cholestatic picture (elevated alkaline phosphatase) was seen alone in 43% of cases and combined with parenchymal inflammation (elevated serum transaminases) in another 34% of cases. Parenchymatous changes alone were seen in only 24% of cases.[2] Severe liver function test abnormalities are defined when three or four tests with three or more times the upper limit of normal persist for at least 3 months, and such profile suggests fibrosis.

Ultrasonography of liver sarcoidosis shows uneven internal echo, intrahepatic mass, diffuse lesions, liver enlargement, and characteristics of acute hepatitis.[6] Computed tomography (CT) scan (Fig. 13.1) and magnetic resonance imaging (MRI) may also evidence morphologic abnormalities concerning not only the liver but also the spleen and abdominal lymphadenopathy.[7] Liver stiffness can be determined by fibroscanning and has proved useful to quantitating the level of fibrosis in viral hepatitis.[8] It may also be useful in sarcoidosis, but further study is warranted.

Liver biopsy is very sensitive to detect granulomas,[2] but several other conditions, including methotrexate therapy, can cause liver granulomas.[1,9,10] The examination is particularly critical to distinguish liver sarcoidosis from malignant tumors.[11] Liver biopsy shows that 40%–70% of unselected sarcoidosis patients will have granulomas, including patients with no symptoms, suggesting hepatic sarcoidosis.[2,10,12] Histopathology of lesions in some patients displays cholestasis, inflammatory necrosis, and vascular changes.[13] In most patients, liver sarcoidosis is benign and spontaneously resolves.

TABLE 13.1
Clinical Features of Hepatic Sarcoidosis

Feature	Frequency
Asymptomatic	50%–80%
Abnormal liver function testing (LFT)[2]	30%
Cholestatic alone	43% of those with abnormal LFT
Parenchymous alone	23% of those with abnormal LFT
Combined	34% of those with abnormal LFT
Organomegaly	50% detected on radiologic imaging; 15% detected clinically
Abdominal pain	15%
Pruritis and/or jaundice	<5%
Cirrhosis	7%
Portal hypertension	5%
Liver failure requiring transplant	<0.02% of all liver transplants in the United States

Adapted from Tadros M, Forouhar F, Wu GY. Hepatic sarcoidosis. *J Clin Transl Hepatol*. 2013;1(2):87–93.

Sarcoidosis. https://doi.org/10.1016/B978-0-323-54429-0.00013-6

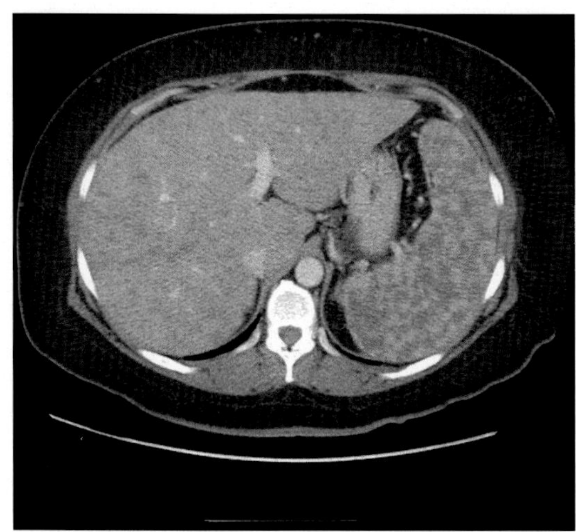

FIG. 13.1 Computed tomography image demonstrating an enlarged spleen and liver from sarcoidosis.

There are still few studies on the impact of sarcoidosis treatment on liver manifestations. Many patients may never require therapy.[14] However, some patients are symptomatic and require treatment.[12] While corticosteroids remain the most common initial therapy, second-line therapy including azathioprine and even methotrexate have been reported as effective.[15] The evolution toward cirrhosis appears very rare but unpredictable.[16]

Reported splenic involvement ranges from 5% to over 70% of cases, depending in part on technique used to detect involvement.[17] Radiologic techniques such as CT scan, MRI, and ultrasound often detect asymptomatic diseases.[6,18,19] Morphologic findings at ultrasound, CT, or MRI are either nodules or splenomegaly (Fig. 13.1). Clinical splenomegaly is observed in 10% of patients.[18] This may induce hypersplenism with splenic sequestration with thrombocytopenia, moderate anemia, and neutropenia. Rarely, splenomegaly is secondary to portal hypertension.

RENAL SARCOIDOSIS

Renal manifestations of sarcoidosis are diverse,[20–23] mainly including hypercalcemia or hypercalciuria, nephrolithiasis, nephrocalcinosis, granulomatous tubulointerstitial nephritis ("renal sarcoidosis" *stricto sensu*), whereas glomerulonephritis and membranous nephropathy are uncommon.[24,25] Renal sarcoidosis occurs in 0.7%–4.3% of cases most often at onset of sarcoidosis but may also occur after a variable delay in 20% of patients, justifying a regular assessment of renal parameters in sarcoidosis patients. Patients with sarcoidosis often overproduce 1,25-dihydroxyvitamin D, leading to increases in intestinal calcium absorption, bone resorption, and urinary calcium, and excessive urinary calcium can result in renal calcification and renal failure.[25,26] Patients with renal sarcoidosis present obvious renal insufficiency, whereas proteinuria, aseptic leukocyturia, and microscopic hematuria are mild or absent. In one prospective study, 190 sarcoidosis patients seen consecutively at a sarcoidosis clinic had spot urine testing for proteinuria. Seven percent had proteinuria, but most of them had known risk factors for proteinuria such as diabetes.[27]

Diagnosis needs confirmation by renal biopsy with evidence of typical granulomatous lesions or sometimes of tubulointerstitial nephritis without granulomas. Table 13.2 summarizes the results of renal biopsies from three studies of sarcoidosis patients. Overall, granulomatous interstitial nephritis was the most common finding, but other pathologic features were identified. A patient with kidney disease in the context of typical sarcoidosis should be highly suspected to have sarcoidosis-associated kidney lesions and should be examined by renal biopsy [12,13]. Granulomatous nephritis without obvious extrarenal manifestations of sarcoidosis needs considering alternative diagnoses such as medication adverse reactions, neoplasia, and autoimmune diseases.[30]

Patients should have corticosteroid treatment immediately after renal sarcoidosis is diagnosed. High dosage of glucocorticosteroids (1 mg/kg/day) is often required to treat granulomatous interstitial nephritis and/or interstitial nephritis. Response to treatment at 1 month is often predictive of long-term response.[20] An incomplete response with persistent renal insufficiency is seen in two-thirds of patients. The dosage should be reduced gradually 8–12 weeks after patients reach the treatment goal. Methotrexate is excreted by the kidney, so its use is limited in renal sarcoidosis. Mycophenolate and azathioprine have been reported as steroid sparing in renal sarcoidosis.[32]

PAROTID GLAND SARCOIDOSIS

Bilateral painless parotid swelling occurs in 2%–5% of patients, usually at onset of sarcoidosis.[33–35] Submaxillary and sublingual (Fig. 13.2) swelling may also be seen. The enlargements are usually hard mass without tenderness on palpation, and patients often have dry mouth.[35] The palpable sarcoidosis nodules underneath the mucous membrane of the lips, cheeks, and tongue can have various sizes, are active, and show dark red

TABLE 13.2
Main Histologic Findings From Renal Biopsy of Patients With Renal Sarcoidosis

	BAGNASCO[28]		LOFFLER[29]		MAHAVES[20]	
First Author	**Number**	**%**	**Number**	**%**	**Number**	**%**
Total	56		27		47	
Granulomatous interstitial nephritis	19	34	8	30	37	79
Interstitial nephritis without granuloma	8	14	12	44	10	21
Diabetic nephropathy	7	13				
Focal segmental glomerulosclerosis	6	11				
Chronic/acute sclerosing changes	6	11				
Immune complex–mediated glomerulonephritis	3	5				
Acute tubular injury	3	5				
Amyloid	1	2				
Membranous glomerulopathy	1	2				
Thin glomerular basement membrane disease	1	2				
Nonspecific changes	1	2				
IgA glomerulonephritis			4	15		
Nephrocalcinosis			3	11		

color, hard mass, and mild tenderness. These nodules are not adhered to the surrounding tissue, and oral examination shows lip and cheek tissue swelling and thickening.

Parotid gland sarcoidosis should be distinguished from Sjögren syndrome.[36] The Heerfordt's syndrome which associates uveitis, parotid swelling, fever, and facial palsy is specific of sarcoidosis.[37] Parotid swelling most often resolves spontaneously in 8–12 weeks independently of the general course of sarcoidosis. Oral and maxillofacial sarcoidosis is rare and can occur at any age.[33] It often develops in the lips, head and neck lymph nodes, jaw bones, oral soft tissue, and parotid gland.[38] The disease at early stage shows mild symptoms or asymptomatic. Local masses and facial and neck lymphadenopathy may be found during routine physical examination when patients have early-stage oral and maxillofacial sarcoidosis. It is challenging to detect small sarcoidosis nodules located in the parotid gland and submandibular gland. If left untreated, those small nodules could grow continuously and thus cause enlargements in the unilateral or bilateral parotid or submandibular gland. The enlargements are usually hard mass without tenderness at palpation, and patients often have dry mouth. The palpable sarcoidosis nodules underneath the mucous membrane of the lips, cheeks, and tongue can have various sizes, are active, and show dark red color, hard mass, and mild tenderness. These nodules are not adhered to the surrounding tissue, and oral examination shows lip and cheek tissue swelling and thickening. Parotid gland sarcoidosis should be distinguished from Sjögren syndrome, and it may be associated with the clinical characteristics and symptoms of Heerfordt's syndrome.[37]

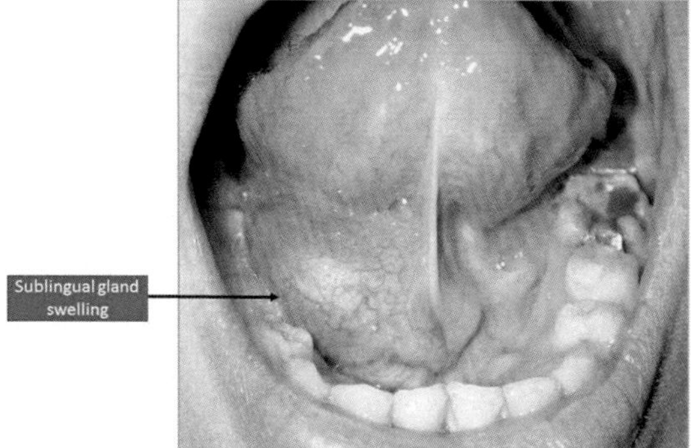

FIG. 13.2 Sublingual gland swelling due to sarcoidosis indicated by *arrow*. (Figure courtesy Dr. Alan Seiden.)

When explicit symptoms and diagnosis of systemic sarcoidosis are unavailable, sarcoidosis initiated at oral and maxillofacial area usually does not

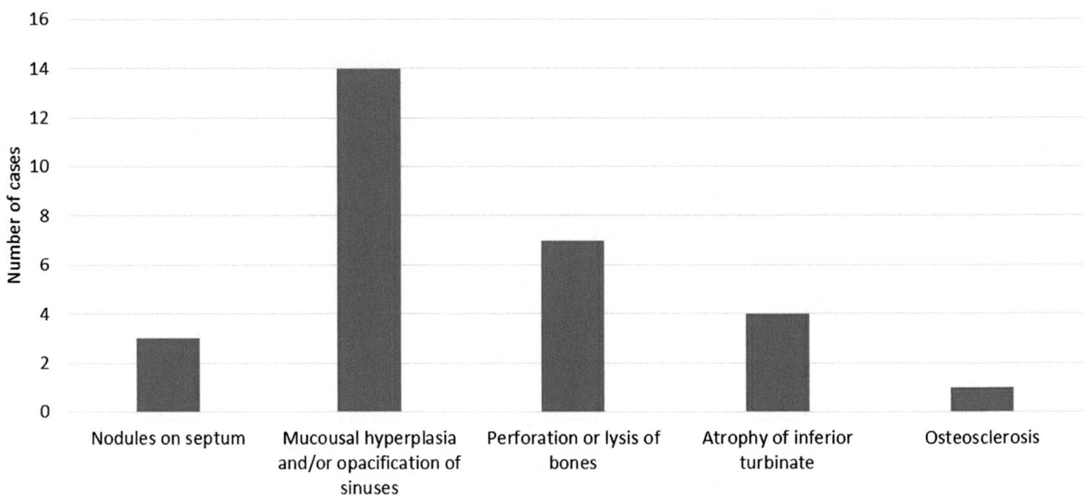

FIG. 13.3 Common manifestations of nasal sarcoidosis found in a series of 15 patients.[31]

present specific symptoms. Thus, these types of sarcoidosis are easily misdiagnosed and mistreated if only clinical symptoms are considered for diagnosis. Biopsy is the reliable method to diagnose oral sarcoidosis. Histopathological examination of lesions in the lymph nodes, labial gland tissue, or skin can be used to diagnose oral sarcoidosis. However, there are other causes of granulomatous involvement in the oral cavity.[39]

SINONASAL AND LARYNGEAL SARCOIDOSIS

Sinonasal sarcoidosis occurs in 1.6% of cases.[40,41] It often precedes other manifestations of sarcoidosis. Symptoms include by decreasing frequency persistent stiffness, anosmia, rhinorrhea, crusting, and epistaxis. Fig. 13.3 demonstrates the common manifestations of nasal sarcoidosis found in one series of 15 patients.[31] Rhinoscopy allows evidencing a typical macroscopic aspects, and biopsy of granulations in the nasal mucosa allows for obtaining easily typical granulomatous lesions (Fig. 13.3A). Sinus CT evidences opacification of the maxillary and ethmoidal sinuses with perforations or lytic lesions in half of the cases (Fig. 13.4). Laryngeal sarcoidosis is rarer and has to be recognized in a patient who presents with hoarseness, inspiratory dyspnea, dysphagia, snoring, and/or sleep apnea. Laryngeal sarcoidosis is often associated to sinonasal involvement. Both are often associated with lupus pernio[42] and longstanding multivisceral sarcoidosis.[43] (Fig. 13.5).

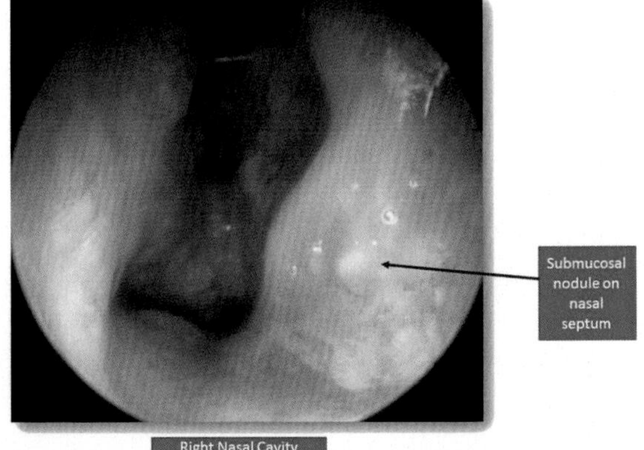

FIG. 13.4 Endoscopic view of right nasal cavity of patient with nasal sarcoidosis. (Figure courtesy Dr. Alan Seiden.)

Treatment with anti-inflammatory agents has been shown to be effective in most cases. Fig. 13.6 summarizes the percentage of patients receiving individual therapies for sinus sarcoidosis. Only one study included patients not receiving systemic therapy.[44] All four studies included patients undergoing surgery as part of their therapy, but this still represented less than a third of all patients.[31,44–46] Many patients required long-term treatment, usually with steroid-sparing agents. In addition to anti-inflammatory treatment of granulomatous disease, one needs to consider the impact of infection. Prior sinus damage, such as bronchiectasis, often leads to symptoms long after the granulomatous disease has resolved. Fig. 13.7 provides a stepwise approach to managing sinus sarcoidosis.

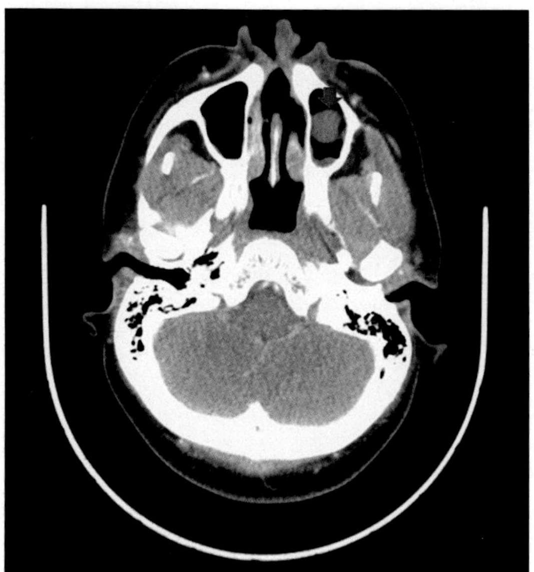

FIG. 13.5 Left maxillary sinus with biopsy confirmed granulomatous tissue (*arrow*) in sarcoidosis patient.

OSSEOUS SARCOIDOSIS

The skeleton may be involved in sarcoidosis following three mechanisms. Both of them, abnormal vitamin D and calcium metabolism and corticosteroid-induced osteoporosis and bone fragility, are considered in another chapter of the book. The third one, osseous sarcoidosis, is detected by either clinical, conventional radiograph, or advanced imaging. The prevalence depends on the method of detection but appears to be below 5%.[48,49] Axial bone involvement is seen in over 80% of cases, with spine disease detected in more than two-thirds of cases from two series (Table 13.3).[49,50] About half of the patients in these series had no symptoms from their bone involvement and did not require specific therapy. Symptomatic disease includes involvement of hands and feet bones (with typically swelling, deformity, redness and stiffness at clinical examination (Fig. 13.8), and cystic lesions or trabeculations of little bones at radiography) in the context of long-term evolution sarcoidosis. Bone involvement is associated with lupus pernio and sinonasal sarcoidosis.[42,43] In one study, 95% of osseous sarcoidosis patients had three or more organs affected compared with 28% of the match sarcoidosis controls ($P<.0001$).[49] In that study, liver, spleen, and extrathoracic lymph node involvement was significantly more common in the osseous sarcoidosis patients. In two series from American bone disease studies, 75%–90% of patients with bone involvement were white.[49,50] (Fig. 13.9).

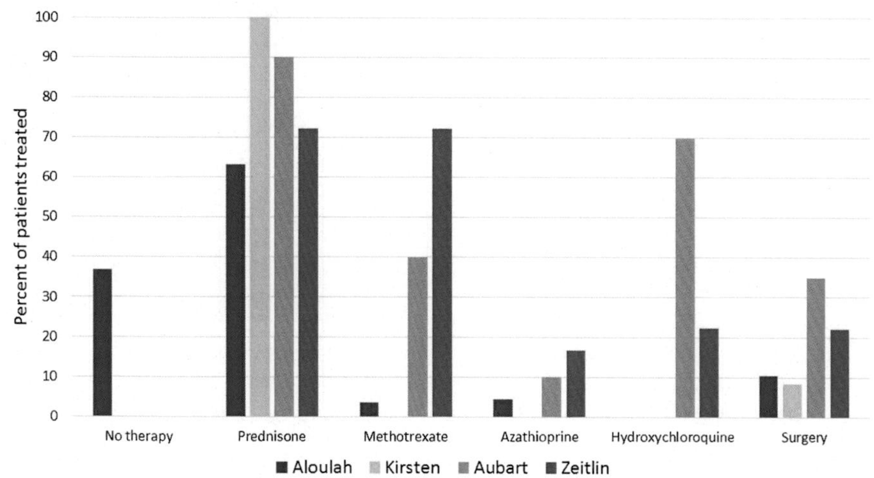

FIG. 13.6 The percentage of patients receiving individual therapies (prednisone, methotrexate, azathioprine, hydroxychloroquine) as well as no treatment or surgery. Only one study reported on patients not receiving systemic therapy.[44] All four studies included patients undergoing surgery as part of their therapy, but this still represented less than a third of all patients.[31,44–46]

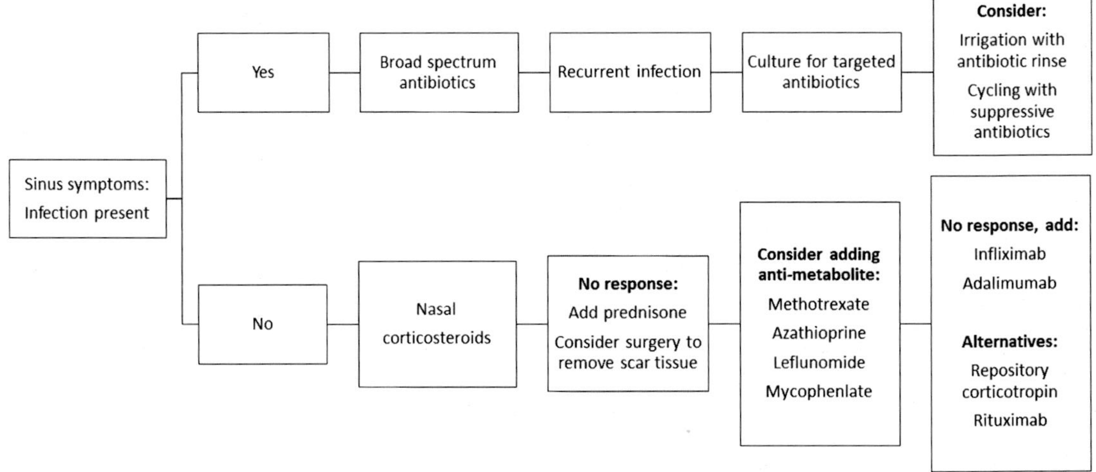

FIG. 13.7 A stepwise approach to management of sinonasal sarcoidosis. Treatment is for the underlying sarcoidosis (top half of the flow chart) as well as management of any infection. Prednisone is the most commonly used oral corticosteroid. Surgical management of residual scarring is usually reserved until after inflammation is controlled. (Adapted from Baughman RP, Seiden A, Lower EE, Sino-nasal sarcoidosis. In: Bernstein JA, eds. *Rhinitis and Related Upper Respiratory Conditions*. New York: Springer; 2018:137–152.)

TABLE 13.3
Location of Bone Invovlement in Osseous Sarcoidosis

Involved Location[a]	Zhou[49]	Sparks[50]
Total number of cases	64	20
Spine/axial	44 (68.8%)[b]	14 (70%)
Sternum	1 (1.6%)	3 (15%)
Scapular	4 (6.3%)	5 (25%)
Clavicle	1 (1.6%)	1 (5%)
Rib	7 (10.9%)	2 (10%)
Pelvis	23 (35.9%)	13 (65%)
Skull	6 (9.4%)	4 (20%)
Femur	9 (14.1%)	5 (25%)
Humerus	3 (4.7%)	6 (30%)
Hands	10 (15.6%)	2 (10%)

[a]Patients could have more than one area affected.
[b]Number affected (% of total).

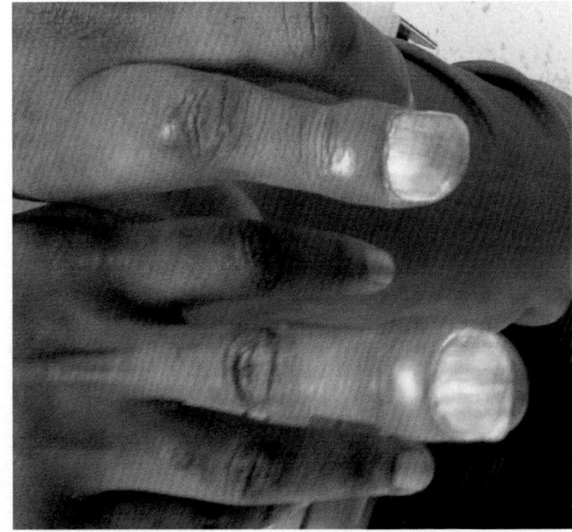

FIG. 13.8 Bone involvement in fingers with swelling and deformity of joints.

The use of advanced imaging of ^{18F}fludeoxyglucose (FDG)–positive emission tomography (PET) (Fig. 13.9) and MRI makes the discovery of osseous sarcoidosis possible far more often.[42,49] In one series of sarcoidosis patients undergoing PET scan for evaluation of the their sarcoidosis, a third had evidence of a bone disease.[51] In half of the cases, PET was performed for diverse extraskeleton indications, and the osseous involvement is fortuitously discovered, whereas in the other half, patients complain of skeleton pains or other symptoms.[51]

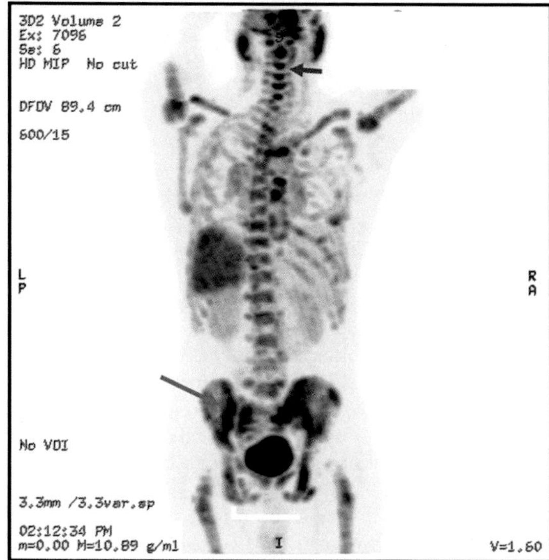

FIG. 13.9 Patient with multiple sites of bone involvement shown by a positive emission tomography scan including spine (*red arrow*) and pelvis (*blue arrow*).

Osseous manifestations at ^{18F}FDG-PET and MRI are not specific, and differential diagnosis with malignancy, particularly metastasis, may be difficult, requiring the use of directed biopsies. Recently, the WASOG instrument indicated that in sarcoidosis patients, only cystic lesions at radiography or positive bone biopsy were considered highly probable diagnosis of bone sarcoidosis, whereas an abnormal PET or MRI in a patient with known sarcoidosis had a probable diagnosis of bone disease.[52]

There is still no recommendation for osseous sarcoidosis treatment. For some authors, treatment is required in symptomatic osseous sarcoidosis, whereas it is determined according to other manifestations in asymptomatic patients. Corticosteroids are usually the first choice, but other agents including immunosuppressive drugs and infliximab and adalimumab have been used.[50,53] In one large series, infliximab was used in a quarter of cases compared with only 5% of a matched control group.[49]

OTHERS (UTERUS, BREAST, TESTICULAR, AND DIGESTIVE TRACT SARCOIDOSIS)

Sarcoidosis in the reproductive system is very rare with usually no deleterious effect on fertility. Sarcoidosis barely affect the male genitourinary system, mainly the epididymis, and a testicular biopsy is required for the diagnosis of sarcoidosis.[54,55] Asymptomatic granuloma can develop in the female genital organs, and the uterus is particularly vulnerable. Breast granuloma, a very rare condition, is very difficult to be distinguished from breast malignancies,[56,57] and surgical biopsy is required to confirm the diagnosis.[58] Digestive tract involvement is infrequent.[3] Main manifestations are weight loss, abdominal pain, vomiting, and bleeding. The stomach is the most frequent localization, whereas ileum and colonic lesions are very rare and needs searching for Crohn's disease.

REFERENCES

1. Tadros M, Forouhar F, Wu GY. Hepatic sarcoidosis. *J Clin Transl Hepatol*. 2013;1(2):87–93.
2. Cremers J, Drent M, Driessen A, et al. Liver-test abnormalities in sarcoidosis. *Eur J Gastroenterol Hepatol*. 2011.
3. Ebert EC, Kierson M, Hagspiel KD. Gastrointestinal and hepatic manifestations of sarcoidosis. *Am J Gastroenterol*. 2008;103(12):3184–3192.
4. Blich M, Edoute Y. Clinical manifestations of sarcoid liver disease. *J Gastroenterol Hepatol*. 2004;19(7):732–737.
5. Tan CB, Rashid S, Rajan D, et al. Hepatic sarcoidosis presenting as portal hypertension and liver cirrhosis: case report and review of the literature. *Case Rep Gastroenterol*. 2012;6(1):183–189.
6. Tana C, Dietrich CF, Schiavone C. Hepatosplenic sarcoidosis: contrast-enhanced ultrasound findings and implications for clinical practice. *BioMed Res Int*. 2014;2014:926203. https://doi.org/10.1155/2014/926203. Epub;%2014 Aug 18:926203.
7. Warshauer DM, Molina PL, Hamman SM, et al. Nodular sarcoidosis of the liver and spleen: analysis of 32 cases. *Radiology*. 1995;195(3):757–762.
8. Sharma P, Dhawan S, Bansal R, et al. Usefulness of transient elastography by FibroScan for the evaluation of liver fibrosis. *Indian J Gastroenterol*. 2014;33(5):445–451.
9. Valla DC, Benhamou JP. Hepatic granulomas and hepatic sarcoidosis. *Clin Liver Dis*. 2000;4(1): 269–26x.
10. Baughman RP, Koehler A, Bejarano PA, et al. Role of liver function tests in detecting methotrexate-induced liver damage in sarcoidosis. *Arch Intern Med*. 2003;163(5): 615–620.
11. Miyamoto R, Sano N, Tadano S, et al. Hepatic sarcoidosis mimicking cholangiocellular carcinoma: a case report and literature review. *Int J Surg Case Rep*. 2017;41:165–168. https://doi.org/10.1016/j.ijscr.2017.10.032. Epub;%2017 Oct 25.:165–168.
12. Kahi CJ, Saxena R, Temkit M, et al. Hepatobiliary disease in sarcoidosis. *Sarcoidosis Vasc Diffuse Lung Dis*. 2006;23(2):117–123.
13. Nakanuma Y, Kouda W, Harada K, et al. Hepatic sarcoidosis with vanishing bile duct syndrome, cirrhosis, and portal phlebosclerosis. Report of an autopsy case. *J Clin Gastroenterol*. 2001;32(2):181–184.

14. Vatti R, Sharma OP. Course of asymptomatic liver involvement in sarcoidosis: role of therapy in selected cases. *Sarcoidosis Vasc Diffuse Lung Dis.* 1997;14(1):73–76.
15. Kennedy PT, Zakaria N, Modawi SB, et al. Natural history of hepatic sarcoidosis and its response to treatment. *Eur J Gastroenterol Hepatol.* 2006;18(7):721–726.
16. Fetzer DT, Rees MA, Dasyam AK, et al. Hepatic sarcoidosis in patients presenting with liver dysfunction: imaging appearance, pathological correlation and disease evolution. *Eur Radiol.* 2016;26:3129–3137.
17. Tetikkurt C, Yanardag H, Pehlivan M, et al. Clinical features and prognostic significance of splenic involvement in sarcoidosis. *Monaldi Arch Chest Dis.* 2017;87(3):893.
18. Judson MA. Hepatic, splenic, and gastrointestinal involvement with sarcoidosis. *Semin Respir Crit Care Med.* 2002;23:529–543.
19. Warshauer DM, Dumbleton SA, Molina PL, et al. Abdominal CT findings in sarcoidosis: radiologic and clinical correlation. *Radiology.* 1994;192(1):93–98.
20. Mahevas M, Lescure FX, Boffa JJ, et al. Renal sarcoidosis: clinical, laboratory, and histologic presentation and outcome in 47 patients. *Medicine (Baltim).* 2009;88(2):98–106.
21. Harzallah A, Kaaroud H, Boubaker K, et al. Acute kidney injury with granulomatous interstitial nephritis and vasculitis revealing sarcoidosis. *Saudi J Kidney Dis Transpl.* 2017;28(5):1157–1161.
22. Horino T, Matsumoto T, Inoue K, et al. A case of acute kidney injury caused by granulomatous interstitial nephritis associated with sarcoidosis. *CEN Case Rep.* 2018;7(1):34–38.
23. Frieder J, Kivelevitch D, Menter A. Symptomatic hypercalcemia and scarring alopecia as presenting features of sarcoidosis. *SAVE Proc.* 2018;31(2):224–226.
24. Rizzato G, Colombo P. Nephrolithiasis as a presenting feature of chronic sarcoidosis: a prospective study. *Sarcoidosis.* 1996;13:167–172.
25. Casella FJ, Allon M. The kidney in sarcoidosis. *J Am Soc Nephrol.* 1993;3(9):1555–1562.
26. Adams JS, Gacad MA. Characterization of 1 alpha-hydroxylation of vitamin D3 sterols by cultured alveolar macrophages from patients with sarcoidosis. *J Exp Med.* 1985;161(4):755–765.
27. Chopra A, Brasher P, Chaudhry H, et al. Proteinuria in sarcoidosis: prevalence and risk factors in a consecutive outpatient cohort. *Sarcoidosis Vasc Diffuse Lung Dis.* 2017;34:142–148.
28. Bagnasco SM, Gottipati S, Kraus E, et al. Sarcoidosis in native and transplanted kidneys: incidence, pathologic findings, and clinical course. *PLoS One.* 2014; %20; 9(10):e110778.
29. Loffler C, Loffler U, Tuleweit A, et al. Renal sarcoidosis: epidemiological and follow-up data in a cohort of 27 patients. *Sarcoidosis Vasc Diffuse Lung Dis.* 2015;31(4):306–315.
30. Shah S, Carter-Monroe N, Atta MG. Granulomatous interstitial nephritis. *Clin Kidney J.* 2015;8(5):516–523.
31. Aubart FC, Ouayoun M, Brauner M, et al. Sinonasal involvement in sarcoidosis: a case-control study of 20 patients. *Medicine (Baltim).* 2006;85(6):365–371.
32. Moudgil A, Przygodzki RM, Kher KK. Successful steroid-sparing treatment of renal limited sarcoidosis with mycophenolate mofetil. *Pediatr Nephrol.* 2006;21(2):281–285.
33. Poate TW, Sharma R, Moutasim KA, et al. Orofacial presentations of sarcoidosis–a case series and review of the literature. *Br Dent J.* 2008;205(8):437–442.
34. James DG, Sharma OP. Parotid gland sarcoidosis. *Sarcoidosis Vasc Diffuse Lung Dis.* 2000;17(1):27–32.
35. Ungprasert P, Crowson CS, Matteson EL. Clinical characteristics of parotid gland sarcoidosis: a population-based study. *JAMA Otolaryngol Head Neck Surg.* 2016;142(5):503–504.
36. Folwaczny M, Sommer A, Sander CA, et al. Parotid sarcoidosis mimicking Sjogren's syndrome: report of a case. *J Oral Maxillofac Surg.* 2002;60(1):117–120.
37. Yang SJ, Salek S, Rosenbaum JT. Ocular sarcoidosis: new diagnostic modalities and treatment. *Curr Opin Pulm Med.* 2017;23(5):458–467.
38. Bouaziz A, Le SJ, Chapelon-Abric C, et al. Oral involvement in sarcoidosis: report of 12 cases. *QJM.* 2012;105(8):755–767.
39. Marcoval J, Vinas M, Bordas X, et al. Orofacial granulomatosis: clinical study of 20 patients. *Oral Surg Oral Med Oral Pathol Oral Radiol.* 2012;113(4):e12–e17.
40. Panselinas E, Halstead L, Schlosser RJ, et al. Clinical manifestations, radiographic findings, treatment options, and outcome in sarcoidosis patients with upper respiratory tract involvement. *South Med J.* 2010;103(9):870–875.
41. Baughman RP, Lower EE, Tami T. Upper airway. 4: sarcoidosis of the upper respiratory tract (SURT). *Thorax.* 2010;65(2):181–186.
42. Neville E, Mills RG, Jash DK, et al. Sarcoidosis of the upper respiratory tract and its association with lupus pernio. *Thorax.* 1976;31(6):660–664.
43. Spiteri MA, Matthey F, Gordon T, et al. Lupus pernio: a clinico-radiological study of thirty-five cases. *Br J Dermatol.* 1985;112(3):315–322.
44. Aloulah M, Manes RP, Ng YH, et al. Sinonasal manifestations of sarcoidosis: a single institution experience with 38 cases. *Int Forum Allergy Rhinol.* 2013;3(7):567–572.
45. Kirsten AM, Watz H, Kirsten D. Sarcoidosis with involvement of the paranasal sinuses - a retrospective analysis of 12 biopsy-proven cases. *BMC Pulm Med.* 2013;13:59:59–13. https://doi.org/10.1186/1471-2466-13-59.
46. Zeitlin JF, Tami TA, Baughman R, et al. Nasal and sinus manifestations of sarcoidosis. *Am J Rhinol.* 2000;14(3):157–161.
47. Baughman RP, Seiden A, Lower EE. Sino-nasal sarcoidosis. In: Bernstein JA, ed. *Rhinitis and Related Upper Respiratory Conditions.* New York: Springer; 2018:137–152.
48. Wilcox A, Bharadwaj P, Sharma OP. Bone sarcoidosis. *Curr Opin Rheumatol.* 2000;12(4):321–330.
49. Zhou Y, Lower EE, Li H, et al. Clinical characteristics of patients with bone sarcoidosis. *Semin Arthritis Rheum.* 2017;47(1):143–148.

50. Sparks JA, McSparron JI, Shah N, et al. Osseous sarcoidosis: clinical characteristics, treatment, and outcomes–experience from a large, academic hospital. *Semin Arthritis Rheum*. 2014;44(3):371–379.
51. Mostard RL, Prompers L, Weijers RE, et al. F-18 FDG PET/CT for detecting bone and bone marrow involvement in sarcoidosis patients. *Clin Nucl Med*. 2012;37(1):21–25.
52. Judson MA, Costabel U, Drent M, et al. The WASOG Sarcoidosis Organ Assessment Instrument: an update of a previous clinical tool. *Sarcoidosis Vasc Diffuse Lung Dis*. 2014;31(1):19–27.
53. Yachoui R, Parker BJ, Nguyen TT. Bone and bone marrow involvement in sarcoidosis. *Rheumatol Int*. 2015;35(11):1917–1924.
54. Kodama K, Hasegawa T, Egawa M, et al. Bilateral epididymal sarcoidosis presenting without radiographic evidence of intrathoracic lesion: review of sarcoidosis involving the male reproductive tract. *Int J Urol*. 2004;11(5):345–348.
55. Babst C, Piller A, Boesch J, et al. Testicular sarcoidosis. *Urol Case Rep*. 2018;17:109–110. https://doi.org/10.1016/j.eucr.2018.01.021. eCollection;%2018 Mar.:109–110.
56. Lower EE, Hawkins HH, Baughman RP. Breast disease in sarcoidosis. *Sarcoidosis Vasc Diffuse Lung Dis*. 2001;18(3):301–306.
57. Mason C, Yang R, Hamilton R, et al. Diagnosis of sarcoidosis from a biopsy of a dilated mammary duct. *SAVE Proc*. 2017;30(2):197–199.
58. Fiorucci F, Conti V, Lucantoni G, et al. Sarcoidosis of the breast: a rare case report and a review. *Eur Rev Med Pharmacol Sci*. 2006;10(2):47–50.

CHAPTER 14

Parasarcoidosis Syndromes

MARC A. JUDSON, MD

INTRODUCTION

Sarcoidosis is a multisystem granulomatous disease that may affect any organ. Sarcoidosis may lead to symptomatic complications through the deposition of granulomas that impairs organ function. In 10%–20% of sarcoidosis cases this granulomatous inflammation of sarcoidosis may lead to the development of fibrosis which results in permanent organ injury.[1,2] However, sarcoidosis may also cause symptoms or dysfunction that is not directly related to granulomatous tissue deposition or fibrosis. These entities are collectively known as parasarcoidosis syndromes,[3] and they are responsible for significant quality-of-life and functional impairment in sarcoidosis patients. Table 14.1 lists common parasarcoidosis syndromes. Most parasarcoidosis syndromes are thought to result from systemic release of inflammatory mediators from the sarcoidosis granuloma. This manuscript will review the manifestations, proposed etiologies, diagnosis, and treatment of the major parasarcoidosis syndromes.

SMALL-FIBER NEUROPATHY

Small-fiber neuropathy (SFN) may occur in up to one-quarter of sarcoidosis patients[4] and may significantly impair the quality of life. SFN affects the unmyelinated C and thinly myelinated A-delta fibers that form nerve endings within the skin. These fibers sense thermal and nociceptive sensations, and pathology of these nerves may lead to a painful neuropathy. In addition, some of these small fibers innervate sweat glands and involuntary muscles that can lead to an autonomic neuropathy.[5]

The painful SFN may result in pain, numbness, vibration or electric shock sensations, and dysesthesias.[6,7] Although these symptoms often begin at the distal end of extremities, they may spread in a patchy, noncontiguous pattern, with patients often complaining of chest tingling, thigh pain, flank numbness, abnormal lip sensations, and facial paresthesias.[5,7] These aforementioned areas may be exquisitely sensitive to extremes in temperature.[5] These symptoms can be severe, and sarcoidosis patients often assess these symptoms as the most concerning aspect of their disease.[5]

The autonomic SFN may cause sweating, anhidrosis, tachycardia, orthostasis, nausea, vomiting, diarrhea, bowel/bladder disturbances, sexual dysfunction, and flushing.[5–8] Autonomic SFN tends to occur in conjunction with a painful SFN and not as an isolated entity.[5]

The immunopathogenesis of sarcoidosis-associated SFN is unknown. Histologically there is significant drop out of small nerve fibers within the skin. However, most often there is no histologic evidence that this relates to granulomatous infiltration of these fibers.[4] It is suspected that inflammatory mediators associated with sarcoidosis may be toxic to the small fibers and/or cause significant ischemia[5]; however, this postulation is currently conjectural. Little is known about the epidemiology of sarcoidosis-associated SFN. Although a large retrospective analysis of 115 American patients with sarcoidosis-associated SFN was not specifically focused on epidemiologic issues, the condition appears to be more common in white females.[8]

The diagnosis of SFN is problematic because currently there is no diagnostic gold standard.[9] Tests that have been used for diagnosis are listed in Table 14.2. Intraepidermal nerve fiber quantification from skin biopsies is probably the most commonly used diagnostic test. It should be noted that conventional peripheral nerve studies to assess large nerve fibers such as nerve conduction studies and needle electromyograms will be negative in patients with SFN.[5]

TABLE 14.1
Parasarcoidosis Syndromes

- Small-fiber neuropathy
  - Painful neuropathy
  - Autonomic neuropathy
- Fatigue
- Vitamin D dysregulation
- Erythema nodosum
- Pain syndromes
- Depression
- Cognitive impairment

Sarcoidosis. https://doi.org/10.1016/B978-0-323-54429-0.00014-8

TABLE 14.2
Potential Diagnostic Tests for Small-Fiber Neuropathy

Diagnostic Test	Test Description	References
Temperature sensation thresholds	Sensation of a difference in temperature applied to the skin sensed by the subject	90,91
Laser-evoked and contact heat–evoked potentials	Detection of brain waves resulting from laser heat stimulus or contact heat stimulus applied to the skin.	92,93
Quantitative sudomotor axon testing (QSART)	Quantification of postganglionic sweat output from axon reflex stimulation using acetylcholine electrophoresis	94
SFN screening list	A 21-item questionnaire that is a sensitive screening test for small-fiber neuropathy	95
Skin biopsy	Intraepidermal nerve fiber quantification from skin biopsy	96,97
In vivo confocal microscopy	Small-fiber quantification using in vivo confocal microscopy	98

The treatment of sarcoidosis-associated SFN is also not standardized. Potential therapies are listed in Table 14.3. As sarcoidosis-associated SFN is thought to be the result of an effect from inflammatory mediators associated with sarcoidosis, antisarcoidosis therapy such as corticosteroids has been recommended[5] and has been shown to be effective on occasion.[10] However, a recent analysis of 115 patients with sarcoidosis-associated SFN found that more than three-quarters of those treated with corticosteroids and/or methotrexate therapy worsened.[8] In contrast, more than two-thirds of the patients improved who received intravenous immunoglobulin (IVIG) and/or anti–tumor necrosis factor alpha (TNFα) therapy (specifically infliximab and adalimumab).[8] Although analgesics and, in particular, drugs used for the treatment of neuropathic pain and dysautonomia such as gabapentin have been advocated for the treatment of sarcoidosis-associated SFN,[5] they were found to be rarely effective in the previously mentioned large retrospective analysis.[8]

We recommend that when a sarcoidosis patient has SFN and concomitant active disease in an organ that requires antigranulomatous therapy, it is reasonable to monitor the effect of this therapy on SFN before considering additional interventions. If the SFN fails to improve and is not severe, therapies listed in Table 14.3 other than IVIG and anti-TNFα drugs are reasonable options. In severe or refractory cases, IVIG and anti-TNFα therapy should be strongly considered. It is important to note that insurance coverage for these latter therapies is often problematic in the United States.

Recently, cibinetide (ARA290), an erythropoietin derivative that is an innate repair receptor agonist that does not stimulate erythropoiesis, was found to be of benefit for sarcoidosis-associated SFN in two

TABLE 14.3
Therapy of Small-Fiber Neuropathy

Noncorticosteroid Therapies	Effectiveness	References
Drugs for neuropathic pain		
Amitriptyline	Poor to fair	5
Nortriptyline		
Desipramine		
Duloxetine		
Anticonvulsants		
Gabapentin		
Pregabalin		
Topiramate		
Lamotrigine		
Carbamazepine		
Oxcarbamazepine		
Topical anesthetics		
5% lidocaine patch		
Capsaicin		
Drugs for nociceptive pain		
Opioids/opiate antagonists	Poor to fair	5
Oxycodone		
Tramadol		
Others		
IVIG	Good to excellent	6
Infliximab		99
Cibinetide		11,100

IVIG, intravenous gamma globulin.

TABLE 14.4
Mechanisms of Fatigue Associated With Sarcoidosis

Mechanism of Sarcoidosis-Associated Fatigue	Associations With Sarcoidosis	References
Sleep disorder	Weight gain from corticosteroids; SURT; ILD	101,102
Adrenal insufficiency	Corticosteroid withdrawal; Schmidt's syndrome; sarcoidosis-induced Addison's disease; hypothalamic-pituitary dysfunction; TASS syndrome	103–106
Hypothyroid state	Autoimmune thyroiditis; high frequency of thyroid disorders	107–110
Depression/mood disorder	High frequency of depression	71,73
Sarcoidosis-induced fatigue	Above causes excluded	

ILD, interstitial lung disease; *SURT*, Sarcoidosis of the upper respiratory tract; *TASS*, thyroiditis, Addison's disease, Sjogren's syndrome, sarcoidosis.

randomized, placebo-controlled phase II trials.[11,12] Cibinetide was shown to increase small nerve fiber density and/or to reduce neuropathic symptoms in these trials. These data suggest that cibinetide shows promise for the treatment of this condition.

FATIGUE

Fatigue is a very common problem in sarcoidosis, occurring in up to 70% of patients.[13] There are many potential causes of fatigue in sarcoidosis (Table 14.4), and the clinician should attempt to determine the specific cause(s) because the treatment of each is different. For the purposes of this discussion, sarcoidosis-associated fatigue includes all common causes of fatigue in sarcoidosis populations (Table 14.4), whereas sarcoidosis-induced fatigue refers to fatigue directly related to sarcoidosis.

Sarcoidosis-induced fatigue is thought to be the consequence of inflammatory mediators associated with the granulomatous inflammation from sarcoidosis.[14] However, this postulation remains conjectural, and one study failed to confirm it.[15] It is possible that sarcoidosis-induced fatigue is not specific for this disease but rather is a general response to a chronic illness. Because, at present, there is no diagnostic test for sarcoidosis-induced fatigue, all the alternative conditions listed in Table 14.4 need to be reasonably excluded before treatment is considered. This point is important to emphasize because in our experience, more than half of all sarcoidosis patients with significant fatigue have evidence for a cause other than sarcoidosis-induced fatigue.

Antigranulomatous therapy has been used for the treatment of sarcoidosis-induced fatigue based on the premise that the condition is related to sarcoidosis-associated inflammation. In patients newly diagnosed with sarcoidosis, corticosteroid therapy was shown to improve fatigue.[16] However, these patients were not specifically treated for fatigue, and they had clinical and radiographic improvement with corticosteroid therapy. Therefore the improvement in fatigue may have been a by-product of improvement in sarcoidosis organ involvement. Although corticosteroid treatment of sarcoidosis-induced fatigue has not been systematically studied, it is the experience of most sarcoidosis clinicians that for chronic fatigue related to sarcoidosis, the risks of corticosteroid treatment outweigh the benefits. Many of the major side effects of corticosteroids are cumulative (e.g., weight gain, osteoporosis, and cataract formation) such that chronic use may cause significant quality-of-life impairment[17] that may offset the quality-of-life benefits of improving fatigue.

Stimulants have been reported to be effective for the treatment of sarcoidosis-induced fatigue including methylphenidate,[18] armodafinil,[19] and dexmethylphenidate,[14] the latter two being demonstrated in double-blind randomized crossover trials. Physical conditioning programs have also been shown to be beneficial for the treatment of fatigue in sarcoidosis,[20–22] although there is a concern that there may have been selection bias in these studies as the subjects elected to participate in an exercise program and may have been more motivated than the comparator groups.[23] TNFα therapy with infliximab and adalimumab have also been found to be reduce fatigue in sarcoidosis cohorts,[24,25] although fatigue was not a primary endpoint of either analysis. A recent systematic review of managing fatigue in sarcoidosis found that although there was evidence for a benefit of neurostimulants, TNFα therapy, and physical conditioning programs, the evidence was limited and requires further investigation.[23]

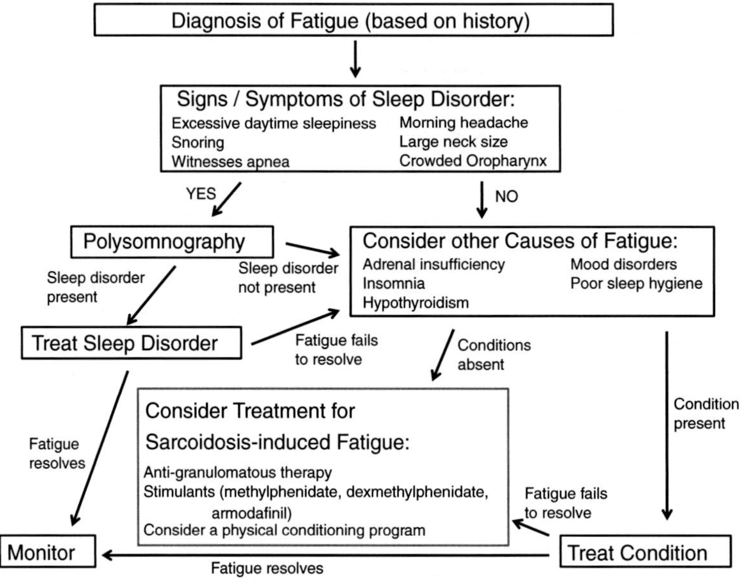

FIG. 14.1 Algorithm for the approach to fatigue in sarcoidosis. (Adapted with permission Judson MA. Quality of life in sarcoidosis. *Semin Respir Crit Care Med*. 2017;38(4):546–558.)

We recommend that a thorough investigation for causes of sarcoidosis-associated fatigue (Table 14.4) be performed on all sarcoidosis patients with significant fatigue. This investigation should include thyroid function studies, blood tests to evaluate the status of the adrenal gland, a screen for sleep disorders and assessment of sleep hygiene, and a psychosocial evaluation. All abnormalities discovered on this evaluation should be corrected to determine if the fatigue then resolves. If this investigation reveals no obvious cause for fatigue or if treatment of potential causes does resolve the fatigue, treatment of sarcoidosis-induced fatigue could be considered. We usually treat sarcoidosis-induced fatigue initially with a trial of a neurostimulant. Primarily because of cost issues, we usually reserve TNFα therapy for those who fail to respond, develop significant side effects, have a contraindication, or refuse to take neurostimulants. We believe initiating a physical conditioning program is a reasonable alternative in motivated patients. An algorithm outlining the approach to sarcoidosis-associated fatigue is shown in Fig. 14.1.

VITAMIN D DYSREGULATION

Vitamin D dysregulation in sarcoidosis results from increased 1-α hydroxylase activity in sarcoidosis macrophages that converts 25-hyroxy vitamin D, the inactive form of vitamin D, to 1,25-dihydroxy vitamin D, the active form of the vitamin.[26–28] This usually results in a low serum 25-hydroxy vitamin D level, while the serum 1,25-dihydroxy vitamin D levels tend to be in the high-normal to elevated range.[29,30] Serum parathyroid hormone (PTH) levels are usually quite low as they are suppressed by the elevated 1,25-dihydroxy vitamin D levels.[31] The elevated serum 1,25-dihydroxy vitamin D levels may cause increased gut absorption and renal excretion of calcium leading to hypercalcemia, hypercalciuria, nephrocalcinosis, nephrolithiasis, acute kidney injury, and chronic kidney disease.[32,33] Because vitamin D dysregulation is directly related to granulomatous inflammation from sarcoidosis, it is often not considered as a parasarcoidosis syndrome but rather as a form of sarcoidosis organ involvement.[34,35] This makes sense from a treatment perspective as corticosteroid therapy and other antisarcoidosis therapies are very effective for sarcoidosis-induced vitamin D dysregulation.[33] However, because the pathological lesions associated with sarcoidosis-induced vitamin D dysregulation do not routinely reveal granulomatous inflammation, this entity meets the criteria of a parasarcoidosis syndrome.

Vitamin D dysregulation from sarcoidosis causes hypercalciuria three times more commonly than hypercalcemia.[33,36,37] Vitamin D dysregulation is one of the few manifestations of sarcoidosis which tends to be more common in white than black patients.[2,38]

It is recommended to assess the vitamin D status of all sarcoidosis patients as part of general medical care

TABLE 14.5
Risk Factors for Complications of Vitamin D Dysregulation From Calcium or Vitamin D Supplementation in Sarcoidosis Patients

- Previous history of sarcoidosis-induced vitamin D dysregulation
- Previous history of calcium nephrolithiasis, hypercalcemia, hypercalciuria, renal insufficiency, and unexplained hematuria
- Previous history of a low 25-hydroxy vitamin D level

and to screen for potential vitamin D dysregulation. Both 25-hydroxy vitamin D and 1,25-dihydroxy vitamin D serum levels should be measured[29] because in a cross-sectional study of 261 sarcoidosis patients, 80% had low 25-hydroxy vitamin D levels, whereas only one patient had a low serum 1,25-dihydroxy vitamin D.[30] We recommend also obtaining a serum PTH level as it should be low in sarcoidosis-induced vitamin D dysregulation and high in primary hyperparathyroidism.

Significant hypercalcemia, nephrolithiasis, and/or renal insufficiency from sarcoidosis-induced vitamin D dysregulation is usually responsive to corticosteroids.[33] Hydroxychloroquine[39,40] and other antisarcoidosis drugs[41] may also be useful. Vigorous hydration and a diet high in citrate (an inhibitor of calcium stone formation) may be useful adjunctive therapy.[39]

Because corticosteroids are frequently used in sarcoidosis, bone fragility is a significant problem for these patients. It is recommended that to avoid the development of osteoporosis, bisphosphonates and/or calcium and vitamin D supplementation is advised in patients receiving daily prednisone at a dose of 7.5 mg or higher.[42] However, the use of vitamin D supplementation to prevent or treat bone fragility is problematic in sarcoidosis because of potential sarcoidosis-induced vitamin D dysregulation. The data concerning the effect of vitamin D supplementation in sarcoidosis cohorts are inconsistent. Some studies have shown that hypercalcemia rarely[43] or never[44] developed, whereas others have shown that hypercalcemia is common.[45] These inconsistences are problematic to resolve as some of these studies were retrospective and some prospective, and the supplementation doses varied.

We believe that the approach to the prevention and treatment of bone fragility in sarcoidosis patients is similar to that in other individuals with certain exceptions. A sarcoidosis patient with any of the features listed in Table 14.5 is at high risk of developing a complication of vitamin D dysregulation with vitamin D and/or calcium supplementation. These patients should be given

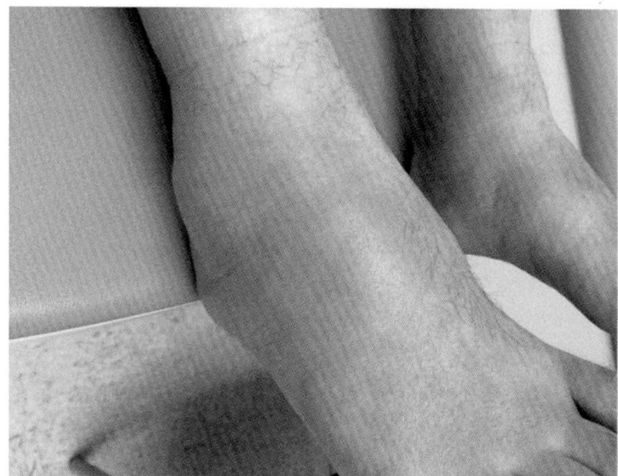

FIG. 14.2 Erythema nodosum skin lesion in a sarcoidosis patient. The patient has an indurated, erythematous, tender areas on the dorsum of his right foot.

bisphosphonates as primary therapy. We believe that these patients can still be given calcium and vitamin D supplementation, but if this is done, we recommend that high doses be avoided and that such patients be monitored iteratively to determine the effect of the therapy on renal function, serum calcium, vitamin D levels, and urinary calcium when appropriate. Furthermore, if such a high-risk patient receives corticosteroids or other effective antisarcoidosis therapies, this may improve or resolve sarcoidosis-induced vitamin D dysregulation and allow even normal doses of vitamin D and calcium to be administered. Again, iterative monitoring with dose escalation can be attempted in these situations.

ERYTHEMA NODOSUM

Erythema nodosum is a nonspecific skin lesion associated with sarcoidosis. Specific sarcoidosis skin lesions are the result of granulomatous inflammation of the skin, whereas nonspecific sarcoidosis skin lesions develop from a reactive process without granuloma formation.[46] As such, nonspecific sarcoidosis skin lesions represent a parasarcoidosis syndrome.

Erythema nodosum is the most common nonspecific sarcoidosis skin lesion, with up to 35% of sarcoidosis cases presenting with such lesions.[47] Erythema nodosum presents as tender erythematous nodules, usually on extensor surfaces such as the shins and ankles (Fig. 14.2). Erythema nodosum is a component of Lofgren's syndrome that consists of a combination of erythema nodosum, bilateral hilar adenopathy on chest radiograph, fever, and ankle arthritis/periarthritis.[48,49] Lofgren's syndrome is a common presenting manifestation of sarcoidosis.[50,51] Frequently, only some of the manifestations of Lofgren's syndrome occur in a sarcoidosis patient, including rare initial presentations of sarcoidosis with erythema nodosum without other manifestations of Lofgren's syndrome.[48] Erythema nodosum is thought to be more common in white than black sarcoidosis patients[52] and is particularly common in Scandinavians where it may be seen in up to one-third of sarcoidosis patients.[53]

Erythema nodosum, with or without other manifestations of Lofgren's syndrome, portends a good prognosis.[54] In particular, sarcoidosis patients with erythema nodosum skin lesions have much better prognosis of their sarcoidosis than patients with sarcoidosis-specific skin lesions.[55] Analysis of the HLA-DRB1*03 haplotype may further delineate the prognosis of Lofgren's syndrome. In a cohort of 275 Swedish sarcoidosis patients followed up for at least 2 years, 81% had resolving disease, whereas 19% had nonresolving or relapsing disease.[49] However, 95% of those with an HLA-DRB1*03-positive haplotype had resolving disease compared with only 51% of those who were HLA-DRB1*03 negative. These data have supported the clinical use of this HLA haplotype as a prognostic biomarker in Swedish sarcoidosis patients with Lofgren's syndrome.

The treatment of erythema nodosum from sarcoidosis is often merged with the treatment for sarcoidosis-related Lofgren's syndrome as they concomitantly occur in more than 90% of cases.[48] Very often the pain from an acute arthritis/periarthritis from Lofgren's syndrome is more debilitating to the sarcoidosis patient than the discomfort from erythema nodosum skin lesions.[56] This arthritis/periarthritis is commonly bilateral and most often affects the ankles, although the knees, wrists, elbows, and small joints of the hands may be involved.[57] Although Lofgren's syndrome is usually a self-limiting condition that typically lasts less than 3 months,[48,57,58] and nonsteroidal antiinflammatory agents (NAIDS) have been recommended as the drugs of choice,[48,56] it is our experience as well as that of others[59] that the periarthritis of Lofgren's syndrome responds poorly to NAIDS and requires short-term corticosteroid therapy.

PAIN SYNDROMES

Pain is reported in more than 70% of patients with sarcoidosis.[60] There are a myriad of causes of sarcoidosis-associated pain, and many of these causes are not directly related to tissue deposition of granulomas, which classifies them as parasarcoidosis syndromes. Two of these painful sarcoidosis syndromes have already been discussed: SFN and an acute periarthritis associated with Lofgren's syndrome.

Chest pain may occur with pulmonary sarcoidosis.[61] The location of the chest pain does not correlate with the severity of mediastinal adenopathy or the location on intrathoracic pulmonary granulomatous lesions,[61] suggesting that this is a parasarcoidosis syndrome. The pain is usually pleuritic and substernal or infrascapular in location.[61] Sarcoidosis-associated chest pain appears to be related to the presence of cough and is postulated to be the result of musculoskeletal pain induced by coughing.[61]

Sarcoiliitis and spondyloarthritis may be more frequent in sarcoidosis than in the general population,[62,63] although it is unknown if this relates to granulomatous inflammation in these locations or a nonspecific inflammatory reaction. Carpel tunnel syndrome also appears to be more frequent in sarcoidosis than in the general population.[64,65] Although at least one case report has been published of carpel tunnel syndrome developing in a sarcoidosis patients with biopsy-proven granulomatous inflammation of the flexor retinaculum,[66] many of these cases may have nongranulomatous causes.

In addition to physiologic causes of pain, sarcoidosis-associated pain may be related to psychological and emotional issues. Pain has been associated with fatigue in sarcoidosis.[67] Pain may also be related to depression or immobility.[68]

The treatment of sarcoidosis-associated pain depends on its cause. The treatment of SFN-associated pain and of erythema nodosum/Lofgren's syndrome has previously been discussed. Pain associated with fatigue or depression may respond to treatment of these conditions. In general, it is not advised to treat nonspecific chronic pain from sarcoidosis with corticosteroids. The management of chronic pain from sarcoidosis is complex and similar to management of chronic pain from other causes that involve careful assessment and interventions that may include pharmacotherapy, behavior modification, physical therapy, and psychosocial interventions.[69]

DEPRESSION

Depression is extremely common in sarcoidosis and reported in 25%–60% of patients.[70–73] It is controversial whether depression should be considered as a parasarcoidosis syndrome. Sarcoidosis patients may be depressed from a psychological response to the physical impairment from granulomatous infiltration of organs, side effects of antisarcoidosis medications, and the psychosocial burden of living with a chronic disease.[74] None of these mechanisms are specific for sarcoidosis. It is also possible that inflammatory mediators related to the granulomatous inflammation of sarcoidosis result in a depressed state, but such a mechanism specific to sarcoidosis remains unproven.

Depression is common in sarcoidosis patients who are female,[71] have decreased access to medical care,[71] and are receiving corticosteroid therapy.[75] Extrapolating from various studies, depression may be more common in black sarcoidosis patients than in white ones.[71–73]

The treatment of sarcoidosis-related depression needs to be individualized. Sarcoidosis patients should be monitored for depression. Depression needs to be distinguished from fatigue and dyspnea as these three conditions have been associated with each other, are often problematic to differentiate, and require discordant therapies.

COGNITIVE IMPAIRMENT

Cognitive impairment has been increasingly recognized as common problem in sarcoidosis cohorts. Sarcoidosis patients have a higher frequency of cognitive failure than control subjects (35% vs. 14%).[76] However, it is not known if sarcoidosis-associated cognitive failure is the result of a parasarcoidosis syndrome. Approximately 20% of neurosarcoidosis patients develop significant cognitive and behavioral manifestations.[77] Although a rigorous analysis of cognitive and behavioral effects of neurosarcoidosis has not been performed, several case reports have described neurosarcoidosis associated with hallucinations,[78] psychosis,[79,80] delirium,[81] aphasia,[78] cognitive decline/dementia,[82–84] amnestic syndrome,[85] schizophrenia,[86] depression,[87] and bipolar disorder.[88] In addition to neurosarcoidosis, cognitive impairment in sarcoidosis may result from antisarcoidosis medicine side effects and the psychosocial burdens of chronic disease.

Notwithstanding the aforementioned potential causes of cognitive impairment in sarcoidosis patients, there is evidence that at least some cases of cognitive impairment in sarcoidosis are the result of a parasarcoidosis syndrome. An analysis of 343 sarcoidosis found that 35% had evidence of cognitive impairment on the basis of a cognitive impairment questionnaire and that those that were treated with infliximab had a statistically significant improvement in their cognitive score as opposed to those who were not receiving antisarcoidosis medication or received corticosteroids and/or methotrexate.[76] These data suggest that the inflammation of sarcoidosis may induce a decline in cognition that is reversed by infliximab, although these patients were receiving infliximab for other sarcoidosis-related symptoms and not specifically for cognitive decline. It is also interesting that other antisarcoidosis medications (corticosteroids and methotrexate) failed to improve cognition of this cohort.

We recommend that sarcoidosis patients with cognitive decline be evaluated similarly to other patients with a physical examination and a detailed medical, psychosocial, behavioral, and medication history. If the history and physical examination fail to reveal an obvious explanation for the cognitive decline and the cognitive impairment is temporally related to onset or activity of sarcoidosis, then a brain magnetic resonance imaging (MRI) study with gadolinium contrast should be considered to assess for neurosarcoidosis.[89] If the brain MRI is consistent with neurosarcoidosis, antisarcoidosis treatment should be strongly considered. If the evaluation aforementioned fails to uncover a cause for the cognitive decline and it is temporally related to the clinical course of sarcoidosis, an empiric limited treatment trial of antisarcoidosis agents could be considered for a presumed parasarcoidosis syndrome. Despite the previously mentioned study that infliximab was superior to other antisarcoidosis medications for this condition, we believe that currently there is inadequate evidence to support a specific pharmacotherapy regimen.

SUMMARY

Parasarcoidosis syndromes are common conditions that affect a large proportion of sarcoidosis. These syndromes often have a profound impact of the sarcoidosis patient's quality of life. These syndromes do not necessarily respond to anti-granulomatous therapy. Optimal therapy of sarcoidosis patients requires not only an evaluation for sarcoidosis organ involvement but also the presence of parasarcoidosis syndromes.

REFERENCES

1. Moller DR. Pulmonary fibrosis of sarcoidosis. New approaches, old ideas. *Am J Respir Cell Mol Biol.* 2003;29(suppl 3):S37–S41.
2. Judson MA, Boan AD, Lackland DT. The clinical course of sarcoidosis: presentation, diagnosis, and treatment in a large white and black cohort in the United States. *Sarcoidosis Vasc Diffuse Lung Dis.* 2012;29(2):119–127.
3. Judson MA. The three tiers of screening for sarcoidosis organ involvement. *Respir Med.* 2016;113:42–49.
4. Bakkers M, Merkies IS, Lauria G, et al. Intraepidermal nerve fiber density and its application in sarcoidosis. *Neurology.* 2009;73(14):1142–1148.
5. Tavee J, Culver D. Sarcoidosis and small-fiber neuropathy. *Curr Pain Headache Rep.* 2011;15(3):201–206.

6. Parambil JG, Tavee JO, Zhou L, Pearson KS, Culver DA. Efficacy of intravenous immunoglobulin for small fiber neuropathy associated with sarcoidosis. *Respir Med.* 2011;105(1):101–105.
7. Hoitsma E, Marziniak M, Faber CG, et al. Small fibre neuropathy in sarcoidosis. *Lancet.* 2002;359(9323):2085–2086.
8. Tavee JO, Karwa K, Ahmed Z, Thompson N, Parambil J, Culver DA. Sarcoidosis-associated small fiber neuropathy in a large cohort: clinical aspects and response to IVIG and anti-TNF alpha treatment. *Respir Med.* 2017;126:135–138.
9. Devigili G, Tugnoli V, Penza P, et al. The diagnostic criteria for small fibre neuropathy: from symptoms to neuropathology. *Brain.* 2008;131(Pt 7):1912–1925.
10. Saito H, Yamaguchi T, Adachi Y, et al. Neurological symptoms of sarcoidosis-induced small fiber neuropathy effectively relieved with high-dose steroid pulse therapy. *Intern Med (Tokyo, Jpn).* 2015;54(10):1281–1286.
11. Heij L, Niesters M, Swartjes M, et al. Safety and efficacy of ARA 290 in sarcoidosis patients with symptoms of small fiber neuropathy: a randomized, double-blind pilot study. *Mol Med (Cambridge, Mass).* 2012;18:1430–1436.
12. Culver DA, Dahan A, Bajorunas D, et al. Cibinetide improves corneal nerve fiber abundance in patients with sarcoidosis-associated small nerve fiber loss and neuropathic pain. *Investig Ophthalmol Vis Sci.* 2017;58(6): Bio52–Bio60.
13. Drent M, Lower EE, De Vries J. Sarcoidosis-associated fatigue. *Eur Respir J.* 2012;40(1):255–263.
14. Lower EE, Harman S, Baughman RP. Double-blind, randomized trial of dexmethylphenidate hydrochloride for the treatment of sarcoidosis-associated fatigue. *Chest.* 2008;133(5):1189–1195.
15. De Vries J, Drent M, Van Heck GL, Wouters EF. Quality of life in sarcoidosis: a comparison between members of a patient organisation and a random sample. *Sarcoidosis Vasc Diffuse Lung Dis.* 1998;15(2):183–188.
16. Aggarwal AN, Sahu KK, Gupta D. Fatigue and health-related quality of life in patients with pulmonary sarcoidosis treated by oral Corticosteroids. *Sarcoidosis Vasc Diffuse Lung Dis.* 2016;33(2):124–129.
17. Judson MA, Chaudhry H, Louis A, Lee K, Yucel R. The effect of corticosteroids on quality of life in a sarcoidosis clinic: the results of a propensity analysis. *Respir Med.* 2015;109(4):526–531.
18. Wagner MT, Marion SD, Judson MA. The effects of fatigue and treatment with methylphenidate on sustained attention in sarcoidosis. *Sarcoidosis Vasc Diffuse Lung Dis.* 2005;22(3):235.
19. Lower EE, Malhotra A, Surdulescu V, Baughman RP. Armodafinil for sarcoidosis-associated fatigue: a double-blind, placebo-controlled, crossover trial. *J Pain Symptom Manag.* 2013;45(2):159–169.
20. Strookappe B, Swigris J, De Vries J, Elfferich M, Knevel T, Drent M. Benefits of physical training in sarcoidosis. *Lung.* 2015;193(5):701–708.
21. Strookappe B, Elfferich M, Swigris J, et al. Benefits of physical training in patients with idiopathic or end-stage sarcoidosis-related pulmonary fibrosis: a pilot study. *Sarcoidosis Vasc Diffuse Lung Dis.* 2015;32(1):43–52.
22. Marcellis R, Van der Veeke M, Mesters I, et al. Does physical training reduce fatigue in sarcoidosis? *Sarcoidosis Vasc Diffuse Lung Dis.* 2015;32(1):53–62.
23. Atkins C, Wilson AM. Managing fatigue in sarcoidosis - a systematic review of the evidence. *Chron Respir Dis.* 2017;14(2):161–173.
24. Wijnen PA, Cremers JP, Nelemans PJ, et al. Association of the TNF-alpha G-308A polymorphism with TNF-inhibitor response in sarcoidosis. *Eur Respir J.* 2014;43(6): 1730–1739.
25. Erckens RJ, Mostard RL, Wijnen PA, Schouten JS, Drent M. Adalimumab successful in sarcoidosis patients with refractory chronic non-infectious uveitis. *Graefes Arch Clin Exp Ophthalmol.* 2012;250(5):713–720.
26. Bell NH, Stern PH, Pantzer E, Sinha TK, DeLuca HF. Evidence that increased circulating 1 alpha, 25-dihydroxyvitamin D is the probable cause for abnormal calcium metabolism in sarcoidosis. *J Clin Investig.* 1979;64(1):218–225.
27. Adams JS, Gacad MA. Characterization of 1 alpha-hydroxylation of vitamin D3 sterols by cultured alveolar macrophages from patients with sarcoidosis. *J Exp Med.* 1985;161(4):755–765.
28. Adams JS, Sharma OP, Gacad MA, Singer FR. Metabolism of 25-hydroxyvitamin D3 by cultured pulmonary alveolar macrophages in sarcoidosis. *J Clin Investig.* 1983;72(5):1856–1860.
29. Burke RR, Rybicki BA, Rao DS. Calcium and vitamin D in sarcoidosis: how to assess and manage. *Semin Respir Crit Care Med.* 2010;31(4):474–484.
30. Baughman RP, Janovcik J, Ray M, et al. Calcium and vitamin D metabolism in sarcoidosis. *Sarcoidosis Vasc Diffuse Lung Dis.* 2013;30(2):113–120.
31. Vucinic V, Skodric-Trifunovic V, Ignjatovic S. How to diagnose and manage difficult problems of calcium metabolism in sarcoidosis: an evidence-based review. *Curr Opin Pulm Med.* 2011;17(5):297–302.
32. Rizzato G, Colombo P. Nephrolithiasis as a presenting feature of chronic sarcoidosis: a prospective study. *Sarcoidosis Vasc Diffuse Lung Dis.* 1996;13(2):167–172.
33. Sharma OP. Renal sarcoidosis and hypercalcemia. *Eur Respir J Monogr.* 2005;32:220–232.
34. Judson MA, Costabel U, Drent M, et al. The WASOG Sarcoidosis Organ Assessment Instrument: an update of a previous clinical tool. *Sarcoidosis Vasc Diffuse Lung Dis.* 2014;31(1):19–27.
35. Judson MA, Baughman RP, Teirstein AS, Terrin ML, Yeager Jr H. Defining organ involvement in sarcoidosis: the access proposed instrument. ACCESS research group. A case control etiologic study of sarcoidosis. *Sarcoidosis Vasc Diffuse Lung Dis.* 1999;16(1):75–86.
36. Casella FJ, Allon M. The kidney in sarcoidosis. *J Am Soc Nephrol.* 1993;3(9):1555–1562.

37. Berliner AR, Haas M, Choi MJ. Sarcoidosis: the nephrologist's perspective. *Am J Kidney Dis*. 2006;48(5):856–870.
38. Baughman RP, Teirstein AS, Judson MA, et al. Clinical characteristics of patients in a case control study of sarcoidosis. *Am J Respir Crit Care Med*. 2001;164(10 Pt 1):1885–1889.
39. Sharma OP. Hypercalcemia in granulomatous disorders: a clinical review. *Curr Opin Pulm Med*. 2000;6(5):442–447.
40. Barre PE, Gascon-Barre M, Meakins JL, Goltzman D. Hydroxychloroquine treatment of hypercalcemia in a patient with sarcoidosis undergoing hemodialysis. *Am J Med*. 1987;82(6):1259–1262.
41. Huffstutter JG, Huffstutter JE. Hypercalcemia from sarcoidosis successfully treated with infliximab. *Sarcoidosis Vasc Diffuse Lung Dis*. 2012;29(1):51–52.
42. Majumdar SR, Lix LM, Yogendran M, Morin SN, Metge CJ, Leslie WD. Population-based trends in osteoporosis management after new initiations of long-term systemic glucocorticoids (1998–2008). *J Clin Endocrinol Metabol*. 2012;97(4):1236–1242.
43. Bolland MJ, Wilsher ML, Grey A, et al. Randomised controlled trial of vitamin D supplementation in sarcoidosis. *BMJ Open*. 2013;3(10):e003562.
44. Kamphuis LS, Bonte-Mineur F, van Laar JA, van Hagen PM, van Daele PL. Calcium and vitamin D in sarcoidosis: is supplementation safe? *J Bone Miner Res*. 2014;29(11):2498–2503.
45. Sodhi A, Aldrich T. Vitamin D supplementation: not so simple in sarcoidosis. *Am J Med Sci*. 2016;352(3):252–257.
46. Haimovic A, Sanchez M, Judson MA, Prystowsky S. Sarcoidosis: a comprehensive review and update for the dermatologist: part I. Cutaneous disease. *J Am Acad Dermatol*. 2012;66(5):699.e691-e618; quiz 717–698.
47. Mana J, Rubio-Rivas M, Villalba N, et al. Multidisciplinary approach and long-term follow-up in a series of 640 consecutive patients with sarcoidosis: cohort study of a 40-year clinical experience at a tertiary referral center in Barcelona, Spain. *Medicine*. 2017;96(29):e7595.
48. Mana J, Gomez-Vaquero C, Montero A, et al. Lofgren's syndrome revisited: a study of 186 patients. *Am J Med*. 1999;107(3):240–245.
49. Grunewald J, Eklund A. Lofgren's syndrome: human leukocyte antigen strongly influences the disease course. *Am J Respir Crit Care Med*. 2009;179(4):307–312.
50. Lofgren S, Lundback H. The bilateral hilar lymphoma syndrome; a study of the relation to tuberculosis and sarcoidosis in 212 cases. *Acta Medica Scandinavica*. 1952;142(4):265–273.
51. Lofgren S, Lundback H. The bilateral hilar lymphoma syndrome; a study of the relation to age and sex in 212 cases. *Acta Medica Scandinavica*. 1952;142(4):259–264.
52. Hunninghake GW, Costabel U, Ando M, et al. ATS/ERS/WASOG statement on sarcoidosis. American Thoracic Society/European respiratory Society/World association of sarcoidosis and other granulomatous disorders. *Sarcoidosis Vasc Diffuse Lung Dis*. 1999;16(2):149–173.
53. Hillerdal G, Nou E, Osterman K, Schmekel B. Sarcoidosis: epidemiology and prognosis. A 15-year European study. *Am Rev Respir Dis*. 1984;130(1):29–32.
54. Lofgren S. Primary pulmonary sarcoidosis. I. Early signs and symptoms. *Acta Medica Scandinavica*. 1953;145(6):424–431.
55. Neville E, Walker AN, James DG. Prognostic factors predicting the outcome of sarcoidosis: an analysis of 818 patients. *Q J Med*. 1983;52(208):525–533.
56. Torralba KD, Quismorio Jr FP. Sarcoid arthritis: a review of clinical features, pathology and therapy. *Sarcoidosis Vasc Diffuse Lung Dis*. 2003;20(2):95–103.
57. Gran JT, Bohmer E. Acute sarcoid arthritis: a favourable outcome? A retrospective survey of 49 patients with review of the literature. *Scand J Rheumatol*. 1996;25(2):70–73.
58. Glennas A, Kvien TK, Melby K, et al. Acute sarcoid arthritis: occurrence, seasonal onset, clinical features and outcome. *Br J Rheumatol*. 1995;34(1):45–50.
59. Israel HL. Periarticular ankle sarcoidosis and Lofgren's syndrome. *Sarcoidosis*. 1994;11(suppl 1):379–388.
60. Hoitsma E, De Vries J, van Santen-Hoeufft M, Faber CG, Drent M. Impact of pain in a Dutch sarcoidosis patient population. *Sarcoidosis Vasc Diffuse Lung Dis*. 2003;20(1):33–39.
61. Highland KB, Retalis P, Coppage L, Schabel SI, Judson MA. Is there an anatomic explanation for chest pain in patients with pulmonary sarcoidosis? *South Med J*. 1997;90(9):911–914.
62. Kobak S, Sever F, Ince O, Orman M. The prevalence of sacroiliitis and spondyloarthritis in patients with sarcoidosis. *Int J Rheumatol*. 2014;2014:289454.
63. Erb N, Cushley MJ, Kassimos DG, Shave RM, Kitas GD. An assessment of back pain and the prevalence of sacroiliitis in sarcoidosis. *Chest*. 2005;127(1):192–196.
64. Yanardag H, Pamuk ON, Kiziltan M, Yildiz H, Demirey S, Karayel T. An increased frequency of carpal tunnel syndrome in sarcoidosis. Results of a study based on nerve conduction study. Universitas Carolina, Facultas Medica Hradec Kralove *Acta Med (Hradec Kralove)*. 2003;46(4):201–204.
65. Niemer GW, Bolster MB, Buxbaum L, Judson MA. Carpal tunnel syndrome in sarcoidosis. *Sarcoidosis Vasc Diffuse Lung Dis*. 2001;18(3):296–300.
66. Kersting-Sommerhoff B, Hof N, Golder W, Becker K, Werber KD. [MRI of the wrist joint: "granulomatous tenovaginitis of the sarcoidosis type"–a rare cause of carpal tunnel syndrome]. *Rontgenpraxis Zeitschrift fur radiologische Technik*. 1995;48(7):206–208.
67. De Vries J, Wirnsberger RM. Fatigue, quality of life and health status in sarcoidosis. *Eur Respir Mon*. 2005;32:92–104.
68. Gvozdenovic BS, Mihailovic-Vucinic V, Ilic-Dudvarski A, Zugic V, Judson MA. Differences in symptom severity and health status impairment between patients with pulmonary and pulmonary plus extrapulmonary sarcoidosis. *Respir Med*. 2008;102(11):1636–1642.

69. Ashburn MA, Staats PS. Management of chronic pain. *Lancet*. 1999;353(9167):1865–1869.
70. Cox CE, Donohue JF, Brown CD, Kataria YP, Judson MA. Health-related quality of life of persons with sarcoidosis. *Chest*. 2004;125(3):997–1004.
71. Chang B, Steimel J, Moller DR, et al. Depression in sarcoidosis. *Am J Respir Crit Care Med*. 2001;163(2): 329–334.
72. Korenromp IH, Grutters JC, van den Bosch JM, Zanen P, Kavelaars A, Heijnen CJ. Reduced Th2 cytokine production by sarcoidosis patients in clinical remission with chronic fatigue. *Brain Behav Immun*. 2011;25(7): 1498–1502.
73. Yeager H, Rossman MD, Baughman RP, et al. Pulmonary and psychosocial findings at enrollment in the ACCESS study. *Sarcoidosis Vasc Diffuse Lung Dis*. 2005;22(2):147–153.
74. Judson MA. Quality of life in sarcoidosis. *Semin Respir Crit Care Med*. 2017;38(4):546–558.
75. Cox CE, Donohue JF, Brown CD, Kataria YP, Judson MA. The Sarcoidosis Health Questionnaire: a new measure of health-related quality of life. *Am J Respir Crit Care Med*. 2003;168(3):323–329.
76. Elfferich MD, Nelemans PJ, Ponds RW, De Vries J, Wijnen PA, Drent M. Everyday cognitive failure in sarcoidosis: the prevalence and the effect of anti-TNF-alpha treatment. *Respir Int Rev Thorac Dis*. 2010;80(3):212–219.
77. Joseph FG, Scolding NJ. Neurosarcoidosis: a study of 30 new cases. *J Neurol Neurosurg Psychiatry*. 2009;80(3):297–304.
78. Hayashi T, Onodera J, Nagata T, Mochizuki H, Itoyama Y. [A case of biopsy-proven sarcoid meningoencephalitis presented with hallucination, nominal aphasia and dementia]. *Rinsho shinkeigaku Clin Neurol*. 1995;35(9):1008–1011.
79. Bona JR, Fackler SM, Fendley MJ, Nemeroff CB. Neurosarcoidosis as a cause of refractory psychosis: a complicated case report. *Am J Psychiatr*. 1998;155(8):1106–1108.
80. O'Brien GM, Baughman RP, Broderick JP, Arnold L, Lower EE. Paranoid psychosis due to neurosarcoidosis. *Sarcoidosis*. 1994;11(1):34–36.
81. Bourgeois JA, Maddock RJ, Rogers L, Greco CM, Mangrulkar RS, Saint S. Neurosarcoidosis and delirium. *Psychosomatics*. 2005;46(2):148–150.
82. Friedman SH, Gould DJ. Neurosarcoidosis presenting as psychosis and dementia: a case report. *Int J Psychiatry Med*. 2002;32(4):401–403.
83. Titlic M, Dolic K, Besenski N. Mild cognitive disorder as clinical manifestation of pituitary stalk neurosarcoidosis: case report. *Acta Clin Croat*. 2011;50(4):581–587.
84. Oh J, Stokes K, Tyndel F, Freedman M. Progressive cognitive decline in a patient with isolated chronic neurosarcoidosis. *Neurol*. 2010;16(1):50–53.
85. Willigers H, Koehler PJ. Amnesic syndrome caused by neurosarcoidosis. *Clin Neurol Neurosurg*. 1993;95(2):131–135.
86. Sabaawi M, Gutierrez-Nunez J, Fragala MR. Neurosarcoidosis presenting as schizophreniform disorder. *Int J Psychiatry Med*. 1992;22(3):269–274.
87. Stiller J, Goodman A, Komhi LM, Sacher M, Bender MB. Neurosarcoidosis presenting as major depression. *J Neurol Neurosurg Psychiatry*. 1984;47(9):1050–1051.
88. McLoughlin D, McKeon P. Bipolar disorder and cerebral sarcoidosis. *Br J Psychiatry J Mental Sci*. 1991;158: 410–413.
89. Nozaki K, Judson MA. Neurosarcoidosis: clinical manifestations, diagnosis and treatment. *Presse Med*. 2012;41(6 Pt 2):e331–e348.
90. Reulen JP, Lansbergen MD, Verstraete E, Spaans F. Comparison of thermal threshold tests to assess small nerve fiber function: limits vs. levels. *Clin Neurophysiol*. 2003;114(3):556–563.
91. Hoitsma E, Drent M, Verstraete E, et al. Abnormal warm and cold sensation thresholds suggestive of small-fibre neuropathy in sarcoidosis. *Clin Neurophysiol*. 2003;114(12):2326–2333.
92. Truini A, Galeotti F, Romaniello A, Virtuoso M, Iannetti GD, Cruccu G. Laser-evoked potentials: normative values. *Clin Neurophysiol*. 2005;116(4):821–826.
93. Atherton DD, Facer P, Roberts KM, et al. Use of the novel Contact Heat Evoked Potential Stimulator (CHEPS) for the assessment of small fibre neuropathy: correlations with skin flare responses and intra-epidermal nerve fibre counts. *BMC Neurol*. 2007;7:21.
94. Low PA, Caskey PE, Tuck RR, Fealey RD, Dyck PJ. Quantitative sudomotor axon reflex test in normal and neuropathic subjects. *Ann Neurol*. 1983;14(5):573–580.
95. Hoitsma E, De Vries J, Drent M. The small fiber neuropathy screening list: construction and cross-validation in sarcoidosis. *Respir Med*. 2011;105(1):95–100.
96. Lauria G, Cornblath DR, Johansson O, et al. EFNS guidelines on the use of skin biopsy in the diagnosis of peripheral neuropathy. *Eur J Neurol*. 2005;12(10): 747–758.
97. Ebenezer GJ, Hauer P, Gibbons C, McArthur JC, Polydefkis M. Assessment of epidermal nerve fibers: a new diagnostic and predictive tool for peripheral neuropathies. *J Neuropathol Exp Neurol*. 2007;66(12):1059–1073.
98. Oudejans LC, Niesters M, Brines M, Dahan A, van Velzen M. Quantification of small fiber pathology in patients with sarcoidosis and chronic pain using cornea confocal microscopy and skin biopsies. *J Pain Res*. 2017;10:2057–2065.
99. Hoitsma E, Faber CG, van Santen-Hoeufft M, De Vries J, Reulen JP, Drent M. Improvement of small fiber neuropathy in a sarcoidosis patient after treatment with infliximab. *Sarcoidosis Vasc Diffuse Lung Dis*. 2006;23(1):73–77.
100. Dahan A, Dunne A, Swartjes M, et al. ARA 290 improves symptoms in patients with sarcoidosis-associated small nerve fiber loss and increases corneal nerve fiber density. *Mol Med (Cambridge, Mass)*. 2013;19:334–345.

101. Lal C, Medarov BI, Judson MA. Interrelationship between sleep-disordered breathing and sarcoidosis. *Chest*. 2015;148(4):1105–1114.
102. Series F, Cormier Y, Lampron N, La Forge J. Increasing the functional residual capacity may reverse obstructive sleep apnea. *Sleep*. 1988;11(4):349–353.
103. Watson JP, Lewis RA. Schmidt's syndrome associated with sarcoidosis. *Postgrad Med*. 1996;72(849):435–436.
104. Takahashi K, Kagami S, Kawashima H, Kashiwakuma D, Suzuki Y, Iwamoto I. Sarcoidosis presenting addison's disease. *Intern Med (Tokyo, Jpn)*. 2016;55(9):1223–1228.
105. Verhage TL, Godfried MH, Alberts C. Hypothalamic-pituitary dysfunction with adrenal insufficiency and hyperprolactinaemia in sarcoidosis. A case report. *Sarcoidosis*. 1990;7(2):139–141.
106. Seinfeld ED, Sharma OP. TASS syndrome: unusual association of thyroiditis, Addison's disease, Sjogren's syndrome and sarcoidosis. *J R Soc Med*. 1983;76(10):883–885.
107. Wu CH, Chung PI, Wu CY, et al. Comorbid autoimmune diseases in patients with sarcoidosis: a nationwide case-control study in Taiwan. *J Dermatol*. 2017;44(4):423–430.
108. Malli F, Bargiota A, Theodoridou K, et al. Increased primary autoimmune thyroid diseases and thyroid antibodies in sarcoidosis: evidence for an under-recognised extrathoracic involvement in sarcoidosis? *Hormones (Basel)*. 2012;11(4):436–443.
109. Isern V, Lora-Tamayo J, Capdevila O, Villabona C, Mana J. Sarcoidosis and autoimmune thyroid disease. A case series of ten patients. *Sarcoidosis Vasc Diffuse Lung Dis*. 2007;24(2):148–152.
110. Martusewicz-Boros MM, Boros PW, Wiatr E, Roszkowski-Sliz K. What comorbidities accompany sarcoidosis? A large cohort (n=1779) patients analysis. *Sarcoidosis Vasc Diffuse Lung Dis*. 2015;32(2):115–120.

CHAPTER 15

Evaluation of Pulmonary Sarcoidosis

DOMINIQUE VALEYRE, MD • FLORENCE JENY, MD • DIANE BOUVRY, MD • YURDAGÜL UZUNHAN, MD, PHD • HILARIO NUNES, MD, PHD • JEAN-FRANÇOIS BERNAUDIN, MD, PHD

There is no desire more natural than that of knowledge. We try all ways that can lead us to it; where reason is wanting, we therein employ experience, which is a means much more weak and cheap; but truth is so great a thing that we ought not to disdain any mediation that will guide us to it.

MICHEL DE MONTAIGNE, LES ESSAIS, III, 13.

INTRODUCTION

Because of its frequency and major impact in morbidity, pulmonary involvement occupies a special place in the natural history of sarcoidosis.[1–8] Moreover, therapeutic decisions are often based on the pulmonary sarcoidosis evolution.[9] Recommendations have been proposed for the evaluation of pulmonary disease in patients with sarcoidosis in the 1999 statement on sarcoidosis.[10] In the last decade, several interesting works on best means and criteria to assess events during follow-up have been published. There is a need to update how to optimize the monitoring of pulmonary sarcoidosis.

The evaluation of pulmonary disease is tightly woven into the fabric of the whole book "Sarcoidosis" (Fig. 15.1). Therefore, we will often have to refer to other chapters, namely imaging (see Sverzellati's chapter), bronchoscopy (Benzaquen), pathology (Bernaudin), quality of life (Birring), pulmonary hypertension (Nunes), diagnosis (Wuyts), and treatment (Baughman) (Fig. 15.1). Monitoring pulmonary sarcoidosis is less evidence based than the topics in other chapters, and it notably relies on clinical experience, justifying the above-mentioned Montaigne's citation.

The evaluation of pulmonary disease serves several goals: (1) to assess the severity and the evolution of the disease progression, stability, or improvement, with a particular attention paid on symptoms and quality of life (QOL); (2) to evaluate the response to treatment; (3) to schedule further surveys; and (4) to determine whether criteria of recovery are met.

Monitoring pulmonary disease is facilitated by a thorough knowledge of the different patterns of sarcoidosis evolution that have been reported[1,3,11] and of the most valid currently available criteria to determine the disease status and evolution.

This chapter, intended to be very practical, consists of four sections: (1) What is the impact of pulmonary sarcoidosis and its assessment at diagnosis workup? (2) How to monitor the pulmonary disease outcome to fulfill the goals designed for the patient's care, what periodicity in the follow-up, and which investigations to be recommended? (3) What are the different patterns of pulmonary sarcoidosis outcome? (4) Specific situations. However, we gave no indications for anti-inflammatory treatments (see Baughman's chapter) nor how to monitor patients registered for transplantation.

WHAT IS THE IMPACT OF PULMONARY SARCOIDOSIS AND HOW TO ASSESS IT AT DIAGNOSIS WORKUP?

Although the intrathoracic involvement at diagnosis is generally obvious on imaging for about 90%–95% of sarcoidosis patients,[1–4] respiratory symptoms such as dry cough in 27%–49%, dyspnea in 18%–51%, and thoracic pain in 9%–23%, are present in 30% to more than 50% of patients.[1,3,12,13] Chronic dyspnea remains the most frequent manifestation, only noted in patients with a delayed diagnosis of sarcoidosis in whom the pulmonary involvement is already advanced.[8] Fortuitous discovery by a routine thoracic imaging in asymptomatic cases is now less frequent than in ancient series of patients (in only 8.4% versus 34%, respectively).[1,4] Many cases are discovered in the presence of

Sarcoidosis. https://doi.org/10.1016/B978-0-323-54429-0.00015-X

nonrespiratory clinically evident manifestations as erythema nodosum (particularly in Northern Europe and for females), extrapulmonary localizations as eye, skin, and lymph node involvement (particularly in Blacks), and general symptoms. It must be stressed that an initial exclusively extrapulmonary disease—uveitis, skin lesions, central nervous system or cranial nerve or nasosinusal involvement—may precede by months to years a lung involvement often unveiled through periodic chest X-rays every 6–12 months. In exceptional cases, sarcoidosis has been incidentally discovered, thanks to fluodeoxyglucose positron emission tomography (^{18F}FDG-PET) performed during cancer follow-up.[14]

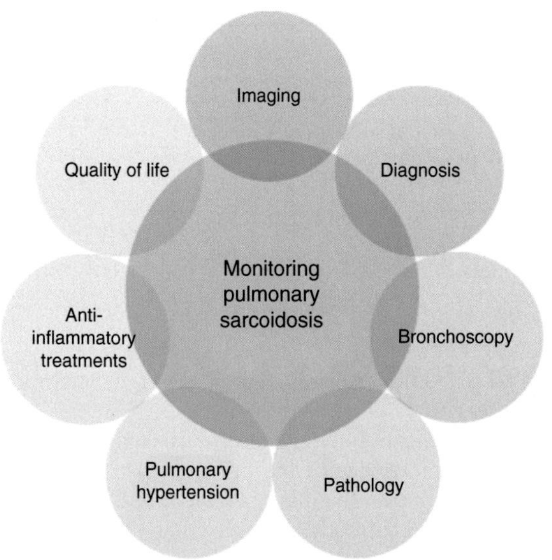

FIG. 15.1 Spectrum of monitoring pulmonary sarcoidosis.

Diagnosis Workup

At diagnosis workup, a full clinical investigation (symptoms and physical examination), imaging (chest radiography), and pulmonary function tests (spirometry and diffusion capacity of carbon monoxide) are recommended. Thoracic CT is available in most cases in routine medical practice (Table 15.1).[10,15]

Dyspnea must be assessed (for example, with *Medical Research Council* (MRC) *Dyspnea Scale* or *New York Heart Association* (NYHA) functional class) as well as fatigue (with Fatigue Assessment Scale) because it may be associated to exertional dyspnea even though other factors may be involved, and finally QOL

TABLE 15.1
Pulmonary Investigation Schedule

Investigations	Diagnosis Workup	Follow-up Visits (3–6 months)	Events
Respiratory symptoms	Always	Always	Always
Physical examination	Always	Always	Always
Fatigue, QOL	Always	When required	Always
Chest X-ray	Always	Always	Always
Thoracic CT (no contrast)	Almost always	No	When unclear findings
Thoracic CT (contrast)	Sometimes	No	Possible pulmonary embolism
^{18F}FDG-PET	Very rarely	No	For specific therapeutic questions
Bronchial endoscopy	Almost always	No	For hemoptysis, airflow obstruction, unclear exacerbation
Spirometry	Always	Every visit	Always
DLCO	Always	Every 6–12 months	Always
Echocardiography	Almost always	When required	When required
6MWT	When required	When required	Often
CPET	When required	No	Sometimes
Right heart catheterization	Rarely	For evaluation of therapy	When pulmonary hypertension is suspected or before transplantation registration

6MWT, 6-minute walk test; *CPET*, cardiopulmonary exercising test; *CT*, computed tomography; *FDG-PET*, fluodeoxyglucose positron emission tomography; *DLCO*, diffusion capacity of carbon monoxide; *QOL*, quality of life.

(St George Respiratory Questionnaire).[16] At physical examination, crackles are heard in 4% of patients, and finger clubbing is observed in 2%.[3] The proportions of patients with either stage 1 or stage 2 versus stage 3 or stage 4 in more recent series compared with earlier ones are similar; these proportions are found also when comparing primary care settings to referral centers. As a matter of fact, chest X-ray staging showed stage 1 in 40%–60% of patients and stage 2 in 22%–37%, whereas stages 3 and 4 remain rare in all series.[1–4] In most patients, pulmonary function tests were normal or near normal (force vital capacity [FVC] > 80% in 69%–84%, FEV1 > 80% in 62%–78.4%; diffusion capacity of carbon monoxide [DLCO] > 80% in 69.7% of patients).[1,2] Volume restriction or airflow limitation indicate lung and airway involvement, whereas a disproportionate decrease of diffusion capacity of carbon monoxide compared with that of forced vital capacity suggests the possibility of pulmonary hypertension (PH). The 6-min walk test (6MWT) distance in symptomatic patients may be often reduced and is correlated with results of the St George respiratory questionnaire and forced vital capacity assessments.[17]

Thoracic CT, in addition to useful information for diagnosis (see Sverzellati's chapter), might also be a promising tool to quantify disease activity in the lung parenchyma through a CT Activity Score (CTAS) and an abbreviated CTAS as shown by their association with further FVC change under treatment.[18] These results should be confirmed in another study. Thoracic CT is particularly helpful for the rare patients diagnosed with a badly tolerated or advanced pulmonary sarcoidosis with fibrosis[19,20] (see Sverzellati's chapter). CT can show the respective contributions of granulomatous and fibrous lesions to the pulmonary disease.

Bronchoscopy, which allows to visualize proximal bronchi and to document granulomas in the bronchial mucosa, is particularly useful in patients with airflow obstruction and, in conjunction with thoracic CT, may help decipher the multiple mechanisms of airflow obstruction in sarcoidosis (bronchial mucosal nodules, localized bronchial stenosis, extrinsic compression by lymph nodes or distortion, and bronchial narrowing and distortion secondary to lung fibrosis).[21–25]

HOW TO MONITOR PULMONARY DISEASE OUTCOME TO FULFILL THE GOALS DESIGNED FOR THE PATIENT'S CARE, AT WHAT FREQUENCY, WHICH INVESTIGATIONS, WHAT ARE THE CRITERIA OF PROGRESSION OR IMPROVEMENT?

Goals

The goals designed for monitoring pulmonary disease are multiple and depend on the context: (1) to detect on time any severity, progression, or improvement or any unexpected event that is important for the patients' care; (2) to specify all events and determine their pathophysiological substratum and estimate the expected response if a treatment is needed; (3) to evaluate the response to initial treatment and then the control of disease during tapering or after withdrawal of medications; (4) to schedule further surveys; and (5) to determine whether criteria of recovery are met. The appropriate expected delayed onset of action of drugs has to be taken into account to assess their efficacy. The fastest response is obtained with corticosteroids, within 4 weeks for newly treated patients,[16,26] whereas a longer time, often 2–8 months, is needed with immunosuppressive drugs or hydroxychloroquine.

Visits, Agenda, and Modalities

The monitoring should be more intense in the first 2 years after presentation.[10] The monitoring of lung involvement is based on consecutive medical appointments for clinical examination (dyspnea and fatigue scores), chest radiography, and pulmonary function survey. Serial serum angiotensin-converting enzyme evaluation has not proved to be useful in most patients with active pulmonary sarcoidosis. Scheduling these appointments depends on sarcoidosis history, severity, and treatments. Every 3-month appointments are usually recommended, but the frequency may vary between 6 weeks and 6 months.[10] Because of risk of radiation despite improved technology that reduces radiation level and lack of evidence supporting additional clinical value, routine repeated CTs are not recommended. When repeated CTs are indicated, adapted radiation doses should be used. Performing an additional CT during the evolution of the disease should be based on an important question concerning the interpretation of an unclear finding on chest X-ray or pulmonary function tests.

What are the Criteria of Progression or Improvement and What is the Underlying Mechanism of Progression?

When symptoms, chest X-ray, and pulmonary function evolve in concordance, either improvement, stability, or progression, the evolution assessment is easy. However, these three criteria may not be strictly concordant. Sometimes, when there is a discrepancy between symptoms and pulmonary function tests, other tests may be needed, such as 6MWT, cardiopulmonary exercising test, and cardiac investigations. Comparison of lung infiltration between two serial chest X-rays is not always reliable as shown by

TABLE 15.2
Mechanisms of Dyspnea in Pulmonary Sarcoidosis

Site	Mechanisms	Investigations
Lung infiltration	Lung granulomatosis and/or fibrosis	Pulmonary function; chest X-ray; thoracic CT (suspicion of fibrosis)
Lower airways	Diffuse or localized granulomatous bronchial stenosis; pulmonary fibrosis; extrinsic compression by lymphadenopathy; bronchial hyperreactivity	Thoracic CT; bronchoscopy with bronchial biopsy; Carbachol test for searching bronchial hyperreactiveness
Upper airways	Laryngeal sarcoidosis	Laryngoscopy; forced inspiratory volume in 1 s
Pulmonary hypertension	See Nunes' chapter	
Cardiac involvement	Cardiac sarcoidosis	Echocardiography; MRI; ^{18F}FDG-PET; Holter ECG
Autonomic disturbance	Small-fiber neuropathy	CPET; Holter ECG
Neuro-muscular causes	Muscular involvement	CPET; EMG
Comorbidity	Asthma and pulmonary embolism	History; Carbachol test; thoracic CT with contrast

CPET, cardiopulmonary exercising test; *CT*, computed tomography; *ECG*, electrocardiography; *EMG*, electromyography; *FDG-PET*, fluodeoxyglucose positron emission tomography; *MRI*, magnetic resonance imaging.

poor interobserver agreement .[27,28] The assessment of pulmonary infiltration evolution is less sensitive than symptoms and pulmonary function tests. In a study, serial chest radiography and serial spirometry were used to investigate pulmonary disease outcome, the serial CT being the morphologic reference.[28] Forced vital capacity was the most reliable tool with a good agreement, whereas the agreement was only moderate with chest radiography.[28] In practice, there is often only a slight change in pulmonary function results between two visits, and comparing current to earlier results may be useful to detect more significant differences. Contrary to idiopathic pulmonary fibrosis, there is no clear threshold to indicate a progression or an improvement, and many sarcoidosis specialists use idiopathic pulmonary fibrosis criteria which include not only a variation of FVC or DLCO larger than 10% and 15%, respectively, of the predicted values but also relative variations by comparison with initial results or marginal variations.[29] An important point is to follow the patients' symptoms, particularly dyspnea and fatigue, to assess QOL, which are very important for therapeutic decisions. Another important point is to determine the best time to assess a response to medications. The Broos' prospective study allowed to estimate the delay before response with corticosteroids in newly treated patients. This study, based on daily home spirometry, showed a 90% of total FVC increase at day 18, reaching a plateau at day 24[16]; such data were similar to Goldstein's[26] and Judson's studies where a response after an exacerbation with return to baseline values of FVC and FEV1 was obtained after only 3 weeks with 20 mg/d of prednisone.[30] Interestingly, in Broos' study, a significant improvement reaching a plateau was also shown at 1 month for dyspnea score MRC, fatigue score Fatigue Assessment Scale, and KSQ-lung scores .[16] Thus, a control 4 weeks after initiating or modifying a treatment appears adapted. It is important to note that such delay is applicable in newly treated patients with a recent disease in most cases, but data are missing concerning initiation of treatments in patients with long-standing sarcoidosis.

The pathophysiological mechanism of dyspnea must always be specified. Although in most cases a worsening dyspnea is linked to sarcoidosis because of the restriction on pulmonary volumes, one must know that multiple other mechanisms may potentially be involved and must be deciphered when things are not clear (Table 15.2). An airflow obstruction due to sarcoidosis is easy to document a decreased FEV1/FVC ratio. It is not rare, and many underlying mechanisms, often associated, have to be discussed. Knowing the main mechanism of airflow obstruction allows to determine the expected response to therapy. Schematically, a significant response is expected when airflow obstruction is combined with diffuse granulomatous involvement of bronchi,[23,24] whereas no response on FEV1 is expected when airflow obstruction is the consequence of upper lobe pulmonary fibrosis, with central bronchial distortions and stenosis .[23] Cardiac sarcoidosis may be a cause of dyspnea, often associated with abnormalities found in cardiac investigations by electrocardiography and echocardiography, as well as magnetic resonance imaging and ^{18F}FDG-PET if necessary. A laryngeal sarcoidosis may also be a cause of dyspnea, particularly when routine pulmonary function tests and radiography are normal or near normal; the diagnosis relies on laryngoscopy and the measure of maximal inspiratory volume in 1 s, which is decreased.[31] Precapillary PH is seldom encountered at diagnosis but may be a significant mechanism particularly when dyspnea persists despite treatment, FVC% of predicted value to DLCO% of predicted value ratio is higher than 1.4–1.5, or when 6 MWT is abnormal with no satisfying explanation (see Nunes' chapter).

OUTCOME OF PULMONARY SARCOIDOSIS

The Different Patterns of Pulmonary Sarcoidosis Evolution

The clinical evolution of sarcoidosis is quite variable.[11] However, there are still too few studies on a long period of clinical observation.[3,11,32] The World Association of Sarcoidosis and Other Granulomatous Disorders Task Force has classified the outcome of 500 patients from 10 worldwide centers in nine categories according to duration, symptoms, and need for treatment. A disease was considered persistent if lasting more than 5 years. Persistent cases were then subdivided according to treatment (never treated, treatment < 1 year, or currently treated) with or without worsening in the prior year and presence or absence of symptoms.[11] Resolution in less than 5 years occurred spontaneously after a <12-month treatment or in patients with only a minimal disease less than 25% of the maximal disease estimated according to chest X-ray or pulmonary function. All patients could be classified in the study. Around 38% of them had no persistent disease, whereas 43% had a persistent disease while still under systemic therapy with 32% either symptomatic or worsening in spite of it. The factors associated with active sarcoidosis persisting for more than 5 years were as follows: (1) older than 40 years, (2) being African American, (3) presence of pulmonary involvement on chest radiography or splenic involvement at diagnosis, (4) lupus pernio, and (5) a need for treatment.[1,11] The longer the sarcoidosis, the less probable a spontaneous resolution is expected in the following years. Improvement of half of patients with abnormal X-ray at 3 years occurs in the following 2 years, whereas a negligible improvement of abnormal X-ray at 5 years can be expected during the further 5 years.[33] Löfgren's syndrome and stage 1 are indicators of a good outcome with more than 80% and 60% of spontaneous remissions, respectively.[1,4,34] In the recent Catalan series from Maña, there were 42.6% spontaneous remissions without treatment, 45.3% with a need for systemic treatments for more than 3 months,[1] and 28.1% showed persistent (more than 5 years) active disease, 2/3 with mild disease and 1/3 with more significant, sometimes severe disease.[1]

Differences according to geography or race have been reported with, for example, a better outcome for Japanese than for Finish patients, with recovery in 76% and 47%, respectively, at 5 years.[35]

How to Investigate Patients at the Individual Level?

Survey of untreated patients

Often, and this is especially the case in primary care settings, newly diagnosed patients have a high probability of spontaneous resolution, for example "Löfgren's" syndrome or asymptomatic stage 1 or stage 2" benefit from repeated medical appointments with chest X-ray and pulmonary function tests. For asymptomatic patients, treatment should be initiated only in patients with confirmed pulmonary disease progression. A visit must be scheduled in case of any new clinical event including suspicion of a new extrapulmonary localization.

Survey of treated patients and response assessment

Most treated patients are treated at workup either because of symptomatic badly tolerated pulmonary sarcoidosis or extrapulmonary involvement or severe hypercalcemia. An evaluation with report of symptoms and pulmonary function tests and biomarkers may be initiated at 1 month and, according to treatment doses, at 3 months (with chest X-ray) and every 3 months. A significant response helps confirm sarcoidosis diagnosis, whereas the absence of improvement creates the need to reconsider diagnosis and to ask why no response is obtained. In one study, a decrease of two serum biomarkers—angiotensin-converting enzyme and soluble interleukin-2 receptor—was observed during methotrexate therapy in sarcoidosis patients, and this decrease was significantly correlated with improvement of pulmonary function.[36] During serial visits, the investigations will focus on whether the disease is under control or the suspicion of relapse while tapering the treatment or after its withdrawal.

How to diagnose exacerbations or relapses

Exacerbations are defined as a worsening of pulmonary symptoms thought to be related to sarcoidosis. Exacerbations are mainly recognized in patients having received a previous corticosteroid treatment in referral centers. Most relapses occur in treated patients either during the phase of decreasing treatment or within 3 years after stopping therapy[11] with 11.3%–74% of relapses, most relapses occurring in the 2–6 months after treatment withdrawal.[1,37] Exacerbations are often confirmed by a spirometric decline of FVC or FEV1 > 10% from baseline values.[27] The lung profusion score at chest X-ray is weakly correlated with the decline of FVC and FEV1, and its serial change has a poor efficiency for detecting pulmonary exacerbations.[27] However, chest X-ray may be useful to exclude alternative causes of pulmonary symptoms such as infection or heart failure. A further response to corticosteroids is also a good way to confirm it.[27,38] The distinct interest of monitoring biomarkers is still not clearly defined, but it might be interesting to evaluate whether it could help detect a biological relapse before a perceptible clinical deterioration allowing the adjustment of treatment and reduce true relapses. However, studies have not yet demonstrated that biomarkers might be sufficiently sensitive and specific for that purpose.

Recurrence of sarcoidosis and recovery

After spontaneous remission, a recurrence of sarcoidosis is very rare, 1.7% of cases,[1] and recovery is considered highly probable. In treated patients, some authors recommend a follow-up of 3 to 5 years with no sarcoidosis relapse after treatment withdrawal before confirming sarcoidosis healing because relapse occurs in 50%–80% of these cases.[10,11]

SPECIAL SITUATIONS

Pulmonary Fibrosis

Pulmonary fibrosis, observed from 1.5% to 5.4% of cases at presentation to 20% during follow-up, is an irreversible process occurring in a subset of patients with most often a persistent disease lasting more than 6 years.[8] Pulmonary fibrosis may be suspected in the presence of typical findings on CT (see Sverzellati's chapter) or when the best earlier pulmonary function cannot be reached under optimal treatment. There are three main pulmonary fibrosis patterns with different pulmonary function profiles: (1) bronchial distortion, mainly central, in 47% of patients (with often an airflow obstruction over the restrictive pattern); (2) honeycombing, mainly peripheral in upper lobes in 29% of patients (with severe restrictive impairment and very low DLCO); and (3) linear hiloperipheral pattern (often with well-preserved pulmonary function). It is important to classify patients with pulmonary fibrosis according to the extent of fibrosis and the presence or absence of an active disease in the lung. CT allows to measure the lung fibrosis extent >20% or <20%. ^{18F}FDG-PET is helpful when pulmonary fibrosis is obvious despite normal serum biomarkers such as serum angiotensin-converting enzyme or soluble interleukin-2 receptor because it can accurately assess the presence of active inflammatory lesions and predict the response to treatment.[39] Some cases present a limited-extent fibrosis without significant pulmonary function impairment and no more activity, a kind of burnout harmless disease with no need for treatment and only spaced follow-up. Advanced pulmonary sarcoidosis is characterized by significant pulmonary fibrosis and pulmonary function impairment, sometimes PH, with or without coexistent active lesions. Two studies have recently demonstrated that poor survival was associated either to a pulmonary fibrosis extent >20% at CT or PH (measured by catheterization or pulmonary artery/aorta (PA/Ao) diameter ratio >1 at CT).[40,41] For one of the studies only, Composite Physiologic Index which integrates pulmonary function impairment parameters was also predictive of a poor survival when >40.[40] Both of these studies evaluated patients for PH, and PH was found to be an independent predictor of mortality.[41] How to best monitor patients with fibrotic pulmonary sarcoidosis has still not been evidenced. By comparison to patients without fibrosis, physicians need to take into account the very important fact that clinical symptoms, imaging, and pulmonary function are all impacted by the addition of fibrotic and inflammatory components in the lung. It has been shown that a response can be expected when active lesions are still present. When a treatment is initiated or doses are increased, one must keep in mind that often test results will not return to normal because of residual fibrosis. In our opinion, it is important to determine what are the best clinical, imaging, and pulmonary function results that can be reachable in the course of initial treatment when the active lesions have been controlled. These values of best results may be used as points of reference for further evaluation. Taking into account symptoms, QOL, chest radiography, and pulmonary function plus 6 MWT and echocardiography at least every year is minimum. CT may be repeated in case of complications such as PH, suspicion of chronic pulmonary aspergillosis (CPA), or unclear new clinical, radiological, or pulmonary function findings; CT may also be used for assessing the response to treatment (control of active lesions). Cardiopulmonary exercise testing may be required in case of discrepancy between symptoms (dyspnea or fatigue) and pulmonary function test results. Even when pulmonary sarcoidosis is advanced, it is important to specify whether the disease is in progression, stabilized, or improved and the impact of its treatment. In some patients, controlling activity will be sufficient to inhibit the progression of the disease, whereas in some cases, there may be a progression of fibrosis in the long run despite an anti-inflammatory treatment which has apparently been proven to work.

Chronic Pulmonary Aspergillosis

CPA is a rare but severe complication in 2% of sarcoidosis patients.[42] Patients are usually symptomatic with hemoptysis in 37% of cases, weight loss in 40%, and fatigue in 45%. CPA occurs mainly in advanced pulmonary sarcoidosis. Diagnosis relies most often on the evidence of chronic cavitary pulmonary aspergillosis or aspergilloma phenotype on CT and evidence of serum Aspergillus-specific IgG and fungal culture of sputum or bronchoscopic specimens.[42] Follow-up will have to integrate survey of CPA per se.

Other Complications Associated to Pulmonary Fibrosis

Acute worsening

Acute worsening involves exacerbation of dyspnea and occurs at a mean frequency of 3 times per year.[43] It may be due to specific sarcoidosis flare up but also due to extrainfection, which often happens in patients with bronchiectasis secondary to fibrotic pulmonary lesions, bronchospasm, pulmonary embolism, or cardiac insufficiency.[43,44]

Pneumothorax

In sarcoidosis patients, a pneumothorax is most often seen in patients with pulmonary fibrosis (8.5% of patients). Relapses are possible.

Pulmonary Hypertension

Precapillary PH is rarely observed at diagnosis workup. It often occurs lately, 59–313 months after sarcoidosis diagnosis in the context of stage 4 for 72% of patients. PH must be sought in patients with persistent dyspnea, as 83% of them have NYHA functional class III or IV dyspnea, FVC% of predicted value to DLCO% of predicted value over 1.4–1.5, a pulmonary artery/aorta diameter ratio > 1 at CT, abnormal 6MWT distance, or PH suspicion at echocardiography. Only right catheterization can confirm PH diagnosis and eliminate postcapillary PH. PH follow-up is specifically discussed in Nunes' chapter.

Comorbidities

All events are not due to sarcoidosis and may be caused by bacterial, viral, or nontuberculous mycobacterial infections, pulmonary embolism or cardiac diseases which need to be differentiated from specific exacerbations.[45] In the presence of macronodules or lymphadenopathy, lung carcinoma and lymphomas must be recognized in patients with sarcoidosis. Associated autoimmune diseases such as Sjögen's syndrome may also be the cause for diagnosis' confusions.[46] Sleep apnea obstructive syndrome is abnormally prevalent in sarcoidosis and may impact symptoms, particularly fatigue and QOL.

Pregnancy

A particular situation is pregnancy because a flare up of the disease may follow parturition,[47] and a doctor's appointment within 6 months after delivery is recommended.[10]

CONCLUSION

Evaluation of pulmonary disease along evolution is crucial for optimizing care of patients with sarcoidosis. A thorough evaluation is needed to tailor at best treatments in a personalized care. For that purpose, well-planned visits with adequate investigations and well-defined criteria to assess evolution trend are necessary. Knowledge of various evolution patterns observed in sarcoidosis is useful for physician in charge of sarcoidosis patients. Complications such as pulmonary fibrosis or PH for the most noteworthy have to be detected.

REFERENCES

1. Mañá J, Rubio-Rivas M, Villalba N, et al. Multidisciplinary approach and long-term follow-up in a series of 640 consecutive patients with sarcoidosis: cohort study of a 40-year clinical experience at a tertiary referral center in Barcelona, Spain. *Medicine (Baltim)*. 2017;96(29):e7595.
2. Baughman RP, Teirstein AS, Judson MA, et al. Clinical characteristics of patients in a case control study of sarcoidosis. *Am J Respir Crit Care Med*. 2001;164(10):1885–1889.
3. Chappell AG, Cheung WY, Hutchings HA. Sarcoidosis: a long-term follow up study. *Sarcoidosis Vasc Diffuse Lung Dis Off J WASOG World Assoc Sarcoidosis Granulomatous Disord*. 2000;17(2):167–173.

4. Siltzbach LE, James DG, Neville E, et al. Course and prognosis of sarcoidosis around the world. *Am J Med.* 1974;57(6):847–852.
5. Perry A, Vuitch F. Causes of death in patients with sarcoidosis. A morphologic study of 38 autopsies with clinicopathologic correlations. *Arch Pathol Lab Med.* 1995;119(2):167–172.
6. Swigris JJ, Olson AL, Huie TJ, et al. Sarcoidosis-related mortality in the United States from 1988 to 2007. *Am J Respir Crit Care Med.* 2011;183(11):1524–1530.
7. Jamilloux Y, Maucort-Boulch D, Kerever S, et al. Sarcoidosis-related mortality in France: a multiple-cause-of-death analysis. *Eur Respir J.* 2016;48(6):1700–1709.
8. Nardi A, Brillet P-Y, Letoumelin P, et al. Stage IV sarcoidosis: comparison of survival with the general population and causes of death. *Eur Respir J.* 2011;38(6):1368–1373.
9. Valeyre D, Prasse A, Nunes H, Uzunhan Y, Brillet P-Y, Müller-Quernheim J. Sarcoidosis. *Lancet.* 2014;383(9923):1155–1167.
10. Hunninghake GW, Costabel U, Ando M, et al. ATS/ERS/WASOG statement on sarcoidosis. American thoracic Society/European Respiratory Society/World Association of sarcoidosis and other granulomatous Disorders. *Sarcoidosis Vasc Diffuse Lung Dis Off J WASOG.* 1999;16(2):149–173.
11. Baughman RP, Nagai S, Balter M, et al. Defining the clinical outcome status (COS) in sarcoidosis: results of WASOG Task Force. *Sarcoidosis Vasc Diffuse Lung Dis Off J WASOG World Assoc Sarcoidosis Granulomatous Disord.* 2011;28(1):56–64.
12. Judson MA, Thompson BW, Rabin DL, et al. The diagnostic pathway to sarcoidosis. *Chest.* 2003;123(2):406–412.
13. Zhou Y, Lower EE, Li H, Baughman RP. Clinical management of pulmonary sarcoidosis. *Expert Rev Respir Med.* 2016;10(5):577–591.
14. Chowdhury FU, Sheerin F, Bradley KM, Gleeson FV. Sarcoid-like reaction to malignancy on whole-body integrated (18)F-FDG PET/CT: prevalence and disease pattern. *Clin Radiol.* 2009;64(7):675–681.
15. Valeyre D, Bernaudin J-F, Jeny F, et al. Pulmonary sarcoidosis. *Clin Chest Med.* 2015;36(4):631–641.
16. Broos CE, Wapenaar M, Looman CWN, et al. Daily home spirometry to detect early steroid treatment effects in newly treated pulmonary sarcoidosis. *Eur Respir J.* 2018;51(1).
17. Baughman RP, Sparkman BK, Lower EE. Six-minute walk test and health status assessment in sarcoidosis. *Chest.* 2007;132(1):207–213.
18. Benamore R, Kendrick YR, Repapi E, et al. CTAS: a CT score to quantify disease activity in pulmonary sarcoidosis. *Thorax.* 2016;71(12):1161–1163.
19. Criado E, Sánchez M, Ramírez J, et al. Pulmonary sarcoidosis: typical and atypical manifestations at high-resolution CT with pathologic correlation. *Radiogr Rev Publ Radiol Soc N Am Inc.* 2010;30(6):1567–1586.
20. Nunes H, Brillet P-Y, Valeyre D, Brauner MW, Wells AU. Imaging in sarcoidosis. *Semin Respir Crit Care Med.* 2007;28(1):102–120.
21. Nunes H, Uzunhan Y, Gille T, Lamberto C, Valeyre D, Brillet P-Y. Imaging of sarcoidosis of the airways and lung parenchyma and correlation with lung function. *Eur Respir J.* 2012;40(3):750–765.
22. Chambellan A, Turbie P, Nunes H, Brauner M, Battesti J-P, Valeyre D. Endoluminal stenosis of proximal bronchi in sarcoidosis: bronchoscopy, function, and evolution. *Chest.* 2005;127(2):472–481.
23. Naccache J-M, Lavolé A, Nunes H, et al. High-resolution computed tomographic imaging of airways in sarcoidosis patients with airflow obstruction. *J Comput Assist Tomogr.* 2008;32(6):905–912.
24. Lavergne F, Clerici C, Sadoun D, Brauner M, Battesti JP, Valeyre D. Airway obstruction in bronchial sarcoidosis: outcome with treatment. *Chest.* 1999;116(5):1194–1199.
25. Baughman RP, Lower EE, Tami T. Upper airway. 4: sarcoidosis of the upper respiratory tract (SURT). *Thorax.* 2010;65(2):181–186.
26. Goldstein DS, Williams MH. Rate of improvement of pulmonary function in sarcoidosis during treatment with corticosteroids. *Thorax.* 1986;41(6):473–474.
27. Judson MA, Gilbert GE, Rodgers JK, Greer CF, Schabel SI. The utility of the chest radiograph in diagnosing exacerbations of pulmonary sarcoidosis. *Respirol Carlton Vic.* 2008;13(1):97–102.
28. Zappala CJ, Desai SR, Copley SJ, et al. Accuracy of individual variables in the monitoring of long-term change in pulmonary sarcoidosis as judged by serial high-resolution CT scan data. *Chest.* 2014;145(1):101–107.
29. Richeldi L, Ryerson CJ, Lee JS, et al. Relative versus absolute change in forced vital capacity in idiopathic pulmonary fibrosis. *Thorax.* 2012;67(5):407–411.
30. McKinzie BP, Bullington WM, Mazur JE, Judson MA. Efficacy of short-course, low-dose corticosteroid therapy for acute pulmonary sarcoidosis exacerbations. *Am J Med Sci.* 2010;339(1):1–4.
31. Duchemann B, Lavolé A, Naccache J-M, et al. Laryngeal sarcoidosis: a case-control study. *Sarcoidosis Vasc Diffuse Lung Dis Off J WASOG World Assoc Sarcoidosis Granulomatous Disord.* 2014;31(3):227–234.
32. Johns CJ, Michele TM. The clinical management of sarcoidosis. A 50-year experience at the Johns Hopkins Hospital. *Medicine (Baltim).* 1999;78(2):65–111.
33. Nagai S, Shigematsu M, Hamada K, Izumi T. Clinical courses and prognoses of pulmonary sarcoidosis. *Curr Opin Pulm Med.* 1999;5(5):293–298.
34. James DG, Thomson AD, Willcox A. Erythema nodosum as a manifestation of sarcoidosis. *Lancet Lond Engl.* 1956;271(6936):218–221.
35. Pietinalho A, Ohmichi M, Löfroos AB, Hiraga Y, Selroos O. The prognosis of pulmonary sarcoidosis in Finland and Hokkaido, Japan. A comparative five-year study of biopsy-proven cases. *Sarcoidosis Vasc Diffuse Lung Dis Off J WASOG.* 2000;17(2):158–166.

36. Vorselaars ADM, van Moorsel CHM, Zanen P, et al. ACE and sIL-2R correlate with lung function improvement in sarcoidosis during methotrexate therapy. *Respir Med.* 2015;109(2):279–285.
37. Rizzato G, Montemurro L, Colombo P. The late follow-up of chronic sarcoid patients previously treated with corticosteroids. *Sarcoidosis Vasc Diffuse Lung Dis Off J WASOG World Assoc Sarcoidosis Granulomatous Disord.* 1998;15(1):52–58.
38. Zappala CJ, Desai SR, Copley SJ, et al. Optimal scoring of serial change on chest radiography in sarcoidosis. *Sarcoidosis Vasc Diffuse Lung Dis Off J WASOG World Assoc Sarcoidosis Granulomatous Disord.* 2011;28(2):130–138.
39. Mostard RLM, Vöö S, van Kroonenburgh MJPG, et al. Inflammatory activity assessment by F18 FDG-PET/CT in persistent symptomatic sarcoidosis. *Respir Med.* 2011;105(12):1917–1924.
40. Walsh SL, Wells AU, Sverzellati N, et al. An integrated clinicoradiological staging system for pulmonary sarcoidosis: a case-cohort study. *Lancet Respir Med.* 2014;2(2):123–130.
41. Kirkil G, Lower EE, Baughman RP. Predictors of mortality in pulmonary sarcoidosis. *Chest.* 2018;153(1):105–113.
42. Uzunhan Y, Nunes H, Jeny F, et al. Chronic pulmonary aspergillosis complicating sarcoidosis. *Eur Respir J.* 2017;49(6).
43. Baughman RP, Lower EE. Frequency of acute worsening events in fibrotic pulmonary sarcoidosis patients. *Respir Med.* 2013;107(12):2009–2013.
44. Panselinas E, Judson MA. Acute pulmonary exacerbations of sarcoidosis. *Chest.* 2012;142(4):827–836.
45. Martusewicz-Boros MM, Boros PW, Wiatr E, Roszkowski-Śliż K. What comorbidities accompany sarcoidosis? A large cohort (n=1779) patients analysis. *Sarcoidosis Vasc Diffuse Lung Dis Off J WASOG World Assoc Sarcoidosis Granulomatous Disord.* 2015;32(2):115–120.
46. Wu C-H, Chung P-I, Wu C-Y, et al. Comorbid autoimmune diseases in patients with sarcoidosis: a nationwide case-control study in Taiwan. *J Dermatol.* 2017;44(4):423–430.
47. King TE. Restrictive lung disease in pregnancy. *Clin Chest Med.* 1992;13(4):607–622.

CHAPTER 16

Roentgenogram, CT, and MRI

MILANESE GIANLUCA, MD • SILVA MARIO, MD, PHD • SVERZELLATI NICOLA, MD, PHD

INTRODUCTION

Chest X-ray (CXR) is a cornerstone technique for both diagnosis and follow-up of subjects with sarcoidosis. In the appropriate clinical setting the presence of typical imaging findings is sufficient for diagnosing sarcoidosis obviating the need of invasive procedures. CXR has been extensively used to diagnose the disease, to evaluate its prognosis, and to monitor patients during therapy or follow-up.[1]

Beyond CXR, high-resolution computed tomography (HRCT) is routinely performed in clinical practice, following the mitigated concerns about radiation exposure. Indeed, HRCT can be obtained by substantially reducing radiation exposure, comparable to a few CXRs.[2] As compared to a CXR, HRCT is more sensitive to subtler abnormalities, including detection of complications and comorbidities. Furthermore, HRCT provides consistent guidance for transbronchial biopsies.[1,3] Recently, thoracic magnetic resonance imaging (MRI) was shown to be potentially diagnostic, displaying substantial correlation with HRCT for pulmonary sarcoidosis—especially when evaluating upper lobes abnormalities—encouraging its use in younger patients.[4]

Imaging plays a pivotal role for the diagnosis and management of patients with sarcoidosis, and this chapter focuses on the thoracic manifestations of the disease, both typical and atypical.

CHEST RADIOGRAPHY

Imaging Findings

Lymph node involvement

Bilateral, symmetrical hilar, and paratracheal lymphadenopathy represent the most typical finding, which can be sufficient for the diagnosis of sarcoidosis within the appropriate clinical scenario.[5,6]

Lymph node enlargement widely varies from minimal to massive, usually displaying a lobulated outline. Symmetry is a key finding as it may differentiate sarcoidosis from other diseases causing mediastinal widening, such as tuberculosis, histoplasmosis, lymphoproliferative disorders, and lymph nodal metastasis. However, some overlapping exists among these disorders, and diagnosis should rely on further diagnostic tests when the clinical findings are more ambiguous.[1,6,7]

Moreover, other lymph nodes locations involvement (e.g., paratracheal and aortopulmonary window) can be detected on CXR.[6] The recognition of typical calcification patterns such as eggshell-like calcifications increases the diagnostic confidence.

Lung involvement

Upper lobes–predominant nodular or reticulonodular opacities are the most frequent lung abnormalities. Sarcoidosis, however, may also manifest as ground glass opacity (GGO), patchy well-defined consolidation, and reticular opacities consistent with pulmonary fibrosis. The latter becomes more obvious when signs of pulmonary volume loss (e.g., hilar retraction, fissures displacement), spiculated consolidation, and coarse linear bands are present.[6–9]

The radiological diagnosis of sarcoidosis may be challenging when atypical findings are spotted on CXR or HRCT. These atypical imaging features may involve different thoracic structures, including lymph nodes, pulmonary parenchyma, airways, and pleura (Table 16.1).[6,10]

Staging Systems

Several CXR-based staging systems have been proposed in the last 5 decades. The system developed by Scadding in 1961 is still the most widely used one, eventually because of its simplicity, straightforward intelligibility, and clinical yield.[11,12] The Scadding staging system for sarcoidosis is based on a 5-stage classification scheme as follows (see Figs. 16.1–16.4)[13]:

- Stage 0: CXR does not display findings consistent with sarcoidosis
- Stage I: hilar and/or mediastinal adenopathy
- Stage II: parenchymal abnormalities associated with hilar and/or mediastinal adenopathy
- Stage III: parenchymal abnormalities without adenopathy
- Stage IV: pulmonary fibrosis

Sarcoidosis. https://doi.org/10.1016/B978-0-323-54429-0.00016-1

TABLE 16.1
Atypical Findings of Sarcoidosis Detectable on CXR or HRCT

Hilar lymph node enlargement
• Unilateral
• Asymmetric
Uncommon sites of lymph node enlargement
• Anterior mediastinal
• Middle mediastinal without hilar lymph nodes enlargement
• Posterior mediastinal
• Paracardiac
• Internal mammary
• Paravertebral
• Retrocrural
Parenchyma
• Unilateral
• Lower lobe predominant
• Patchy consolidations
• Necrotizing or cavitary lesions
• Honeycomb alterations
• "Galaxy" sign
• "Reverse halo" sign
• Ground glass opacities
• Miliary-like distribution pattern
Airway
• Atelectasis
• Air trapping
Pleura
• Pleural effusion
• Pleural thickening
• Pleural calcifications
• Pleural plaque-like opacities
• Pneumothorax
Skeletal involvement

CXR, chest radiograph; *HRCT*, high-resolution computed tomography.

The staging system was demonstrated to carry significant prognostic information as spontaneous remission could occur in about 60%–90%, 40%–70%, 10%–20%, and 0% of patients with stage I, II, III, and IV, respectively.[1,14,15]

The radiologic follow-up of sarcoidosis may show alterations of the baseline CXR findings. The detection of such changes is of paramount clinical relevance because the evidence of deteriorating CXRs has been considered a sign of active sarcoidosis, notably when progression is seen through more advanced stages.[16] However, it is to be underscored that the reliability of the CXR staging system is limited by its intrinsic interobserver variability, mostly for the interpretation CXR findings, representing pulmonary fibrosis (e.g., stage IV).[3,14,17,18] More recently, Muers developed a radiographic staging system based on the evaluation of both extent and profusion of four parenchymal components (reticulonodular, mass, confluent, and fibrosis), which showed a better interobserver agreement than the abovementioned system.[14]

Complications

CXR represents the first-line imaging for patients with suspected complications.

CXR may detect aspergillomas, atelectasis, malignancies, and pneumothorax.[6] Aspergillomas are masses of fungal mycelia colonizing preexisting pulmonary cavities; they appear as soft tissue masses within the lung cavity. Typically the aspergilloma is separated from the cavity by an antigravitational air crescent (Monod sign), and it is mobilized by different postures. Aspergillomas affect 3%–12% of patients with advanced sarcoidosis.[8,19–22] Lobar atelectasis secondary to a bronchial occlusion (either by endobronchial disease or extraluminal compression by an enlarged lymph node) may involve any lobe—although a predilection for the right middle lobe was noted—and can be assessed on CXR.[23]

Although relatively insensitive, the dilation of either pulmonary trunk or main pulmonary arteries, as well as peripheral vascular pruning (i.e., disproportionately small peripheral vessels), represents CXR findings associated with pulmonary hypertension.[24] Of note, the assessment of central vascular abnormalities may be particularly challenging when enlarged hilar and mediastinal lymph nodes are present.[1] The prevalence of CXR signs of sarcoidosis-associated pulmonary hypertension (SAPH) ranges 5%–15%. Although SAPH more commonly affects subjects with advanced stage disease, it cannot be overemphasized that about 30% of patients can develop SAPH in the absence of parenchymal fibrosis. Hence CXR without signs of fibrosis does not necessarily rule out SAPH.[25,26]

COMPUTED TOMOGRAPHY

For patients with an established diagnosis of sarcoidosis, undertaking an HRCT scan has little advantage compared with CXR. Nevertheless, a baseline HRCT may be helpful for the interpretation of subsequent ambiguous changes also for these patients. Subjects with either atypical clinical or CXR findings (e.g., asymmetrical lymph node enlargement or subtle parenchymal abnormalities) should undergo HRCT scanning.[3,8,27]

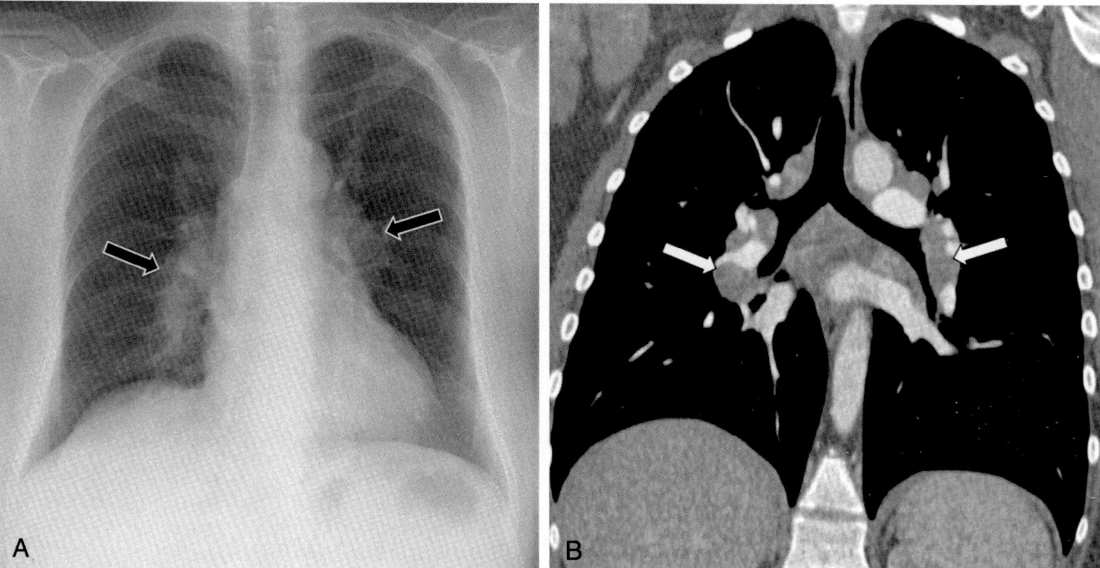

FIG. 16.1 Stage I Sarcoidosis. **(A)** Frontal view of CXR. Bilaterally enlarged hilar lymph nodes are depicted as lobulated structures with smooth margins (*black arrows*). **(B)** A multiplanar reformatted coronal CT image obtained after intravenous injection of iodinated contrast agent highlights multiple enlarged mediastinal and hilar lymph nodes (*white arrows*). *CT*, computed tomography; *CXR*, chest radiograph.

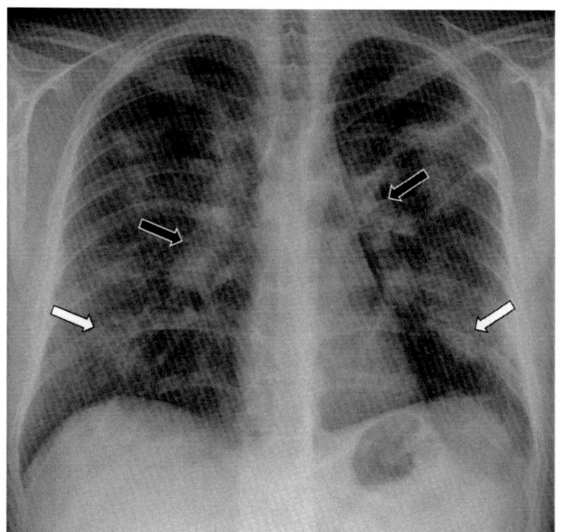

FIG. 16.2 Stage II sarcoidosis. Frontal view of CXR showing bilateral hilar lymph node enlargement (*black arrows*), associated with diffuse parenchymal opacities (*white arrows*). *CXR*, chest radiograph.

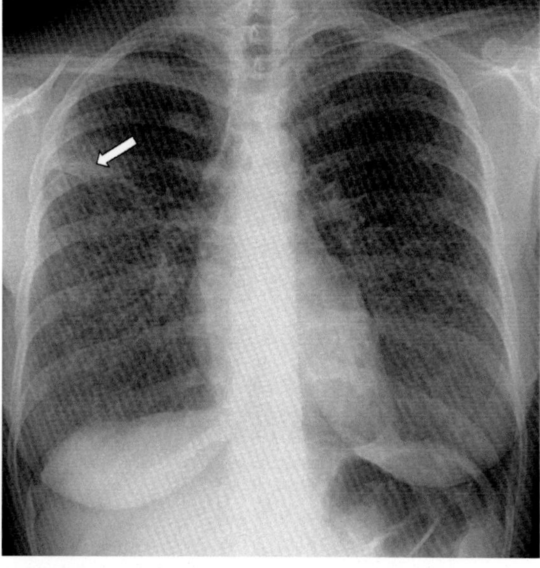

FIG. 16.3 Stage III sarcoidosis. Frontal view of CXR showing bilateral reticulonodular opacities. A right upper lobe consolidation can be observed (*white arrow*). *CXR*, chest radiograph.

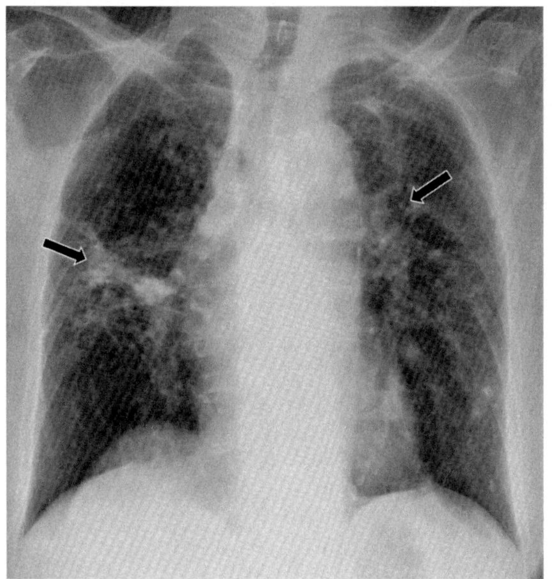

FIG. 16.4 Stage IV sarcoidosis. Frontal view of CXR showing bilateral peri-hilar consolidations (*black arrows*), reticulonodular opacities, and imaging features of parenchymal distortion. *CXR*, chest radiograph.

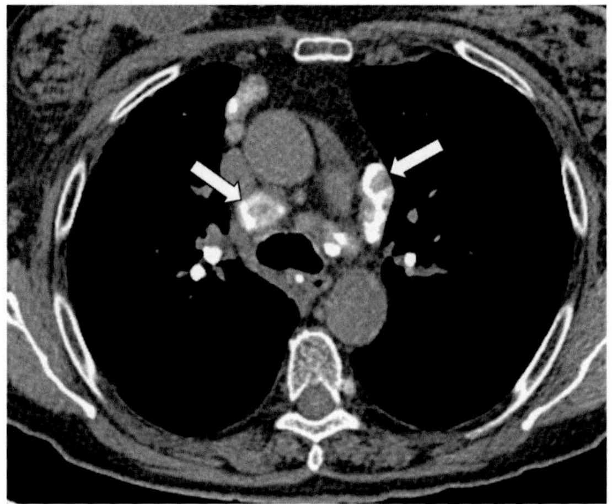

FIG. 16.5 Eggshell lymph node calcification pattern in sarcoidosis. Axial HRCT image (mediastinal window) showing bilaterally enlarged lymph nodes with peripheral calcifications showing remarkably high density and peel-predominant distribution within the lymph node *(white arrows)*. *HRCT*, high-resolution computed tomography.

Imaging Findings

Lymph node involvement

The most common lymphadenopathy pattern is represented by the bilateral, symmetrical, hilar, and mediastinal paratracheal lymph node enlargement.[20] The most commonly involved mediastinal lymph node stations are as follows: right paratracheal, aortopulmonary, tracheobronchial, distal bronchopulmonary, and subcarinal. These lymph node stations are usually easily accessible by bronchoscopy, allowing a high diagnostic yield of transbronchial needle aspiration.[21,28] HRCT is more sensitive than CXR in the evaluation of atypical lymph node enlargement (e.g., internal mammary, retrocrural, and posterior mediastinal lymph nodes) as well as in the depiction of the calcification pattern.[3] Lymph nodal calcification may display various morphology, including eggshell-, "icing sugar"–, punctate, and popcorn-like patterns. The "icing sugar" pattern is highly suggestive for sarcoidosis and appears as amorphous calcifications within enlarged lymph nodes.[20] For the other calcification patterns there is a wider range of differential, notably between sarcoidosis and silicosis in case of eggshell calcification pattern. In sarcoidosis, lymph node calcifications have been related with a chronic condition, with an occurrence of 3% and 20% after 5 and 10 years, respectively (Fig. 16.5).[29]

Lung involvement

In the adequate clinical context the presence of bilateral symmetrically enlarged hilar lymph nodes along with well-defined perilymphatic micronodules is virtually diagnostic for sarcoidosis.[21] Nodules usually range from 2 to 5 mm in diameter, either with smooth or irregular margins, and they predominate in the upper and middle zones.[1]

The perilymphatic distribution reflects the close relation of the disease with the lymphatic system. Hence nodules are usually both centrilobular and clustered along bronchovascular bundles, interlobular septa. Notably the involvement of interlobar fissures with irregularly thickening or beaded outline is a common tip to differentiate sarcoidosis from other diseases with nodular pattern.[1] The subcostal subpleural regions are also involved, although less than the other regions, and it is to be differentiated from silicosis in that coalescent nodules may appear as "pseudo plaques".[30]

Solid nodules can have odd distribution within the lung parenchyma, either resulting in clusters of innumerable individual nodules or coalescing into ill-defined lesions (i.e., nodules, or masses when greater than 3 cm). Compared to other diseases, such findings are most typically bilateral in sarcoidosis. The "sarcoid galaxy" sign defines the presence of a main focal consolidation surrounded by small nodules that indeed recall the shape of an astronomic galaxy (Fig. 16.6).[20] The "reverse halo" sign consists of a ring-shaped consolidation surrounding a central area of GGO. The reverse halo represents a quite unusual manifestation of sarcoidosis, and it is more commonly associated with organizing pneumonia.[31] Sometimes the massive profusion of tiny nodules may resemble a miliary pattern challenging the differential diagnosis with either tuberculosis or pulmonary metastases.

Small sarcoid nodules below the spatial resolution of HRCT may produce an amorphous GGO pattern, which may either resolve or progress toward fibrosis (Fig. 16.7).[21] Fine pulmonary fibrosis should be suspected when abundant GGO is associated with HRCT

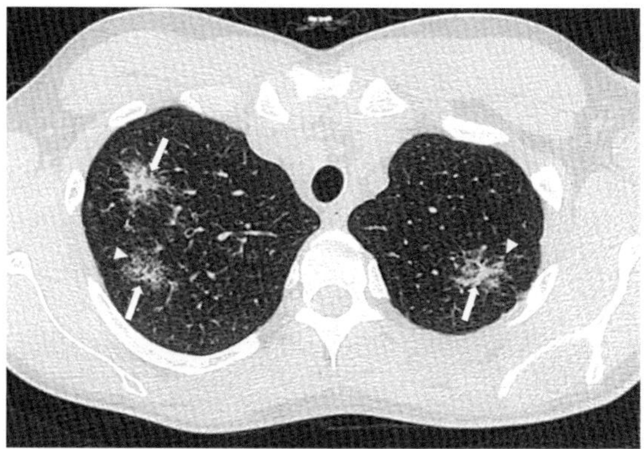

FIG. 16.6 Sarcoid galaxy sign. Axial image of an HRCT (lung window) showing three ill-defined lesions (*white arrows*) surrounded by smaller nodules (*white arrowheads*). HRCT, high-resolution computed tomography.

signs of architectural distortion (hilar/fissural retraction, cysts, and traction bronchiectasis). Not surprisingly, GGO at diagnosis is associated with worse prognosis.[32] Although in the majority of cases sarcoidosis remains stable or resolves, and lung fibrosis may be supervening in up to 20% of patients, with significant impact on the patients prognosis (Fig. 16.8).[20] Hence it is essential that radiologists differentiate between potentially reversible (nodules, septal lines, and consolidations) and irreversible HRCT abnormalities.[21] The signs of pulmonary fibrosis on HRCT are as follows: coarse reticular opacities radiating posterolaterally from the hilum toward the periphery, displacement of fissure and bronchovascular bundles, and honeycombing (mainly located in the subpleural regions of the upper and middle lung zones) (Fig. 16.9).[21] The differential diagnosis with other upper zones–predominant fibrosing diseases (chronic hypersensitivity pneumonitis, and pleuroparenchymal fibroelastosis) is easier when adenopathies are present. In rare cases, honeycombing may be located within lower lung zones, thus mimicking usual interstitial pneumonia (UIP) and idiopathic pulmonary fibrosis. Atypical HRCT manifestations of sarcoidosis may be present in about 25%–30% of individuals (Table 16.1),[33,34] and sarcoidosis is indeed named "the great mimicker" or "the great pretender" (Table 16.2).[1,35]

Pleural involvement is quite exceptional in sarcoidosis; frequency is reported from 1% to 4%. In particular, pleural effusion (frequency about 1.9%) has been reported in association with cases of extensive

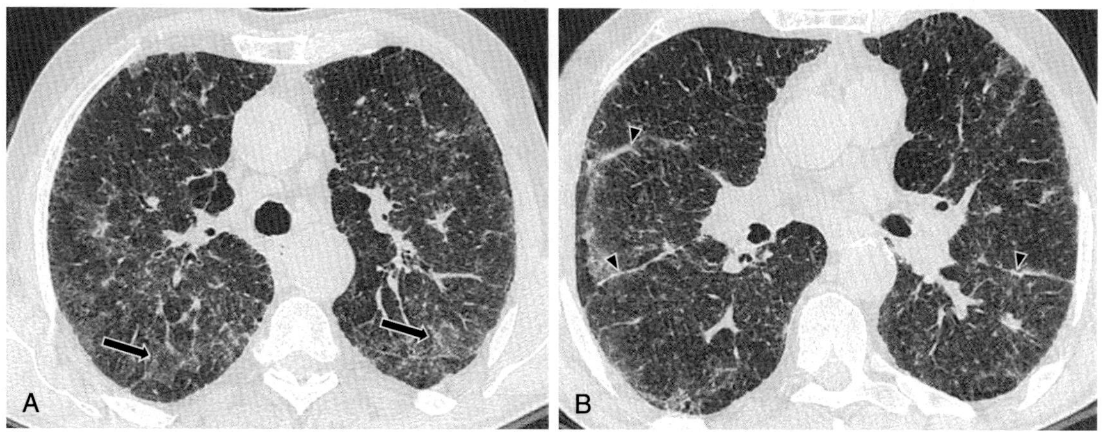

FIG. 16.7 Axial HRCT images (lung window). **(A)** Innumerable small sarcoid nodules representing interstitial granulomas beyond the spatial resolution of HRCT are seen as amorphous ground glass opacity pattern (*black arrows*). **(B)** A caudal image shows fissural involvement (*black arrowheads*). *HRCT*, high-resolution computed tomography.

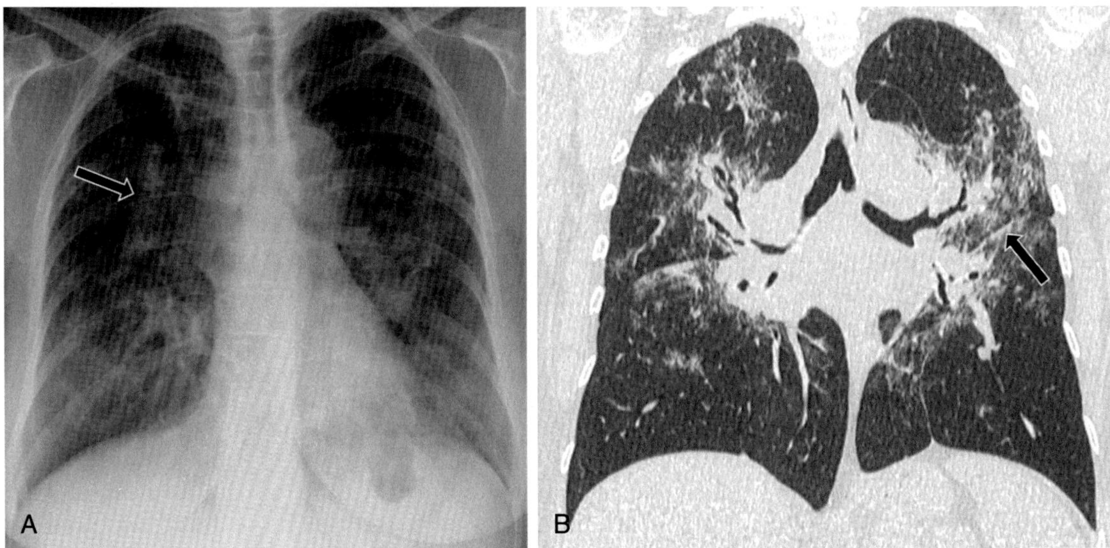

FIG. 16.8 Fibrotic sarcoidosis. **(A)** Frontal view of CXR showing fibrotic masses, with bilateral peri-hilar distribution and mediastinal widening. **(B)** Coronal HRCT image highlighting fibrotic masses associated with perilymphatic nodules (*black arrow*) and signs of parenchymal distortion (cranial displacement of fissure and traction bronchiectasis). *CXR*, chest radiograph; *HRCT*, high-resolution computed tomography.

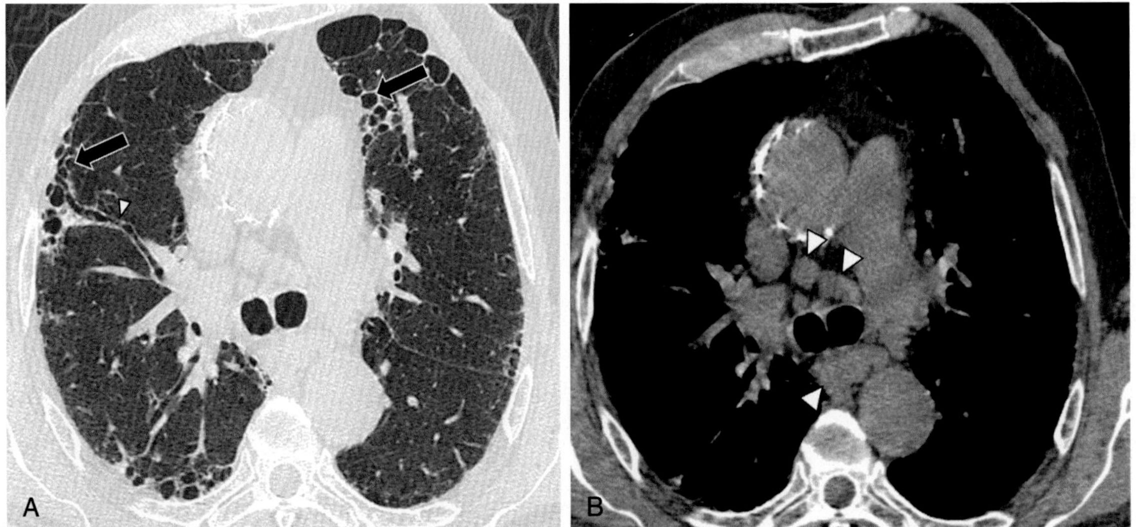

FIG. 16.9 Sarcoidosis with usual interstitial pneumonia (UIP) pattern. **(A)** Areas of honeycombing (*black arrows*) are associated with traction bronchiectasis (*white arrowhead*). **(B)** Mediastinal window showing enlarged lymph nodes in the station 4R and 4L (*white arrowheads*). The patient underwent a skin biopsy of the forehead, with histologic evidence of nonnecrotizing granulomatous dermatitis.

pulmonary or systemic disease.[29] Pleural effusion can be either unilateral or bilateral, small or massive, and the association with sarcoidosis can be suggested by parenchymal or lymph nodal involvement. However, the presence of unilateral pleural effusion in sarcoidosis should always be investigated to rule out malignancy. Pneumothorax is usually associated with extensive parenchymal disease and is caused by the rupture of subpleural bullae or the necrosis of a subpleural sarcoidotic granuloma.[23] There are reports

TABLE 16.2
List of Diseases That Most Frequently Overlap Sarcoidosis on High-Resolution Computed Tomography

Lymphangitic carcinomatosis
- Patchy distribution
- Nodular septal thickening ("beaded appearance") outlining the secondary pulmonary lobule
- Pleural effusion, usually unilateral

Silicosis
- Upper lobe fibrotic consolidations (progressive massive fibrosis)

Lymphoproliferative disorders
- Asymmetrical, unilateral lymph node enlargement

Chronic hypersensitivity pneumonia (HP)
- Centrilobular nodules

Pleuroparenchymal fibroelastosis (PPFE)
- Upper and middle lung zones irregular pleural thickening
- Subpleural fibrosis

Idiopathic pulmonary fibrosis
- Subpleural disease, anterior in upper lobes or posterior in lower lobes ("propeller blade")
- Disseminated dendriform pulmonary ossification

Tuberculosis (TB)
- Tree-in-bud or random nodules
- Unilateral lymph node enlargement
- Dense lymph node calcifications
- Parenchymal consolidation

Aluminosis
- Small ill-defined centrilobular opacities predominant in the upper lung zones

The table reports the most useful imaging features consistent with alternative diagnoses.

of an increased occurrence of cancer in patients with sarcoidosis. Therefore the detection of large masses—especially within the first 5 years of follow-up—should prompt a careful investigation until the exclusion of an underlying malignancy (Fig. 16.10).[1,36]

Airway Involvement

In sarcoidosis, airways obstruction may be caused by various mechanisms such as intrinsic granulomatous luminal narrowing (peribronchovascular thickening), extrinsic lymphadenopathy compression, and small airway obstruction. The latter can be defined by the presence of areas of decreased parenchymal attenuation, namely "mosaic attenuation" pattern, associated with decreased number and size of pulmonary vessels.[34,37,38] Notably an expiratory scan is useful to confirm air trapping as the cause of the mosaic attenuation.[39] Sarcoidosis may cause tracheal stenosis (smooth, irregular, nodular, or mass-like) and tracheomalacia, the latter because of the loss of elastic and cartilaginous structures.[8,20,40]

Complications

Aspergillomas present as sponge-like masses characterized by irregular airspaces, typically described as an antigravitational air crescent. The coalescent fungal hyphae are mobile within the fungus ball being the solid component subject to localization variation according to the patient position (e.g., supine and prone CT scanning result in different location of the fungus ball within the cavity). The detection of a pleural surface thickening adjacent to the cavity wall represents an early sign of aspergilloma formation and may be apparent on both CXR or HRCT.[41]

The intravenous administration of contrast media may provide information regarding the obstruction or compression of pulmonary vessels by mediastinal lymphadenopathy or fibrosis and findings suggestive for pulmonary venoocclusive disease (PVOD).[42] Findings consistent with PVOD—enlarged main pulmonary artery and right heart chambers, smooth interlobular septal thickening, GGO, and pleural and/or pericardial effusion—were found in 85.7% of patients suffering from pulmonary hypertension in nonfibrotic sarcoidosis.[25]

Functional and Prognostic Evaluation

HRCT may reveal abnormalities without clinical significance; thus its specificity should be weighted in the specific clinical scenario.[21] Notably, the staging of sarcoidosis was developed based on CXR findings, and pulmonary involvement evaluated on HRCT should not be mixed with the aforementioned classification.[43] When evaluating morphologic changes on paired CXR and paired HRCT scans in patients with sarcoidosis, changes depicted on serial HRCT demonstrated a higher agreement with pulmonary function test trends than CXR changes in the definition of disease improvement or progression.[44] Changes in forced vital capacity were moderately correlated with HRCT changes.[45] In particular, an inverse correlation was found between the micronodules profusion and lung function.[18] A composite score for disease activity (CT Activity Score (CTAS))—including the visual assessment of the extent of GGO, interlobular septal thickening, consolidation and nodularity—was shown to predict response to

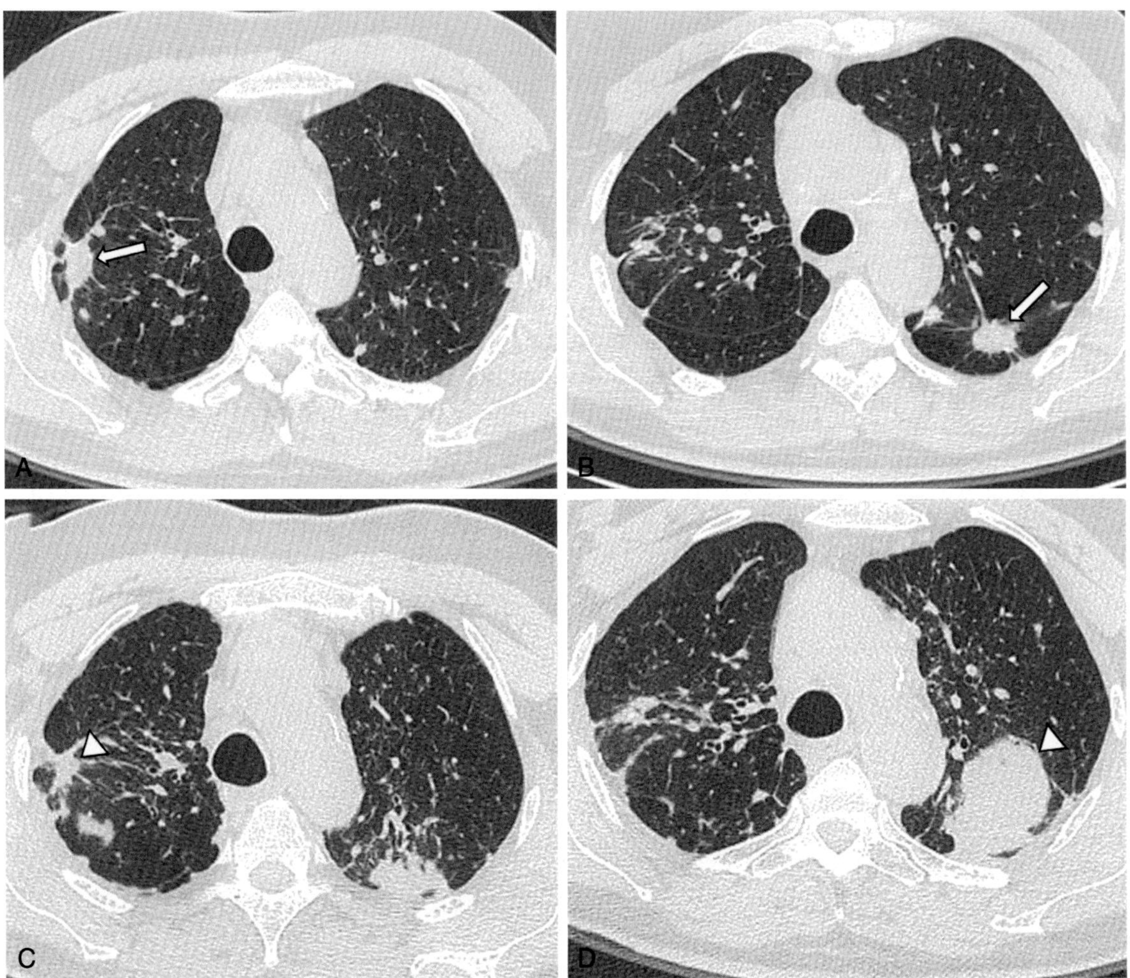

FIG. 16.10 **(A–B)** Axial HRCT images at different anatomical levels showing various nodular lesions (*white arrows*) in a subject suffering from sarcoidosis. **(C–D)** Axial HRCT images at the same anatomical levels of A and B, 4 years later. The nodule shown in A did not grow (*white arrowhead* in **C**), whereas the nodule shown in **B** grew significantly (*white arrowhead* in **D**), histologically confirmed as neoplastic lesion. This case shows the different potential evolution of HRCT findings with similar HRCT features at the baseline scan. *HRCT*, high-resolution computed tomography.

treatment.[46] A computer-based approach calculating the lung texture score was also shown to significantly correlate with pulmonary function indexes.[47]

An HRCT score was developed for prediction of mortality in sarcoidosis and tested in a large cohort of patients. The score integrated the composite physiologic index (CPI, a weighted index of pulmonary function variables correlating with the extent of interstitial lung disease on HRCT) and two imaging variables, namely the extent of fibrosis and the main pulmonary artery diameter to ascending aorta diameter ratio. The composite HRCT-CPI score is easy to calculate and may be helpful to differentiate between subjects at different mortality risk.[48]

MAGNETIC RESONANCE IMAGING

Compared to HRCT, MRI allows more specific tissue characterization and is not associated with ionizing radiation burden. On the other hand, MRI suffers from reduced spatial resolution and intrinsic technical limitation related to the abundance of interfaces between air and soft tissue (significant deterioration of the electromagnetic field).[49] Hence thoracic MRI was tested specifically for the mediastinal compartment and for the detection of major parenchymal abnormalities in a number of diseases, including sarcoidosis.[50]

Imaging Findings

Lymph node involvement

Inflammatory and metastatic lymph nodes may display similar imaging features on MRI, including low signal intensity on T1-weighted (T1w) images and high signal intensity on T2-weighted (T2w) images, whereas normal lymph nodes are usually hypointense on T1w and isointense or slightly hyperintense on T2w images. Some studies reported that diffusion-weighted imaging and apparent diffusion coefficient (ADC) values may be used to differentiate between lymphoma or malignant tumors involving hilar lymph nodes and sarcoidosis. In particular, ADC values are quantitative parameters (expressed in mm^2/s) reflecting the degree of diffusion of water molecules within different tissues. Indeed, most lymphomas are hypercellular with a contracted extracellular space, thus limiting the diffusion of water molecules, which ultimately decreases the ADC values, while ADC values are less perturbed in patients with sarcoidosis (e.g., higher values than in metastatic lymph nodes).[51,52]

Recently, lymph nodes appearing as centrally hypointense signal structures—reflecting focal fibrosis—with peripheral hyperintense signal ("dark lymph node" sign) were demonstrated in subjects with sarcoidosis on T2w fast spin-echo and post-gadolinium 3D gradient-echo sequences.[53]

Lung involvement

MRI parenchymal findings were shown to correlate with CT findings. However, MRI is less sensitive for the detection of parenchymal opacification, reticulation, nodules, and masses, mostly when located in the lower pulmonary zones (particularly susceptible to motion artefacts because of diaphragm and heart motion).[4] In pediatric patients, fast sequences (with an average scan time of about 10 min) could accurately demonstrate the presence of lymph nodal enlargement, cardiac findings, and—moderate-to-severe—chronic interstitial parenchymal changes. MRI was considered comparable with HRCT regarding the detection of stages I, II, and IV.[54]

On MRI, late enhancement after the intravenous administration of paramagnetic contrast media allows the detection of fibrotic tissue. In patients with sarcoidosis, late-enhanced MRI with individual nulling of the pulmonary blood pool signals correlated significantly with the extent of fibrotic sarcoid, as measured on HRCT.[49] Currently, MRI has been proposed as an imaging technique applicable during the follow-up of patients who have simultaneously undergone CT and MRI scan to prospectively evaluate changes on MRI to be confronted with prior CT.[4]

Future directions

MRI could represent a promising imaging technique, particularly for pediatric patients. The development of fast sequence protocols with high spatial resolution will be particularly beneficial for young individuals suffering from sarcoidosis, whose disease could therefore be monitored without the risk related to ionizing radiation.

REFERENCES

1. Silva M, Nunes H, Valeyre D, Sverzellati N. Imaging of sarcoidosis. *Clin Rev Allergy Immunol.* 2015;49(1):45–53.
2. Larke FJ, Kruger RL, Cagnon CH, et al. Estimated radiation dose associated with low-dose chest CT of average-size participants in the National Lung Screening Trial. *AJR Am J Roentgenol.* 2011;197(5):1165–1169.
3. Greco FG, Spagnolo P, Muri M, et al. The value of chest radiograph and computed tomography in pulmonary sarcoidosis. *Sarcoidosis Vasc Diffuse Lung Dis.* 2014;31(2):108–116.
4. Chung JH, Little BP, Forssen AV, et al. Proton MRI in the evaluation of pulmonary sarcoidosis: comparison to chest CT. *Eur J Radiol.* 2013;82(12):2378–2385.
5. Baughman RP, Teirstein AS, Judson MA, et al. Clinical characteristics of patients in a case control study of sarcoidosis. *Am J Respir Crit Care Med.* 2001;164(10 Pt 1):1885–1889.
6. Nunes H, Brillet PY, Valeyre D, Brauner MW, Wells AU. Imaging in sarcoidosis. *Semin Respir Crit Care Med.* 2007;28(1):102–120.
7. Calandriello L, Walsh SLF. Imaging for sarcoidosis. *Semin Respir Crit Care Med.* 2017;38(4):417–436.
8. Nishino M, Lee KS, Itoh H, Hatabu H. The spectrum of pulmonary sarcoidosis: variations of high-resolution CT findings and clues for specific diagnosis. *Eur J Radiol.* 2010;73(1):66–73.
9. Nunes H, Soler P, Valeyre D. Pulmonary sarcoidosis. *Allergy.* 2005;60(5):565–582.
10. Al-Jahdali H, Rajiah P, Koteyar SS, Allen C, Khan AN. Atypical radiological manifestations of thoracic sarcoidosis: a review and pictorial essay. *Ann Thorac Med.* 2013;8(4):186–196.
11. Scadding JG. Prognosis of intrathoracic sarcoidosis in England. A review of 136 cases after five years' observation. *Br Med J.* 1961;2(5261):1165–1172.
12. DeRemee RA. The roentgenographic staging of sarcoidosis. Historic and contemporary perspectives. *Chest.* 1983;83(1):128–133.

13. Little BP. Sarcoidosis: overview of pulmonary manifestations and imaging. *Semin Roentgenol*. 2015;50(1):52–64.
14. Baughman RP, Shipley R, Desai S, et al. Changes in chest roentgenogram of sarcoidosis patients during a clinical trial of infliximab therapy: comparison of different methods of evaluation. *Chest*. 2009;136(2):526–535.
15. Aleksoniene R, Zeleckiene I, Mataciunas M, et al. Relationship between radiologic patterns, pulmonary function values and bronchoalveolar lavage fluid cells in newly diagnosed sarcoidosis. *J Thorac Dis*. 2017;9(1):88–95.
16. Consensus conference: activity of sarcoidosis. Third WASOG meeting, Los Angeles, USA, September 8–11, 1993. *Eur Respir J*. 1994;7(3):624–627.
17. Valeyre D, Prasse A, Nunes H, Uzunhan Y, Brillet PY, Muller-Quernheim J. Sarcoidosis. *Lancet*. 2014;383(9923): 1155–1167.
18. Ors F, Gumus S, Aydogan M, Sari S, Verim S, Deniz O. HRCT findings of pulmonary sarcoidosis; relation to pulmonary function tests. *Multidiscip Respir Med*. 2013;8(1):8.
19. Uzunhan Y, Nunes H, Jeny F, et al. Chronic pulmonary aspergillosis complicating sarcoidosis. *Eur Respir J*. 2017;49(6).
20. Criado E, Sanchez M, Ramirez J, et al. Pulmonary sarcoidosis: typical and atypical manifestations at high-resolution CT with pathologic correlation. *Radiographics*. 2010;30(6):1567–1586.
21. Spagnolo P, Sverzellati N, Wells AU, Hansell DM. Imaging aspects of the diagnosis of sarcoidosis. *Eur Radiol*. 2014;24(4):807–816.
22. Denning DW, Pleuvry A, Cole DC. Global burden of chronic pulmonary aspergillosis complicating sarcoidosis. *Eur Respir J*. 2013;41(3):621–626.
23. Rockoff SD, Rohatgi PK. Unusual manifestations of thoracic sarcoidosis. *AJR Am J Roentgenol*. 1985;144(3): 513–528.
24. Baughman RP, Culver DA, Judson MA. A concise review of pulmonary sarcoidosis. *Am J Respir Crit Care Med*. 2011;183(5):573–581.
25. Nunes H, Humbert M, Capron F, et al. Pulmonary hypertension associated with sarcoidosis: mechanisms, haemodynamics and prognosis. *Thorax*. 2006;61(1):68–74.
26. Corte TJ, Wells AU, Nicholson AG, Hansell DM, Wort SJ. Pulmonary hypertension in sarcoidosis: a review. *Respirology*. 2011;16(1):69–77.
27. Kouranos V, Hansell DM, Sharma R, Wells AU. Advances in imaging of cardiopulmonary involvement in sarcoidosis. *Curr Opin Pulm Med*. 2015;21(5):538–545.
28. Trisolini R, Anevlavis S, Tinelli C, Orlandi P, Patelli M. CT pattern of lymphadenopathy in untreated patients undergoing bronchoscopy for suspected sarcoidosis. *Respir Med*. 2013;107(6):897–903.
29. Park HJ, Jung JI, Chung MH, et al. Typical and atypical manifestations of intrathoracic sarcoidosis. *Korean J Radiol*. 2009;10(6):623–631.
30. Hansell DM, Bankier AA, MacMahon H, McLoud TC, Muller NL, Remy J. Fleischner Society: glossary of terms for thoracic imaging. *Radiology*. 2008;246(3):697–722.
31. Kumazoe H, Matsunaga K, Nagata N, et al. "Reversed halo sign" of high-resolution computed tomography in pulmonary sarcoidosis. *J Thorac Imag*. 2009;24(1):66–68.
32. Akira M, Kozuka T, Inoue Y, Sakatani M. Long-term follow-up CT scan evaluation in patients with pulmonary sarcoidosis. *Chest*. 2005;127(1):185–191.
33. Polverosi R, Russo R, Coran A, et al. Typical and atypical pattern of pulmonary sarcoidosis at high-resolution CT: relation to clinical evolution and therapeutic procedures. *Radiol Med*. 2014;119(6):384–392.
34. Cozzi D, Bargagli E, Calabro AG, et al. Atypical HRCT manifestations of pulmonary sarcoidosis. *Radiol Med*. 2018;123(3):174–184. https://doi.org/10.1007/s11547-017-0830-y. Epub 2017 Nov 9.
35. Hawtin KE, Roddie ME, Mauri FA, Copley SJ. Pulmonary sarcoidosis: the 'great pretender'. *Clin Radiol*. 2010;65(8):642–650.
36. Bonifazi M, Bravi F, Gasparini S, et al. Sarcoidosis and cancer risk: systematic review and meta-analysis of observational studies. *Chest*. 2015;147(3):778–791.
37. Terasaki H, Fujimoto K, Muller NL, et al. Pulmonary sarcoidosis: comparison of findings of inspiratory and expiratory high-resolution CT and pulmonary function tests between smokers and nonsmokers. *AJR Am J Roentgenol*. 2005;185(2):333–338.
38. Naccache JM, Lavole A, Nunes H, et al. High-resolution computed tomographic imaging of airways in sarcoidosis patients with airflow obstruction. *J Comput Assist Tomogr*. 2008;32(6):905–912.
39. Kligerman SJ, Henry T, Lin CT, Franks TJ, Galvin JR. Mosaic attenuation: etiology, methods of differentiation, and pitfalls. *Radiographics*. 2015;35(5):1360–1380.
40. Brandstetter RD, Messina MS, Sprince NL, Grillo HC. Tracheal stenosis due to sarcoidosis. *Chest*. 1981;80(5):656.
41. Sansom HE, Baque-Juston M, Wells AU, Hansell DM. Lateral cavity wall thickening as an early radiographic sign of mycetoma formation. *Eur Radiol*. 2000;10(2):387–390.
42. Frazier AA, Franks TJ, Mohammed TL, Ozbudak IH, Galvin JR. From the Archives of the AFIP: pulmonary veno-occlusive disease and pulmonary capillary hemangiomatosis. *Radiographics*. 2007;27(3):867–882.
43. Wessendorf TE, Bonella F, Costabel U. Diagnosis of sarcoidosis. *Clin Rev Allergy Immunol*. 2015;49(1):54–62.
44. Zappala CJ, Desai SR, Copley SJ, et al. Accuracy of individual variables in the monitoring of long-term change in pulmonary sarcoidosis as judged by serial high-resolution CT scan data. *Chest*. 2014;145(1):101–107.
45. Gafa G, Sverzellati N, Bonati E, et al. Follow-up in pulmonary sarcoidosis: comparison between HRCT and pulmonary function tests. *Radiol Med*. 2012;117(6):968–978.
46. Benamore R, Kendrick YR, Repapi E, et al. CTAS: a CT score to quantify disease activity in pulmonary sarcoidosis. *Thorax*. 2016;71(12):1161–1163.
47. Erdal BS, Crouser ED, Yildiz V, et al. Quantitative computerized two-point correlation analysis of lung CT scans correlates with pulmonary function in pulmonary sarcoidosis. *Chest*. 2012;142(6):1589–1597.

48. Walsh SLF, Wells AU, Sverzellati N, et al. An integrated clinicoradiological staging system for pulmonary sarcoidosis: a case-cohort study. *Lancet Respirat Med.* 2014;2(2):123–130.
49. Brady D, Lavelle LP, McEvoy SH, et al. Assessing fibrosis in pulmonary sarcoidosis: late-enhanced MRI compared to anatomic HRCT imaging. *QJM.* 2016;109(4):257–264.
50. Biederer J, Beer M, Hirsch W, et al. MRI of the lung (2/3). Why... when... how? *Insights Imag.* 2012;3(4):355–371.
51. Gumustas S, Inan N, Akansel G, Basyigit I, Ciftci E. Differentiation of lymphoma versus sarcoidosis in the setting of mediastinal-hilar lymphadenopathy: assessment with diffusion-weighted MR imaging. *Sarcoidosis Vasc Diffuse Lung Dis.* 2013;30(1):52–59.
52. Kosucu P, Tekinbas C, Erol M, et al. Mediastinal lymph nodes: assessment with diffusion-weighted MR imaging. *J Magn Reson Imag.* 2009;30(2):292–297.
53. Chung JH, Cox CW, Forssen AV, Biederer J, Puderbach M, Lynch DA. The dark lymph node sign on magnetic resonance imaging: a novel finding in patients with sarcoidosis. *J Thorac Imag.* 2014;29(2):125–129.
54. Gorkem SB, Kose S, Lee EY, Doganay S, Coskun AS, Kose M. Thoracic MRI evaluation of sarcoidosis in children. *Pediatr Pulmonol.* 2017;52(4):494–499.

CHAPTER 17

Nuclear Imaging

R.G.M. KEIJSERS, MD, PHD • JAN C. GRUTTERS, MD

INTRODUCTION

In sarcoidosis treatment, clinicians might struggle with determining the presence of disease activity. Symptoms, deteriorating pulmonary function, chest radiography, and biomarkers can be sufficient, but in some patients, additional information is indispensable.

By using molecular imaging techniques, the biological process at cellular and molecular level can be visualized. Imaging the actual state of a multisystem disease process throughout the body is of significant clinical relevance, given the possibility of personalizing patient care (Figure 17.1). In sarcoidosis, several nuclear techniques are available for imaging the disease process in an organ-specific manner of which fludeoxyglucose–positron emission tomography/computed tomography (FDG-PET/CT) is currently the most sensitive. FDG-PET/CT scanning has several potential benefits in sarcoidosis (Table 17.1).

FLUDEOXYGLUCOSE–POSITRON EMISSION TOMOGRAPHY/COMPUTED TOMOGRAPHY

The glucose analog on fluodeoxyglucose (FDG) is a positron emitter which annihilates with an electron in the tissue, thereby sending two gamma photons of both 511 kilo electron volt (keV). These two gamma photons are detected by the positron emission tomography (PET) camera, and three-dimensional images are reconstructed. The simultaneously obtained computed tomography (CT) image is used for attenuation correction and provides anatomical information as well.

In granuloma formation such as sarcoidosis, several cell types are involved, such as lymphocytes, macrophages, and fibroblasts. These cells all demonstrate FDG uptake, although it is suggested that fibroblasts contribute less to the total FDG uptake in the inflammatory process.

FDG-PET/CT Preparation and Protocol

FDG-PET/CT is performed in accordance with the joint guideline of the Society of Nuclear Medicine and European Association of Nuclear Medicine.[1] FDG dosage depends on the PET/CT system, time per bed position, and the patient's body weight. In state-of-the-art cameras, a quadratic dose regimen can be used.[2] This results in a slightly higher dosage for patients above 75 kg of bodyweight (165 pounds) but improves the image quality.

The effective radiation dose of FDG-PET/CT is determined by several parameters. Using 200 megabecquerel (MBq), the effective radiation dose of FDG is 3.8 millisievert (mSv). CT dosage needs to be added. However, CT parameters may vary based on the requested image quality. In most PET studies, low-dose CT for attenuation correction and anatomical mapping or high-end CT with intravenous contrast is performed. CT parameters will be optimized depending on the patient's body weight, resulting in a higher dosage with increasing body weight. The radiation from the CT scan may therefore range from approximately 5 to 20 mSv.

Physiologic uptake of FDG in the myocyte influences the accuracy of FDG-PET/CT in assessing cardiac sarcoidosis (CS). To reduce the glucose metabolism in the myocyte, the patient should be prepared with a high fat and low carbohydrate diet. This diet induces the use of fatty acids instead of glucose. This reduced physiologic uptake of FDG in the myocyte enables the imaging of pathologic uptake, such as granulomas. Therefore, the carbohydrate-restricted diet improves the sensitivity of FDG-PET/CT in detecting active CS.[3]

Additional unfractionated heparin administration 15 min before FDG injection favors the cardiac glucose metabolism suppression.[4] Therefore, a dosage of 50 IE per kg bodyweight is recommended, with a maximum of 5000 IE.

Given the clinical relevance, evaluating the presence of active CS is important. Therefore, any patient with (suspected) sarcoidosis referred for FDG-PET/CT should be prepared with a carbohydrate-restricted diet and unfractionated heparin.

FDG-PET/CT Compared to Biomarkers, Symptoms, and Pulmonary Function Tests

Various studies over the last decade have shown the crucial role of FDG-PET/CT in sarcoidosis care, especially in organ-specific assessment of disease activity.[5,6] As an imaging tool for active disease, FDG-PET/CT was compared with several other markers of sarcoidosis activity and showed its additional value.

Sarcoidosis. https://doi.org/10.1016/B978-0-323-54429-0.00017-3

Angiotensin-converting enzyme (ACE) is produced by the epitheloid cells and macrophages and is thought to represent the total granuloma load.[7] It is a frequently used marker, particularly for treatment monitoring.[8,9]

Soluble interleukin-2 receptor (sIL-2R) is associated with cellular immune reactions and might therefore be increased in sarcoidosis. Its sensitivity is approximately 70% and higher in patients with parenchymal involvement.[10,11] However, sIL-2R does not correlate with the radiographic changes, and conflicting results have been documented about the correlation between sIL-2R and lung functional outcome.[11,12]

In sarcoidosis, several important biomarkers have been correlated with FDG-PET. In patients recently diagnosed with sarcoidosis and increased metabolic activity on FDG-PET, ACE was increased in only 36%, whereas sIL-2R was increased in 47%.[13] In 89 patients with chronic sarcoidosis and persistent disabling symptoms, 65 (73%) demonstrated active disease on FDG-PET/CT. Only 22% showed an elevated ACE level, whereas sIL-2R was increased in 68%. Remarkably, none of the 24 patients without metabolic activity on FDG-PET/CT had an increased ACE or sIL-2R.[14] Similar results were found in 90 patients with chronic disease and persistent symptoms. In 74 patients (82%), FDG-PET/CT revealed inflammation. In the group with positive FDG-PET/CT lesions, 38 patients (51%) had normal ACE levels.[15]

The prognostic value of FDG-PET in pulmonary involvement was evaluated in 43 patients, and the change in pulmonary function tests (PFTs) after 12 months was observed.[16] In 16 patients without parenchymal disease activity and no treatment, no changes in PFT were found. In 11 untreated patients with diffuse parenchymal disease activity, a significant decrease in diffusion capacity of the lung for carbon monoxide (DLCO) was observed. On the other hand, in 16 treated patients with diffuse parenchymal disease activity, a significant increase in PFT was found.

FDG-PET/CT and Chest Radiography

Evaluating 188 FDG-PET studies in sarcoidosis patients, active pulmonary disease occurred in two-thirds of patients with radiographic stage II and III sarcoidosis. Negative pulmonary FDG-PET was common in patients with radiographic stage 0, I, and IV sarcoidosis.[17]

In the majority of 89 sarcoidosis patients with persistent disabling symptoms, inflammatory activity was found by FDG-PET/CT, even in patients with signs of fibrosis. Of the 15 patients with radiological stage IV disease, 14 demonstrated active inflammation (93%).[14] Additional analysis of pulmonary disease in 26 patients with fibrotic changes on high-resolution computerized tomography revealed increased pulmonary metabolic activity in 22 (85%).[18]

FDG-PET/CT in Treatment Monitoring

FDG-PET/CT can be used for treatment monitoring in sarcoidosis. In 12 patients treated with infliximab, reduction in metabolic activity imaged by FDG-PET correlated with signs of clinical improvement. This finding supports the hypothesis that FDG uptake represents granulomatous inflammation, and FDG-PET might have predictive value in treatment response.[19]

The results of FDG-PET/CT after corticosteroid treatment were evaluated in 27 symptomatic patients, and the metabolic response was correlated with disease relapse. Fourteen patients were classified as metabolic responder (8 complete responders and six partial responders on FDG-PET), whereas 13 were nonresponders. In the responder group, the relapse rate was significantly lower (14.2%) than that in the nonresponder group (61.5%). Remarkably, none of the eight patients with a complete metabolic response showed recurrent disease.[20]

In a prospective analysis of 47 patients treated with infliximab, a relapse was found in 29 (61.7%). A maximum standardized uptake value (SUV_{max}) of ≥6.0 in mediastinal lymph nodes as well as sIL-2R levels ≥ 4000 pg/mL at baseline were found to significantly predict relapse rate in sarcoidosis patients after discontinuation of therapy.[21]

In a limited number of patients, FDG-PET/CT was evaluated in a prospective study analyzing the steroid-sparing effect of repository corticotropin.[22] Of the PET studies available in 15 patients, there was a significant fall in pulmonary SUV. However, the metabolic change did not correlate with DLCO or forced vital capacity.

MOLECULAR IMAGING IN CARDIAC SARCOIDOSIS

CS may give rise to conduction abnormalities, ventricular tachycardia (VT) or fibrillation, sudden cardiac death, and heart failure due to inflamed and scarred myocardium.

Determining the presence of CS is therefore extremely relevant. A cardiac device may be required, depending on the conduction abnormality, functional impairment, or arrhythmia. Additional immunosuppressive therapy is necessary when active CS is present.

Disease presence and activity can be evaluated by molecular imaging techniques. Currently, cardiac magnetic resonance (CMR) imaging with late gadolinium enhancement (LGE) and FDG-PET/CT seem to be the appropriate techniques in CS imaging. CMR reveals damaged myocardium and provides functional data such as the end diastolic volume and left ventricular ejection fraction. Acute inflammation may be detected by T2-weighted CMR revealing edema. However, this sequence is to date unreliable in CS. FDG-PET/CT on the other hand indicates the presence of disease activity in CS, especially when there is correlation with late enhancement on CMR (Figure 17.2 and 17.3).

FDG-PET/CT in CS

The diagnostic performance of FDG PET in (CS) depends on the used imaging technique and patient preparation. Systematic reviews for the accuracy of FDG-PET/CT in diagnosing CS demonstrated a sensitivity of 81%–89% and a specificity of 78%–82%.[3,23]

Subanalysis demonstrated an improved diagnostic odds ratio of FDG-PET/CT due to preparation by fasting and heparin, but not by a carbohydrate-restricted diet.[3] However, expert panels recommend to prepare patients with a carbohydrate-restricted diet.[24] Such a diet increases the interobserver agreement of image interpretation and therefore the overall detection of CS.[25]

It is suggested that in CS patients with VT, FDG uptake is significantly higher than in those with advanced atrioventricular block and asymptomatic patients. These results may imply that the degree of myocardial involvement on FDG-PET/CT is related to the clinical presentation.[26] Besides the ability of FDG-PET/CT to detect CS, it simultaneously reveals extrathoracic disease activity. Therefore, FDG-PET/CT is of additional value compared with CMR in CS evaluation because the scanning field of CMR is limited.[27,28]

FDG-PET/CT and Myocardial Blood Flow

Sarcoid-mediated inflammation in the myocardium is associated with a regional impairment of the coronary flow.[29] In CS analysis, FDG-PET/CT for imaging inflammation and Rubidium-82 for imaging myocardial perfusion can be combined. This approach can be used for risk analysis because patients with an increased FDG uptake and a focal perfusion defect are at higher risk of death or VT.[30] The combined imaging of metabolic activity and myocardial perfusion is now recommended by the Society of Nuclear Medicine and American Society of Nuclear Cardiology.[24]

FDG-PET/CT in Monitoring

FDG-PET/CT can be used to monitor the effect of immunosuppressive therapy in active CS. An increased or unchanged FDG uptake after steroid therapy may be associated with poor clinical outcome, indicating a role for FDG-PET/CT in therapeutic decision-making.[31,32]

In addition, a reduction in the intensity and extent of myocardial inflammation on FDG-PET appeared to be associated with an improvement in ejection fraction of the left ventricle.[33] Focal FDG uptake in the interventricular septum was associated with complete heart block recovery after corticosteroids, especially when magnetic resonance imaging shows thinning of the interventricular septum.[34]

Hybrid CMR/PET in CS

Hybrid CMR/PET imaging can simultaneously assess the damaged myocardium on LGE images and disease activity on PET. This technique provides accurate coregistration and therefore improves the diagnostic accuracy. At the same time, comprehensive cardiac function can be assessed, extracardiac disease activity can be determined, patient efficacy is increased, and the radiation dose is reduced.[35]

In patients without LGE and FDG uptake, CS is unlikely. Matching LGE and FDG uptake is considered as active CS. Patients with LGE and no FDG uptake are considered of having CS but without currently active disease. To date, the challenge lays in patients without LGE and FDG uptake (Table 17.2).

TABLE 17.1
FDG-PET/CT Imaging in Sarcoidosis Appears Particularly Useful in Evaluation of Organ Involvement (Staging), in Evaluating (Organ Specific) Disease Activity (Inflammation), and in Monitoring Treatment Response

FDG-PET/CT IN SARCOIDOSIS FOR EVALUATING:
1. Organ involvement
2. Organ-specific disease activity
3. Treatment response
4. Lesions for biopsy

FDG-PET/CT, fludeoxyglucose–positron emission tomography/computed tomography.

TABLE 17.2
FDG-PET/CT Imaging in Sarcoidosis Appears Particularly Useful in Evaluation of Organ Involvement (Staging), in Evaluating (Organ Specific) Disease Activity (Inflammation), and in Monitoring Treatment Response

CMR WITH LGE AND FDG-PET/CT IN EVALUATING CS	
LGE – and PET –	No CS
LGE + and PET +	Active CS
LGE + and PET –	Inactive CS
LGE – and PET +	Possible active CS though physiologic uptake needs to be excluded

CMR, cardiac magnetic resonance; *CS*, cardiac sarcoidosis; *FDG-PET/CT*, fluorodeoxyglucose positron emission tomography/computed tomography; *LGE*, late gadolinium enhancement.

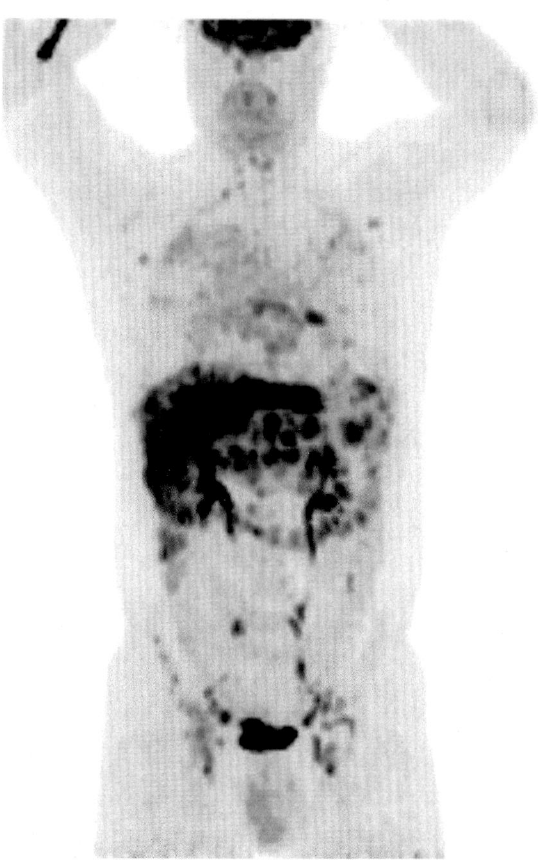

FIG. 17.1 FDG-PET/CT of active sarcoidosis in the lung parenchyma, thoracic and extrathoracic lymph nodes, anterior left ventricle wall, spleen, liver, and skeleton. *FDG-PET/CT*, fluorodeoxyglucose positron emission tomography/computed tomography.

Diffuse FDG uptake in the myocardium or increased activity in all basal segments is considered physiologic. However, focal (on diffuse) activity should be interpreted with caution because it might indeed represent active CS. Early myocardial inflammation might then be detectable by FDG-PET, but not by CMR.

FUTURE RADIONUCLIDE IMAGING IN SARCOIDOSIS ACTIVITY

As false-positive FDG uptake remains a diagnostic challenge in CS as well as neurosarcoidosis, there is an ongoing search for new PET tracers. A potential tracer is fluorothymidine (FLT) demonstrating a low physiologic uptake in the myocardium. A recent study in 20 patients demonstrated that FLT-PET/CT can detect CS. However, FDG-PET/CT was inconclusive in 4 (20%) due to diffuse uptake, whereas all FLT-PET/CT studies were assessable. At the same time, FLT-PET/CT is easier to perform because it requires no special diet before imaging.[36] Both FLT-PET/CT and FDG-PET/CT detected all extracardiac lesions.

Somatostatin receptor–based PET/CT imaging appears feasible as well and might provide a more specific alternative for visualizing active CS.[37] Especially the tracer Gallium-68 (Ga-68) [1,4,7,10-tetraazacyclododecane-1,4,7,10-tetraaceticacid]-1-Nal3-octreotide (DOTANOC) looks very promising as an alternative CS PET tracer, showing 100% accuracy in a small series of patients with suspected CS.[38] In a study comparing PET/CT and Gallium-67 (Ga-67) citrate scintigraphy, the Ga-68 DOTANOC appeared more sensitive. It revealed active disease in 19 out of 20 patients, whereas 17 patients demonstrated active disease in Ga-67 scintigraphy. In addition, Ga-68 DOTANOC visualized more lesions in lymph nodes, uvea, and muscles (Figure 17.4).[39]

CONCLUSIONS

FDG-PET/CT currently appears to be the most sensitive technique for evaluating disease activity in sarcoidosis. The use of this technique might be considered in clinically suspected sarcoidosis with normal chest radiography and serum biomarkers. It is also of use in detecting inflammatory lesions in symptomatic patients with chronic sarcoidosis and normal routine findings as well as in finding occult organs or tissues for biopsy.

In addition, FDG-PET/CT can be used for risk assessment in pulmonary sarcoidosis and might identify patients that could benefit from (supplementary) anti-inflammatory therapy. In organ-specific monitoring of granulomatous inflammation, FDG-PET/CT can be used in both cardiac and extra-CS.

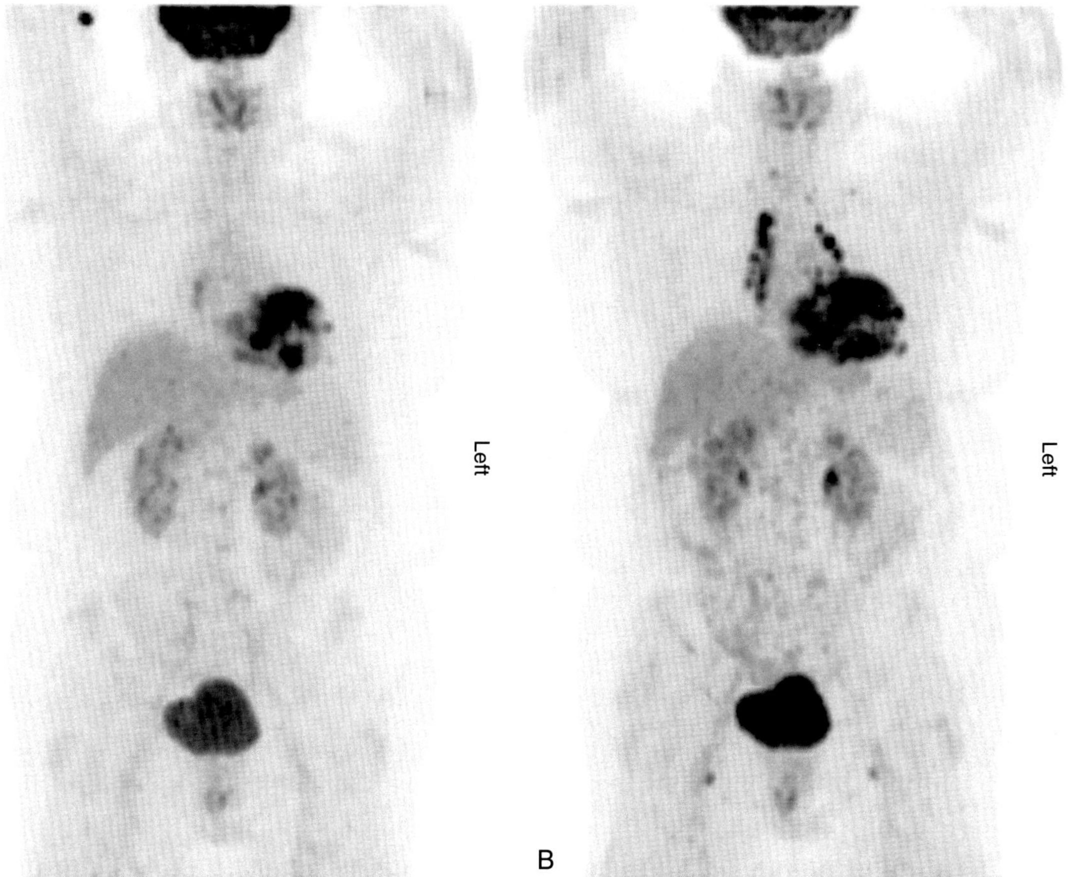

FIG. 17.2 FDG-PET/CT and cardiac MRI of a 65-year-old female presenting with a complete atrioventricular block, left bundle branch block, and normal left ventricular ejection fraction. A pacemaker was implanted. Because she developed ventricular tachycardia, cardiac sarcoidosis was suspected. FDG-PET/CT showed focal activity throughout the LV walls, as well as RV wall, and most active in the interventricular septum. No other disease activity was found by FDG-PET/CT, and HRCT was normal. ACE was slightly increased, and sIL-2R was normal. BAL was performed revealing increased CD4+ lymphocytes and an elevated CD4/CD8 ratio. Prednisone was started. After 6 months, the LVEF decreased, and metabolic activity was further increased. Remarkably, active lymph nodes were seen in the mediastinum and hila, supporting the diagnosis of sarcoidosis. *BAL*, bronchoalveolar lavage; *FDG-PET/CT*, fluorodeoxyglucose positron emission tomography/computed tomography; *HRCT*, high-resolution computerized tomography; *MRI*, magnetic resonance imaging; *sIL-2R*, serum soluble interleukin two receptor. *LV*, left ventricle; *RV*, right ventricle; *LVEF*, left ventricular ejection fraction.

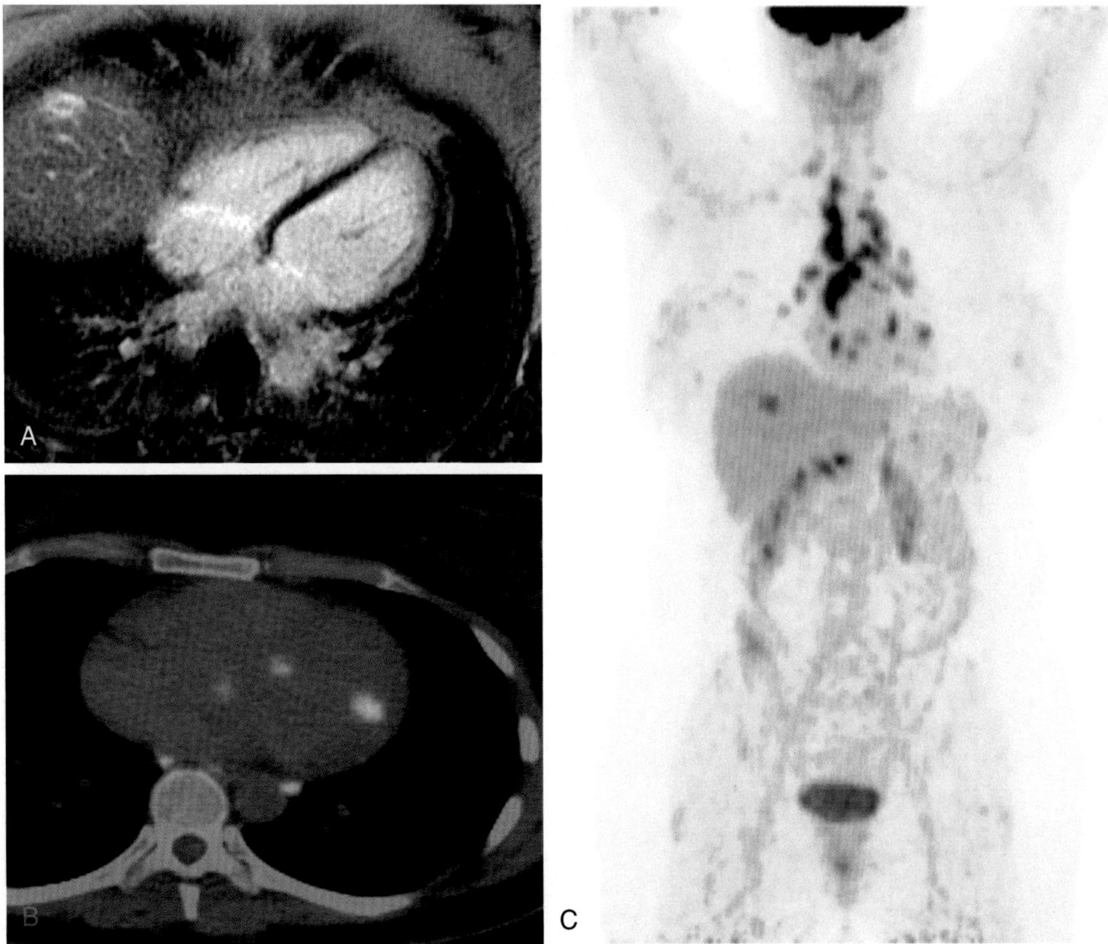

FIG. 17.3 A 45-year-old female presented with collapse and a third-degree AV block during exercise. Because of the suspicion of cardiac sarcoidosis, MRI was performed. Cardiac MRI showed no late gadolinium enhancement and a normal left ventricular ejection fraction. **(A)** FDG-PET/CT at the same time revealed focal increased activity in the interventricular septum and the lateral wall. **(B and C)** In addition, active thoracic and extrathoracic lymphadenopathy with liver and spleen involvement was observed. *AV,* atrial ventricular; *FDG-PET/CT*, fluorodeoxyglucose positron emission tomography/computed tomography; *MRI*, magnetic resonance imaging.

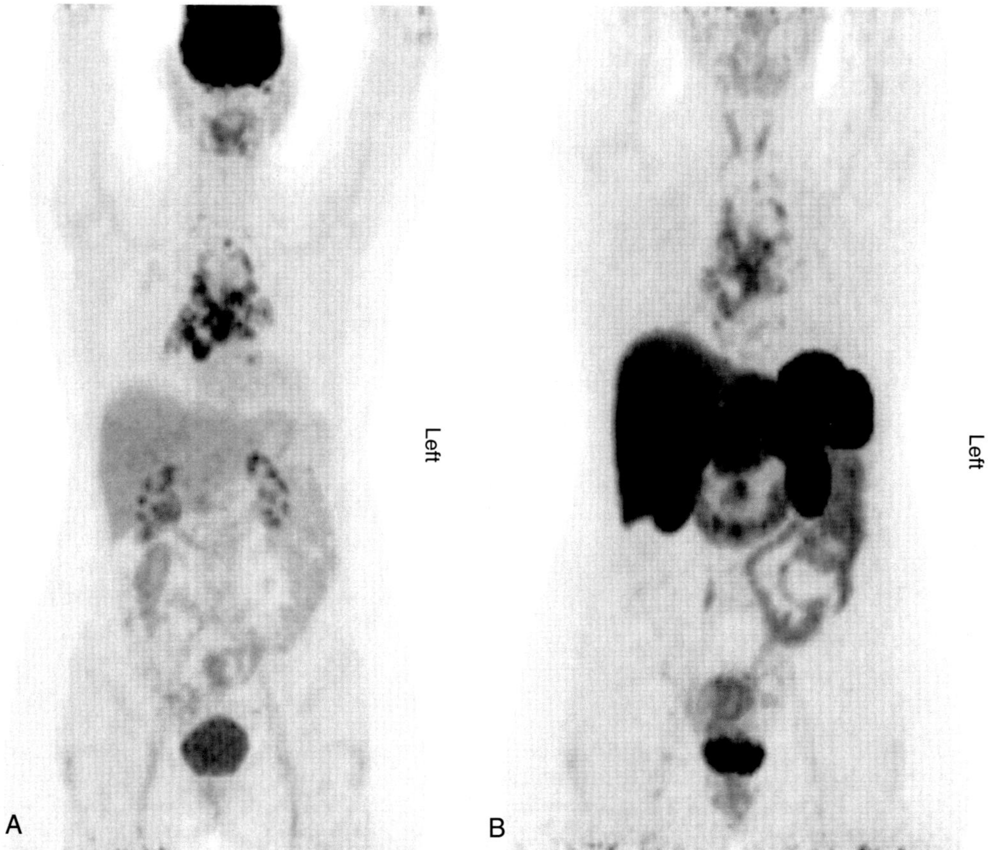

FIG. 17.4 **(A)** FDG-PET/CT of a 50-year-old sarcoidosis patient with active lymph nodes in the mediastinum and hila. **(B)** Additional Gallium-68 DOTANOC PET/CT was performed 1 week later, demonstrating a similar uptake pattern, although the uptake seems less intense. *FDG-PET/CT*, fluorodeoxyglucose positron emission tomography/computed tomography.

REFERENCES

1. Jamar F, Buscombe J, Chiti A, et al. EANM/SNMMI guideline for 18F-FDG use in inflammation and infection. *J Nucl Med*. 2013;54(4):647–658.
2. Boellaard R, Delgado-Bolton R, Oyen WJ, et al. FDG PET/CT: EANM procedure guidelines for tumour imaging: version 2.0. *Eur J Nucl Med Mol Imaging*. 2015;42(2):328–354.
3. Tang R, Wang JT, Wang L, et al. Impact of patient preparation on the diagnostic performance of 18F-FDG PET in cardiac sarcoidosis: a systematic review and meta-analysis. *Clin Nucl Med*. 2016;41(7):e327–e339.
4. Scholtens AM, Verberne HJ, Budde RP, Lam MG. Additional heparin preadministration improves cardiac glucose metabolism suppression over low-carbohydrate diet alone in (1)(8)F-FDG PET imaging. *J Nucl Med*. 2016;57(4):568–573.
5. Adams H, Keijsers RG, Korenromp IH, Grutters JC. FDG PET for gauging of sarcoid disease activity. *Semin Respir Crit Care Med*. 2014;35(3):352–361.
6. Keijsers RG, Veltkamp M, Grutters JC. Chest imaging. *Clin Chest Med*. 2015;36(4):603–619.
7. Gilbert S, Steinbrech DS, Landas SK, Hunninghake GW. Amounts of angiotensin-converting enzyme mRNA reflect the burden of granulomas in granulomatous lung disease. *Am Rev Respir Dis*. 1993;148(2):483–486.
8. Rust M, Bergmann L, Kuhn T, et al. Prognostic value of chest radiograph, serum-angiotensin-converting enzyme and T helper cell count in blood and in bronchoalveolar lavage of patients with pulmonary sarcoidosis. *Respiration*. 1985;48(3):231–236.
9. Hollinger WM, Staton Jr GW, Fajman WA, Gilman MJ, Pine JR, Check IJ. Prediction of therapeutic response in steroid-treated pulmonary sarcoidosis. Evaluation of clinical parameters, bronchoalveolar lavage, gallium-67 lung scanning, and serum angiotensin-converting enzyme levels. *Am Rev Respir Dis*. 1985;132(1):65–69.
10. Bons JA, Drent M, Bouwman FG, Mariman EC, van Dieijen-Visser MP, Wodzig WK. Potential biomarkers for diagnosis of sarcoidosis using proteomics in serum. *Respir Med*. 2007;101(8):1687–1695.

11. Rothkrantz-Kos S, van Dieijen-Visser MP, Mulder PG, Drent M. Potential usefulness of inflammatory markers to monitor respiratory functional impairment in sarcoidosis. *Clin Chem.* 2003;49(9):1510–1517.
12. Grutters JC, Fellrath JM, Mulder L, Janssen R, van den Bosch JM, van Velzen-Blad H. Serum soluble interleukin-2 receptor measurement in patients with sarcoidosis: a clinical evaluation. *Chest.* 2003;124(1):186–195.
13. Keijsers RG, Verzijlbergen FJ, Oyen WJ, et al. 18F-FDG PET, genotype-corrected ACE and sIL-2R in newly diagnosed sarcoidosis. *Eur J Nucl Med Mol Imaging.* 2009;36(7):1131–1137.
14. Mostard RL, Voo S, van Kroonenburgh MJ, et al. Inflammatory activity assessment by F18 FDG-PET/CT in persistent symptomatic sarcoidosis. *Respir Med.* 2011;105(12):1917–1924.
15. Sobic-Saranovic D, Grozdic I, Videnovic-Ivanov J, et al. The utility of 18F-FDG PET/CT for diagnosis and adjustment of therapy in patients with active chronic sarcoidosis. *J Nucl Med.* 2012;53(10):1543–1549.
16. Keijsers RG, Verzijlbergen EJ, van den Bosch JM, et al. 18F-FDG PET as a predictor of pulmonary function in sarcoidosis. *Sarcoidosis Vasc Diffuse Lung Dis.* 2011;28(2):123–129.
17. Teirstein AS, Machac J, Almeida O, Lu P, Padilla ML, Iannuzzi MC. Results of 188 whole-body fluorodeoxyglucose positron emission tomography scans in 137 patients with sarcoidosis. *Chest.* 2007;132(6):1949–1953.
18. Mostard RL, Verschakelen JA, van Kroonenburgh MJ, et al. Severity of pulmonary involvement and (18)F-FDG PET activity in sarcoidosis. *Respir Med.* 2013;107(3):439–447.
19. Keijsers RG, Verzijlbergen JF, van Diepen DM, van den Bosch JM, Grutters JC. 18F-FDG PET in sarcoidosis: an observational study in 12 patients treated with infliximab. *Sarcoidosis Vasc Diffuse Lung Dis.* 2008;25(2):143–149.
20. Maturu VN, Rayamajhi SJ, Agarwal R, Aggarwal AN, Gupta D, Mittal BR. Role of serial F-18 FDG PET/CT scans in assessing treatment response and predicting relapses in patients with symptomatic sarcoidosis. *Sarcoidosis Vasc Diffuse Lung Dis.* 2016;33(4):372–380.
21. Vorselaars AD, van Moorsel CH, Zanen P, et al. ACE and sIL-2R correlate with lung function improvement in sarcoidosis during methotrexate therapy. *Respir Med.* 2015;109(2):279–285.
22. Baughman RP, Sweiss N, Keijsers R, et al. Repository corticotropin for chronic pulmonary sarcoidosis. *Lung.* 2017;195(3):313–322.
23. Youssef G, Leung E, Mylonas I, et al. The use of 18F-FDG PET in the diagnosis of cardiac sarcoidosis: a systematic review and metaanalysis including the Ontario experience. *J Nucl Med.* 2012;53(2):241–248.
24. Chareonthaitawee P, Beanlands RS, Chen W, et al. Joint SNMMI-ASNC expert consensus document on the role of (18)F-FDG PET/CT in cardiac sarcoid detection and therapy monitoring. *J Nucl Cardiol.* 2017;24(5):1741–1758.
25. Ohira H, Ardle BM, deKemp RA, et al. Inter- and intraobserver agreement of 18F-FDG PET/CT image interpretation in patients referred for assessment of cardiac sarcoidosis. *J Nucl Med.* 2017;58(8):1324–1329.
26. Mc Ardle BA, Birnie DH, Klein R, et al. Is there an association between clinical presentation and the location and extent of myocardial involvement of cardiac sarcoidosis as assessed by (1)(8)F- fluorodoexyglucose positron emission tomography? *Circ Cardiovasc Imaging.* 2013;6(5):617–626.
27. Patel DC, Gunasekaran SS, Goettl C, Sweiss NJ, Lu Y. FDG PET-CT findings of extra-thoracic sarcoid are associated with cardiac sarcoid: a rationale for using FGD PET-CT for cardiac sarcoid evaluation. *J Nucl Cardiol.* 2017.
28. Ishiyama M, Soine LA, Vesselle HJ. Semi-quantitative metabolic values on FDG PET/CT including extracardiac sites of disease as a predictor of treatment course in patients with cardiac sarcoidosis. *EJNMMI Res.* 2017;7(1):67. 6017-0315-y.
29. Kruse MJ, Kovell L, Kasper EK, et al. Myocardial blood flow and inflammatory cardiac sarcoidosis. *JACC Cardiovasc Imaging.* 2017;10(2):157–167.
30. Blankstein R, Osborne M, Naya M, et al. Cardiac positron emission tomography enhances prognostic assessments of patients with suspected cardiac sarcoidosis. *J Am Coll Cardiol.* 2014;63(4):329–336.
31. Shelke AB, Aurangabadkar HU, Bradfield JS, Ali Z, Kumar KS, Narasimhan C. Serial FDG-PET scans help to identify steroid resistance in cardiac sarcoidosis. *Int J Cardiol.* 2017;228:717–722.
32. Lee PI, Cheng G, Alavi A. The role of serial FDG PET for assessing therapeutic response in patients with cardiac sarcoidosis. *J Nucl Cardiol.* 2017;24(1):19–28.
33. Osborne MT, Hulten EA, Singh A, et al. Reduction in (1)(8)F-fluorodeoxyglucose uptake on serial cardiac positron emission tomography is associated with improved left ventricular ejection fraction in patients with cardiac sarcoidosis. *J Nucl Cardiol.* 2014;21(1):166–174.
34. Orii M, Hirata K, Tanimoto T, et al. Comparison of cardiac MRI and 18F-FDG positron emission tomography manifestations and regional response to corticosteroid therapy in newly diagnosed cardiac sarcoidosis with complete heart block. *Heart Rhythm.* 2015;12(12):2477–2485.
35. Dweck MR, Abgral R, Trivieri MG, et al. Hybrid magnetic resonance imaging and positron emission tomography with fluorodeoxyglucose to diagnose active cardiac sarcoidosis. *JACC Cardiovasc Imaging.* 2017.
36. Norikane T, Yamamoto Y, Maeda Y, Noma T, Dobashi H, Nishiyama Y. Comparative evaluation of 18F-FLT and 18F-FDG for detecting cardiac and extra-cardiac thoracic involvement in patients with newly diagnosed sarcoidosis. *EJNMMI Res.* 2017;7(1):69-017-0321-0.
37. Lapa C, Reiter T, Kircher M, et al. Somatostatin receptor based PET/CT in patients with the suspicion of cardiac sarcoidosis: an initial comparison to cardiac MRI. *Oncotarget.* 2016;7(47):77807–77814.
38. Gormsen LC, Haraldsen A, Kramer S, Dias AH, Kim WY, Borghammer P. A dual tracer (68)Ga-DOTANOC PET/CT and (18)F-FDG PET/CT pilot study for detection of cardiac sarcoidosis. *EJNMMI Res.* 2016;6(1):52-016-0207-6. Epub 2016 Jun 17.
39. Nobashi T, Nakamoto Y, Kubo T, et al. The utility of PET/CT with (68)Ga-DOTATOC in sarcoidosis: comparison with (67)Ga-scintigraphy. *Ann Nucl Med.* 2016;30(8):544–552.

CHAPTER 18

Quality of Life

TIMOTHY TULLY, MB BCH BAO MRCP • AMIT S. PATEL, MD, FRCP • SURINDER S. BIRRING, MD

ABBREVIATIONS

6MWT 6 Minute Walk Test
BDI Beck Depression Inventory
Borg Borg Dyspnoea Scale
CES-D Centre for Epidemiologic Studies Depression Scale; Cognitive Depression Index
CPI Composite Physiologic Index
CXR Chest X-Ray
DLCO Diffusion Capacity for Carbon Monoxide
FAS Fatigue Assessment Scale
FEV Forced Expiratory Volume
FVC Forced Vital Capacity
HAD Hospital Anxiety and Depression Scale
HRCT High Resolution Computed Tomography
HRQOL Health Related Quality of Life
KSQ Kings Sarcoidosis Questionnaire
LCQ Leicester Cough Questionnaire
MRC Medical Research Council Dyspnoea Scale
MRI Magnetic Resonance Imaging
NPS Neuropathic Pain Scale
PET Positron Emission Tomography
PFI Patient Reported Outcomes Measurement Information Systems (PROMIS) Fatigue Instrument
SAT Sarcoidosis Assessment Tool
SF36 Medical Outcomes Study 36-Item Short Form-36
SGRQ St. George's Respiratory Questionnaire
SHQ Sarcoidosis Health Questionnaire
VAS Visual Analogue Scale
WHOQOL-100 World Health Organisation Quality of Life Assessment Instrument-100

The goal is a good life all the way 'til the very end. We need to ask people what their priorities are – especially when they have a serious illness or frailty. If we don't ask, our care and what we do to people isn't aligned with what matters most to them and then you get suffering

DR. ATUL GUWANDE[1]

INTRODUCTION TO HEALTH-RELATED QUALITY OF LIFE

Sarcoidosis is a systemic disorder of unknown etiology which most frequently affects the lungs. Other organs involved include the skin, eyes, musculoskeletal system, nervous system, heart, liver, and kidneys. Patient-reported symptoms not only relate to the organ affected but also include the impact of medications and psychological and social well-being.[2] Fatigue and sleep disturbance are also well-recognized symptoms.[3] With advances in medical care, patients with chronic disease can expect to live longer lives and subsequently accumulate an array of symptoms that can be progressive and detrimental to their health-related quality of life (HRQOL).

The World Health Organization described quality of life (QOL) in 1947 as "a state of complete

Sarcoidosis. https://doi.org/10.1016/B978-0-323-54429-0.00018-5

physical, mental and social well-being, and not merely the absence of disease and infirmity".[4] This definition is not all encompassing however, and QOL is specific to an individual. As a result, its meaning can depend on psychological, social, spiritual, or physical aspects of life or, indeed, a combination of many of these aspects within the context of the culture and customs in which people live. From a health point of view, one has to be more specific in terms of QOL, and so the term health-related quality of life (HRQOL) is used as a means to describe a patient's perception of the impact of health or disease on their QOL.[5] This generally encompasses three domains: physical function, mental status, and ability to engage in normative social interactions.[6] Specifically in sarcoidosis, these domains revolve around a general health status, medications, and organ-specific impact.[7] Health status is a complementary concept, which refers to the impact of disease on patients' physical, psychological, and social functioning.[8] Functional status, another concept, refers to the subjective ability to perform in physical, social, and mental activities of daily living (See Fig. 18.1).

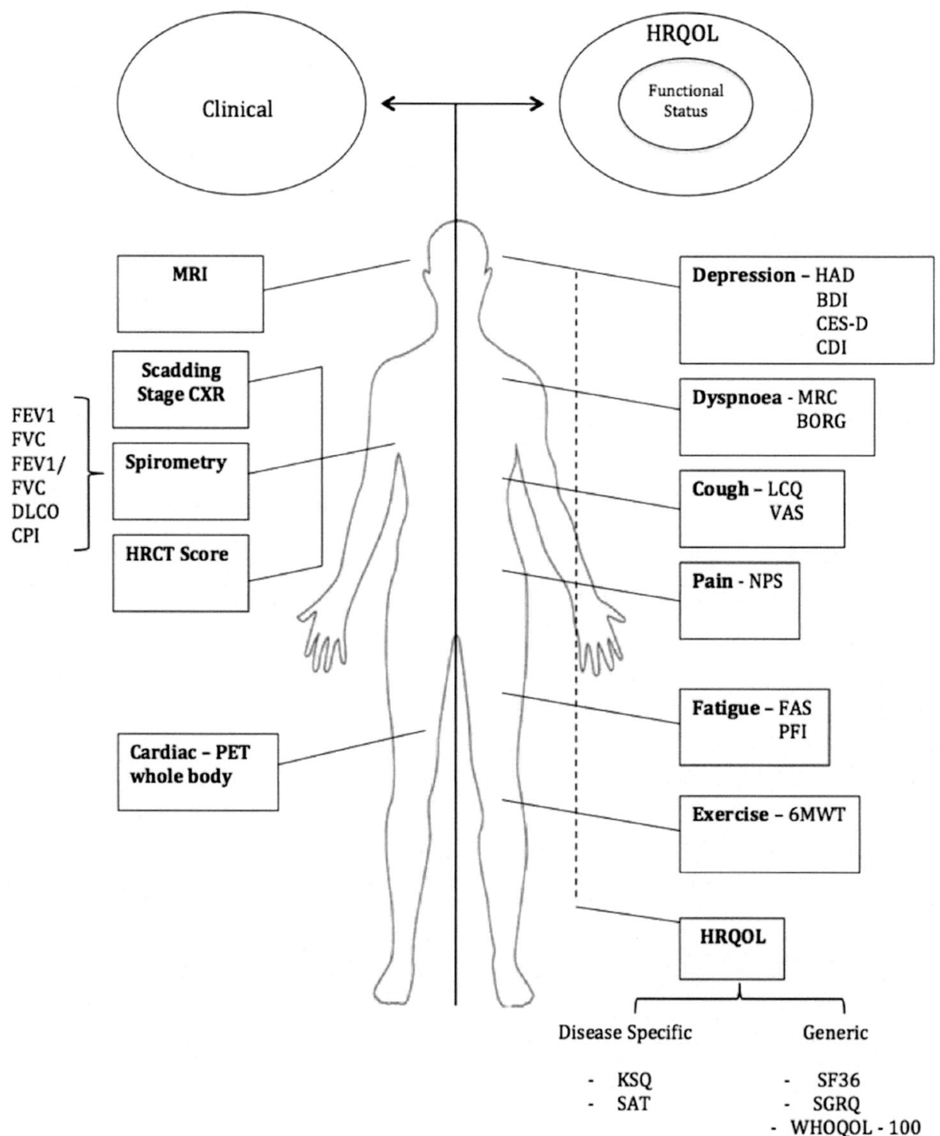

FIG. 18.1 Outcome Measures in Sarcoidosis.

Interactions between patients and clinicians are often infrequent. When the focus is on the measurement of physiological variables, this can fail to capture the impact on a patient's HRQOL.[9] Thus the assessment of HRQOL is an important aspect of patient care. Over the past 20 years there have been great advances in how HRQOL is measured in sarcoidosis, progressing from using generic tools of HRQOL measurement such as the Short Form-36 (SF-36) to pulmonary-specific questionnaires such as St. George's Respiratory Questionnaire (SGRQ) and more recently to sarcoidosis-specific questionnaires such as the Kings Sarcoidosis Questionnaire (KSQ, 2012) and the Sarcoidosis Assessment Tool (SAT, 2013). These questionnaires continue to be tested, challenged, and developed to gain a better understanding of this condition and its impact on patients. There is accumulating evidence that sarcoidosis HRQOL assessment tools are valid and reliable, reflect important clinical changes, and have become more concise and easier to understand and administer.[10,11]

PATIENT-REPORTED OUTCOME (PRO)

A patient-reported outcome (PRO) is any report of the status of a patient's health condition which comes directly from the patient, without interpretation of the patient's response by a clinician or anyone else.[12] HRQOL in sarcoidosis can be measured using Patient-Reported Outcome Measures (PROMs). These tools, in the form of questionnaires, are self-administered by the patient. PROMs should follow a recognized framework of design and use methods such as cognitive patient interviewing to generate items and further validated methods to select items important and relevant to patients with sarcoidosis.[13,14] These tools must be carefully designed and validated, including their translations for cross-cultural use.[15]

PROMs must assess patients' subjective feeling of well-being, of physical symptoms such as pain and fatigue, and of how they perceive the impact of their disease at any particular stage of their life. PROMs must pass through a methodical and exhaustive process before being approved by regulatory agencies such as the Food and Drug Administration in the United States of America.[16]

VALIDATION OF HRQOL ASSESSMENT TOOLS

Examining the validity of instruments is to examine whether an instrument measures what it is intended to measure. It is a core component in the development of PROMs. Different aspects of validity must be assessed when developing tools for the assessment of health status. Examining validity typically includes examining content validity, criterion validity, and construct validity. The intricacies of validation are summarized here. Repeatability and responsiveness are also important aspects in the development of HRQOL questionnaires but are beyond the scope of this chapter.

Content validity measures the extent to which the items in the instrument are sensible and represent the concepts of interest.[17] The target population and the measurement aims need to be clearly defined. Items in the instrument must comprehensively cover the relevant issues. For example, if symptoms of a certain condition are being assessed, then excluding some major relevant symptoms may result in undetected differences between patients. Measuring item coverage is not statistically possible and depends on ensuring robust and thorough processes such as literature review, patient interviews, and multidisciplinary team discussions.[18]

Criterion validity involves assessing an instrument against the perceived gold standard. In HRQOL the instruments measure postulated constructs that are experimental and subjective.[19] Instruments can be measured against other measures that may be argued to be the best measures at that time. This usually involves comparing a new instrument against one or more well-established instruments.

Construct validity assesses the degree to which an instrument measures the construct that it was designed to measure. A construct is a theoretically derived domain that is to be measured. One of the simplest methods of examining construct validity is to examine results of known group validity.[18] An example of this would be the expectation perhaps that individuals with advanced lung disease would have a poorer HRQOL than those with earlier disease. If the instrument is unable to distinguish between groups, then it is unlikely to be particularly useful.

The minimal clinical important difference (MCID) is mentioned later on in this chapter when referring to the sarcoidosis-specific HRQOL questionnaires. The MCID is a patient-derived score that reflects changes in a clinical intervention which is meaningful for the patient.[20]

GENERIC HRQOL ASSESSMENT TOOLS USED IN SARCOIDOSIS

Generic HRQOL assessment tools such as the Medical Outcomes Study 36-Item SF-36 and the World Health Organization Quality of Life Assessment

TABLE 18.1
A Comparison of HRQOL Questionnaires Used in Sarcoidosis

ITEM	KSQ	SAT	SHQ	SGRQ	SF36
Sarcoid modules	+	+	–	-	–
Lung items	+	+	+	+	–
Skin items	+	+	+	–	–
Eye items	+	–	+	–	–
Fatigue item	+	+	+	–	+
Internal consistency (Cronbach's α coefficient)	0.93	≥0.87	≥0.84		
Repeatability (ICC)	>0.9	Not studied	Not studied		
Correlation with FVC (Pearson)	0.45–0.49[a]	−0.23 (Spearman)	0.19[a]	−0.45[a]	0.31[a]

Note: + indicates yes, and – indicates no (related to original study).
FVC, Forced Vital Capacity; *HRQOL*, Health-Related Quality of Life; *ICC*, Intraclass Correlation Coefficient; *KSQ*, Kings Sarcoidosis Questionnaire; *SAT*, Sarcoidosis Assessment Tool; *SGRQ*, St. George's Respiratory Questionnaire; *SHQ*, Sarcoidosis Health Questionnaire; *SF36*, Short Form-36.
[a]= $P < .05$.

Instrument-100 (WHOQOL-100) have been used to assess HRQOL in sarcoidosis. The emphasis of these tools is on physical, emotional, and social functioning (Table 18.1).

Short Form-36

The SF-36 is a validated HRQOL tool that can be used in a wide spectrum of medical conditions. It has been translated and validated in many languages and cultures. The SF-36 covers eight different dimensions of HRQOL: physical functioning, social functioning, role limitations due to physical functioning (role functioning—physical), bodily gain, general mental health, role limitations due to emotional functioning (role functioning—emotional), vitality (energy and fatigue), and general health perception. Scores can be summed together from all domains with differing weightings to contribute to two summary scores, a physical component score and a mental component score.[21]

SF-36 has been well studied in sarcoidosis. Cox et al. studied HRQOL in 111 sarcoidosis patients in an outpatient setting in North and South Carolina in 2002. There were statistically significant and clinically important reductions in SF-36 scores of patients who were prescribed oral corticosteroids.[9] Brancaleone et al. assessed the impact of inspiratory muscle impairment on exercise tolerance and HRQOL because it has been suggested that impaired inspiration in sarcoidosis, caused by subclinical granulomatous skeletal muscle involvement, is an important factor causing dyspnea and reduced walking capacity.[22] The study supported this theory, reporting significantly lower HRQOL in all subscores of SF-36.[23] Bourbannais et al. investigated clinical markers predictive of poor HRQOL in 162 sarcoidosis patients. Using a composite model containing the distance saturation product and the Borg Dyspnoea Scale score at the end of a 6-min walk test (6MWT) they showed a significant association with SF-36 HRQOL scores. A limitation of this study was that there was very little racial diversity as almost all of the patients were African American women.[24] In another large prospective study, Bourbannais et al. investigated gender differences in HRQOL using SF-36 and reported that women have lower HRQOL scores and a greater degree of functional impairment than men. In this study the authors also showed that reduction in diffusion capacity for carbon monoxide (DLCO) and the 6MWT distance are predictors of lower HRQOL.[25] Judson et al. studied the efficacy of thalidomide in pulmonary sarcoidosis and found no effect on SF36-HRQOL.[26] These studies show SF36 to be a well-studied measure of HRQOL in sarcoidosis across a wide spectrum of patients. A limitation of SF-36 is that is not sarcoidosis specific and so does not directly address symptoms and problems that are frequent and important to patients with sarcoidosis.

World Health Organization Quality of Life Assessment-100

The World Health Organization Quality of Life Assessment (WHOQOL-100) was developed simultaneously across 15 international field centers and includes 24 facets relating to QOL, which are grouped into four larger domains: physical, psychological, social relationships, and environment. It also includes one facet examining overall QOL and general health perceptions.[27] The WHOQOL-100 has been used in large sarcoidosis studies in the Netherlands to demonstrate that patients with pain perceived a lower HRQOL.[28] HRQOL was compared with QOL of patients with rheumatoid arthritis and was found to be less severe.[29] As with SF-36, this questionnaire is not disease specific. It is a lengthy questionnaire containing 100 items. The WHOQOL-10 covers a wide range of topics that other tools do not assess such as perception about appearance and detailed questions on mood and sexuality. As a result, it can take longer (up to 2–3 times longer) to complete than other questionnaires.

St George's Respiratory Questionnaire

Pulmonary-specific questionnaires have also been tested in sarcoidosis, namely SGRQ.[30] The SGRQ was developed in 1991 to assess three domains of health in chronic obstructive pulmonary disease (COPD) patients: symptoms, activity, and impacts. The questionnaire has 50 items with 76 weighted responses. Recall ranges from 1 month to 3 months to 1 year depending on the time frame of a study. The total scale is 0–100; lower score indicates a better HRQOL.[31] It was developed and validated in both asthma and COPD patients, although it has also been validated for use in patients with bronchiectasis and interstitial lung disease (ILD) and has been applied to patients with sarcoidosis.[32] The activity component of SGRQ has been shown to be an independent predictor of the 6MWD.[33] SGRQ total scores demonstrating impaired HRQOL are also associated with dyspnea assessed by the Nijmegen questionnaire.[34] A case-control study of the effect of obesity on PROs in 184 sarcoidosis patients used SGRQ to demonstrate a significant impact on HRQOL.[35] There have been conflicting reports of an association between SGRQ and lung function, ranging from none to moderate. Chang et al. demonstrated a significant correlation between SGRQ and forced vital capacity (FVC) and Forced Expiratory Volume 1 (FEV1) and DLCO in a cross-sectional study of 50 patients with ILD including sarcoidosis patients.[36] A significant correlation with FVC and FEV1 has also been reported by Antoniou et al. in a study from Greece; however the correlation was relatively weak ($r = 0.4$).[37] Cox et al. however reported no correlation between SGRQ and spirometry.[9] Gvozdenovic et al. reported that patients with multisystem sarcoidosis have a worse SGRQ activities score than patients with pulmonary sarcoidosis alone.[38]

Fatigue Questionnaires

It is important to assess fatigue in sarcoidosis; it is reported in 50%–70% of patients.[39] A number of questionnaires are available to assess fatigue. The Fatigue Assessment Scale (FAS) is a 10-item sarcoidosis-specific PRO questionnaire. It is commonly used in clinical studies and is a well-validated and reliable fatigue measure in sarcoidosis.[40]

There are other questionnaires available such as the Functional Assessment of the Chronic Illness Therapy-Fatigue, the Visual Analog Scale (VAS), and the WHOQOL-100.[41] The Patient-Reported Outcome Measurement Information Systems (PROMIS) is another option that was developed to provide a comprehensive item bank for PROs used to assess chronic disease.[42] Kalanis et al. studied an alternative PRO fatigue instrument. They developed the Patient-Reported Outcomes Measurement Information Systems (PROMIS) Fatigue Instrument (PFI). A total of 107 consecutive sarcoidosis patients underwent a comparison of PFI versus FAS. Using Cronbach's alpha, PFI demonstrated a superior internal consistency (0.96 vs. 0.74).[43]

Fatigue items are incorporated into HRQOL questionnaires commonly used in sarcoidosis. SF-36 asks patients questions about feeling worn out and tired. The SHQ asks about energy, effort, and concentration. The KSQ asks about tiredness and its impact on social activities. The SAT has a fatigue module similar to the PFI developed from PROMIS items. The SGRQ however does not directly ask about fatigue. Fatigue is addressed in more detail in another chapter in this book.

Dyspnea, Cough, and Depression

Dyspnea and cough may contribute to the patients suffering in sarcoidosis. The Medical Research Council Breathlessness Questionnaire and the Borg scale have been used as assessment tools in sarcoidosis clinical trials and are brief and effective tools.[44,45] Cough items are included in the SGRQ, SHQ, KSQ, and SAT but are not reported as an outcome. Cough-related HRQOL can be assessed using the Leicester Cough Questionnaire (LCQ).[46] The LCQ is a 19-item questionnaire that is the most widely used and validated outcome measure for cough. In sarcoidosis the LCQ was associated with 24-hour objectively measured cough frequency. The severity of cough can simply be quantified using a 0–100 mm VAS.[47]

Depression has been reported to occur in 25%–66% of sarcoidosis patients.[33] A specific PRO to assess depression in sarcoidosis has not been developed. As such, generic depression assessment tools such as the Hospital Anxiety and Depression Scale, the Beck

Depression Inventory (BDI), the Center for Epidemiologic Studies-Depression Scale (CES-D), and the Cognitive Depression Index have been used in sarcoidosis.[48] Assessment of depression in sarcoidosis is complex and closely linked to fatigue and dyspnea, often with all three occurring simultaneously.[11]

SARCOIDOSIS-SPECIFIC HRQOL ASSESSMENT TOOLS

Generic measures of HRQOL may not be sufficiently sensitive to detect the impact of a condition on HRQOL.[49] Sarcoidosis-specific HRQOL assessment tools have been developed to address this limitation.

Sarcoidosis Health Questionnaire

The Sarcoidosis Health Questionnaire (SHQ) was developed and validated in a two-part study in the United States in 2003. The clinicians aimed to produce a self-completed questionnaire to measure HRQOL in patients with varying disease burden and organ involvement.[8] Twenty-nine of 151 questionnaire items were selected for the final version by the order of importance rated by patients. These items were initially generated after detailed discussions with patients, support groups, and sarcoidosis experts and a review of the literature. They focused on three domains: Daily Functioning, Physical Functioning, and Emotional Functioning. The questionnaire was validated (criterion, convergent, and divergent validity) in part two of the development study with a different group of patients. Reliability was demonstrated with Cronbach's coefficient values of 0.84–0.92 (acceptable values for a PRO range from >0.75) for the health domains. The SHQ has been translated and validated in Serbia, Japan, and the Netherlands.[50] It was translated into Hindi and used in a study by Aggarwal et al. in India.[51]

The SHQ has since been used as an HRQOL outcome measure in several sarcoidosis studies. In 2015 Judson et al. studied the effects of corticosteroid therapy. Patients taking higher doses of corticosteroids (>500 mg total in previous year) demonstrated worse HRQOL in the daily functioning domain.[52] Aggarwal et al. used the SHQ again in 2016 to study the effects of corticosteroids on HRQOL in [50] patients. Their results showed that all domains of SHQ significantly improved after 6 months of treatment with prednisolone using standardized dosing.[50] Two sarcoidosis studies have looked at the effects of gender on HRQOL. Female patients were found to have a statistically significant lower HRQOL score and a greater degree of functional impairment than men.[24,53] Bourbonnais et al. aimed to identify clinical markers predictive of a poorer HRQOL in sarcoidosis. They assessed a composite model of the distance saturation product and the Borg Dyspnoea Scale score at the end of a 6MWT. This model predicted SHQ scores.[23]

There are limitations to the SHQ. The questionnaire's responsiveness to change in HRQOL over time has not been fully tested. There is no established clinically important difference score. Perhaps the most important limitation is the SHQ is a "one size fits all" questionnaire. It cannot be specifically tailored to the organ involved and does not focus on treatment side effects. It may be insensitive to changes in specific organs such as skin or eyes.

The Kings Sarcoidosis Questionnaire

The KSQ was developed in 2012 in a cohort of patients attending secondary and tertiary sarcoidosis clinics.[7] Its development consisted of item generation, item reduction, and Rasch analysis (Item Response Theory) to create unidimensional scales. The KSQ consists of modules: General health status, Lung, Skin, Eye and Medications. This allows the flexibility to generate "total" scores for a combination of modules, such as general health status and lung for patients with predominantly pulmonary involvement. Hence the KSQ allows for individualized HRQOL scoring that depends on specific patient organ involvement. The questionnaire also includes a fatigue item and is the only sarcoidosis questionnaire to score eye disease as a module. The KSQ has been validated. Internal consistency, assessed using Cronbach's coefficient, was high (0.93 for general health status). Interclass correlation coefficients suggested good repeatability in a subgroup of 39 patients in the study (>0.9). The KSQ also has the expected construct validity, with a good correlation with the SGRQ and moderate correlation with lung function.[7]

The KSQ has been translated into 15 languages using validated methods; this should facilitate international and cross-cultural studies.[54] The KSQ has been used in a study of 67 sarcoidosis patients in Serbia with the study team obtaining similar validity characteristics to the original English KSQ, suggesting that the KSQ can be adapted across cultures.[55] The KSQ was also used in a Dutch study, which determined construct validity, internal consistency, and repeatability comparable to KSQ validity characteristics in the original version.[56] The minimal important difference (MID) for modules General health status, Lung, Medication, and the combined KSQ Lung and general health status modules has been reported.[57]

The KSQ has been used in a number of studies since its development which demonstrates it is responsive and effective in clinical trials. The KSQ was a secondary outcome measure in a study of repository corticotropin (RCI) by Baughman et al. for chronic pulmonary sarcoidosis (Acthar Gel in Chronic Pulmonary Sarcoidosis).[58] This was a double-blind prospective study, comparing two doses of RCI in patients already taking corticosteroids. At 6 months there was a decrease in the dose of corticosteroids and a statistically significant improvement in KSQ HRQOL scores. As expected, there was a poor correlation of HRQOL with pulmonary function tests. It can therefore be concluded that HRQOL and lung function measure different domains of sarcoidosis, and to understand the impact of this condition, HRQOL has to be assessed with the appropriate tool.[59] The KSQ was also used as a measure in a randomized, placebo-controlled trial Roflumilast to prevent Exacerbations in Fibrotic Sarcoidosis (REFS).[60] This study enrolled patients with a history of two or more acute worsening events in the previous year. They were reviewed every 3 months for 1 year. There was a statistically significant improvement in the KSQ Lung domain for the treatment group.[60] The Registry for Advanced Sarcoidosis-associated Pulmonary Hypertension (Re-SAPH) is an international registry, which has enrolled 180 patients with a median follow-up of 300 days. The aim of the registry is to better categorize the phenotypes of advanced sarcoidosis.[61] The KSQ is being used in HRQOL analysis in this patient group. The KSQ is also currently being used as an outcome measure in a number of clinical trials.[62]

The Sarcoidosis Assessment Tool

The SAT was developed by the same authors as the SHQ, principally to address the inability to tailor the SHQ for patients with multiorgan disease. The SAT was developed in patients participating in a double-blind, placebo-controlled clinical trial evaluating the safety and efficacy of treatment with ustekinumab and golimumab in patients with chronic sarcoidosis.[63] The SAT selected items from the PROMIS item bank as well as introduced new sarcoidosis-specific items. The SAT, similar to the KSQ, was also developed using item response theory, which is based on the relationship between an individuals' performances on a test item and the test takers' levels of performance on an overall measure of the ability that item was designed to measure. The SAT components include physical functioning, satisfaction with roles and activities, fatigue, pain, sleep disturbance, lung concerns, skin concerns, and skin stigma. The questionnaire is valid; it has good internal consistency, construct validity, and reliability. It can be used to assess fatigue, and the MID has been established.[33] A key difference in SAT compared with KSQ is that there are no overall/total or combination scores from the SAT, so each module is analyzed individually.

The SAT has been evaluated in a study of corticosteroid therapy in sarcoidosis.[39] Patients taking higher doses of corticosteroids (>500 mg total in previous year) demonstrated worse HRQOL. The SAT is a further advancement in HRQOL assessment in sarcoidosis.

CONCLUSIONS AND FUTURE WORK

Sarcoidosis has a significant impact on the HRQOL of patients. The assessment of HRQOL is important as it reflects the patients' perception of their illness. The HRQOL is a global measure of the patient's health, encompassing the wide range of disease phenotypes that are typical of sarcoidosis. They also capture the impact of side effects of therapy. The assessment of HRQOL is increasingly requested by regulators such as the FDA and European Medicines Agency to license new treatments and is required by organizations such as National Institute for Clinical Excellence in the UK to guide decisions regarding their reimbursement. The HRQOL is not captured by standard assessments such as chest radiograph, lung function, and symptom scales. Therefore standardized and validated methods are required to capture it. The KSQ and SAT are two disease-specific HRQOL tools. They have been developed using Rasch Analysis, a psychometric method used to create linear and unidimensional scales. They are both well validated and have good construct validity, internal consistency, and repeatability. Clinical trials using the KSQ demonstrate that HRQOL measures are responsive and useful in assessing the efficacy of therapy. Measuring the HRQOL in the clinic may facilitate patients and their clinician to make more informed decisions about treatments by offering a unique insight into sarcoidosis not captured by other assessments.

REFERENCES

1. Gawande A. *Interview for "Being Mortal: Medicine and what Matters in the End"*. Surgeon, Harvard Medical School Professor; September 2017.
2. Victorson DE, Cella D, Grund H, Judson MA. A conceptual model of health-related quality of life in sarcoidosis. *Qual Life Res*. 2014;23(1):89–101.
3. Wirnsberger RM, De Vries J, Breteler MHM, Van Heck GL, Wouters EFM, Drent M. Evaluation of quality of life in sarcoidosis patients. *Respir Med*. 1998;92(5):750–756.

4. World Health Organization. The constitution of the World Health Organization. *WHO Chron*. 1947;1:29.
5. Swigris JJ, Kuschner WG, Jacobs SS, Wilson SR, Gould MK. Health-related quality of life in patients with idiopathic pulmonary fibrosis: a systematic review. *Thorax*. 2005;60(7):588–594.
6. Spitzer WO. State of science 1986: quality of life and functional status as target variables for research. *J Chronic Dis*. 1987;40(6):465–471.
7. Patel AS, Siegert RJ, Creamer D, et al. The development and validation of the King's Sarcoidosis Questionnaire for the assessment of health status. *Thorax*. 2012. pp.thoraxjnl-2012.
8. Cox CE, Donohue JF, Brown CD, Kataria YP, Judson MA. The Sarcoidosis Health Questionnaire: a new measure of health-related quality of life. *Am J Respir Crit Care Med*. 2003;168(3):323–329.
9. Cox CE, Donohue JF, Brown CD, Kataria YP, Judson MA. Health-related quality of life of persons with sarcoidosis. *Chest*. 2004;125:997–1004.
10. Wilson IB, Cleary PD. Linking clinical variables with health-related quality of life: a conceptual model of patient outcomes. *JAMA*. 1995;273(1):59–65.
11. Judson. Quality of life in sarcoidosis. *Semin Respir Crit Care Med*. 2017;38(4):546–558.
12. US Department of Health and Human Services FDA Center for Drug Evaluation and Research, US Department of Health and Human Services FDA Center for Biologics Evaluation and Research and US Department of Health and Human Services FDA Center for Devices and Radiological Health. Guidance for industry: patient-reported outcome measures: use in medical product development to support labeling claims: draft guidance. *Health Qual Life Outcome*. 2006;4:1–20.
13. Victorson DE, Choi S, Judson MA, Cella D. Development and testing of item response theory-based item banks and short forms for eye, skin and lung problems in sarcoidosis. *Qual Life Res*. 2014;23(4):1301–1313.
14. Younossi ZM, Guyatt G, Kiwi M, Boparai N, King D. Development of a disease specific questionnaire to measure health related quality of life in patients with chronic liver disease. *Gut*. 1999;45(2):295–300.
15. Gibbons CJ, Skevington SM, WHOQOL Group. Adjusting for cross-cultural differences in computer-adaptive tests of quality of life. *Qual Life Res*. 2017:1–13.
16. Food and Drug Administration, Center for Drug Evaluation and Research. *Guidance for industry: qualification process for Drug development tools silver*. Spring, MD: US Department of Health and Human Services; 2010.
17. Guyatt GH, Feeny DH, Patrick DL. Measuring health-related quality of life. *Ann Intern Med*. 1993;118(8): 622–629.
18. Terwee CB, Bot SD, de Boer MR, et al. Quality criteria were proposed for measurement properties of health status questionnaires. *J Clin Epidemiol*. 2007;60:34–42.
19. Fayers PM, Machin D. *Quality of Life: Assessment, Analysis and Interpretation*. 1 ed. Wiley; 2000.
20. Cook CE. Clinimetrics corner: the minimal clinically important change score (MCID): a necessary pretense. *J Man Manip Ther*. 2008;16(4):82E–83E.
21. Ware Jr JE, Sherbourne CD. The MOS 36-item short-form health survey (SF-36): I. Conceptual framework and item selection. *Medical Care*. 1992:473–483.
22. Douglas AC, Macleod JG, Matthews JD. Symptomatic sarcoidosis of skeletal muscle. *J Neurol Neurosurg Psychiatr*. 1973;36(6):1034–1040.
23. Brancaleone P, Perez T, Robin S, Neviere R, Wallaert B. Clinical impact of inspiratory muscle impairment in sarcoidosis. *Sarcoidosis Vasc Diffuse Lung Dis*. 2004;21(3):219–227.
24. Bourbonnais JM, Malaisamy S, Dalal BD, Samarakoon PC, Parikh SR, Samavati L. Distance saturation product predicts health-related quality of life among sarcoidosis patients. *Health Qual Life Outcome*. 2012;10(1):67.
25. Bourbonnais JM, Samavati L. Effect of gender on health related quality of life in sarcoidosis. *Sarcoidosis Vasc Diffuse Lung Dis*. 2010;27(2):96–102.
26. Judson MA, Silvestri J, Hartung C, Byars T, Cox CE. The effect of thalidomide on corticosteroid-dependent pulmonary sarcoidosis. *Sarcoidosis Vasc Diffuse Lung Dis*. 2006;23(1):51–57.
27. Power M, Bullinger M, Harper A. The World Health Organization WHOQOL-100: tests of the universality of quality of life in 15 different cultural groups worldwide. *Health Psychol*. 1999;18(5):495.
28. Hoitsma E, et al. Impact of pain in a Dutch sarcoidosis patient population. *Sarcoidosis Vasc Diffuse Lung Dis*. 2003;20(1):33–39.
29. Wirnsberger RM, et al. Impairment of quality of life: rheumatoid arthritis versus sarcoidosis. *Neth J Med*. 1999;54(3):86–95.
30. Drake WP, Richmond BW, Oswald-Richter K, et al. Effects of broad-spectrum antimycobacterial therapy on chronic pulmonary sarcoidosis. *Sarcoidosis Vasc Diffuse Lung Dis*. 2013;30(3):201.
31. Jones PW, Quirk FH, Baveystock CM. The St George's respiratory questionnaire. *Respir Med*. 1991;85:25–31.
32. Wilson CB, Jones PW, O'leary CJ, Cole PJ, Wilson R. Validation of the St. George's respiratory questionnaire in bronchiectasis. *Am J Respir Crit Care Med*. 1997;156(2):536–541.
33. Baughman RP, Sparkman BK, Lower EE. Six-minute walk test and health status assessment in sarcoidosis. *Chest*. 2007;132(1):207–213.
34. Boer S, Kolbe J, Wilsher ML. The relationships among dyspnoea, health-related quality of life and psychological factors in sarcoidosis. *Respirology*. 2014;19(7):1019–1024.
35. Gvozdenovic BS, Mihailovic-Vucinic V, Vukovic M, et al. Effect of obesity on patient-reported outcomes in sarcoidosis. *Int J Tubercul Lung Dis*. 2013;17(4):559–564.
36. Chang JA, Curtis JR, Patrick DL, Raghu G. Assessment of health-related quality of life in patients with interstitial lung disease. *Chest*. 1999;116(5):1175–1182.
37. Antoniou KM, Tzanakis N, Tzouvelekis A, et al. Quality of life in patients with active sarcoidosis in Greece. *Eur J Intern Med*. 2006;17(6):421–426.

38. Gvozdenovic BS, Mihailovic-Vucinic V, Ilic-Dudvarski A, Zugic V, Judson MA. Differences in symptom severity and health status impairment between patients with pulmonary and pulmonary plus extrapulmonary sarcoidosis. *Respir Med*. 2008;102(11):1636–1642.
39. Drent M, Lower EE, De Vries J. Sarcoidosis-associated fatigue. *Eur Respir J*. 2012;40.
40. Vries J, Michielsen H, Heck GL, Drent M. Measuring fatigue in sarcoidosis: the fatigue assessment scale (FAS). *Br J Health Psychol*. 2004;9(3):279–291.
41. de Kleijn WP, De Vries J, Lower EE, Elfferich MD, Baughman RP, Drent M. Fatigue in sarcoidosis: a systematic review. *Curr Opin Pulm Med*. 2009;15(5):499–506.
42. Cella D, et al. The Patient-Reported Outcomes Measurement Information System (PROMIS) developed and tested its first wave of adult self-reported health outcome item banks: 2005–2008. *J Clin Epidemiol*. 2010;63(11):1179–1194.
43. Kalkanis A, Yucel RM, Judson MA. The internal consistency of PRO fatigue instruments in sarcoidosis: superiority of the PFI over the FAS. *Sarcoidosis Vasc Diffuse Lung Dis*. 2013;30(1):60–64.
44. Baughman RP, et al. Clinical characteristics of patients in a case control study of sarcoidosis. *Am J Respir Crit Care Med*. 2001;164(10):1885–1889.
45. Yeager H, et al. Pulmonary and psychosocial findings at enrollment in the ACCESS study. *Sarcoidosis Vasc Diffuse Lung Dis*. 2005;22(2):147–153.
46. Birring SS, et al. Development of a symptom specific health status measure for patients with chronic cough: Leicester Cough Questionnaire (LCQ). *Thorax*. 2003;58(4):339–343.
47. Sinha A, Lee KK, Rafferty GF, et al. Predictors of objective cough frequency in pulmonary sarcoidosis. *Eur Respir J*. 2016;47(5):1461–1471.
48. Drent M, Wirnsberger RM, Breteler MH, Kock LM, de Vries J, Wouters EF. Quality of life and depressive symptoms in patients suffering from sarcoidosis. *Sarcoidosis Vasc Diffuse Lung Dis*. 1998;15(1):59–66.
49. Jones PW. Quality of life measurement for patients with diseases of the airways. *Thorax*. 1991;46(9):676.
50. Tanizawa K, et al. Validation of the Japanese version of the sarcoidosis health questionnaire: a cross-sectional study. *Health Qual Life Outcome*. 2011;9(1):34.
51. Aggarwal, Nath A, Kant Sahu K, Gupta D. "Fatigue and health-related quality of life in patients with pulmonary sarcoidosis treated by oral Corticosteroids. *Sarcoidosis Vasc Diffuse Lung Dis*. 2016;33(2):124–129.
52. Judson MA, et al. The effect of corticosteroids on quality of life in a sarcoidosis clinic: the results of a propensity analysis. *Respir Med*. 2015;109(4):526–531.
53. Milić M, Goranović T, Holjevac JK. Health related quality of life regarding to gender in sarcoidosis. *Coll Antropol*. 2009;33(3):837–840.
54. Fletcher H, et al. Standardised translation of the King's sarcoidosis questionnaire (ksq) into eleven languages. *Am J Respir Crit Care Med*. 2017;195:A4759.
55. Gvozdenovic BS, Patel AS, Birring SS, Vucinic V, Vukovic M. *Impact of Gender on Disease Activity, Pulmonary Function and Health Status in Sarcoidosis Patients-King's Sarcoidosis Questionnaire (KSQ)*; 2013.
56. Van Manen MJ, Wapenaar M, Strookappe B, et al. Validation of the King's sarcoidosis questionnaire (KSQ) in a Dutch sarcoidosis population. *Sarcoidosis Vasc Diffuse Lung Dis*. 2016;33(1):75–82.
57. Patel AS, et al. *Assessing Sarcoidosis: The Kings Sarcoidosis Questionnaire and the Minimal Important Difference*; 2012:P699.
58. https://clinicaltrials.gov/ct2/show/NCT02188017?term=baughman&cond=sarcoid&draw=2&rank=1.
59. Baughman RP, et al. Repository corticotropin for chronic pulmonary sarcoidosis. *Lung*. 2017;195(3):313–322.
60. Birring S, Judson MA, Culver DA, et al. A double blind, placebo controlled study of roflumilast to prevent acute events in fibrotic sarcoidosis. *Am J Respir Crit Care Med*. 2017;195:A4752.
61. Sauer WH, et al. High-risk sarcoidosis. Current concepts and research imperatives. *Annal Am Thoracic Soc*. 2017;14(suppl 6):S437–S444.
62. https://clinicaltrials.gov/ct2/results?cond=&term=KINGS+SARCOIDOSIS+QUESTIONNAIRE&cntry=&state=&city=&dist=.
63. Judson MA, et al. Validation and important differences for the sarcoidosis assessment tool. A new patient-reported outcome measure. *Am J Res Critical Care Med*. 2015;191(7):786–795.

CHAPTER 19

Biomarkers in Sarcoidosis

MILOU C. SCHIMMELPENNINK, MD • ADRIANE D.M. VORSELAARS, MD, PHD • JAN C. GRUTTERS, MD

SERUM AND BAL BIOMARKERS IN PULMONARY AND EXTRAPULMONARY SARCOIDOSIS

The definition of a biomarker according to the National Institutes of Health Biomarkers Definitions Working Group is "A characteristic that can be objectively measured and evaluated as an indicator of normal biological processes, pathogenic processes, or pharmacologic responses to a therapeutic intervention".[1] In sarcoidosis care, biomarkers can be useful in many ways: to diagnose sarcoidosis, to predict prognosis and determine severity, to evaluate the response to therapy, or to predict relapse. The ideal biomarker is highly sensitive and is not related to other diseases. Furthermore, it should be reproducible, not very invasive to the patient, and ideally it should be low priced. Unfortunately, none of the currently used biomarkers in sarcoidosis care fulfill all these criteria.[2]

The best way to determine the diagnostic value of a biomarker is by determining the area under the receiver operating characteristic (ROC) curve (AUC). An AUC of 0.9–1.0 is considered excellent, 0.80–0.90 is good, 0.70–0.80 is fair, 0.60–0.70 is poor, and 0.50–0.60 is bad.

The following biomarkers for sarcoidosis most commonly used around the world ('conventional biomarkers') will be discussed: serum angiotensin-converting enzyme (sACE), serum soluble interleukin-2 receptor (sIL-2R), serum and urinary calcium, serum lysozyme, bronchoalveolar lavage (BAL) lymphocytosis, and BAL lymphocyte subset parameters (Table 19.1).

In addition, we will highlight some recent developments and potential biomarkers for future use.

CONVENTIONAL BIOMARKERS

Serum Angiotensin-1–Converting Enzyme

sACE converts blood angiotensin I into angiotensin II during circulation through the lungs.[3] In sarcoidosis, increased ACE levels is the result of additional production by activated macrophages and epithelioid cells in the granulomas.[4–6] As such, serum levels of ACE in sarcoidosis are thought to reflect the total-body burden of granulomas.[7]

Clinical sensitivity of an elevated sACE level for pulmonary sarcoidosis roughly varies between 41% and 83%,[8–10] with the following AUCs: 0.656 (poor), 0.643 (poor), and 0.790 (fair) (Table 19.1). Importantly the sensitivity of sACE depends on the clinical manifestations of sarcoidosis. In patients with sarcoid uveitis, the sensitivity of sACE lies between 22% and 54%,[11,12] with the following AUCs: 0.650 (poor) and 0.608 (poor). In patients diagnosed with neurosarcoidosis, the sensitivity of sACE lies around 44%;[13] however, AUC could not be estimated because of the lack of a control group.

Of particular importance is that the sensitivity of sACE has been shown to be affected by a common polymorphism in the ACE gene. This genetic polymorphism is characterized by the insertion (I) or deletion (D) of the 287 base-pair fragment in intron 16. Patients with an II genotype have lower levels of sACE than patients with DD genotypes, and patients with ID genotype have intermediate sACE levels.[14] Using I/D-corrected reference intervals, 8.5% of the measurements lead to a different interpretation.[15] Genotype-corrected levels of sACE show improved sensitivity of 69%–83% for diagnosing sarcoidosis.[16,17]

Furthermore, sACE has a limited specificity (Table 19.1). Increased levels of sACE can also be found in other granulomatous disease, such as tuberculosis, histoplasmosis, and leprosy.[18–20]

It is uncertain if sACE reflects the severity of sarcoidosis. Some studies found higher sACE levels and a higher sensitivity of sACE in more advanced radiographic stages of sarcoidosis.[5,21,22] However, other studies did not confirm this correlation.[23–26]

No prognostic value of sACE measurement in sarcoidosis has so far been demonstrated. sACE cannot predict the need for therapy[23] and progression of disease,[27] nor predict relapse after therapy.[28]

However, serial measurements of sACE might provide valuable information on the course of disease in individual patients, (Table 19.5). First, it has been shown that change in serial measurement corresponds to the course of disease as well as to clinical response to systemic therapy.[5,21,29–33] Second, during treatment, the magnitude of change in sACE was found to correlate significantly to the

Sarcoidosis. https://doi.org/10.1016/B978-0-323-54429-0.00019-7

TABLE 19.1
Serum ACE: Sensitivity, Specificity, Severity Biomarker, and Prognosis

Study	Inclusion	Subtype	Control Group	Cutoff Value	Sensitivity	Specificity	Severity	Prognosis	AUC
De Smet 2010[8]	(n = 36) Biopsy proven, except for 1 patient with LS, no corticosteroids during diagnostic workup	Pulmonary	(n = 117) Patients who were evaluated for sarcoidosis, but sarcoidosis was ruled out	34 U/L	83.3%	66.7%			0.79
Popevic 2016[9]	(n = 430) Biopsy-proven sarcoidosis patients. Patients with active sarcoidosis[a]		(n = 264) Healthy controls matched for age and gender.	32 U/L	66%	54%	No differences in sACE levels between different Scadding stages. No correlation between COS[b] categories and sACE		0.643
Sharma 1997[16]	(n = 47) White patients, histologically proven sarcoidosis. No use of steroids, diuretics, or ACE inhibitors at the time of evaluation		(n = 146) Healthy white volunteers	Not genotype corrected: 15–70/L Genotype corrected: II: 4.6–30.6 U/L ID: 10.0–47.6U/L DD 17.9–64.3U/L	51.7% 69%				
Tomita 1997[17]	(n = 207) Biopsy proven, no corticosteroids during evaluation			Not genotype corrected: 8.3–21.4IU/L Genotype-corrected: II: 9–12.5 IU/L DI:10.5–17.1IU/L DD: 11.9–22.5IU/L	60.8% 83%		Increase in sACE was seen in more advanced radiographic stages		
Groen-Hakan 2017[11]	(n = 37) Definitive or presumed ocular sarcoidosis based on the International Workshop on Ocular Sarcoidosis criteria (biopsy or radiologic finding). 36% used immunosuppressive medication and 16% used ACE inhibitor of the whole (sarcoidosis + control) group.	Sarcoid uveitis	(n = 212) Patients with other or unknown causes of uveitis, including patients with probable or possible uveitis	51 U/L	54%	70%			0.65

Gundlach 2016[12]	(n = 42) Patients with intraocular sarcoidosis; definite n = 10, presumed n = 12, probable n = 19, and possible n = 1. ACE inhibitors were taken by 2 patients in the sarcoid group and 1 patient in the control group.	Sarcoid uveitis	(n = 12) Uveitis without sarcoidosis.	82 U/mL	22%	99.5%		[c]0.608
Ungprasert 2016[10]	(n = 251) Histological evidence was required, except for stage I pulmonary sarcoidosis in the absence of other causes. Isolated granulomatous disease of an organ except for skin was also included in the absence of a better alternative. Data concerning use of ACE inhibitors are unknown.		(n = 3277) Residents of Olmsted County who had ACE levels tested but did not have a diagnosis of sarcoidosis.	ACE levels were recorded as high/low/normal according to the reference range for the time the tests were performed.	41.4%	89.9%		[c]0.656
Leonhard 2016[13]	(n = 52) 1 patient with definite, 37 probable, and 14 possible neurosarcoidosis (Zajicek criteria)	Neurosarcoidosis		>70 U/L	44%		Elevated ACE levels were more frequent in patients with neurosarcoidosis and pulmonary sarcoidosis (65%) than patients with only neurosarcoidosis (1%).	

ACE, angiotensin-converting enzyme; *D*, deletion; *I*, insertion; *sACE*, serum angiotensin-converting enzyme.

[a]Active sarcoidosis, defined as the presence of clinical symptoms, with/without pathological X-ray, or asymptomatic patients with absolute and marked roentgenographic worsening, or patients with major manifestations such as recently developed skin lesions, parotid/ocular involvement, peripheral lymphadenopathy, or deterioration of pulmonary function tests.

[b]Clinical outcome status (COS)

[c]Area under the ROC curve was not evaluated in this study; the AUC was estimated by the following formula: $(0.5 \times [\text{sensitivity} \times (1 - \text{specificity})]) + (0.5 \times [\text{specificity} \times (1 - \text{sensitivity})]) + (\text{sensitivity} \times \text{specificity})$.

change in pulmonary function parameters.[30,34] For this reason, serial measurement of sACE still appears useful in the follow-up of disease and assessment of therapeutic response in individual patients. Of note, sACE levels can be influenced by corticosteroids independently, which should be taken into account when evaluating treatment response during corticosteroid therapy.[33]

Also in patients using ACE inhibitors, measurement of sACE levels is not useful.[35]

In summary, diagnostic value of sACE in sarcoidosis is limited (sensitivity/specificity: poor-fair) but has not been properly reevaluated in the context of the D/I gene polymorphism. Furthermore, serial measurement of sACE can be useful in the follow-up of disease, especially in the evaluation of nonsteroid systemic therapy. There is currently no evidence that sACE can serve as a prognostic biomarker and/or marker for staging of severity in sarcoidosis.

Serum Soluble Interleukin-2 Receptor

The sIL-2R is released by activated T lymphocytes and correlates well with CD4+ T lymphocytes in BAL and serum[36] and is therefore regarded as a parameter for activation of T lymphocytes.[37] Although it is mainly produced by T lymphocytes, also small amounts of sIL-2R are produced by B-lymphocytes.[38] Serum sIL-2R binds to interleukin-2 and plays an important role in the immune response.

Sensitivity of serum sIL-2R as a diagnostic biomarker for sarcoidosis lies around 79% (Table 19.2). However, no studies have been performed to the diagnostic accuracy of serum sIL-2R in patients with (pulmonary) sarcoidosis compared with a control group. Therefore no ROC curve analysis could so far be performed. In patients with uveitis the sensitivity of elevated sIL-2R levels to establish underlying sarcoidosis is around 81%–98%,[11,12] with an AUC of 0.76 (fair) and 0.96 (excellent).

Interestingly, patients with extrapulmonary involvement have been shown to have relatively high levels of serum sIL-2R, suggesting a value as staging and/or severity biomarker.[36,39]

Also, increase of serum sIL-2R values appears not to be specific for sarcoidosis as elevated values can also be found in other conditions, including hematologic malignancies, other granulomatous diseases, various autoimmune disorders, and posttransplantation.[40–44]

An important pitfall in using sIL-2R as a biomarker in sarcoidosis is that renal insufficiency may have major impact on levels leading to misinterpretation of test results.[45,46]

Interestingly, serum sIL-2R levels might be useful as a marker of severity of sarcoidosis. Patients with more advanced radiographic stages and progressive disease show higher levels of sIL-2R levels[47–49] (Table 19.2). Rothkrantz-Kos et al.[50] evaluated the diagnostic accuracy of inflammatory markers to predict respiratory severity, defined by diffusion capacity for carbon monoxide (DLCO) <80, force vital capacity (FVC) <80%, or forced expiratory volume 1 (FEV1) <80% of predicted. Serum sIL-2R test had the highest ability to determine pulmonary severity in comparison to ACE.

Serum sIL-2R measurement has also shown usefulness as a prognostic marker. High serum sIL-2R levels can predict the need for therapy in sarcoidosis patients.[50,51] Furthermore, high sIL-2R at initiation of therapy has shown value as a predictor of relapse after therapy with infliximab.[28]

Serial measurement of serum sIL-2R in the follow-up can be useful to assess the evolution of disease activity in sarcoidosis, (Table 19.5). Changes in concentration of serum sIL-2R have been shown to be related to clinical changes and correlate well with changes in pulmonary function parameters and radiological abnormalities[30,36,52,53] (Table 19.6).

In summary, the value of serum sIL-2R as a diagnostic biomarker for sarcoidosis is not yet fully established. However, the diagnostic value of sIL-2R is fair to excellent in patients presenting with uveitis. Serum sIL-2R measurement might also have prognostic value, especially in the context of infliximab therapy. In contrast to sACE, interpretation of serum sIL-2R levels is not confounded by the use of drugs or immunosuppressants. Finally, serial measurements can be useful in the follow-up of patients and to evaluate treatment effect.

Serum Calcium and Urinary Calcium

Sarcoidosis is associated with an altered calcium metabolism. In sarcoidosis, activated macrophages produce 1α-hydroxylase.[54,55] The enzyme 1α-hydroxylase facilitates the hydroxylation of 25-hydroxyvitamin D (inactive form of vitamin D) to 1,25-dihydroxyvitamin D (calcitriol, the biologically active form of vitamin D). Calcitriol is a sterol hormone that stimulates the intestinal absorption of calcium and bone resorption, which can lead to hypercalcemia and hypercalciuria.[56]Thus sarcoidosis patients with hypercalcemia and/or hypercalciuria are classically characterized by increased levels of 1,25-hydroxyvitamin D and decreased levels of 25-hydroxyvitamin.

Measurement of serum calcium and urinary calcium belongs to the standard diagnostic workup of sarcoidosis. Hypercalcemia affects only 3.6%–16% of the patients with extrapulmonary and/or pulmonary sarcoidosis[57–61] (Table 19.3); however, when measuring ionized serum calcium, the biologically active form

TABLE 19.2
Serum sIL-2R: Sensitivity, Specificity, Severity Biomarker, and Prognosis

Study	Inclusion	Subtype	Control Group	Cutoff Value	Sensitivity	Specificity	Severity	Prognosis	AUC
Grutters 2003[36]	(n = 57) Diagnosis was confirmed by histologic evidence. All patients had active disease. No treatment during evaluation.[a]	Only pulmonary sarcoidosis (n = 25); Pulmonary and extrapulmonary disease (n = 21); 1 patient with solely extrapulmonary disease		Normal range given by manufacturer 223–710 U/mL	79%		Patients with pulmonary and extrapulmonary sarcoidosis (excluding erythema nodosum) had higher sIL-2R levels than patients with only pulmonary disease. sIL-2R was not associated with change in lung function during follow-up. Lowest sIL-2R was in Scadding stage III and highest in stage I.	Initial sIL-2R could not predict chronic disease on chest radiograph at 2 years.	
Groen-Hakan 2017[11]	(n = 37) Definitive or presumed ocular sarcoidosis based on the International Workshop on Ocular Sarcoidosis criteria (biopsy or radiologic finding). 36% used immunosuppressive medication of the whole (sarcoidosis + control) group	Sarcoid uveitis	(n = 212) Patients with other causes of uveitis and patients with unknown cause of uveitis, including patients with probable or possible uveitis	4000 pg/mL	81%	64%			0.76
Gundlach 2016[12]	(n = 42) Patients with intraocular sarcoidosis; definite n = 10, presumed n = 12, probable n = 19, possible n = 1.	Sarcoid uveitis	(n = 12) Uveitis without sarcoidosis.	639 U/mL	98%	94%			[c]0.96
Rothkrantz-Kos 2003[50]	(n = 73) Diagnosis was histologically confirmed. Evaluation of markers was in untreated patients. No comorbidities.[b]						sIL-2R had the highest ability to determine pulmonary severity defined by DLCO <80%, FVC <80%, FEV1 <80% of predicted	73% of the untreated nonchronic patients with high values of sIL-2R required eventually treatment, vs. 23% with low sIL-2R	

DLCO, diffusion capacity for carbon monoxide; *FEV1*, forced expiratory volume 1; *FVC*, forced vital capacity; *sIL-2R*, soluble interleukin-2 receptor.
[a]Active disease was defined as: (1) recently developed or increasing cough or dyspnea; and/or (2) presence of compatible systemic symptoms such as cutaneous lesions, eye manifestations, fever, and athralgia; and/or (3) recently developed abnormalities on chest radiograph; and/or (4) T-lymphocytosis in BAL and/or (5) elevated level of serum angiotensin-converting enzyme (sACE).
[b]Sensitivity and specificity to evaluate the diagnostic accuracy of inflammatory markers to predict respiratory severity (RFI) in sarcoidosis.
[c]Area under the ROC curve was not performed in this study, the AUC was estimated by the following formula: $(0.5 \times [\text{sensitivity} \times (1-\text{specificity})]) + (0.5 \times [\text{specificity} \times (1-\text{sensitivity})]) + (\text{sensitivity} \times \text{specificity})$.

TABLE 19.3
Serum Calcium and Urinary Calcium: Sensitivity, Specificity, Severity Biomarker, and Prognosis

Study	Inclusion	Subtype	Cutoff Value	Prevalence Hypercalcemia	Prevalence Hypercalciuria	Renal Insufficiency/ Nephrocalcinosis	Severity	Prognosis
Baughman 2013[57]	Diagnosis was made according to criteria of American Thoracic Society/European Respiratory Society/World Association for Sarcoidosis and Other Granulomatous Disorders (ATS/ERS/WASOG). 1606 patients were seen during 13576 visits.		10.2 mg/dL	6.6% had hypercalcemia, of whom 0.6% patients with hyperparathyroidism and 6% diagnosis with SAHC (sarcoidosis associated hypercalcemia)		42% of the pt with hypercalcemia had renal insufficiency		
Kamphuis 2014[58]	Diagnosis was made according to criteria of ATS/ERS/WASOG. Serum calcium was measured in 293 patients, and urinary calcium was measured in 89 patients. Serum calcium level was corrected for albumin.		Ca >2.65 mmol/L and uCa > 5 mmol/L	8%	27%		No correlation between serum levels of calcium and sarcoidosis stadium on chest X-ray.	
Hamada 1998[62]	(n = 36) In 30 patients, sarcoidosis was histologically proven, and in 6 patients, sarcoidosis was clinically diagnosed. 8 patients received corticosteroids 1 > yr before the study. Patients with hyper/hypoparathyroidism or bone disease were excluded. All patients had normal renal function, except for 2 with histories of nephrolithiasis and slightly reduced creatinine. Calcium was corrected for albumin.		sCa2+: >1.26 mmol/L Serum calcium (adjusted for albumin) > 2.54 mmol/L Hypercalciurea: >0.3 g/day in males and 0.25 mg/day in females.	27.8% 5.6%	 33.3%	A history of nephrolithiasis was in 8.3% of the patients	sCa2+ >1.23 mmol/L suggested extrathoracic involvement with a sensitivity of 50% and a specificity of 100%.	

Darlington 2014[59]	Non-LS (non-Löfgren's syndrome) n = 617. LS (Löfgren's syndrome) n = 383. Diagnosis was made according to criteria of WASOG. Incidence of hypercalcemia and/or renal failure was estimated together.	LS versus non-LS	Hypercalcemia and/or kidney involvement was diagnosed when repeated blood samples with p-calcium >2.60 mmol/L and/or p-creatinine >90umol/L for women and>100umol/L for men.	Non-LS: 3.6% LS: 0%				
Morimoto 2008[60]	Japanese cohort. All patients had histopathological evidence. Calcium was measured in 842 patients and hypercalciuria in 298 patients.		Unknown	7.4%	6.4%			
Rodrigues 2011[72]	(n = 137) Diagnosis was based on histological evidence. Abnormal calcium metabolism evaluated.		Unknown	Incidence of abnormal calcium metabolism 20.4%				Relapse was associated with an abnormal calcium metabolism
Doubkova 2015[61]	Sarcoidosis diagnosis was based on ATS/ERS/WASOG criteria. sCa was measured in 301 patients, and urinary calcium was measured in 253 patients.		Normal range serum Calcium 2.15–2.55 mmol/L Normal range urinary calcium 2.4–7.5 mmol/L	16%	33%			Percentage of patients with spontaneous remission was lower in patients with elevated serum calcium than in patients with normal calcium

of calcium, the incidence of hypercalcemia lies around the 28%[62] (Table 19.3).

Mild-to-moderate elevation of serum calcium is mostly asymptomatic. However, it can cause serious danger when levels rise above 3.0 mmol/L and as such is regarded an absolute indication for treatment.[63] Hypercalcemia and hypercalciuria occur more often in males[60,64] and white patients.[65,66] Hypercalcemia is a rare phenomenon in patients with Löfgren's syndrome.[59]

Hypercalciuria in sarcoidosis has a reported prevalence varying from 6.4% to 33% of patients.[58,60–62] Nephrolithiasis and nephrocalcinosis can be serious consequences of hypercalciuria.[67–69] Moreover, both can lead to renal failure.[57,70,71]

Hypercalcemia and hypercalciuria are both markers reflecting granulomatous inflammatory activity in sarcoidosis. Their presence is also associated with a more worse prognosis, i.e., these patients are less likely to have spontaneous remission and a higher rate of relapses[61,72] (Table 19.3).

In conclusion, serum calcium should be measured as part of the diagnostic workup, and hypercalcemia can be an absolute indication to start systemic therapy. Furthermore, both hypercalcemia and hypercalciuria reflect on-going granulomatous inflammation and can be regarded as biomarkers for disease activity. However, this only applies for a small subset of patients and thus cannot be regarded useful biomarkers for sarcoidosis in general.

Lysozyme

Lysozyme is a low-weight enzyme with antibacterial activity. This enzyme is found in macrophages and epithelioid cells of granulomas in sarcoidosis,[32,73] however not in older lesions.[73] Like with sACE, it has been thought that serum lysozyme levels might reflect the total-body mass of granulomas.[74]

Sensitivity of serum lysozyme for the diagnosis of sarcoidosis lies between 69% and 80%,[34,75,76] Table 19.4, with the following AUCs: 0.695 (poor) and 0.799 (fair). Elevated serum levels of lysozyme are also found in patients with pulmonary tuberculosis, silicosis, and asbestosis,[77–79] limiting the specificity of lysozyme for the diagnosis of sarcoidosis (Table 19.4). Little is known about the value of lysozyme as severity or prognostic biomarker.

Serial measurements of lysozyme might however be useful to measure response to systemic antiinflammatory treatment. For example, monitoring of lysozyme levels has been shown to inversely correlate with change of DLCO during follow-up, (Table 19.5).[76]

Lysozyme is metabolized in the kidneys; thus in patients with renal impairment, serum lysozyme has to be interpreted with caution (Table 19.5).[80]

BAL Fluid Characteristics

In many clinics, BAL is routinely performed in the diagnosis of sarcoidosis.[81] The disease is characterized by an increased percentage of lymphocytes, increased CD4+/CD8+ ratio, and a decreased CD103 + CD4+/CD4+ ratio in BAL fluid. Of general importance is the notion that BAL fluid cell counts can be influenced by smoking.[82] Smoking can even mask the typical BAL fluid characteristics of sarcoidosis patients.

Percentage of Lymphocytes

Various studies on sensitivity of BAL fluid lymphocytosis have shown percentages varying from 71% to 85%.[8,83,84] And, specificity of this cellular characteristic in BAL has been reported to lay between 68% and 93%[8,83–85] (Table 19.6). ROC curve analysis varied between 0.695 and 0.775 (poor to fair).

This is at least in part related to the fact that increased lymphocytes in BAL fluid can also been found in patients with infections, malignancies,[86] and in other interstitial lung diseases such as hypersensitivity pneumonitis,[87] and in cryptogenic organizing pneumonitis.[88]

In literature there is no consensus if this marker reflects the severity of sarcoidosis. There are reports on higher percentage of lymphocytes in patients with acute presentation of disease,[89] which is associated with a favorable course of disease.[90] However, in other studies, no such correlation was found.[49,82]

Furthermore, the percentage of lymphocytes in BAL fluid is also found not to be predictive for disease outcome in sarcoidosis.[91,92]

In summary, percentage of lymphocytes in BAL fluid can be used as a diagnostic marker for sarcoidosis. However, its test performance has to be qualified as poor to fair. Furthermore, lymphocytosis is not informative in terms of disease severity and/or has no predictive value.

CD4+/CD8+ Ratio

Determining CD4+/CD8+ ratio can be helpful in the diagnosis of sarcoidosis. Sarcoidosis is characterized by an increased CD4/CD8 ratio (>3.5), compared with other interstitial lung diseases. Sensitivity of the CD4+/CD8+ ratio lies between 54% and 80%,[8,83–86,93–95] whereas the specificity varies from 59% to 80%[8,83–86,93,94] (Table 19.6). The area under the ROC curve for CD4+/CD8+ ratio for diagnosing sarcoidosis varies

TABLE 19.4
Serum Lysozyme: Sensitivity, Specificity, Severity Biomarker, and Prognosis

Study	Inclusion	Subtype	Control Group	Cutoff Value	Sensitivity	Specificity	Severity	Prognosis	AUC
Prior 1990[34]	(n = 25) Histologically proven sarcoidosis, all with radiographic evidence of lung involvement	Pulmonary sarcoidosis		Normal range: 0.4–1.5 mg/L	80%		Patients with higher lysozyme levels had higher radiographic profusion scores and more impaired FVC and DLCO	Pretreatment lysozyme did not correlate with change in lung function and radiographic profusion score after corticosteroids.	
Tomita 1999[76]	(n = 110) Sarcoidosis was diagnosed based on clinical picture and the presence of epithelioid cell granulomas in biopsies from the lung, skin, or lymph nodes. All subjects had normal renal function.		(n = 30) Patients with other granulomatous disease: summer-type hypersensitivity pneumonitis (n = 7), pulmonary tuberculosis (n = 20), pulmonary aspergillosis (n = 3).	11.0 μg/mL	79%	60%	Maximum lysozyme increases with the number of organs involved. Lysozyme levels were significantly higher in patients with more advanced radiographic stages.		[a]0.695
Turton 1979[75]	(n = 72) Patients with definite sarcoidosis where the clinical diagnosis has been confirmed histologically by tissue biopsy or the kveim test.		(n = 64) with various other diseases affecting the lungs, post-primary pulmonary tuberculosis (n = 8), old pulmonary tuberculosis (n = 4), cryptogenic fibrosing alveolitis (n = 26), asthma (n = 8), carcinoma of the bronchus (n = 8)	Normal range 0.9–2.6 units.	69%	90.7%			[a]0.7985
Leonhard 2016[13]	The whole cohort consisted of 1 patient with definite, 37 probable, and 14 possible neurosarcoidosis (Zajicek criteria). Lysozyme was measured in 26 patients	Neurosarcoidosis		>3.5 mg/L	46%				

DLCO, diffusion capacity for carbon monoxide; *FVC*, forced vital capacity.
[a]Area under the ROC curve was not performed in this study, the AUC was estimated by the following formula: (0.5 × (sensitivity × (1−specificity))) + (0.5 × (specificity × (1−sensitivity))) + (sensitivity × specificity).

TABLE 19.5
Serial Measurement of Biomarkers

Study	Inclusion	Subtype	Duration of Follow-up	Change in Biomarker	Correlation with Course
ACE					
Vorselaars 2015[30]	(n = 114) Sarcoidosis patients started on second-line treatment with methotrexate. sACE was measured before and after methotrexate.	76 patients with pulmonary treatment indication and 38 patients with an extrapulmonary treatment indication.	6 months	Mean ACE decreased from 71.4 U/L to 54.2 U/L	In patients with pulmonary treatment indication, sACE correlated with ΔVC, ΔFEV1, and ΔDLCO after methotrexate therapy
Baughman 1983[33]	(n = 36, 55 observations) Diagnosis was biopsy proven in all patients. After first measurement initiation of 40 mg/day prednisone. Thereafter, tapering of prednisone.	Pulmonary sarcoidosis	7 weeks of treatment with prednisone, than tapering of prednisone in the following 7–10 months. Mean duration of follow-up of 4.2 months after institution or change in steroid dose	–	In 6 of 13 patients with clinical deterioration, a rise in ACE was seen. In 10 of 21 patients with clinical improvement, a fall in ACE levels was seen. In patients with no change in clinical scale, 13 patients had a rise and 7 had a fall in ACE. Strong negative relationship in change of steroid dose and change in ACE level.
SIL-2R					
Thi Hong Nguyen 2017[52]	Skin lesions were assessed by skin biopsy. In 44 pt at least 2 measurements were determined	Cutaneous sarcoidosis. In 36% of the patients was pulmonary involvement			Changes in sIL-2R correlated with clinical progress in 90.1%
Vorselaars 2015[30]	(n = 114) Sarcoidosis patients started on second-line treatment with methotrexate	76 patients with pulmonary treatment indication and 38 patients with an extrapulmonary treatment indication.	6 months	Mean sIL-2R decreased from 4840 pg/ml to 2290 pg/mL	Significant correlation was found between ΔsIL-2R and ΔFVC, ΔDLCO after methotrexate therapy in patients with a pulmonary treatment indication.
Grutters 2003[36]	(n = 14) Diagnosis was confirmed by histologic evidence. All patients had active disease.		2 years		Positive correlation between change in sIL-2R and change in radiographic stage, which remained significant after correction for treatment. The initial sIL-2R level correlated inversely to the extent of change in the follow-up sIL-3r level

Lawrence 1988[53]	(n=5) Diagnosis was confirmed with biopsy in conjunction with negative histories, cultures, serologic, and cytologic studies for other causes of granuloma formation. All patients were treated for 6 weeks with 40 mg of prednisolone		6 weeks	Mean sIL-2R decreased from 1499U/mL to 476U/mL	All patients showed clinical improvement measured with pulmonary function and chest re-ontgenograph, corresponding with a decrease in sIL-2R.
CALCIUM					
Baughman 2013[57]	Diagnosis was made according to criteria of ATS/ERS/WASOG.				81/86 (94%) patients' hypercalcemia improved, with normalization in 91%. In 9% withdrawal of calcium and vitamin D supplementation normalized the hypercalcemia.
LYSOZYME					
Prior 1990[34]	(n=25) Histologically proven sarcoidosis, all with radiographic evidence of lung involvement. Serum lysozyme was measured before treatment and after prednisolone treatment (40 mg daily for 1–2 months followed by gradual tapering to 15 mg daily over the subsequent months)	Pulmonary sarcoidosis	Median duration of 13 months, (range 3–49) months		Fall in lysozyme after corticosteroid treatment correlates with the improvement in DLCO.

DLCO, diffusion capacity for carbon monoxide; *FEV1*, forced expiratory volume 1; *FVC*, forced vital capacity; *sIL-2R*, soluble interleukin-2 receptor.

TABLE 19.6
BAL Biomarkers Lymphocytes (%), CD4+/CD8+ Ratio, CD103+CD4+/CD4+ Ratio: Sensitivity, Specificity, and Severity Biomarker

Study	Inclusion	Subtype	Control Group	Cutoff value	Sensitivity	Specificity	Severity	AUC
Tanriverdi 2016[83]	(n = 68) Diagnosis was confirmed by biopsy. None of the patients received steroids before BAL.	Sarcoidosis patients with diffuse parenchymal lung disease	(n = 72) Nonsarcoidosis patients with diffuse parenchymal lung diseases (DPLD): CTD-ILD (n = 20), pneumoconiosis (n = 14), IPF (n = 12), infections (n = 5), other ILD (n = 16), malignancy (n = 4).	9.40%	85%	72%		0.776
De Smet 2010[8]	(n = 36) All biopsy proven, except 1 patient with LS. None of the patients received corticosteroids during diagnostic workup.	Pulmonary sarcoidosis	(n = 117) Patients with clinical suspicion of pulmonary sarcoidosis but who turned out to have another diagnosis	18%	75%	74%		0.77
Hyldgaard 2012[84]	(n = 17) All patients had biopsy confirmed sarcoidosis.		(n = 73) Patients with other pulmonary diseases (EAA, IPF, NSIP, DIP,LIP ILD associated with collagen vascular disease, unclassified interstitial lung disease, TBC, aspergillosis, and other nongranulomatous lung disease)	13%	71%	68%		[a]0.695
CD4+/CD8+ RATIO								
Tanriverdi 2016[83]	(n = 68) Diagnosis was confirmed by biopsy. None of the patients received steroids before BAL.	Sarcoidosis patients with diffuse parenchymal lung disease	(n = 72) Nonsarcoidosis patients with diffuse parenchymal lung diseases (DPLD): CTD-ILD, pneumoconiosis, IPF, infections, PAP, COP, NSIP, malignancy.	1.34	76%	79%		0.844
De Smet 2010[8]	(n = 36) All biopsy proven, except 1 patient with LS. None of the patients received corticosteroids during diagnostic workup.	Pulmonary sarcoidosis	(n = 117) Patients with clinical suspicion of pulmonary sarcoidosis but who turned out to have another diagnosis	2.62	67%	82%		0.79
Suchankova 2013[85]	(n = 26) Sarcoidosis diagnosis was based on ATS/ERS/WASOG criteria. No subjects received corticosteroids before BAL.	Pulmonary sarcoidosis	(n = 27): IPF (n = 12); CTD-related ILD (n = 7); drug-induced ILD (n = 3); NSIP (n = 3); and radiation-induced ILD (n = 12).	3.5	68%	94%		[a]0.81
Heron 2008[93]	(n = 119) Sarcoidosis diagnosis was based on ATS/ERS/WASOG criteria. No subjects received corticosteroids before BAL.	Pulmonary sarcoidosis	(N = 63) other ILD: HP (n = 22); IPF (n = 8); other interstitial pneumonia (n = 3); infection (n = 13); systemic disease (n = 8); malignancy (n = 6); other (n = 3)	2.5	73%	67%		0.81

Danila 2009[94]	(n=318) Diagnosis was confirmed according to ATS/ERS/WASOG. Diagnosis was biopsy proven in 98 patients, in other patients, final diagnosis was based on typical picture and radiographic symptoms (e.g., Löfgren's syndrome).	Pulmonary Sarcoidosis	(n=185): 55 healthy controls and 130 patients with other disorders who underwent BAL.	3.5	80%	90%	Sensitivity of CD4+/CD8+ ratio decreases in higher radiological stages. Optimal cutoff points for CD4+/CD8+ ratio is 3.5 in asymptomatic and 4.0 in symptomatic patients.	0.936
Hyldgaard 2012[84]	(n=19) All patients had biopsy confirmed sarcoidosis.		(n=83) Patients with other pulmonary diseases (EAA, IPF, NSIP, DIP,LIP ILD associated with collagen vascular disease, unclassified interstitial lung disease, TBC, aspergillosis, and other nongranulomatous lung disease)	3.8	68%	73%		[a]0.705
Winterbauer 1993[86]	(n=27) Diagnostic criteria were a compatible clinical picture, demonstration of multiple noncaseating granuloma or a positive Kveim test, and exclusion of other diseases capable of mimicking sarcoidosis. All patients had>16% lymphoycytes. None of the patients had received corticosteroids.		Nonsarcoidosis ILD (n=28): IPF n=10, drug-induced pneumonitis n=7, collagen vascular disease n=4, radiation pneumonitis n=4, berylliosis n=1, BOOP n=1.	4	59%	96%		[a]0.775
CD103+CD4+/CD4+								
Heron 2008[93]	(n=119) Diagnosis was based on ATS/ERS/WASOG criteria. No subjects received corticosteroids prior to BAL. Only patients with alveolar lymphocytosis, defined by≥10% lymphocytes in BAL, were included.	Pulmonary sarcoidosis	(N=63) other ILD: HP (n=22); IPF (n=8); Other interstitial pneumonia (n=3); infection (n=13); systemic disease (n=8); malignancy (n=6); other (n=3)					0.79
Hyldgaard 2012[84]	(n=19) All patients had biopsy confirmed sarcoidosis.		(n=82) Patients with other pulmonary diseases (EAA, IPF, NSIP, DIP,LIP ILD associated with collagen vascular disease, unclassified interstitial lung disease, TBC, aspergillosis, and other nongranulomatous lung disease)	<0.22	63%	76%	No correlation between CD103+CD4+/CD4+ ratio and radiographic staging.	[a]0.695
Mota 2012[97]	(n=41) Diagnosis was confirmed according to ATS/ERS/WASOG.		(n=45) Other ILD: HP, IPF, NSIP, COP, SLE, RA, scleroderma, drug-induced lung disease, and silicosis.	0.45	81%	78%		0.86

ILD, interstitial lung disease; IPF, idiopathic pulmonary fibrosis; SLE, systemic lupus erythematosus; RA, rheumatoid arthritis; HP, hypersensitivity pneumonia; BAL, bronchoalveolar lavage; NSIP, nonspecific interstitial pneumonia; DIP, desquamative interstitial pneumonia; LIP, lymphoid interstitial pneumonia; COP, cryptogenic organizing pneumonia; EAA, extrinsic allergic alveolitis; TBC, tuberculosis; BOOP, bronchiolitis obliterans with organizing pneumonia; PAP, pulmonary alveolar proteinosis; CTD, connective tissue disease.

[a]Area under the ROC curve was not performed in this study, the AUC was estimated by the following formula: (0.5 × (sensitivity × (1−specificity))) + (0.5 × (specificity × (1−sensitivity))) + (sensitivity × specificity).

between 0.705 and 0.936, which means that this is a fair-excellent biomarker for diagnosing sarcoidosis.

The ratio appears to have value as an indicator for the severity of the disease/extend of organ involvement. Some studies found higher CD4+/CD8+ ratio and higher sensitivity of CD4+/CD8+ ratio in less advanced Scadding stages.[90,94] Furthermore, a higher CD4+/CD8+ ratio is found in patients who carry HLA-DRB1*03, a genotype that is correlated with favorable outcome in sarcoidosis.[96] In addition, many studies have reported relatively high CD4+/CD8+ ratio in patients with acute onset sarcoidosis. This clinical phenotype usually has a favorable prognosis.[61,82,89,90,96] Therefore measurement of CD4+/CD8+ ratio in BAL fluid also appears to have some prognostic value.

In summary, CD4+/CD8+ ratio can be classified as a fair-to-excellent diagnostic marker for sarcoidosis. Furthermore, it has an association with disease severity and outcome, although this has limited clinical value.

CD103+CD4+/CD4+ Ratio

Typically in sarcoidosis a decreased CD103+CD4+/CD4+ ratio (<0.2) in BAL fluid is found.[93] Such a decreased CD103+CD4+/CD4+ ratio has a sensitivity of circa 63%–81% and a specificity of 76%–78%,[84,97] with an AUC of 0.695 and 0.790 (poor to fair) (Table 19.6). Interestingly, it has been shown that the combined use of the CD4+/CD8+ ratio and the CD103+CD4+/CD4+ ratio increases the specificity for diagnosing sarcoidosis to 91%.[93]

It is thought that CD103 positive cells are involved in fibrogenic inflammation.[98] By this means, in more advanced radiologic stages of sarcoidosis, a higher proportion of CD4+ T lymphocytes express CD103.[93,97] Indicating that patients with relatively high CD103+CD4+/CD4+ ratio might have a worse prognosis.

In summary, especially the combination of CD4+/CD8+ ratio and CD103+CD4+/CD4+ ratio can be regarded as a specific biomarker for diagnosis of sarcoidosis. CD103+CD4+/CD4+ ratio might be a severity and prognostic biomarker, but this will need further research.

POTENTIAL BIOMARKERS

Chitotriosidase

Chitotriosidase is an enzyme produced by activated macrophages which plays a role in the defense against fungi, insects, and nematodes.[99] Chitotriosidase can determine disease activity in sarcoidosis with a sensitivity that lies between 89% and 100%[100–102] and a specificity of circa 93%.[100]

Chitotriosidase also appears to be an indicator of the severity of sarcoidosis.[47,100,102] Patients with Löfgren's syndrome and with stable disease have lower levels of chitotriosidase,[100,103] whereas patients with persistent disease on steroids have the highest levels.[100]

Serial measurements of chitotriosidase seem to correlate well with the clinical course of disease.[101,103] However, like in sACE, it is possible that treatment with corticosteroids can lower chitotriosidase levels irrespective of the lowering of disease activity.[101,102]

Th17-Cells and Tregs

Recently, increased amounts of Th17 (CCR4+/CXCR3-) CD4+ T cells have been found in the BAL fluid and the peripheral blood of sarcoidosis patients.[104,105] Th17 CD4+ T cells play a role in many inflammatory diseases. Interestingly, higher BAL fluid Th17.1 cell proportions (i.e., interferon-γ–producing Th17 cells) have been described in patients developing chronic disease than in patients with resolving disease, indicating a potential cellular biomarker to predict disease course in sarcoidosis.[106] Paradoxically, higher frequency of Th17.1 cells has also been observed in Lofgren syndrome, which usually has a favorable outcome.[107]

Another T cell subset, regulatory T cells (Tregs), has been found increased in blood of sarcoidosis patients, most prominently in those developing chronic disease.[108] However, before such potential cellular biomarkers can be acceptable for clinical use, further research is required.

Serum Amyloid A

Serum amyloid A (SAA) is a family of proteins produced in the liver which are elevated in an acute-phase response. SAA3 is a member of this family that can be produced extrahepatically in inflammatory tissue by macrophages.[109] SAA depositions are found in the granulomas in sarcoidosis patients.[110] Elevated levels of serum SAA have been found in sarcoidosis,[110,111] and higher levels were shown in patients with more active disease.[39] Furthermore, data exist showing that serum SAA levels correlate with severity of lung function impairment and need for systemic therapy.[111]

Chemokines

Chemokines are a family of chemoattractant proteins, and certain chemokine actions can stimulate the migration of T cells to inflammatory sites.[112]

Increased amounts of IFN-γ–inducible chemokines CXCL9, 10, and 11 and the receptor CXCR3 have been found in the BAL and serum of patients with sarcoidosis.[113–118] As CXCL9 and CXC10 are involved in the migration of Th1 lymphocytes, they might potentially be useful as biomarkers for disease severity and prognosis. Interestingly, CXCL9 and CXCL10 were shown to be inversely correlated with the FVC% and DLCO% of predicted.[119] Furthermore, blood transcriptomic signature reflecting CXCL9 can predict disease outcome longitudinally.[120]

Future Purposes: Omics

To identify novel biomarkers, new techniques have been used applying omic technologies, which means profiling of sets of molecules.[121]

Gene expression analysis on tissue of sarcoidosis patients mostly reveals overexpression of genes engaging T-helper one response.[122] Especially MMP-12 and ADAMDEC1 transcripts were highly expressed in lung tissue. MMP-12 plays a role in lung remodeling and lung fibrosis; thus this marker can possibly be interesting as a prognostic marker for fibrosing phenotypes of sarcoidosis.[122] One study identified a blood gene signature to diagnose sarcoidosis with 92% sensitivity and 92% specificity.[123] Other studies found that gene expression signatures in biopsies[122,124] and blood[125] of sarcoidosis patients were able to identify patients with a self-limiting disease from patients with more complicated sarcoidosis, also suggesting potential prognostic biomarkers.

Furthermore, proteomic profiling is an interesting development that might reveal new biomarkers in sarcoidosis. A recent study used microarrays built on protein fragments to detect sarcoidosis-associated antigens. This study found four proteins as potential sarcoidosis-associated autoimmune targets.[126] Another study performed a breath analysis by applying electronic nose technology. Interestingly, in the acquired breath prints containing exhaled molecular profiles, untreated pulmonary sarcoidosis patients could be differentiated from health controls.[127]

CONCLUSION

Commonly used markers in sarcoidosis are serum ACE, sIL-2R, calcium, lysozyme, and urine calcium and cellular parameters in BAL. None of them actually would qualify as an adequate diagnostic, prognostic, and/or staging biomarker. However, still the (combined) use of these markers can be helpful in the appropriate clinical context. A promising horizon is recent publications on gene expression/protein signatures in sarcoidosis. This technology can provide new insights into this enigmatic disease and help the development of novel biomarkers.

REFERENCES

1. Biomarkers Definitions Working Group. Biomarkers and surrogate endpoints: preferred definitions and conceptual framework. *Clin Pharmacol Ther.* 2001;69(3):89–95. https://doi.org/S0009-9236(01)63448-9 [pii].
2. Consensus conference: activity of sarcoidosis. Third WASOG meeting, Los Angeles, USA, September 8–11, 1993. *Eur Respir J.* 1994;7(3):624–627.
3. Ryan JW, Smith U, Niemeyer RS, Angiotensin I. Metabolism by plasma membrane of lung. *Science.* 1972;176(4030):64–66.
4. Okabe T, Suzuki A, Ishikawa H, Yotsumoto H, Ohsawa N. Cells originating from sarcoid granulomas in vitro. *Am Rev Respir Dis.* 1981;124(5):608–612.
5. Lieberman J. The specificity and nature of serum-angiotensin-converting enzyme (serum ACE) elevations in sarcoidosis. *Ann N Y Acad Sci.* 1976;278:488–497.
6. Silverstein E, Pertschuk LP, Friedland J. Immunofluorescent localization of angiotensin converting enzyme in epithelioid and giant cells of sarcoidosis granulomas. *Proc Natl Acad Sci U S A.* 1979;76(12):6646–6648.
7. Muthuswamy PP, Lopez-Majano V, Ranginwala M, Trainor WD. Serum angiotensin-converting enzyme (SACE) activity as an indicator of total body granuloma load and prognosis in sarcoidosis. *Sarcoidosis.* 1987;4(2):142–148.
8. De Smet D, Martens GA, Berghe BV, et al. Use of likelihood ratios improves interpretation of laboratory testing for pulmonary sarcoidosis. *Am J Clin Pathol.* 2010;134(6):939–947. https://doi.org/10.1309/AJCPNC7STHG0FWMP.
9. Popevic S, Sumarac Z, Jovanovic D, et al. Verifying sarcoidosis activity: chitotriosidase versus ACE in sarcoidosis - a case-control study. *J Med Biochem.* 2016;35(4):390–400. https://doi.org/10.1515/jomb-2016-0017.
10. Ungprasert P, Carmona EM, Crowson CS, Matteson EL. Diagnostic utility of angiotensin-converting enzyme in sarcoidosis: a population-based study. *Lung.* 2016;194(1):91–95. https://doi.org/10.1007/s00408-015-9826-3.
11. Groen-Hakan F, Eurelings L, ten Berge JC, et al. Diagnostic value of serum-soluble interleukin 2 receptor levels vs angiotensin-converting enzyme in patients with sarcoidosis-associated uveitis. *JAMA Ophthalmol.* 2017;135(12):1352–1358. https://doi.org/10.1001/jamaophthalmol.2017.4771.
12. Gundlach E, Hoffmann MM, Prasse A, Heinzelmann S, Ness T. Interleukin-2 receptor and angiotensin-converting enzyme as markers for ocular sarcoidosis. *PLoS One.* 2016;11(1):e0147258. https://doi.org/10.1371/journal.pone.0147258.
13. Leonhard SE, Fritz D, Eftimov F, van der Kooi AJ, van de Beek D, Brouwer MC. Neurosarcoidosis in a tertiary referral center: a cross-sectional cohort study. *Medicine (Baltim).* 2016;95(14):e3277. https://doi.org/10.1097/MD.0000000000003277.

14. Rigat B, Hubert C, Alhenc-Gelas F, Cambien F, Corvol P, Soubrier F. An insertion/deletion polymorphism in the angiotensin I-converting enzyme gene accounting for half the variance of serum enzyme levels. *J Clin Invest.* 1990;86(4):1343–1346.
15. Kruit A, Grutters JC, Gerritsen WB, et al. ACE I/D-corrected Z-scores to identify normal and elevated ACE activity in sarcoidosis. *Respir Med.* 2007;101(3):510–515.
16. Sharma P, Smith I, Maguire G, Stewart S, Shneerson J, Brown MJ. Clinical value of ACE genotyping in diagnosis of sarcoidosis. *Lancet.* 1997;349(9065):1602–1603. https://doi.org/S0140-6736(05)61631-5 [pii].
17. Tomita H, Ina Y, Sugiura Y, et al. Polymorphism in the angiotensin-converting enzyme (ACE) gene and sarcoidosis. *Am J Respir Crit Care Med.* 1997;156(1):255–259.
18. Brice EA, Friedlander W, Bateman ED, Kirsch RE. Serum angiotensin-converting enzyme activity, concentration, and specific activity in granulomatous interstitial lung disease, tuberculosis, and COPD. *Chest.* 1995;107(3): 706–710.
19. Ryder KW, Jay SJ, Kiblawi SO, Hull MT. Serum angiotensin converting enzyme activity in patients with histoplasmosis. *J Am Med Assoc.* 1983;249(14):1888–1889.
20. Lieberman J, Rea TH. Serum angiotensin-converting enzyme in leprosy and coccidioidomycosis. *Ann Intern Med.* 1977;87(4):423–425.
21. Rohrbach MS, Deremee RA. Serum angiotensin converting enzyme activity in sarcoidosis as measured by a simple radiochemical assay. *Am Rev Respir Dis.* 1979;119(5):761–767.
22. Rohatgi PK, Ryan JW. Simple radioassay for measuring serum activity of angiotensin-converting enzyme in sarcoidosis. *Chest.* 1980;78(1):69–76.
23. Lieberman J, Schleissner LA, Nosal A, Sastre A, Mishkin FS. Clinical correlations of serum angiotensin-converting enzyme (ACE) in sarcoidosis. A longitudinal study of serum ACE, 67gallium scans, chest roentgenograms, and pulmonary function. *Chest.* 1983;84(5): 522–528.
24. Bunting PS, Szalai JP, Katic M. Diagnostic aspects of angiotensin converting enzyme in pulmonary sarcoidosis. *Clin Biochem.* 1987;20(3):213–219.
25. Studdy P, Bird R, James DG. Serum angiotensin-converting enzyme (SACE) in sarcoidosis and other granulomatous disorders. *Lancet.* 1978;2(8104–5):1331–1334.
26. Specks U, Martin 2nd WJ, Rohrbach MS. Bronchoalveolar lavage fluid angiotensin-converting enzyme in interstitial lung diseases. *Am Rev Respir Dis.* 1990;141(1):117–123.
27. Ziegenhagen MW, Benner UK, Zissel G, Zabel P, Schlaak M, Muller-Quernheim J. Sarcoidosis: TNF-alpha release from alveolar macrophages and serum level of sIL-2R are prognostic markers. *Am J Respir Crit Care Med.* 1997;156(5):1586–1592. https://doi.org/10.1164/ajrccm.156.5.97-02050.
28. Vorselaars AD, Verwoerd A, van Moorsel CH, Keijsers RG, Rijkers GT, Grutters JC. Prediction of relapse after discontinuation of infliximab therapy in severe sarcoidosis. *Eur Respir J.* 2014;43(2):602–609. https://doi.org/10.1183/09031936.00055213.
29. Klech H, Kohn H, Kummer F, Mostbeck A. Assessment of activity in sarcoidosis. sensitivity and specificity of 67Gallium scintigraphy, serum ACE levels, chest roentgenography, and blood lymphocyte subpopulations. *Chest.* 1982;82(6):732–738.
30. Vorselaars AD, van Moorsel CH, Zanen P, et al. ACE and sIL-2R correlate with lung function improvement in sarcoidosis during methotrexate therapy. *Respir Med.* 2015;109(2):279–285.
31. Vorselaars AD, Crommelin HA, Deneer VH, et al. Effectiveness of infliximab in refractory FDG PET-positive sarcoidosis. *Eur Respir J.* 2015;46(1):175–185. https://doi.org/10.1183/09031936.00227014.
32. Silverstein E, Friedland J, Ackerman T. Elevation of granulomatous lymph-node and serum lysozyme in sarcoidosis and correlation with angiotensin-converting enzyme. *Am J Clin Pathol.* 1977;68(2):219–224.
33. Baughman RP, Ploysongsang Y, Roberts RD, Srivastava L. Effects of sarcoid and steroids on angiotensin-converting enzyme. *Am Rev Respir Dis.* 1983;128(4):631–633.
34. Prior C, Barbee RA, Evans PM, et al. Lavage versus serum measurements of lysozyme, angiotensin converting enzyme and other inflammatory markers in pulmonary sarcoidosis. *Eur Respir J.* 1990;3(10):1146–1154.
35. Krasowski MD, Savage J, Ehlers A, et al. Ordering of the serum angiotensin-converting enzyme test in patients receiving angiotensin-converting enzyme inhibitor therapy: an avoidable but common error. *Chest.* 2015;148(6):1447–1453.
36. Grutters JC, Fellrath JM, Mulder L, Janssen R, van den Bosch JM, van Velzen-Blad H. Serum soluble interleukin-2 receptor measurement in patients with sarcoidosis: a clinical evaluation. *Chest.* 2003;124(1):186–195. https://doi.org/S0012-3692(15)36009-8.
37. Rubin LA, Kurman CC, Fritz ME, et al. Soluble interleukin 2 receptors are released from activated human lymphoid cells in vitro. *J Immunol.* 1985;135(5): 3172–3177.
38. Nelson DL, Rubin LA, Kurman CC, Fritz ME, Boutin B. An analysis of the cellular requirements for the production of soluble interleukin-2 receptors in vitro. *J Clin Immunol.* 1986;6(2):114–120.
39. Gungor S, Ozseker F, Yalcinsoy M, et al. Conventional markers in determination of activity of sarcoidosis. *Int Immunopharmacol.* 2015;25(1):174–179. https://doi.org/10.1016/j.intimp.2015.01.015.
40. Rubin LA, Nelson DL. The soluble interleukin-2 receptor: biology, function, and clinical application. *Ann Intern Med.* 1990;113(8):619–627.
41. Greene WC, Leonard WJ, Depper JM, Nelson DL, Waldmann TA. The human interleukin-2 receptor: normal and abnormal expression in T cells and in leukemias induced by the human T-lymphotropic retroviruses. *Ann Intern Med.* 1986;105(4):560–572.
42. Brown AE, Rieder KT, Webster HK. Prolonged elevations of soluble interleukin-2 receptors in tuberculosis. *Am Rev Respir Dis.* 1989;139(4):1036–1038. https://doi.org/10.1164/ajrccm/139.4.1036.

43. Tung KS, Umland E, Matzner P, et al. Soluble serum interleukin 2 receptor levels in leprosy patients. *Clin Exp Immunol.* 1987;69(1):10–15.
44. Wolf RE, Brelsford WG. Soluble interleukin-2 receptors in systemic lupus erythematosus. *Arthritis Rheum.* 1988;31(6):729–735.
45. Verwoerd A, Vorselaars AD, van Moorsel CH, Bos WJ, van Velzen-Blad H, Grutters JC. Discrepant elevation of sIL-2R levels in sarcoidosis patients with renal insufficiency. *Eur Respir J.* 2015;46(1):277–280. https://doi.org/10.1183/09031936.00005315.
46. Takamatsu T, Yasuda N, Ohno T, Kanoh T, Uchino H, Fujisawa A. Soluble interleukin-2 receptors in the serum of patients with chronic renal failure. *Tohoku J Exp Med.* 1988;155(4):343–347.
47. Bargagli E, Bianchi N, Margollicci M, et al. Chitotriosidase and soluble IL-2 receptor: comparison of two markers of sarcoidosis severity. *Scand J Clin Lab Invest.* 2008;68(6):479–483. https://doi.org/10.1080/00365510701854975.
48. Ina Y, Takada K, Sato T, Yamamoto M, Noda M, Morishita M. Soluble interleukin 2 receptors in patients with sarcoidosis. possible origin. *Chest.* 1992;102(4):1128–1133. https://doi.org/S0012-3692(16)34292-1.
49. Ziegenhagen MW, Rothe ME, Schlaak M, Muller-Quernheim J. Bronchoalveolar and serological parameters reflecting the severity of sarcoidosis. *Eur Respir J.* 2003;21(3):407–413.
50. Rothkrantz-Kos S, van Dieijen-Visser MP, Mulder PG, Drent M. Potential usefulness of inflammatory markers to monitor respiratory functional impairment in sarcoidosis. *Clin Chem.* 2003;49(9):1510–1517.
51. Prasse A, Katic C, Germann M, Buchwald A, Zissel G, Muller-Quernheim J. Phenotyping sarcoidosis from a pulmonary perspective. *Am J Respir Crit Care Med.* 2008;177(3):330–336. https://doi.org/200705-742OC [pii].
52. Thi Hong Nguyen C, Kambe N, Kishimoto I, Ueda-Hayakawa I, Okamoto H. Serum soluble interleukin-2 receptor level is more sensitive than angiotensin-converting enzyme or lysozyme for diagnosis of sarcoidosis and may be a marker of multiple organ involvement. *J Dermatol.* 2017;44(7):789–797. https://doi.org/10.1111/1346-8138.13792.
53. Lawrence EC, Brousseau KP, Berger MB, Kurman CC, Marcon L, Nelson DL. Elevated concentrations of soluble interleukin-2 receptors in serum samples and bronchoalveolar lavage fluids in active sarcoidosis. *Am Rev Respir Dis.* 1988;137(4):759–764. https://doi.org/10.1164/ajrccm/137.4.759.
54. Adams JS, Singer FR, Gacad MA, et al. Isolation and structural identification of 1,25-dihydroxy vitamin D3 produced by cultured alveolar macrophages in sarcoidosis. *J Clin Endocrinol Metab.* 1985;60(5):960–966. https://doi.org/10.1210/jcem-60-5-960.
55. Bell NH, Stern PH, Pantzer E, Sinha TK, DeLuca HF. Evidence that increased circulating 1 alpha, 25-dihydroxy vitamin D is the probable cause for abnormal calcium metabolism in sarcoidosis. *J Clin Invest.* 1979;64(1):218–225. https://doi.org/10.1172/JCI109442.
56. Jones G, Strugnell SA, DeLuca HF. Current understanding of the molecular actions of vitamin D. *Physiol Rev.* 1998;78(4):1193–1231.
57. Baughman RP, Janovcik J, Ray M, Sweiss N, Lower EE. Calcium and vitamin D metabolism in sarcoidosis. *Sarcoidosis Vasc Diffuse Lung Dis.* 2013;30(2):113–120.
58. Kamphuis LS, Bonte-Mineur F, van Laar JA, van Hagen PM, van Daele PL. Calcium and vitamin D in sarcoidosis: is supplementation safe? *J Bone Miner Res.* 2014;29(11):2498–2503. https://doi.org/10.1002/jbmr.2262.
59. Darlington P, Gabrielsen A, Sorensson P, et al. HLA-alleles associated with increased risk for extra-pulmonary involvement in sarcoidosis. *Tissue Antigens.* 2014;83(4):267–272. https://doi.org/10.1111/tan.12326.
60. Morimoto T, Azuma A, Abe S, et al. Epidemiology of sarcoidosis in Japan. *Eur Respir J.* 2008;31(2):372–379. https://doi.org/09031936.00075307 [pii].
61. Doubkova M, Pospisil Z, Skrickova J, Doubek M. Prognostic markers of sarcoidosis: an analysis of patients from everyday pneumological practice. *Clin Respir J.* 2015;9(4):443–449. https://doi.org/10.1111/crj.12160.
62. Hamada K, Nagai S, Tsutsumi T, Izumi T. Ionized calcium and 1,25-dihydroxy vitamin D concentration in serum of patients with sarcoidosis. *Eur Respir J.* 1998;11(5):1015–1020.
63. Bilezikian JP. Management of acute hypercalcemia. *N Engl J Med.* 1992;326(18):1196–1203. https://doi.org/10.1056/NEJM199204303261806.
64. Zurkova M, Kolek V, Tomankova T, Kriegova E. Extrapulmonary involvement in patients with sarcoidosis and comparison of routine laboratory and clinical data to pulmonary involvement. *Biomed Pap Med Fac Univ Palacky Olomouc Czech Repub.* 2014;158(4):613–620. https://doi.org/10.5507/bp.2014.026.
65. Judson MA, Boan AD, Lackland DT. The clinical course of sarcoidosis: presentation, diagnosis, and treatment in a large white and black cohort in the United States. *Sarcoidosis Vasc Diffuse Lung Dis.* 2012;29(2):119–127.
66. Baughman RP, Teirstein AS, Judson MA, et al. Clinical characteristics of patients in a case control study of sarcoidosis. *Am J Respir Crit Care Med.* 2001;164(10 Pt 1):1885–1889. https://doi.org/10.1164/ajrccm.164.10.2104046.
67. Rizzato G, Colombo P. Nephrolithiasis as a presenting feature of chronic sarcoidosis: a prospective study. *Sarcoidosis Vasc Diffuse Lung Dis.* 1996;13(2):167–172.
68. Capolongo G, Xu LH, Accardo M, et al. Vitamin-D status and mineral metabolism in two ethnic populations with sarcoidosis. *J Investig Med.* 2016;64(5):1025–1034. https://doi.org/10.1136/jim-2016-000101.
69. Lebacq E, Desmet V, Verhaegen H. Renal involvement in sarcoidosis. *Postgrad Med J.* 1970;46(538):526–529.
70. Loffler C, Loffler U, Tuleweit A, Waldherr R, Uppenkamp M, Bergner R. Renal sarcoidosis: epidemiological and follow-up data in a cohort of 27 patients. *Sarcoidosis Vasc Diffuse Lung Dis.* 2015;31(4):306–315.
71. Mahfoudhi M, Mamlouk H, Turki S, Kheder A. Systemic sarcoidosis complicated of acute renal failure: about 12 cases. *Pan Afr Med J.* 2015;22:75. https://doi.org/10.11604/pamj.2015.22.75.6237.

72. Rodrigues SC, Rocha NA, Lima MS, et al. Factor analysis of sarcoidosis phenotypes at two referral centers in Brazil. *Sarcoidosis Vasc Diffuse Lung Dis*. 2011;28(1):34–43.
73. Selroos OB. Biochemical markers in sarcoidosis. *Crit Rev Clin Lab Sci*. 1986;24(3):185–216. https://doi.org/10.3109/10408368609110273.
74. Selroos O, Klockars M. Serum lysozyme in sarcoidosis. evaluation of its usefulness in determination of disease activity. *Scand J Respir Dis*. 1977;58(2):110–116.
75. Turton CW, Grundy E, Firth G, Mitchell D, Rigden BG, Turner-Warwick M. Value of measuring serum angiotensin I converting enzyme and serum lysozyme in the management of sarcoidosis. *Thorax*. 1979;34(1):57–62.
76. Tomita H, Sato S, Matsuda R, et al. Serum lysozyme levels and clinical features of sarcoidosis. *Lung*. 1999;177(3):161–167.
77. Gronhagen-Riska C, Kurppa K, Fyhrquist F, Selroos O. Angiotensin-converting enzyme and lysozyme in silicosis and asbestosis. *Scand J Respir Dis*. 1978;59(4):228–231.
78. Koskinen H, Nordman H, Froseth B. Serum lysozyme concentration in silicosis patients and workers exposed to silica dust. *Eur J Respir Dis*. 1984;65(7):481–485.
79. Perillie PE, Khan K, Finch SC. Serum lysozyme in pulmonary tuberculosis. *Am J Med Sci*. 1973;265(4):297–302.
80. Pruzanski W, Platts ME. Serum and urinary proteins, lysozyme (muramidase), and renal dysfunction in mono- and myelomonocytic leukemia. *J Clin Invest*. 1970;49(9): 1694–1708. https://doi.org/10.1172/JCI106387.
81. Statement on sarcoidosis. Joint statement of the american thoracic society (ATS), the european respiratory society (ERS) and the world association of sarcoidosis and other granulomatous disorders (WASOG) adopted by the ATS board of directors and by the ERS executive committee, february 1999. *Am J Respir Crit Care Med*. 1999;160(2):736–755.
82. Drent M, van Velzen-Blad H, Diamant M, Hoogsteden HC, van den Bosch JM. Relationship between presentation of sarcoidosis and T lymphocyte profile. A study in bronchoalveolar lavage fluid. *Chest*. 1993;104(3):795–800. https://doi.org/S0012-3692(16)32081-5 [pii].
83. Tanriverdi H, Uygur F, Ornek T, et al. Comparison of the diagnostic value of different lymphocyte subpopulations in bronchoalveolar lavage fluid in patients with biopsy proven sarcoidosis. *Sarcoidosis Vasc Diffuse Lung Dis*. 2016;32(4):305–312.
84. Hyldgaard C, Kaae S, Riddervold M, Hoffmann HJ, Hilberg O. Value of s-ACE, BAL lymphocytosis, and CD4+/CD8+ and CD103+CD4+/CD4+ T-cell ratios in diagnosis of sarcoidosis. *Eur Respir J*. 2012;39(4):1037–1039. https://doi.org/10.1183/09031936.00144311.
85. Suchankova M, Bucova M, Tibenska E, et al. Triggering receptor expressed on myeloid cells-1 and 2 in bronchoalveolar lavage fluid in pulmonary sarcoidosis. *Respirology*. 2013;18(3):455–462. https://doi.org/10.1111/resp.12028.
86. Winterbauer RH, Lammert J, Selland M, Wu R, Corley D, Springmeyer SC. Bronchoalveolar lavage cell populations in the diagnosis of sarcoidosis. *Chest*. 1993;104(2):352–361. https://doi.org/S0012-3692(16)35339-9.
87. D'Ippolito R, Chetta A, Foresi A, et al. Induced sputum and bronchoalveolar lavage from patients with hypersensitivity pneumonitis. *Respir Med*. 2004;98(10):977–983.
88. King TE Jr , Mortenson RL. Cryptogenic organizing pneumonitis. the north american experience. *Chest*. 1992;102(suppl 1):8S–13S.
89. Ward K, O'Connor C, Odlum C, Fitzgerald MX. Prognostic value of bronchoalveolar lavage in sarcoidosis: the critical influence of disease presentation. *Thorax*. 1989;44(1):6–12.
90. Verstraeten A, Demedts M, Verwilghen J, et al. Predictive value of bronchoalveolar lavage in pulmonary sarcoidosis. *Chest*. 1990;98(3):560–567. https://doi.org/S0012-3692(16)32081-5 [pii].
91. Bjermer L, Rosenhall L, Angstrom T, Hallgren R. Predictive value of bronchoalveolar lavage cell analysis in sarcoidosis. *Thorax*. 1988;43(4):284–288.
92. Laviolette M, La Forge J, Tennina S, Boulet LP. Prognostic value of bronchoalveolar lavage lymphocyte count in recently diagnosed pulmonary sarcoidosis. *Chest*. 1991;100(2):380–384. https://doi.org/S0012-3692(16)32081-5 [pii].
93. Heron M, Slieker WA, Zanen P, et al. Evaluation of CD103 as a cellular marker for the diagnosis of pulmonary sarcoidosis. *Clin Immunol*. 2008;126(3):338–344. https://doi.org/10.1016/j.clim.2007.11.005.
94. Danila E, Norkuniene J, Jurgauskiene L, Malickaite R. Diagnostic role of BAL fluid CD4/CD8 ratio in different radiographic and clinical forms of pulmonary sarcoidosis. *Clin Respir J*. 2009;3(4):214–221. https://doi.org/10.1111/j.1752-699X.2008.00126.x.
95. von Bartheld MB, Dekkers OM, Szlubowski A, et al. Endosonography vs conventional bronchoscopy for the diagnosis of sarcoidosis: the GRANULOMA randomized clinical trial. *J Am Med Assoc*. 2013;309(23):2457–2464. https://doi.org/10.1001/jama.2013.5823.
96. Planck A, Eklund A, Grunewald J. Inflammatory BAL-fluid and serum parameters in HLA DR17 positive vs. DR17 negative patients with pulmonary sarcoidosis. *Sarcoidosis Vasc Diffuse Lung Dis*. 2001;18(1):64–69.
97. Mota PC, Morais A, Palmares C, et al. Diagnostic value of CD103 expression in bronchoalveolar lymphocytes in sarcoidosis. *Respir Med*. 2012;106(7):1014–1020. https://doi.org/10.1016/j.rmed.2012.03.020.
98. Braun RK, Foerster M, Grahmann PR, Haefner D, Workalemahu G, Kroegel C. Phenotypic and molecular characterization of CD103+ CD4+ T cells in bronchoalveolar lavage from patients with interstitial lung diseases. *Cytometry B Clin Cytom*. 2003;54(1):19–27. https://doi.org/10.1002/cyto.b.10021.
99. van Eijk M, van Roomen CP, Renkema GH, et al. Characterization of human phagocyte-derived chitotriosidase, a component of innate immunity. *Int Immunol*. 2005;17(11):1505–1512. https://doi.org/dxh328.

100. Bargagli E, Bennett D, Maggiorelli C, et al. Human chitotriosidase: a sensitive biomarker of sarcoidosis. *J Clin Immunol.* 2013;33(1):264–270. https://doi.org/10.1007/s10875-012-9754-4.
101. Boot RG, Hollak CE, Verhoek M, Alberts C, Jonkers RE, Aerts JM. Plasma chitotriosidase and CCL18 as surrogate markers for granulomatous macrophages in sarcoidosis. *Clin Chim Acta.* 2010;411(1–2):31–36. https://doi.org/10.1016/j.cca.2009.09.034.
102. Tercelj M, Salobir B, Simcic S, Wraber B, Zupancic M, Rylander R. Chitotriosidase activity in sarcoidosis and some other pulmonary diseases. *Scand J Clin Lab Invest.* 2009;69(5):575–578. https://doi.org/10.1080/00365510902829362.
103. Harlander M, Salobir B, Zupancic M, Dolensek M, Bavcar Vodovnik T, Tercelj M. Serial chitotriosidase measurements in sarcoidosis–two to five year follow-up study. *Respir Med.* 2014;108(5):775–782. https://doi.org/10.1016/j.rmed.2014.02.002.
104. Ostadkarampour M, Eklund A, Moller D, et al. Higher levels of interleukin IL-17 and antigen-specific IL-17 responses in pulmonary sarcoidosis patients with lofgren's syndrome. *Clin Exp Immunol.* 2014;178(2):342–352. https://doi.org/10.1111/cei.12403.
105. Ten Berge B, Paats MS, Bergen IM, et al. Increased IL-17A expression in granulomas and in circulating memory T cells in sarcoidosis. *Rheumatology.* 2012;51(1):37–46. https://doi.org/10.1093/rheumatology/ker316.
106. Miedema JR, Kaiser Y, Broos CE, Wijsenbeek MS, Grunewald J, Kool M. Th17-lineage cells in pulmonary sarcoidosis and lofgren's syndrome: friend or foe?. *J Autoimmun.* 2018. https://doi.org/S0896-8411(17)30805-3 [pii]
107. Kaiser Y, Lepzien R, Kullberg S, Eklund A, Smed-Sorensen A, Grunewald J. Expanded lung T-bet+ROR gammaT+ CD4+ T-cells in sarcoidosis patients with a favourable disease phenotype. *Eur Respir J.* 2016;48(2):484–494. https://doi.org/10.1183/13993003.00092-2016.
108. Broos CE, van Nimwegen M, Kleinjan A, et al. Impaired survival of regulatory T cells in pulmonary sarcoidosis. *Respir Res.* 2015;16(108). 015-0265-8. https://doi.org/10.1186/s12931-015-0265-8.
109. Meek RL, Eriksen N, Benditt EP. Murine serum amyloid A3 is a high density apolipoprotein and is secreted by macrophages. *Proc Natl Acad Sci U S A.* 1992;89(17):7949–7952.
110. Zhang Y, Chen X, Hu Y, et al. Preliminary characterizations of a serum biomarker for sarcoidosis by comparative proteomic approach with tandem-mass spectrometry in ethnic han Chinese patients. *Respir Res.* 2013;14:18–9921. https://doi.org/10.1186/1465-9921-14-18.
111. Bargagli E, Magi B, Olivieri C, Bianchi N, Landi C, Rottoli P. Analysis of serum amyloid A in sarcoidosis patients. *Respir Med.* 2011;105(5):775–780. https://doi.org/10.1016/j.rmed.2010.12.010.
112. Baggiolini M, Dewald B, Moser B. Human chemokines: an update. *Annu Rev Immunol.* 1997;15:675–705. https://doi.org/10.1146/annurev.immunol.15.1.675.
113. Agostini C, Cabrelle A, Calabrese F, et al. Role for CXCR6 and its ligand CXCL16 in the pathogenesis of T-cell alveolitis in sarcoidosis. *Am J Respir Crit Care Med.* 2005;172(10):1290–1298. https://doi.org/200501-142OC [pii].
114. Agostini C, Cassatella M, Zambello R, et al. Involvement of the IP-10 chemokine in sarcoid granulomatous reactions. *J Immunol.* 1998;161(11):6413–6420.
115. Katchar K, Eklund A, Grunewald J. Expression of Th1 markers by lung accumulated T cells in pulmonary sarcoidosis. *J Intern Med.* 2003;254(6):564–571. https://doi.org/1230 [pii].
116. Miotto D, Christodoulopoulos P, Olivenstein R, et al. Expression of IFN-gamma-inducible protein; monocyte chemotactic proteins 1, 3, and 4; and eotaxin in TH1- and TH2-mediated lung diseases. *J Allergy Clin Immunol.* 2001;107(4):664–670. https://doi.org/S0091-6749(01)23352-1 [pii].
117. Nishioka Y, Manabe K, Kishi J, et al. CXCL9 and 11 in patients with pulmonary sarcoidosis: a role of alveolar macrophages. *Clin Exp Immunol.* 2007;149(2):317–326. https://doi.org/CEI3423 [pii].
118. Piotrowski WJ, Mlynarski W, Fendler W, et al. Chemokine receptor CXCR3 ligands in bronchoalveolar lavage fluid: associations with radiological pattern, clinical course, and prognosis in sarcoidosis. *Pol Arch Med Wewn.* 2014;124(7–8):395–402. https://doi.org/AOP_14_044 [pii].
119. Su R, Nguyen ML, Agarwal MR, et al. Interferon-inducible chemokines reflect severity and progression in sarcoidosis. *Respir Res.* 2013;14:121–9921. https://doi.org/10.1186/1465-9921-14-121.
120. Su R, Li MM, Bhakta NR, et al. Longitudinal analysis of sarcoidosis blood transcriptomic signatures and disease outcomes. *Eur Respir J.* 2014;44(4):985–993. https://doi.org/10.1183/09031936.00039714.
121. Crouser ED, Fingerlin TE, Yang IV, et al. Application of "omics" and systems biology to sarcoidosis research. *Ann Am Thorac Soc.* 2017;14(Suppl 6):S445–S451. https://doi.org/10.1513/AnnalsATS.201707-567OT.
122. Crouser ED, Culver DA, Knox KS, et al. Gene expression profiling identifies MMP-12 and ADAMDEC1 as potential pathogenic mediators of pulmonary sarcoidosis. *Am J Respir Crit Care Med.* 2009;179(10):929–938. https://doi.org/10.1164/rccm.200803-490OC.
123. Koth LL, Solberg OD, Peng JC, Bhakta NR, Nguyen CP, Woodruff PG. Sarcoidosis blood transcriptome reflects lung inflammation and overlaps with tuberculosis. *Am J Respir Crit Care Med.* 2011;184(10):1153–1163. https://doi.org/10.1164/rccm.201106-1143OC.
124. Lockstone HE, Sanderson S, Kulakova N, et al. Gene set analysis of lung samples provides insight into pathogenesis of progressive, fibrotic pulmonary sarcoidosis. *Am J Respir Crit Care Med.* 2010;181(12):1367–1375. https://doi.org/10.1164/rccm.200912-1855OC.

125. Zhou T, Zhang W, Sweiss NJ, et al. Peripheral blood gene expression as a novel genomic biomarker in complicated sarcoidosis. *PLoS One*. 2012;7(9):e44818. https://doi.org/10.1371/journal.pone.0044818.
126. Haggmark A, Hamsten C, Wiklundh E, et al. Proteomic profiling reveals autoimmune targets in sarcoidosis. *Am J Respir Crit Care Med*. 2015;191(5):574–583. https://doi.org/10.1164/rccm.201407-1341OC.
127. Dragonieri S, Brinkman P, Mouw E, et al. An electronic nose discriminates exhaled breath of patients with untreated pulmonary sarcoidosis from controls. *Respir Med*. 2013;107(7):1073–1078. https://doi.org/10.1016/j.rmed.2013.03.011.

CHAPTER 20

Antiinflammatory Therapy

ROBERT PHILLIP BAUGHMAN, MD • W. ENNIS JAMES, MD

INTRODUCTION

Overall treatment of sarcoidosis includes modulating the inflammatory response of the granuloma, dealing with the resulting fibrosis, or managing the noninflammatory manifestations of the disease. For the most part the fibrosis seen in sarcoidosis is best left alone. In some cases the damage can be removed, such as removing a cataract. In other cases one has to deal with the consequences of the damage, such as an aspergilloma in an area of bronchiectasis. Elsewhere in this book, manifestations that usually do not respond to antiinflammatory therapy are discussed.

In treating the inflammation of sarcoidosis, several possible targets have been identified. These include general targets such as the CD4-positive lymphocyte and the macrophage, as well as specific targets such as tumor necrosis factor (TNF). Over the years, treatments have focused on the initial inflammatory reaction leading to the granuloma formation (Fig. 20.1). Glucocorticoids are the classic agents that inhibit both macrophage and lymphocyte activation.[1,2] They are the prototype drugs for treating sarcoidosis. However, they have significant side effects associated with long-term use, and alternatives have been sought for years.

Cytotoxic drugs such as methotrexate and leflunomide inhibit inflammatory response of macrophages and other inflammatory cells in two ways. The first is by inhibiting the release of one or more cytokines from macrophages. For example, methotrexate at low doses has antiinflammatory activity which is complex, but includes potentiation of adenosine signaling.[3] At high doses, methotrexate is toxic to the bone marrow. Although leukopenia is an acknowledged toxicity of methotrexate, it is not a requirement for drug effectiveness. The second way in which cytotoxic agents such as azathioprine and mycophenolate inhibit inflammation is by inhibiting macrophage and lymphocyte function. Azathioprine and, to a lesser extent, mycophenolate both cause bone marrow suppression. However, this does not appear to have a role in their treatment as antiinflammatory agents.

Other drugs have direct effect on one or more cytokines generated by macrophages and other inflammatory cells. Thalidomide and pentoxifylline (a phosphodiesteare-4 inhibitor) reduce TNF release by macrophages.[4,5] Hydroxychloroquine also inhibits the inflammatory response of the activated macrophage.

Monoclonal antibodies against inflammatory cytokines have revolutionized the approach to treatment of inflammatory diseases such as rheumatoid arthritis and Crohn's disease. In sarcoidosis, anti-TNF antibodies have proved to be effective in patients who still have active disease despite glucocorticoids and other treatments.[6,7]

One key aspect of sarcoidosis is that more than half of the time, the granulomatous reaction resolves.[8] In nearly half of the patients, systemic treatment is not required.[8,9] In fact, the use of systemic therapy in the first 6 months is associated with a higher risk for long-term treatment of the sarcoidosis.[10,11] As we better understand the cause for persistent disease, we may develop more treatments to lead to resolution of the condition.

INDIVIDUAL TREATMENTS OF SARCOIDOSIS

The first question is always whether to start therapy. At least half of the patients never require systemic therapy.[10,12] The decision to start therapy should be based on one of the two reasons: to avoid danger or to improve quality of life.[13] Table 20.1 lists some examples for each of the two broad categories. The decision about which therapy to use and when to use it is a step-wise approach, summarized in Fig. 20.2. Based on the level of evidence in the literature and the strength of that evidence, we graded the level of support for individual therapies. This was a modification of prior

Sarcoidosis. https://doi.org/10.1016/B978-0-323-54429-0.00020-3

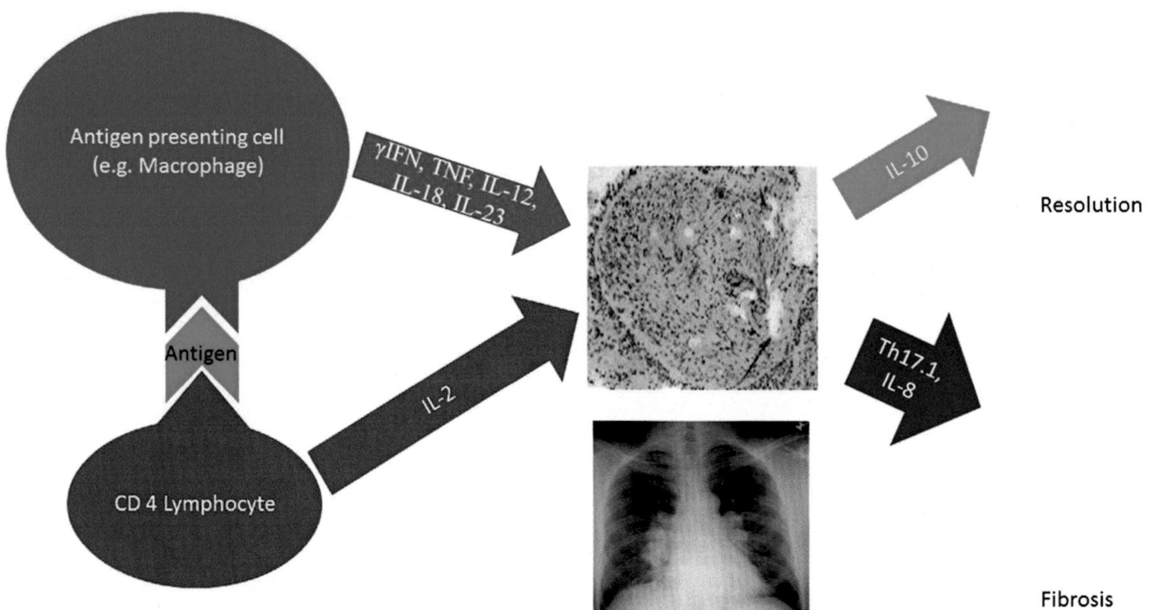

FIG. 20.1 The inflammatory response of sarcoidosis and potential targets for immunomodulatory therapy. *IL*, interleukin; *IFN*, interferon; *TNF*, tumor necrosis factor.

TABLE 20.1
Reasons to Treat in Sarcoidosis

DANGER OF ORGAN FAILURE

• Respiratory
  • Pulmonary fibrosis
  • Pulmonary hypertension

• Cardiac
• Neurologic
• Liver
• Ocular
• Renal
• Hypercalcemia
QUALITY OF LIFE

• Pulmonary
  • Cough
  • Dyspnea

• Cosmetically important skin lesions
• Nephrolithiasis
• Fatigue[a]
• Small-fiber neuropathy[a]

[a]Not likely to respond to antiinflammatory therapy alone.
Adapted from REF.

grading systems.[14] We will now discuss the specific levels of therapy.

FIRST LINE

The oral corticosteroids prednisone and prednisolone are the most commonly used drugs in treating sarcoidosis. There have been several studies of glucocorticoids (GCs) for treating pulmonary and extrapulmonary disease.[15,16] However, there are major limitations for most of these trials including lack of placebo control, variation of dosing and duration of treatment, and variable end points used.[17,18] Despite these limitations, there have been at least five randomized, placebo-controlled trials leading to sufficient evidence to support the use of GCs in pulmonary sarcoidosis (Table 20.2).

The use of GCs in extrapulmonary disease has also been reported. However, for advanced disease such as cardiac, neurologic, or lupus pernio, the long-term use of GCs may lead to more toxicity than benefit. For cardiac disease, there are no randomized, placebo-controlled trials demonstrating efficacy. However, there have been several case series demonstrating evidence for GCs in treating cardiac sarcoidosis. For patients with cardiomyopathy, improvement in left ventricular ejection fraction (LVEF) has been reported.[19–22] Some studies have reported that patients with a low LVEF

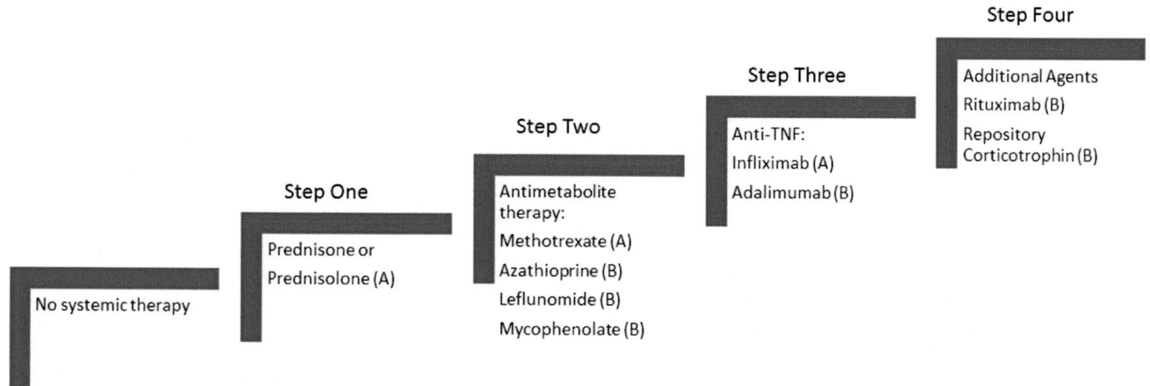

FIG. 20.2 A step-wise approach to therapy for sarcoidosis. Based on level of evidence the recommendation for treatment were graded as: **(A)**: at least one double-blind placebo-controlled trial demonstrating efficacy; **(B)**: at least one prospective or two or more retrospective studies demonstrating efficacy; **(C)**: at least one retrospective study demonstrating effectiveness. *CLEAR*, concurrent levofloxacin, ethambutol, azithromycin, and rifampin; *TNF*, tumor necrosis factor.

TABLE 20.2
Evidence for the Use of Glucocorticoids for Pulmonary Sarcoidosis

Outcome	Studies	Number of Patients Studied	Treatment Duration	Duration Follow-Up	Treatment Effect	Quality of Evidence[a]
Radiographic improvement	5 RCTs[8,146–150]	569	3 mo–2 y	6 mo–3.5 y	Supports CS use	Inconsistent results and risk of bias
Improvement in FVC	3 RCTs[8,146–148]	409	3 mo–2 y	18 mo–4 y	Supports CS use	Inconsistent results across studies
Improvement in DLCO	2 RCTs[8,146,147]	228	3 mo–2 y	4–5 y	Supports CS use	Inconsistent results and risk of bias

CS, corticosteroids; *DLCO*, diffusing capacity for carbon monoxide; *FVC*, forced vital capacity; *RCT*, randomized clinical trials.
Adapted from James WE, Baughman R. Treatment of sarcoidosis: grading the evidence. *Expert Rev Clin Pharmacol.* 2018;1–11.
[a]See text.

(less than 40%) were unlikely to respond to GC therapy,[23] but this was not observed in other studies.[19,20] In one study the positive effect of GCs on LVEF waned over time.[24] For neurologic disease, GC therapy alone was effective in about a third of patients.[25,26] For lupus pernio, GC therapy was associated with reduction of skin lesions, but total regression was far less frequent than with other agents.[27]

The dose and duration of GC use are unclear. The trials in Table 20.2 used different doses and durations of therapy. For example, the usual initial dose of prednisone for pulmonary sarcoidosis had been 20–40 mg a day.[28] However, a recent study found no relationship between the dose of prednisone and the improvement in force vital capacity (FVC) for patients treated for the first time for pulmonary sarcoidosis.[29] In another study the dose of 20 mg or more of prednisone was associated with improvement in acute deterioration of pulmonary sarcoidosis.[30] In cardiac sarcoidosis there was no difference in improvement in LVEF for those treated with more or less than 30 mg/day of prednisone.[23] All of these studies were retrospective and did not allow for variation of response to prednisone for the individual patient. However, these studies support the recommendation that the initial dose of prednisone be 20–30 mg a day or its equivalent. Neurologic disease may be refractory to that low dose,[25,26] and recommendations are usually made to use a higher initial dose for neurosarcoidosis.[31]

The concept of an induction dose for a minimal duration has been a basic premise of sarcoidosis treatment.[32,33] The duration of this induction phase is often 1–3 months.[28] However, there is increasing evidence that the duration of this induction phase can be much shorter. In treating acute deterioration of pulmonary sarcoidosis, it was noted that treatment for as little as 2 weeks reversed the process.[30] In a prospective study of daily pulmonary function testing after initiation of GC therapy, Broos et al. found that improvement in FVC leveled off by 2 weeks.[34] These studies suggest that tapering of GC therapy can be done within a month of starting treatment.

Because GC therapy in sarcoidosis is often for months to years,[33] patients are at risk for toxicity. GC toxicity has been noted in sarcoidosis and other conditions. These include weigh gain, diabetes, hypertension, mood swings, insomnia, osteoporosis, gastroesophageal reflux, cataracts, glaucoma, and acne. Past studies found that patients receiving the equivalent of 10 mg a day or more of prednisone were more likely to report these effects.[35] For many clinicians, patients who were able to be maintained on 10 mg or less of prednisone a day were considered on a "safe" dose of prednisone and did not require steroid-sparing therapy unless the patient had specific GC-associated toxicity.[28,32] For many patients with sarcoidosis, long-term therapy with this stable dose of prednisone had become the standard form of therapy.[36,37]

Recent studies have pointed out that toxicity can occur even at low doses of corticosteroids, especially with prolonged therapy. One study found that weight gain, a marker for steroid toxicity, was encountered even at doses as little as 5 mg a day of prednisone when patients were on more than a few months of therapy.[29] Others have noted increase risk for multiple toxicities. In a recent retrospective study comparing GC versus no GC therapy, the overall rate of complications which could be made worse was twice as high as those receiving GC (Fig. 20.3).[38] In analyzing patient-reported outcomes, significantly worse scores were reported for patients receiving the equivalent of more than 5 mg prednisone a day for more than 6 months.[39] These reports are not surprising because the cumulative risk of GC toxicity for long-term therapy has been well established in rheumatoid arthritis and other chronic inflammatory conditions.

SECOND LINE

As shown in Fig. 20.2, there are several drugs that have been studied as second-line therapy for sarcoidosis. For the most part, these immunomodulators are cytotoxic

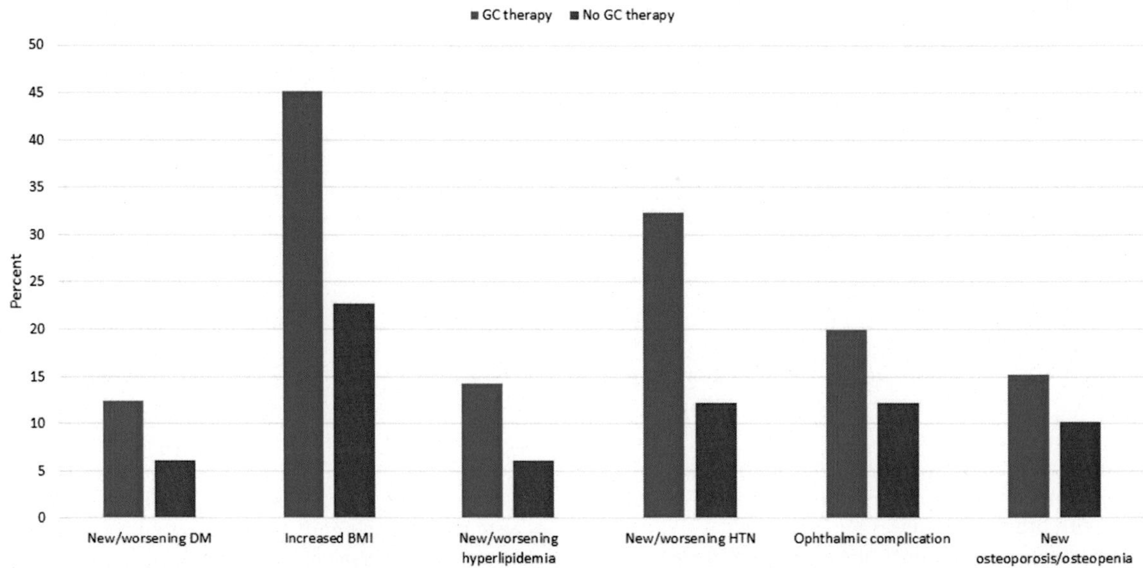

FIG. 20.3 Rate of complications seen in sarcoidosis patients observed on glucocorticoid (GC) therapy or not. *DM*, diabetes mellitus; *BMI*, body mass index; *HTN*, hypertension. *Significant difference between GC and No GC therapy, *P* = .01. (Adapted from the study by Khan NA, Donatelli CV, Tonelli AR, et al. Toxicity risk from glucocorticoids in sarcoidosis patients. *Respir Med*. 2017;132:9–14. https://doi.org/10.1016/j.rmed.2017.09.003.)

agents. Many of these cytotoxic agents had been used for chronic sarcodiosis.[40,41] Early studies limited the use of these drugs to short periods of time, mostly because of concerns regarding toxicity. Today, prolonged use of these drugs is common. Several reports have found that these drugs have similar rate of response but different toxicities.[42–44]

Methotrexate: The first drug widely used for prolonged therapy in sarcoidosis was methotrexate.[45] Early reports indicated that the drug could be used for patients in up to 2 years without difficulty in chronic sarcoidosis.[46] Table 20.3 summarizes the evidence supporting the use of methotrexate for pulmonary sarcoidosis. Several studies reported on the effect of therapy on pulmonary function. To date, there has been one double-blind, placebo-controlled trial demonstrating that methotrexate was steroid sparing.[47] That study did not demonstrate an improvement in pulmonary function with the addition of methotrexate to prednisone therapy. However, the study was able to demonstrate a significant reduction in prednisone dose after 6 months of therapy which was associated with a significant reduction in weight gain compared with the placebo group.

Methotrexate has also been reported as effective in nonpulmonary sarcoidosis. In particular, it has been effective in two-thirds of patients with neurologic disease, including patients failing prednisone alone.[25] In a study of cardiac sarcoidosis comparing methotrexate and low-dose prednisone with prednisone alone, the investigators found both drugs were equally effective. However, the effectiveness of prednisone waned over time, whereas methotrexate's effectiveness persisted for 3 years.[24] For ocular disease, methotrexate has also been an effective steroid-sparing agent.[48] Methotrexate is often used in combination with other agents to minimize the dosage of prednisone and other GC in management of sarcoidosis. Fig. 20.4 demonstrates the outcome of methotrexate therapy for 365 patients with ocular sarcoidosis treated at one center.[48] The figure demonstrates that methotrexate is usually well tolerated. However, treatment is often with multiple agents. The goal is to minimize toxicity by using the lowest effective dose of each drug.

The recommended dose of methotrexate is between 10 and 15 mg once a week.[49] This dose is lower than that used in rheumatoid arthritis or psoriasis. It reflects the concern regarding bone marrow suppression of the drug. It is not clear that higher doses have additional benefit in sarcoidosis. Nausea is a dose-related toxicity of methotrexate. Use of folic acid supplements reduced methotrexate-associated toxicity in one randomized placebo-controlled trial.[50] However, another study failed to demonstrate changes in the rate of gastrointestinal toxicity for those taking 10 mg or less a week.[51] Some clinicians advocate subcutaneous injection of methotrexate to reduce toxicity,[49] although this has not been systematically studied in sarcoidosis.

Leukopenia and anemia are other commonly encountered toxicity risks in sarcoidosis.[52,53] However, the use of low doses of methotrexate with routine monitoring can minimize the risk for bone marrow toxicity from methotrexate.[49] Liver toxicity is another recognized potential complication of methotrexate.[54] Screening for methotrexate hepatotoxicity in high-risk patients by routine liver biopsy has been advocated by some groups.[55] In one study of a 100 liver biopsies of patients receiving methotrexate for two or more years, the risk for liver toxicity was low.[56] Current recommendations are monitoring liver function tests for patients

TABLE 20.3
Evidence for Use of Methotrexate in Pulmonary Sarcoidosis

Outcome	Studies	Number of Patients	Treatment Duration	Treatment Effect	Quality of Evidence
Reduction of steroid dose (MTX vs. placebo)	1 RCT[47]	15	12 months	Favors MTX	High
Improvement in FVC	3 obs studies[43,46,151] No change RCT[47]	385	6 mo–2 y	Favors MTX	Low
Improvement in FEV1	1 obs study[151]	186	6 mo–2 y	Favors MTX	Low
Improvement in DLCO	2 obs studies[43,151]	331	6 mo–2 y	Favors MTX	Low

DLCO, diffusing capacity for carbon monoxide; *FEV1*, Forced expiratory volume 1 s; *FVC*, forced vital capacity; *MTX*, methotrexate; *obs*, observational; *RCT*, randomized clinical trial.
Adapted from James WE, Baughman R. Treatment of sarcoidosis: grading the evidence. *Expert Rev Clin Pharmacol.* 2018;1–11.

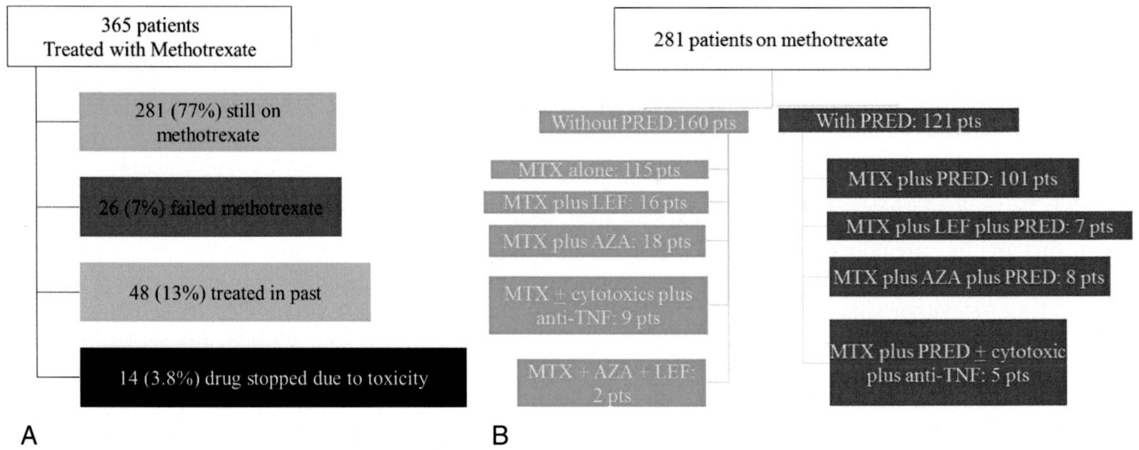

FIG. 20.4 Results of methotrexate therapy in a cohort of ocular sarcoidosis patients treated at University of Cincinnati.[48] Fig. 20.3A shows the outcome over time of patients started on methotrexate. Fig. 20.3B shows the final treatment regimens for those patients still on methotrexate at time of final evaluation.

TABLE 20.4
Evidence for Use of Azathioprine for Pulmonary Sarcoidosis

Outcome	Studies	Participants	Treatment Duration	Treatment Effect	Quality of Evidence
Steroid dose reduction	1 obs study[43]	55	2y	Favors AZA	Low
Radiographic improvement	3 obs study[58–60]	30	6m	Favors AZA	Very low
Improvement in FVC/FEV1/ DLCO	2 obs study[43,58]	66	2y	Favors AZA	Low

AZA, azathioprine; *CS*, corticosteroids; *DLCO*, diffusing capacity for carbon monoxide; *FEV1*, Forced expiratory volume in 1 s; *FVC*, forced vital capacity; *MTX*, methotrexate; *obs*, observational.
Adapted from James WE, Baughman R. Treatment of sarcoidosis: grading the evidence. *Expert Rev Clin Pharmacol*. 2018;1–11.

on methotrexate. Patients with new and persistent (two or more tests) elevations of the transaminases should have drug discontinued.[49] Methotrexate can also cause a hypersensitivity pneumonitis.[57] As more cytotoxic agents have become available, the willingness to go to another drug has made it less necessary to fully evaluate patients with potential hepatic or pulmonary toxicity.

Azathioprine has been another widely used cytotoxic agent, although there is limited evidence to support its effectiveness in sarcoidosis (Table 20.4). Azathioprine has mostly been reported as second-line therapy. One report found significant improvement in inflammatory markers, including bronchoalveolar lavage (BAL) findings with azathioprine therapy.[58] A large retrospective study found that azathioprine could be steroid sparing and associated with improvement in pulmonary function studies.[43] In that study, azathioprine was associated with more drug discontinuations than a group of patients treated with methotrexate. Other studies have demonstrated some radiographic improvement for patients treated with azathioprine,[59] but others did not find significant response with azathioprine.[60]

The usual dose of azathioprine is 50–200 mg daily. The dose is determined by drug toxicity. Leukopenia can be a significant problem, especially in those with thiopurine S-methyltransferase (TPMT) deficiency. Some have advocated measurements of TPMT in all patients, whereas others have advocated selective testing.[61] In any case, one should check the complete blood count after starting azathioprine to look for bone marrow toxicity. Bone marrow suppression is more common with azathioprine than methotrexate. There is an increased risk for infections requiring antibiotics in patients treated with azathioprine versus methotrexate.[43] Other

TABLE 20.5
Evidence for Use of Leflunomide and Mycophenolate for Pulmonary Sarcoidosis

Outcome	Studies	Number of Patients Studied	Treatment Duration	Duration of Follow-Up	Treatment Effect	Quality of Evidence
LEFLUNOMIDE						
Steroid dose reduction	1 obs study[67]	33	≥6 mo	>6 mo	Favors leflunomide	Low
Improvement in FVC	2 obs studies[67,68]	49	≥6 mo	>6 mo	Favors leflunomide	Low
MYCOPHENOLATE						
Steroid dose reduction	2 obs studies[32,33]	47	≥6 mo	>6 mo	Favors mycophenolate	Low
Improvement in FVC	2 obs studies[32,33]	47	6–33 mo	6–33 mo	Equivocal	Very low

DLCO, diffusing capacity for carbon monoxide; *FEV1*, Forced expiratory volume in 1 s; *FVC*, forced vital capacity; *obs*, observational; m, month.
Adapted from James WE, Baughman R. Treatment of sarcoidosis: grading the evidence. *Expert Rev Clin Pharmacol*. 2018;1–11.

problems with azathioprine include nausea, vomiting, hepatotoxicity, and increased risk for nonmelanoma skin cancers.[62,63] A recent study examining risk for myelodysplastic syndrome and/or acute myeloid leukemia in treating patients with autoimmune diseases found that azathioprine use was associated with an unadjusted odds ratio of 7.05, whereas methotrexate was associated with an odds ratio of 0.60.[64] In comparing antimetabolite agents for chronic inflammatory indications, methotrexate was significantly better tolerated than azathioprine.[65,66]

Leflunomide has also been reported as effective in treating pulmonary and extrapulmonary sarcoidosis. The two largest series were observational studies (Table 20.5).[67,68] These studies included patients with extrapulmonary disease, especially ocular disease.[68] Toxicity was similar to that encountered with methotrexate. However, several patients in both series had been switched from methotrexate to leflunomide because of intolerance to methotrexate. The most common reasons to switch were gastrointestinal nausea and cough. Leflunomide can lead to pulmonary toxicity,[69] but the rate is much lower than that encountered with methotrexate. Leflunomide therapy is associated with peripheral neuropathy,[70] which is not a problem with methotrexate.

There has been reported synergism in giving leflunomide with methotrexate.[71] The combination was not associated with increased toxicity compared with methotrexate alone. In some cases, concurrent leflunomide and methotrexate were effective in treating sarcoidosis.[68]

Mycophenolate has also been used in patients with sarcoidosis.[44,72] There have been retrospective case series of use in pulmonary sarcoidosis patients (Table 20.5). The drug appears to be as effective as other antimetabolites for pulmonary sarcoidosis. Patients switched from methotrexate to mycophenolate because of methotrexate intolerance did respond to the mycophenolate. However, those switched because of lack of efficacy of methotrexate also failed to respond to mycophenolate.[44]

The role of mycophenolate in extrapulmonary disease depends somewhat on which manifestation is being treated. Uveitis seems fairly responsive to mycophenolate.[73] This is in line with a large retrospective series of antimetabolites for chronic uveitis, in which mycophenolate was superior to methotrexate and azathioprine.[65] Mycophenolate was reported as effective for neurologic disease but not myopathy.[74] For neurologic disease, mycophenolate has been preferred by some specialists because its onset of action appears to be more rapid than methotrexate.[75] However, one retrospective study found that neurosarcoidosis patients treated with mycophenolate were more likely to relapse than those treated with methotrexate.[76]

STEP THREE

As demonstrated in Fig. 20.2, the next step for patients who fail antimetabolite therapy are monoclonal antibodies directed against TNF. Table 20.6 summarizes the use of infliximab and adalimumab for pulmonary

TABLE 20.6
Evidence for Use of Infliximab and Adalimumab for Sarcoidosis

Outcome	Studies	Number of Patients Studied	Treatment Duration	Duration of Follow-Up	Treatment Effect	Quality of Evidence
INFLIXIMAB						
Improvement in FVC	2 RCTs[6,79] 4 obs studies[7,152–154]	236	6 wk–46 mo	12 wk–46 mo	Favors IFX use	Moderate, due to inconsistency
Improvement in chest X-ray	1 RCT[81]	129	6 mo	12 mo	Favors IFX use	High
Improvement in symptoms/QoL	1 RCT[6] 2 obs study[7,154]	209	24 wk–46 mo	24 wk–46 mo	Favors IFX use (RCT-no; obs study-yes)	Low, due to inconsistency and indirectness
Improvement in 6-minute walk distance	1 RCT[80]	138	24 wk	52 wk	Favors IFX use	High
ADALIMUMAB						
Improvement in FVC	4 obs studies[93,94,155,156]	43	12–52 wk	12–52 wk	Favors Ada use	Low, due to inconsistency
Improvement in symptoms/QoL	3 obs studies[93,155,156]	25	12–52 wk	12–52 wk	Favors Ada use	Low, due to inconsistency

Ada, adalimumab; *FVC*, forced vital capacity; *IFX*, infliximab; *obs*, observational; *QoL*, quality of life; *RCT*, randomized clinical trials.
Adapted from James WE, Baughman R. Treatment of sarcoidosis: grading the evidence. *Expert Rev Clin Pharmacol.* 2018;1–11.

sarcoidosis. There are also several other studies using these agents for extrapulmonary disease.

Infliximab is the most widely studied and used anti-TNF monoclonal antibody.[77,78] There have been two double-blind, placebo-controlled trials of infliximab for advanced pulmonary disease.[6,79] The larger one include more than 130 patients and examined multiple end points, including FVC, chest X-ray changes, quality of life (QoL), and 6-minute walk distance.[6] While the overall change in FVC of infliximab versus placebo was only an absolute change of 2.5%, response rate of infliximab versus placebo was larger when certain features were present. These included an FVC% predicted below the median of the study patients, disease being present for more than 2 years, or a C-reactive protein (CRP) that was elevated.[6,80] These results are summarized in Fig. 20.5. Also noted in that study were patients who had a reticulonodular pattern on chest X-ray were more likely to respond to infliximab.[81] Others have noted that the higher the FDG activity in the lung parenchyma, the better the response to infliximab.[7] On the other hand, those patients receiving 20 mg or more of prednisone daily were unlikely to have further improvement in their FVC when treated with infliximab.[82]

Infliximab has proven useful for extrapulmonary disease. For cutaneous sarcoidosis, the response is often rapid and can be quite dramatic.[83] One large retrospective study found infliximab was superior to all other therapies, including prednisone, in inducing a remission of lupus pernio.[84] Others have noted a good initial response but point out disease may relapse when therapy is withdrawn.[85] The efficacy of infliximab for treating chronic cutaneous sarcoidosis was confirmed in a double-blind, placebo-controlled trial.[86]

Another indication for infliximab has been neurologic disease.[75] Two recent studies have demonstrated efficacy in patients who failed other treatments.[87,88] While both of these studies reported a high response rate, they both found that there was significant toxicity, often leading to drug withdrawal. Unfortunately, drug withdrawal was associated with a high rate of recurrence of disease.

Uveitis and retinal vasculitis have been shown to be responsive to anti-TNF therapy.[89,90] This has been verified in smaller series of sarcoidosis-associated uveitis.[91,92] These two anti-TNF antibodies appear to have similar effectiveness for treating refractory uveitis.[90]

Adalimumab has also been reported as effective in treating sarcoidosis (Table 20.6). As a humanized

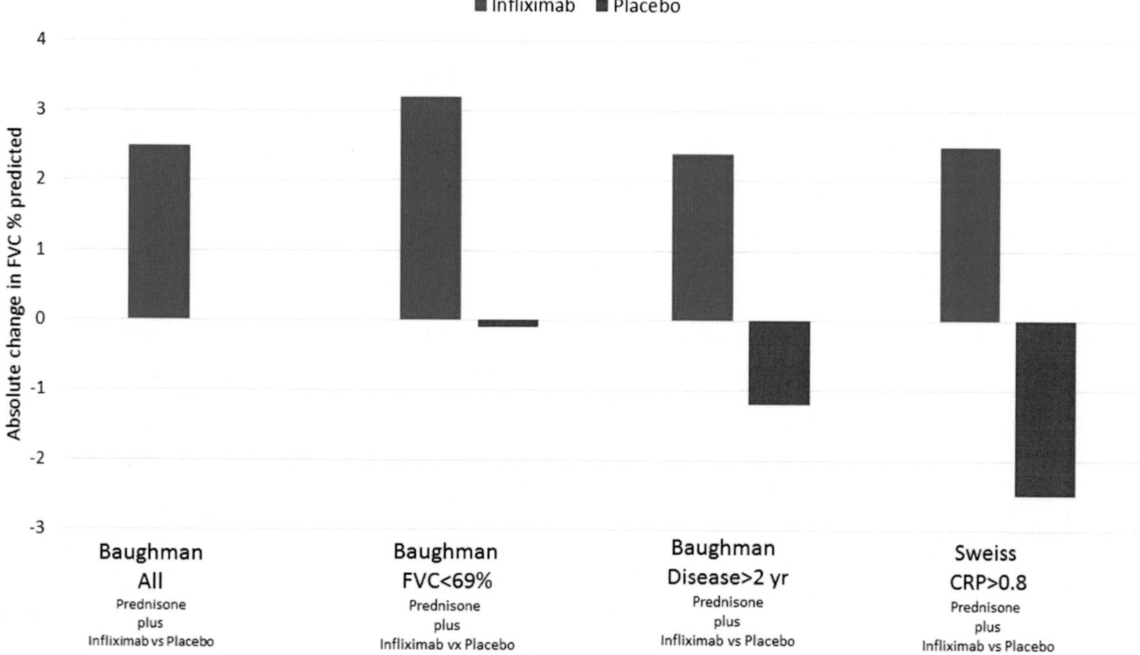

FIG. 20.5 Analysis of a large placebo-controlled trial of infliximab for chronic pulmonary sarcoidosis.[6] Absolute change in FVC% predicted for all patients as well as several subgroups: those below the median of FVC% predicted, disease being present for more than 2 years, or a C-reactive protein (CRP) that was elevated.[6,80] *FVC*, force vital capacity; *TNF*, tumor necrosis factor.

TABLE 20.7
Indications to Consider Anti-TNF Monoclonal Antibody Therapy

• Chronic advanced pulmonary disease
• Evidence for ongoing inflammation
  • Elevated CRP
  • Increased soluble IL-2 receptor
  • Positive PET scan

• Lupus pernio
• Neurologic disease
• Refractory eye disease

CRP, C-reactive protein; *IL-2*, interleukin 2; *PET*, positron emission tomography.
Modified from Drent M, Cremers JP, Jansen TL, et al. Practical eminence and experience-based recommendations for use of TNF-alpha inhibitors in sarcoidosis. *Sarcoidosis Vasc Diffuse Lung Dis*. 2014;31(2):91–107.

monoclonal antibody, it has significantly lower risk for severe allergic reactions than infliximab. For pulmonary disease, there are no randomized trials. One prospective open-label study did demonstrate benefit for the majority of patients treated.[93] In another study, adalimumab was mostly used in patients who had become intolerant to infliximab. In that study, the drug was equally effective to infliximab.[94] In one retrospective study comparing infliximab with adalimumab, patients treated with infliximab had a higher rate and more rapid response than patients treated with adalimumab.[95]

There are additional studies of the use of adalimumab for extrapulmonary disease. In a series of 26 sarcoidosis patients with chronic uveitis, adalimumab was found effective.[96] In large randomized trials of patients with chronic uveitis, including those with sarcoidosis, adalimumab was superior to placebo.[97,98] Infliximab and adalimumab appear to have similar effectiveness for treating refractory uveitis.[90] In a double-blind, randomized trial, adalimumab was shown to be more effective than placebo in treating chronic cutaneous sarcoidosis.[99]

Taken together, these various reports suggest that there are some indications for which an anti-TNF monoclonal antibody such as infliximab or adalimumab should be considered. These are summarized in Table 20.7.[77] While most of these recommendations are based on studies for infliximab, as noted previously, there are several studies supporting the use of adalimumab for sarcoidosis.

The use of other anti-TNF agents for sarcoidosis is less clear. Etanercept is a TNF receptor antagonist. It has been reported as effective in selected cases of sarcoidosis.[100,101] However, it was not found effective as a single agent in treating progressive pulmonary sarcoidosis.[102] In a double-blind, randomized trial, etanercept was not more effective than placebo in treating sarcoidosis-associated uveitis.[103] The lack of efficacy of a TNF receptor in sarcoidosis is similar to the failure of etanercept in treating Crohn's disease, another chronic granulomatous disease.[104] Golimumab is another humanized monoclonal antibody. In a large, double-blind, placebo-controlled trial, golimumab was no more effective than placebo in treating chronic pulmonary sarcoidosis.[105] These studies demonstrate that not all anti-TNF therapies are the same in treating sarcoidosis.

Interestingly, some anti-TNF–treated patients have developed a granulomatous reaction which appears "sarcoid like".[106,107] This seems to occur in less than 1 in 10,000.[106] However, these reports highlight the variable potential causes of a granulomatous reaction. Although TNF may be a crucial cytokine in the formation of granulomas, there are other possible mechanisms of granuloma formation.

FOURTH LINE

Several drugs have been possible alternatives to the anti-TNF therapies (Table 20.8). Some of these are supported by clinical trials for sarcoidosis patients, whereas others have been proposed based on their effectiveness in other pulmonary diseases. Two of the drugs (pirfenidone and nintenanib) have proven useful in treating idiopathic pulmonary fibrosis and are currently being studied in other fibrotic lung diseases.[108,109] This includes a double-blind, placebo-controlled trial of pirfenidone for sarcoidosis-associated pulmonary fibrosis (Clintrials registry NCT03260556). We will not discuss the treatment of sarcoidosis-associated pulmonary hypertension, the focus of another chapter in this book. Most of the drugs listed in Table 20.8 have anti-inflammatory properties.

Rituximab has been used as an alternative biologic agent for rheumatoid arthritis.[110] It has also been reported as effective in treating sarcoidosis. In a prospective, open-label trial of rituximab for refractory pulmonary sarcoidosis, seven of 10 patients had objective improvement of one or more aspects of lung disease.[111] In that study, patients received only the induction therapy of two treatments given 2 weeks apart. Over the year after treatment, all patients had resolution of improvement observed with rituximab therapy. In other reports, rituximab has been used for ocular, cutaneous, cardiac, and pulmonary disease.[112–115] In those

TABLE 20.8
New Treatments for Sarcoidosis

Currently used for sarcoidosis
• Rituximab[a]
• Repository corticotrophin injection (RCI)[a]
Not widely available/used in sarcoidosis
• CLEAR[a]
• Anakinra[a]
• Transdermal nicotine[a]
• Vasoactive intestinal peptide
• Mesenchymal stem cells
• Roflumilast[a]
• Aprelimast[a]
• Somatostatin receptor–directed peptide receptor radionuclide therapy[a]
• Pirfenidone[a]
• Nintenanib[a]

CLEAR, Concurrent Levaquin, Ethambutol, Azythromycin, Rifabutin.
[a]Commercially available in United States.

reports, patients were often placed on maintenance therapy. The frequency and duration of maintenance rituximab therapy is unclear.

It has also been reported that a "sarcoid-like" reaction can occur after treatment with rituximab.[116,117] This may be part of the reduction of IgG levels seen with rituximab therapy. Rituximab can lead to hypogammaglobulinemia. Common variable immune deficiency can lead to a granulomatous disease identical to sarcoidosis.[118] Once again, immune manipulation points out the multiple pathways leading to sarcoidosis.

Repository corticotropin injection (RCI) was first approved by the Food and Drug Administration for treating sarcoidosis in 1952. Although early studies reported that it was very effective for sarcoidosis,[119] it was quickly replaced by prednisone and other oral glucocorticoids when these became available in the late 1950s. However, with the discovery of melanocortin receptors (MCRs) on various inflammatory and other tissue cells,[120] the role of RCI in treating sarcoidosis has been reinvestigated. Treatment has been limited to those with advanced disease who have contraindications or have failed other third-line therapies. In a retrospective study from two centers, two-third of patients were able to tolerate at least 3 months of RCI therapy.[121] For those patients, more than 90% had either significant steroid reduction or improvement of their disease. In a prospective single-blind study of advanced pulmonary disease, RCI was found to be steroid sparing.[122] In addition, it was associated with improvement in lung diffusion, positron emission tomography (PET) scan activity, and health-related quality of life. The most commonly reported side effects have been agitation and edema. These seem to be associated with the increased endogenous cortisol released on the day of the injection. Current regimen is to give 40–80 units twice a week. A double-blind, placebo-controlled trial of this drug for pulmonary sarcoidosis is underway (Clintrials registry NCT03320070).

Other regimens have been proposed based on either small series of case reports or possible mechanisms of action. The combination of levofloxacin, ethambutol, azithromycin, and rifampin (CLEAR) has been studied in patients with advanced skin or pulmonary disease. In a single-masked, randomized trial of cutaneous sarcoidosis, CLEAR was associated with a significant improvement in skin lesions as well as marked reduction of the inflammatory pathway.[123] In an open-label trial of pulmonary sarcoidosis, patients treated with CLEAR for 8 weeks had significant improvement in their FVC.[124] These two studies had significant drop outs because of drug toxicity. A large, double-blind placebo-controlled trial of CLEAR is underway (Clintrials registry NCT02024555). In the present study, rifabutin has been substituted for rifampin to reduce potential toxicity.

Sarcoidosis patients are much less likely to be smokers than the general population. Nicotine has anti-inflammatory activity. Crouser et al. proposed that transdermal nicotine may treat sarcoidosis. In the first trial of pulmonary sarcoidosis, transdermal nicotine did reduce the inflammatory response in the lung but had no significant impact on lung function or chest imaging.[125] A larger double-blind trial is underway (Clintrials registry NCT02265874).

Vasoactive intestinal peptide (VIP) has also been reported to be an immunomodulator in pulmonary sarcoidosis. In an open-label, single-arm trial, Prasse et al. demonstrated that inhaled VIP significantly reduced the inflammatory cells found in the BAL of active sarcoidosis patients.[126] In particular, they demonstrated downregulation of Treg cells. However, there was no impact on pulmonary function in this small study. A larger trial will be required to determine the role of VIP in sarcoidosis.

Phosphodiesterase 4 (PDE-4) inhibition has been shown to inhibit the release of TNF from alveolar macrophages (AMs).[5,127] This is especially true in blocking the increased spontaneous release of TNF of AM retrieved from patients with active sarcoidosis. There have been studies demonstrating some benefit with pentoxifylline, a PDE-4 inhibitor, in sarcoidosis.[128] In a randomized, placebo-controlled trial, pentoxifylline was found to be steroid sparing but did not improve lung function.[129] The gastrointestinal toxicity of pentoxifylline has been a limitation to its widespread use.

Apremilast is a new-generation oral PDE-4 inhibitor approved for treatment of refractory psoriasis and psoriatic arthritis.[130] In an open-label trial of chronic cutaneous sarcoidosis, 12 weeks of aprelimast was found to significantly reduce skin lesions.[131] Roflumilast is another commercially available PDE-4 inhibitor. It was found to reduce the number of acute exacerbations in chronic bronchitis patients.[132] The drug is currently being studied in chronic pulmonary sarcoidosis patients who have recurrent acute events similar to those seen in chronic bronchitis[133] (Clintrials registry NCT01830959).

Radioimaging of sarcoidosis has included gallium, FDG, and somatostatin markers.[134,135] All three have concentrated in areas of active inflammation. Somatostatin receptor–directed therapy has been used to treat neuroendocrine tumors. Lapa et al. reported on the use of somatostatin receptor–directed therapy for treating refractory sarcoidosis.[136,137] While this treatment was effective in the two cases reported, there are several areas of concern. The potential bone marrow suppression is incompletely understood. Also, repeat treatment was needed in at least one case. The overall cost needs to be considered in using this treatment.

Thalidomide was reported as effective for some patients with cutaneous sarcoidosis.[138–140] However, a randomized trial failed to demonstrate a significant difference.[141] These studies used different end points for evaluating skin disease.[142] In a study of pulmonary sarcoidosis, Judson et al. were only able to demonstrate a steroid-sparing effect of thalidomide in a subset of patients.[143]

Placenta-derived mesenchymal-like cells (PDMCs) have been used to "reset" the inflammatory response encountered in Crohn's disease.[144] In a pilot trial of four cases with refractory pulmonary sarcoidosis, PDMCs were found to be persistent in alveolar space for at least a week after treatment.[145] Two of four had some improvement on lung markers with therapy.

CONCLUSION

The decision to treat sarcoidosis should be made on the basis of Wells' law: treat only to avoid danger or to improve quality of life. Over the past 20 years, a range of antiinflammatory therapies have been developed to replace or supplement glucocorticoid therapy. For the patient and physician, a step-wise approach to therapy seems reasonable.

REFERENCES

1. Baughman RP, Lower EE. The effect of corticosteroid or methotrexate therapy on lung lymphocytes and macrophages in sarcoidosis. *Am Rev Respir Dis.* 1990;142:1268–1271.
2. Pinkston P, Saltini C, Muller-Quernheim J, et al. Corticosteroid therapy suppresses spontaneous interleukin 2 release and spontaneous proliferation of lung T lymphocytes of patients with active pulmonary sarcoidosis. *J Immunol.* 1987;139:755–760.
3. Brown PM, Pratt AG, Isaacs JD. Mechanism of action of methotrexate in rheumatoid arthritis, and the search for biomarkers. *Nat Rev Rheumatol.* 2016;12(12):731–742.
4. Tavares JL, Wangoo A, Dilworth P, et al. Thalidomide reduces tumour necrosis factor-alpha production by human alveolar macrophages. *Respir Med.* 1997;91(1):31–39.
5. Tong Z, Dai H, Chen B, et al. Inhibition of cytokine release from alveolar macrophages in pulmonary sarcoidosis by pentoxifylline: comparison with dexamethasone. *Chest.* 2003;124(4):1526–1532.
6. Baughman RP, Drent M, Kavuru M, et al. Infliximab therapy in patients with chronic sarcoidosis and pulmonary involvement. *Am J Respir Crit Care Med.* 2006;174(7):795–802.
7. Vorselaars AD, Crommelin HA, Deneer VH, et al. Effectiveness of infliximab in refractory FDG PET positive sarcoidosis. *Eur Respir J.* 2015;46:175–185.
8. Gibson GJ, Prescott RJ, Muers MF, et al. British Thoracic Society Sarcoidosis study: effects of long term corticosteroid treatment. *Thorax.* 1996;51(3):238–247.
9. Pietinalho A, Lindholm A, Haahtela T, et al. Inhaled budesonide for treatment of pulmonary sarcoidosis. Results of a double-blind, placebo-controlled, multicentre study. *Eur Respir J.* 1996;9(2):suppl 23: 406s.
10. Baughman RP, Judson MA, Teirstein A, et al. Presenting characteristics as predictors of duration of treatment in sarcoidosis. *QJM.* 2006;99(5):307–315.
11. Gottlieb JE, Israel HL, Steiner RM, et al. Outcome in sarcoidosis. The relationship of relapse to corticosteroid therapy. *Chest.* 1997;111(3):623–631.
12. Rizzato G, Montemurro L, Colombo P. The late follow-up of chronic sarcoid patients previously treated with corticosteroids. *Sarcoidosis.* 1998;15:52–58.
13. Baughman RP, Judson MA, Wells AU. The indications for the treatment of sarcoidosis: Wells law. *Sarcoidosis Vasc Diffuse Lung Dis.* 2017;34:280–282.
14. Guyatt G, Gutterman D, Baumann MH, et al. Grading strength of recommendations and quality of evidence in clinical guidelines: report from an American college of chest physicians task force. *Chest.* 2006;129(1):174–181.
15. Baughman RP, Nunes H. Therapy for sarcoidosis: evidence-based recommendations. *Expert Rev Clin Immunol.* 2012;8(1):95–103.
16. Baughman RP, Nunes H, Sweiss NJ, et al. Established and experimental medical therapy of pulmonary sarcoidosis. *Eur Respir J.* 2013;41:1424–1438.

17. Paramothayan NS, Lasserson TJ, Jones PW. Corticosteroids for pulmonary sarcoidosis. *Cochrane Database Syst Rev*. 2005;(2):CD001114.
18. James WE, Baughman R. Treatment of sarcoidosis: grading the evidence. *Expert Rev Clin Pharmacol*. 2018:1–11.
19. Padala SK, Peaslee S, Sidhu MS, et al. Impact of early initiation of corticosteroid therapy on cardiac function and rhythm in patients with cardiac sarcoidosis. *Int J Cardiol*. 2017;227:565–570. https://doi.org/10.1016/j.ijcard.2016.10.101. Epub;%2016 Nov 2.:565–570.
20. Zhou Y, Lower EE, LI HP, et al. Cardiac sarcoidosis: the impact of age and implanted devices on survival. *Chest*. 2017;151(1):139–148.
21. Sugisaki K, Yamaguchi T, Nagai S, et al. Clinical characteristics of 195 Japanese sarcoidosis patients treated with oral corticosteroids. *Sarcoidosis Vasc Diffuse Lung Dis*. 2003;20(3):222–226.
22. Sadek MM, Yung D, Birnie DH, et al. Corticosteroid therapy for cardiac sarcoidosis: a systematic review. *Can J Cardiol*. 2013;29(9):1034–1041.
23. Yazaki Y, Isobe M, Hiroe M, et al. Prognostic determinants of long-term survival in Japanese patients with cardiac sarcoidosis treated with prednisone. *Am J Cardiol*. 2001;88(Nov 1):1006–1010.
24. Nagai S, Yokomatsu T, Tanizawa K, et al. Treatment with methotrexate and low-dose corticosteroids in sarcoidosis patients with cardiac lesions. *Intern Med*. 2014;53(5):427–433.
25. Lower EE, Broderick JP, Brott TG, et al. Diagnosis and management of neurologic sarcoidosis. *Arch Intern Med*. 1997;157:1864–1868.
26. Agbogu BN, Stern BJ, Sewell C, et al. Therapeutic considerations in patients with refractory neurosarcoidosis. *Arch Neurol*. 1995;52:875–879.
27. Stagaki E, Mountford WK, Lackland DT, et al. The treatment of lupus pernio: results of 116 treatment courses in 54 patients. *Chest*. 2009;135(2):468–476.
28. Schutt AC, Bullington WM, Judson MA. Pharmacotherapy for pulmonary sarcoidosis: a Delphi consensus study. *Respir Med*. 2010;104(5):717–723.
29. Broos CE, Poell LHC, Looman CWN, et al. No evidence found for an association between prednisone dose and FVC change in newly-treated pulmonary sarcoidosis. *Respir Med*. 2018;(138S):S31–S37. https://doi.org/10.1016/j.rmed.2017.10.022.
30. McKinzie BP, Bullington WM, Mazur JE, et al. Efficacy of short-course, low-dose corticosteroid therapy for acute pulmonary sarcoidosis exacerbations. *Am J Med Sci*. 2010;339(1):1–4.
31. Scott TF, Yandora K, Valeri A, et al. Aggressive therapy for neurosarcoidosis: long-term follow-up of 48 treated patients. *Arch Neurol*. 2007;64(5):691–696.
32. Hunninghake GW, Costabel U, Ando M, et al. ATS/ERS/WASOG statement on sarcoidosis. American Thoracic Society/European Respiratory Society/World Association of sarcoidosis and other granulomatous disorders. *Sarcoidosis Vasc Diffuse Lung Dis*. 1999;16(Sep):149–173.
33. Judson MA. An approach to the treatment of pulmonary sarcoidosis with corticosteroids: the six phases of treatment. *Chest*. 1999;115(4):1158–1165.
34. Broos CE, Wapenaar M, Looman CWN, et al. Daily home spirometry to detect early steroid treatment effects in newly treated pulmonary sarcoidosis. *Eur Respir J*. 2018;51(1):51-1-2017.
35. Baughman RP, Iannuzzi MC, Lower EE, et al. Use of fluticasone for acute symptomatic pulmonary sarcoidosis. *Sarcoidosis Vasc Diffuse Lung Dis*. 2002;19:198–204.
36. Johns CJ, Michele TM. The clinical management of sarcoidosis: a 50-year experience at the Johns Hopkins hospital. *Medicine*. 1999;78:65–111.
37. Moller DR. Negative clinical trials in sarcoidosis: failed therapies or flawed study design? *Eur Respir J*. 2014;44(5):1123–1126.
38. Khan NA, Donatelli CV, Tonelli AR, et al. Toxicity risk from glucocorticoids in sarcoidosis patients. *Respir Med*. 2017;132:9–14. https://doi.org/10.1016/j.rmed.2017.09.003.
39. Judson MA, Chaudhry H, Louis A, et al. The effect of corticosteroids on quality of life in a sarcoidosis clinic: the results of a propensity analysis. *Respir Med*. 2015;109(4):526–531.
40. Israel HL. The treatment of sarcoidosis. *Postgrad Med J*. 1970;46:537–540.
41. Kataria YP. Chlorambucil in sarcoidosis. *Chest*. 1980;78:36–42.
42. Baughman RP, Lower EE. Alternatives to corticosteroids in the treatment of sarcoidosis. *Sarcoidosis*. 1997;14:121–130.
43. Vorselaars AD, Wuyts WA, Vorselaars VM, et al. Methotrexate versus azathioprine in second line therapy of sarcoidosis. *Chest*. 2013;144:805–812.
44. Hamzeh N, Voelker A, Forssen A, et al. Efficacy of mycophenolate mofetil in sarcoidosis. *Respir Med*. 2014;108:1663–1669.
45. Lower EE, Baughman RP. The use of low dose methotrexate in refractory sarcoidosis. *Am J Med Sci*. 1990;299:153–157.
46. Lower EE, Baughman RP. Prolonged use of methotrexate for sarcoidosis. *Arch Intern Med*. 1995;155:846–851.
47. Baughman RP, Winget DB, Lower EE. Methotrexate is steroid sparing in acute sarcoidosis: results of a double blind, randomized trial. *Sarcoidosis Vasc Diffuse Lung Dis*. 2000;17:60–66.
48. Baughman RP, Lower EE, Ingledue R, et al. Management of ocular sarcoidosis. *Sarcoidosis Vasc Diffuse Lung Dis*. 2012;29:26–33.
49. Cremers JP, Drent M, Bast A, et al. Multinational evidence-based World Association of Sarcoidosis and Other Granulomatous Disorders recommendations for the use of methotrexate in sarcoidosis: integrating systematic literature research and expert opinion of sarcoidologists worldwide. *Curr Opin Pulm Med*. 2013;19:545–561.
50. Morgan SL, Baggott JE, Vaughn WH, et al. Supplementation with folic acid during methotrexate therapy for rheumatoid arthritis. *Ann Intern Med*. 1994;121:833–841.

51. van Ede AE, Laan RF, Rood MJ, et al. Effect of folic or folinic acid supplementation on the toxicity and efficacy of methotrexate in rheumatoid arthritis: a forty-eight week, multicenter, randomized, double-blind, placebo-controlled study. *Arthritis Rheum*. 2001;44(7):1515–1524.
52. Lower EE, Smith JT, Martelo OJ, et al. The anemia of sarcoidosis. *Sarcoidosis*. 1988;5:51–55.
53. Browne PM, Sharma OP, Salkin D. Bone marrow sarcoidosis. *J Am Med Assoc*. 1978;240:43–50.
54. Schnabel A, Gross WL. Low-dose methotrexate in rheumatic diseases–efficacy, side effects, and risk factors for side effects. *Semin Arthritis Rheum*. 1994;23(5):310–327.
55. Thomas JA, Aithal GP. Monitoring liver function during methotrexate therapy for psoriasis: are routine biopsies really necessary? *Am J Clin Dermatol*. 2005;6(6):357–363.
56. Baughman RP, Koehler A, Bejarano PA, et al. Role of liver function tests in detecting methotrexate-induced liver damage in sarcoidosis. *Arch Intern Med*. 2003;163(5): 615–620.
57. Zisman DA, McCune WJ, Tino G, et al. Drug-induced pneumonitis: the role of methotrexate. *Sarcoidosis Vasc Diffuse Lung Dis*. 2001;18(3):243–252.
58. Muller-Quernheim J, Kienast K, Held M, et al. Treatment of chronic sarcoidosis with an azathioprine/prednisolone regimen. *Eur Respir J*. 1999;14(5):1117–1122.
59. Pacheco Y, Marechal C, Marechal F, et al. Azathioprine treatment of chronic pulmonary sarcoidosis. *Sarcoidosis*. 1985;2:107–113.
60. Lewis SJ, Ainslie GM, Bateman ED. Efficacy of azathioprine as second-line treatment in pulmonary sarcoidosis. *Sarcoidosis Vasc Diffuse Lung Dis*. 1999;16:87–92.
61. Hagaman JT, Kinder BW, Eckman MH. Thiopurine S-methyltranferase testing in idiopathic pulmonary fibrosis: a pharmacogenetic cost-effectiveness analysis. *Lung*. 2010;188(2):125–132.
62. Mackenzie KA, Wells JE, Lynn KL, et al. First and subsequent nonmelanoma skin cancers: incidence and predictors in a population of New Zealand renal transplant recipients. *Nephrol Dial Transplant*. 2009.
63. de Jong DJ, Goullet M, Naber TH. Side effects of azathioprine in patients with Crohn's disease. *Eur J Gastroenterol Hepatol*. 2004;16(2):207–212.
64. Ertz-Archambault N, Kosiorek H, Taylor GE, et al. Association of therapy for autoimmune disease with myelodysplastic syndromes and acute myeloid leukemia. *JAMA Oncol*. 2017;3(7):936–943.
65. Galor A, Jabs DA, Leder HA, et al. Comparison of antimetabolite drugs as corticosteroid-sparing therapy for noninfectious ocular inflammation. *Ophthalmology*. 2008;115(10):1826–1832.
66. Jeurissen ME, Boerbooms AM, van de Putte LB, et al. Methotrexate versus azathioprine in the treatment of rheumatoid arthritis. A forty-eight-week randomized, double-blind trial. *Arthritis Rheum*. 1991;34(8):961–972.
67. Sahoo DH, Bandyopadhyay D, Xu M, et al. Effectiveness and safety of leflunomide for pulmonary and extrapulmonary sarcoidosis. *Eur Respir J*. 2011;38:1145–1150.
68. Baughman RP, Lower EE. Leflunomide for chronic sarcoidosis. *Sarcoidosis Vasc Diffuse Lung Dis*. 2004;21:43–48.
69. Raj R, Nugent K. Leflunomide-induced interstitial lung disease (a systematic review). *Sarcoidosis Vasc Diffuse Lung Dis*. 2013;30(3):167–176.
70. Martin K, Bentaberry F, Dumoulin C, et al. Neuropathy associated with leflunomide: a case series. *Ann Rheum Dis*. 2005;64(4):649–650.
71. Kremer JM, Genovese MC, Cannon GW, et al. Concomitant leflunomide therapy in patients with active rheumatoid arthritis despite stable doses of methotrexate. A randomized, double-blind, placebo-controlled trial. *Ann Intern Med*. 2002;137(9):726–733.
72. Brill AK, Ott SR, Geiser T. Effect and safety of mycophenolate mofetil in chronic pulmonary sarcoidosis: a retrospective study. *Respiration*. 2013;86:376–383.
73. Bhat P, Cervantes-Castaneda RA, Doctor PP, et al. Mycophenolate mofetil therapy for sarcoidosis-associated uveitis. *Ocul Immunol Inflamm*. 2009;17(3):185–190.
74. Androdias G, Maillet D, Marignier R, et al. Mycophenolate mofetil may be effective in CNS sarcoidosis but not in sarcoid myopathy. *Neurology*. 2011;76(13):1168–1172.
75. Moravan M, Segal BM. Treatment of CNS sarcoidosis with infliximab and mycophenolate mofetil. *Neurology*. 2009;72(4):337–340.
76. Bitoun S, Bouvry D, Borie R, et al. Treatment of neurosarcoidosis: a comparative study of methotrexate and mycophenolate mofetil. *Neurology*. 2016;87(24):2517–2521.
77. Drent M, Cremers JP, Jansen TL, et al. Practical eminence and experience-based recommendations for use of TNF-alpha inhibitors in sarcoidosis. *Sarcoidosis Vasc Diffuse Lung Dis*. 2014;31(2):91–107.
78. Jamilloux Y, Cohen-Aubart F, Chapelon-Abric C, et al. Efficacy and safety of tumor necrosis factor antagonists in refractory sarcoidosis: a multicenter study of 132 patients. *Semin Arthritis Rheum*. 2017;47(2):288–294.
79. Rossman MD, Newman LS, Baughman RP, et al. A double-blind, randomized, placebo-controlled trial of infliximab in patients with active pulmonary sarcoidosis. *Sarcoidosis Vasc Diffuse Lung Dis*. 2006;23:201–208.
80. Sweiss NJ, Barnathan ES, Lo K, et al. C-reactive protein predicts response to infliximab in patients with chronic sarcoidosis. *Sarcoidosis Vasc Diffuse Lung Dis*. 2010;27:49–56.
81. Baughman RP, Shipley R, Desai S, et al. Changes in chest roentgenogram of sarcoidosis patients during a clinical trial of infliximab therapy: comparison of different methods of evaluation. *Chest*. 2009;136:526–535.
82. Judson MA, Baughman RP, Costabel U, et al. The potential additional benefit of infliximab in patients with chronic pulmonary sarcoidosis already receiving corticosteroids: a retrospective analysis from a randomized clinical trial. *Respir Med*. 2014;108(1):189–194.
83. Baughman RP, Lower EE. Infliximab for refractory sarcoidosis. *Sarcoidosis Vasc Diffuse Lung Dis*. 2001;18:70–74.

84. Stagaki E, Mountford WK, Lackland DT, et al. The treatment of lupus pernio: the results of 116 treatment courses in 54 patients. *Chest*. 2008.
85. Heidelberger V, Ingen-Housz-Oro S, Marquet A, et al. Efficacy and tolerance of anti-tumor necrosis factor alpha agents in cutaneous sarcoidosis: a French study of 46 cases. *JAMA Dermatol*. 2017;153(7):681–685.
86. Baughman RP, Judson MA, Lower EE, et al. Infliximab for chronic cutaneous sarcoidosis: a subset analysis from a double-blind randomized clinical trial. *Sarcoidosis Vasc Diffuse Lung Dis*. 2016;32(4):289–295.
87. Gelfand JM, Bradshaw MJ, Stern BJ, et al. Infliximab for the treatment of CNS sarcoidosis: a multi-institutional series. *Neurology*. 2017;89(20):2092–2100.
88. Cohen AF, Bouvry D, Galanaud D, et al. Long-term outcomes of refractory neurosarcoidosis treated with infliximab. *J Neurol*. 2017;264(5):891–897.
89. Fabiani C, Sota J, Rigante D, et al. Efficacy of adalimumab and infliximab in recalcitrant retinal vasculitis inadequately responsive to other immunomodulatory therapies. *Clin Rheumatol*. 2018:10–4133.
90. Vallet H, Seve P, Biard L, et al. Infliximab versus adalimumab in the treatment of refractory inflammatory uveitis: a multicenter study from the French uveitis network. *Arthritis Rheumatol*. 2016;68(6):1522–1530.
91. Riancho-Zarrabeitia L, Calvo-Rio V, Blanco R, et al. Anti-TNF-alpha therapy in refractory uveitis associated with sarcoidosis: multicenter study of 17 patients. *Semin Arthritis Rheum*. 2015;45(3):361–368.
92. Baughman RP, Bradley DA, Lower EE. Infliximab for chronic ocular inflammation. *Int J Clin Pharmacol Ther*. 2005;43:7–11.
93. Sweiss NJ, Noth I, Mirsaeidi M, et al. Efficacy results of a 52-week trial of adalimumab in the treatment of refractory sarcoidosis. *Sarcoidosis Vasc Diffuse Lung Dis*. 2014;31(1):46–54.
94. Crommelin HA, van der Burg LM, Vorselaars AD, et al. Efficacy of adalimumab in sarcoidosis patients who developed intolerance to infliximab. *Respir Med*. 2016;115:72–77. https://doi.org/10.1016/j.rmed.2016.04.011.
95. Baughman RP. Tumor necrosis factor inhibition in treating sarcoidosis: the American experience. *Revista Portuguesa de Pneumonologia*. 2007;13:S47–S50.
96. Erckens RJ, Mostard RL, Wijnen PA, et al. Adalimumab successful in sarcoidosis patients with refractory chronic non-infectious uveitis. *Graefes Arch Clin Exp Ophthalmol*. 2011.
97. Ramanan AV, Dick AD, Jones AP, et al. Adalimumab plus methotrexate for uveitis in juvenile idiopathic arthritis. *N Engl J Med*. 2017;376(17):1637–1646.
98. Jaffe GJ, Dick AD, Brezin AP, et al. Adalimumab in patients with active noninfectious uveitis. *N Engl J Med*. 2016;375(10):932–943.
99. Pariser RJ, Paul J, Hirano S, et al. A double-blind, randomized, placebo-controlled trial of adalimumab in the treatment of cutaneous sarcoidosis. *J Am Acad Dermatol*. 2013;68(5):765–773.
100. Tuchinda C, Wong HK. Etanercept for chronic progressive cutaneous sarcoidosis. *J Drugs Dermatol*. 2006;5(6):538–540.
101. Khanna D, Liebling MR, Louie JS. Etanercept ameliorates sarcoidosis arthritis and skin disease. *J Rheumatol*. 2003;30(8):1864–1867.
102. Utz JP, Limper AH, Kalra S, et al. Etanercept for the treatment of stage II and III progressive pulmonary sarcoidosis. *Chest*. 2003;124(1):177–185.
103. Baughman RP, Lower EE, Bradley DA, et al. Etanercept for refractory ocular sarcoidosis: results of a double-blind randomized trial. *Chest*. 2005;128(2):1062–1067.
104. Sandborn WJ, Hanauer SB, Katz S, et al. Etanercept for active Crohn's disease: a randomized, double-blind, placebo-controlled trial. *Gastroenterology*. 2001;121(5):1088–1094.
105. Judson MA, Baughman RP, Costabel U, et al. Safety and efficacy of ustekinumab or golimumab in patients with chronic sarcoidosis. *Eur Respir J*. 2014;44:1296–1307.
106. Daien CI, Monnier A, Claudepierre P, et al. Sarcoid-like granulomatosis in patients treated with tumor necrosis factor blockers: 10 cases. *Rheumatology*. 2009;48(8):883–886.
107. Verschueren K, Van EE, Verschueren P, et al. Development of sarcoidosis in etanercept-treated rheumatoid arthritis patients. *Clin Rheumatol*. 2007.
108. King Jr TE, Bradford WZ, Castro-Bernardini S, et al. A phase 3 trial of pirfenidone in patients with idiopathic pulmonary fibrosis. *N Engl J Med*. 2014;370(22):2083–2092.
109. Richeldi L, du Bois RM, Raghu G, et al. Efficacy and safety of nintedanib in idiopathic pulmonary fibrosis. *N Engl J Med*. 2014;370(22):2071–2082.
110. van Vollenhoven RF, Fleischmann RM, Furst DE, et al. Longterm safety of rituximab: final report of the rheumatoid arthritis global clinical trial program over 11 years. *J Rheumatol*. 2015;42(10):1761–1766.
111. Sweiss NJ, Lower EE, Mirsaeidi M, et al. Rituximab in the treatment of refractory pulmonary sarcoidosis. *Eur Respir J*. 2014;43(5):1525–1528.
112. Krause ML, Cooper LT, Chareonthaitawee P, et al. Successful use of rituximab in refractory cardiac sarcoidosis. *Rheumatology*. 2015;55.
113. Lower EE, Baughman RP, Kaufman AH. Rituximab for refractory granulomatous eye disease. *Clin Ophthalmol*. 2012;6:1613–1618.
114. Green S, Partridge E, Idedevbo E, et al. Steroid refractory autoimmune haemolytic anaemia secondary to sarcoidosis successfully treated with rituximab and mycophenolate mofetil. *Case Rep Hematol*. 2016;2016:9495761. https://doi.org/10.1155/2016/9495761.
115. Cinetto F, Compagno N, Scarpa R, et al. Rituximab in refractory sarcoidosis: a single centre experience. *Clin Mol Allergy*. 2015;13(1):19–0025.
116. Pescitelli L, Emmi G, Tripo L, et al. Cutaneous sarcoidosis during rituximab treatment for microscopic polyangiitis: an uncommon adverse effect? *Eur J Dermatol*. 2017;27(6):667–668.

117. Galimberti F, Fernandez AP. Sarcoidosis following successful treatment of pemphigus vulgaris with rituximab: a rituximab-induced reaction further supporting B-cell contribution to sarcoidosis pathogenesis? *Clin Exp Dermatol.* 2016;41(4):413–416.
118. Bouvry D, Mouthon L, Brillet PY, et al. Granulomatosis-associated common variable immunodeficiency disorder: a case-control study versus sarcoidosis. *Eur Respir J.* 2013;41(1):115–122.
119. Salomon A, Appel B, Collins SF, et al. Sarcoidosis: pulmonary and skin studies before and after ACTH and cortisone therapy. *Dis Chest.* 1956;29(3):277–291.
120. Gong R. The renaissance of corticotropin therapy in proteinuric nephropathies. *Nat Rev Nephrol.* 2011;8(2): 122–128.
121. Baughman RP, Barney JB, O'hare L, et al. A retrospective pilot study examining the use of Acthar gel in sarcoidosis patients. *Respir Med.* 2016;110:66–72. https://doi.org/10.1016/j.rmed.2015.11.007.
122. Baughman RP, Sweiss N, Keijsers R, et al. Repository corticotropin for chronic pulmonary sarcoidosis. *Lung.* 2017;195(3):313–322.
123. Drake WP, Oswald-Richter K, Richmond BW, et al. Oral antimycobacterial therapy in chronic cutaneous sarcoidosis: a randomized, single-masked, placebo-controlled study. *JAMA Dermatol.* 2013;149(9):1040–1049.
124. Drake W, Richmond BW, Oswald-Richter K, et al. Effects of broad-spectrum antimycobacterial therapy on chronic pulmonary sarcoidosis. *Sarcoidosis Vasc Diffuse Lung Dis.* 2013;30(3):201–211.
125. Julian MW, Shao G, Schlesinger LS, et al. Nicotine treatment improves TLR2 and TLR9 responsiveness in active pulmonary sarcoidosis. *Chest.* 2013;143:461–470.
126. Prasse A, Zissel G, Lutzen N, et al. Inhaled vasoactive intestinal peptide exerts immunoregulatory effects in sarcoidosis. *Am J Respir Crit Care Med.* 2010;182(4):540–548.
127. Marques LJ, Zheng L, Poulakis N, et al. Pentoxifylline inhibits TNF-alpha production from human alveolar macrophages. *Am J Respir Crit Care Med.* 1999;159(2):508–511.
128. Zabel P, Entzian P, Dalhoff K, et al. Pentoxifylline in treatment of sarcoidosis. *Am J Respir Crit Care Med.* 1997;155:1665–1669.
129. Park MK, Fontana JR, Babaali H, et al. Steroid sparing effects of pentoxifylline in pulmonary sarcoidosis. *Sarcoidosis Vasc Diffuse Lung Dis.* 2009;26:121–131.
130. Papp K, Reich K, Leonardi CL, et al. Apremilast, an oral phosphodiesterase 4 (PDE4) inhibitor, in patients with moderate to severe plaque psoriasis: results of a phase III, randomized, controlled trial (Efficacy and Safety Trial Evaluating the Effects of Apremilast in Psoriasis [ESTEEM] 1). *J Am Acad Dermatol.* 2015;73(1):37–49.
131. Baughman RP, Judson MA, Ingledue R, et al. Efficacy and safety of apremilast in chronic cutaneous sarcoidosis. *Arch Dermatol.* 2012;148:262–264.
132. Martinez FJ, Calverley PM, Goehring UM, et al. Effect of roflumilast on exacerbations in patients with severe chronic obstructive pulmonary disease uncontrolled by combination therapy (REACT): a multicentre randomised controlled trial. *Lancet.* 2015;385(9971): 857–866.
133. Baughman RP, Lower EE. Frequency of acute worsening events in fibrotic pulmonary sarcoidosis patients. *Respir Med.* 2013;107:2009–2013.
134. Keijsers RG, van den Heuvel DA, Grutters JC. Imaging the inflammatory activity of sarcoidosis. *Eur Respir J.* 2013;41(3):743–751.
135. Lebtahi R, Crestani B, Belmatoug N, et al. Somatostatin receptor scintigraphy and gallium scintigraphy in patients with sarcoidosis. *J Nucl Med.* 2001;42(1):21–26.
136. Lapa C, Grigoleit GU, Hanscheid H, et al. Peptide receptor radionuclide therapy for sarcoidosis. *Am J Respir Crit Care Med.* 2016;194(11):1428–1430.
137. Lapa C, Kircher M, Hanscheid H, et al. Peptide receptor radionuclide therapy as a new tool in treatment-refractory sarcoidosis - initial experience in two patients. *Theranostics.* 2018;8(3):644–649.
138. Baughman RP, Judson MA, Teirstein AS, et al. Thalidomide for chronic sarcoidosis. *Chest.* 2002;122:227–232.
139. Nguyen YT, Dupuy A, Cordoliani F, et al. Treatment of cutaneous sarcoidosis with thalidomide. *J Am Acad Dermatol.* 2004;50(2):235–241.
140. Fazzi P, Manni E, Cristofani R, et al. Thalidomide for improving cutaneous and pulmonary sarcoidosis in patients resistant or with contraindications to corticosteroids. *Biomed Pharmacother.* 2012;66(4):300–307.
141. Droitcourt C, Rybojad M, Porcher R, et al. A randomized, investigator-masked, double-blind, placebo-controlled trial on thalidomide in severe cutaneous sarcoidosis. *Chest.* 2014;146(4):1046–1054.
142. Baughman RP, Drent M, Culver DA, et al. Endpoints for clinical trials of sarcoidosis. *Sarcoidosis Vasc Diffuse Lung Dis.* 2012;29:90–98.
143. Judson MA, Silvestri J, Hartung C, et al. The effect of thalidomide on corticosteroid-dependent pulmonary sarcoidosis. *Sarcoidosis Vasc Diffuse Lung Dis.* 2006;23(1):51–57.
144. Melmed GY, Pandak WM, Casey K, et al. Human placenta-derived cells (PDA-001) for the treatment of moderate-to-severe Crohn's disease: a phase 1b/2a study. *Inflamm Bowel Dis.* 2015;21(8):1809–1816.
145. Baughman RP, Culver DA, Jankovic V, et al. Placenta-derived mesenchymal-like cells (PDA-001) as therapy for chronic pulmonary sarcoidosis: a phase 1 study. *Sarcoidosis Vasc Diffuse Lung Dis.* 2015;32:106–114.
146. Pietinalho A, Tukiainen P, Haahtela T, et al. Early treatment of stage II sarcoidosis improves 5-year pulmonary function. *Chest.* 2002;121:24–31.
147. Selroos O, Sellergren TL. Corticosteroid therapy of pulmonary sarcoidosis. *Scand J Resp Dis.* 1979;60: 215–221.

148. Zaki MH, Lyons HA, Leilop L, et al. Corticosteroid therapy in sarcoidosis: a five year controlled follow-up. *NY State J Med*. 1987;87:496–499.
149. James DG, Carstairs LS, Trowell J, et al. Treatment of sarcoidosis: report of a controlled therapeutic trial. *Lancet*. 1967;2:526–528.
150. Israel HL, Fouts DW, Beggs RA. A controlled trial of prednisone treatment of sarcoidosis. *Am Rev Respir Dis*. 1973;107:609–614.
151. Vucinic VM. What is the future of methotrexate in sarcoidosis? A study and review. *Curr Opin Pulm Med*. 2002;8(5):470–476.
152. Panselinas E, Rodgers JK, Judson MA. Clinical outcomes in sarcoidosis after cessation of infliximab treatment. *Respirology*. 2009;14(4):522–528.
153. Vorselaars AD, Verwoerd A, Van Moorsel CH, et al. Prediction of relapse after discontinuation of infliximab therapy in severe sarcoidosis. *Eur Respir J*. 2014;43(2):602–609.
154. Russell E, Luk F, Manocha S, et al. Long term follow-up of infliximab efficacy in pulmonary and extra-pulmonary sarcoidosis refractory to conventional therapy. *Semin Arthritis Rheum*. 2013;43(1):119–124.
155. Milman N, Graudal N, Loft A, et al. Effect of the TNFalpha inhibitor adalimumab in patients with recalcitrant sarcoidosis: a prospective observational study using FDG-PET. *Clin Respir J*. 2011;6:238–247.
156. Minnis PA, Poland M, Keane MP, et al. Adalimumab for refractory pulmonary sarcoidosis. *Ir J Med Sci*. 2016;185(4):969–971.

CHAPTER 21

Sarcoidosis-Associated Disability

MARJOLEIN DRENT, MD, PHD • CELINE HENDRIKS, MSC •
MARJON ELFFERICH, MSC • JOLANDA DE VRIES, PHD

INTRODUCTION

Sarcoidosis is complex and highly variable, with protean clinical manifestations and a wide array of consequences for patients. The course is likewise unpredictable, leading to the moniker "sarcoidoses" to connote that sarcoidosis may be a syndrome rather than a single disease.[1] The clinical manifestation, natural history, and prognosis of sarcoidosis are highly variable, and its course is often unpredictable, depending on the duration of the illness, the organs involved, and fluctuating granulomatous activity.[2] Patients report disabling impairments, especially when they become chronic.[3,4] As a consequence, the interpretation of the severity of sarcoidosis can be complicated by its heterogeneity.[2] Several major concerns of sarcoidosis patients include symptoms that cannot be explained by granulomatous involvement of a particular organ.[3] Apart from pulmonary symptoms (e.g., coughing, breathlessness, and dyspnea on exertion), patients may suffer from a wide range of rather nonspecific disabling symptoms. These symptoms, such as fatigue, fever, anorexia, arthralgia, muscle pain, general and muscle weakness, exercise limitation, and cognitive failure, often do not correspond with objective physical evidence of disease activity.[3] Several studies have reported that neither lung function tests nor chest radiograph abnormalities correlate with nonspecific health complaints, including fatigue or quality of life (QoL). Sarcoidosis-related symptoms may become chronic and affect patients' QoL even after all of the clinically measurable signs of disease activity have disappeared.[5,6] Sarcoidosis-associated chronic fatigue is often troubling to clinicians because it does not relate directly to physiologic abnormalities and is a challenge to treat. Moreover, absence of evidence does not mean evidence of absence.[3,7] It can be argued that when a disease is not overtly dangerous, decisions on treatment of morbidity should be patient-driven because the impact of symptoms on overall QoL is something that can never be fully grasped by anyone other than the patient and immediate family. However, when there is danger from disease (consisting of a higher risk either of mortality or disability due to major organ involvement), the management strategy should ideally be based on medical expertise.[8]

Assessment of Symptom Burden and Disability

Sarcoidosis consists of several overlapping clinical syndromes ('the sarcoidoses'), each with its own specific pathogenesis.[1,2] Physicians generally assess disease activity, severity, and progression in sarcoidosis on the basis of clinical tests, such as serological tests, pulmonary function tests, chest radiographs, and more recently positron emission tomography scans (https://www.ncbi.nlm.nih.gov/pubmed/23018903—comments).[2,9–11] However, these objective clinical parameters correlate poorly with the patients' subjective sense of well-being.[3,12] Moreover, the field of sarcoidosis is rapidly expanding from being solely the bailiwick of chest physicians to intense focus by other specialties, especially cardiology, rheumatology, ophthalmology, and neurology. A phenotyping system centered on the lung is increasingly less relevant.[1] Delineating distinct subgroups, "phenotypes", has been an attempt to simplify prediction about individual patients. Sarcoidosis phenotypes have been used most often to predict prognosis or to cluster patients with similar outcomes.[1,13] A complete evaluation of sarcoidosis could make use of novel phenotypes that are more powerful for prognosis, severity, treatment response, and other clinical characteristics. As these new phenotypes are developed, they must be interpreted and validated within the context of the sarcoidosis clinic and the patient's experience to be acceptable and useful.[1,13] Phenotyping could also be used primarily to stratify patients by clinical features such as extent of organ involvement or by perceived severity. Phenotypic organ-based clusters should assess the severity of sarcoidosis in each organ, which is defined as the degree of organ damage sustained from sarcoidosis. This damage can be estimated subjectively by the intensity of specific organ-related symptoms or objectively by critical localization of lesions, physiologic abnormalities, and the percentage decline from normal capacity. Membership in a given cluster entails higher odds for certain other clinical features, such as

Sarcoidosis. https://doi.org/10.1016/B978-0-323-54429-0.00021-5

acute versus subacute onset, symptoms, and need for therapy.[1,13] Obviously, the interpretation, qualification, and quantification of the severity of sarcoidosis can be complicated by its heterogeneity.[1,6,14] The question whether the burden or localization of the disease contributes to fatigue levels and low energy is highly interesting. It has been shown that patients with both pulmonary and extrapulmonary sarcoidosis report higher fatigue levels than those in whom only the lungs are affected. This suggests a possible additive effect for the troublesome symptom of fatigue.

Fatigue

Although less recognized than exertional dyspnea, fatigue is a very common and frustrating physical symptom. Fatigue is the most frequently described and devastating symptom in sarcoidosis and is globally recognized as a disabling symptom. The reported prevalence varies from 60% to 90% of sarcoidosis patients.[15] Up to 25% of fatigued sarcoidosis patients report extreme fatigue. Several types of fatigue have been described in sarcoidosis.[16,17] One of these types is early morning fatigue, where the patient arises with feelings of inadequate sleep. Another type is intermittent fatigue, where the patient wakes up normally but feels tired after a few hours of activity. After a short rest, the patient is able to resume activity, followed by another period of fatigue. Patients bothered by all-day fatigue have reported the highest level of clinical and psychological problems.[17] About 5% of the patients who appear to be recovered from active sarcoidosis suffer from the so-called postsarcoidosis chronic fatigue syndrome (CFS), first described by James.[7] These sarcoidosis patients may suffer from substantial fatigue even in the absence of other symptoms or disease-related abnormalities.

Cause, risk factors, and diagnosis of fatigue

Fatigue can be nonspecific and hard to objectify and quantify. So far, no organic substrate has been found for sarcoidosis-associated fatigue. The etiology of this fatigue is poorly understood, and there is evidence that it is multifactorial. Active inflammation, cytokine release, depression, altered sleep patterns, overweight, and/or small fiber neuropathy (SFN) all appear to contribute to fatigue.[15,16,18,19] Fatigue can also be a consequence of treatment itself, e.g., as a complication of corticosteroid therapy.

The diagnosis of sarcoidosis-associated fatigue requires an extensive evaluation to identify and treat potentially reversible causes. Despite an exhaustive search for treatable clinical causes of fatigue, however, most patients' complaints of fatigue do not correlate with clinical parameters of disease activity. This means that patients may experience substantial fatigue even without respiratory functional impairment, chest radiograph abnormalities, or markers of diseases activity.[20] Moreover, many patients continue to experience fatigue, causing limitations, even when effective treatment of the sarcoidosis activity is provided.

Predictors of sarcoidosis-associated fatigue

It is important to examine the potential factors that predict and sustain fatigue in sarcoidosis. This may be accomplished by understanding clinical, psychological, and social predictors of fatigue in these patients. The knowledge concerning correlates of the development of fatigue and possible interrelationships is still incomplete. Significant predictors of fatigue include everyday cognitive failure, depressive symptoms, symptoms suggestive of SFN, and, to a lesser extent, dyspnea.[21] Symptoms of fatigue and dyspnea induce exercise limitation, and fatigue may also lead to physical inactivity. Strookappe et al. showed that exercise capacity is also one of the predictors of patients' fatigue.[22] In their study, fatigue was not explained by lung function test results, inflammatory markers, or other clinical parameters. Fatigue, low energy, and exercise limitations affect patients' social life and physical as well as psychological capacities. Decreased physical activity can induce general deconditioning, which in turn contributes to increased perceived physical fatigue and a sense of dyspnea, lack of energy, or exhaustion.

Treatment options of fatigue

Treatment of sarcoidosis obviously is the first option. Often sarcoidosis-associated fatigue is not influenced by the sarcoidosis treatment. Besides, when there is no strict indication to treat sarcoidosis, fatigue can be very devastating for the patient. Some alternative options can be considered. Cognitive behavioral training is an effective behavioral intervention for the CFS, which combines a rehabilitative approach of a graded increase in physical activity with a psychological approach that addresses thoughts and beliefs about CFS which may impair recovery. In line with this, McBride et al. demonstrated subjective and objective performance improvements and suggest that a computerized, home-based cognitive training program may be an effective intervention for patients with CFS.[23] Studies are warranting to evaluate whether this works in sarcoidosis as well. Recent studies have demonstrated the effectiveness of various neurostimulants, including methylphenidate, for the treatment of sarcoidosis-associated fatigue, and these and other agents may be useful adjuncts in its treatment.[24]

Assessment of fatigue

The assessment of sarcoidosis-associated fatigue requires extensive evaluation to identify and treat potentially reversible causes. The severity of fatigue experienced by a patient can be assessed using the Fatigue Assessment Scale (FAS), a 10-item self-report fatigue questionnaire (Table 21.1). The minimum score is 10, and the maximum score is 50. Based on large representative samples of the Dutch population, the cutoff score of the FAS is 21, i.e., scores of >21 are considered to represent fatigue, and a score of ≥35 represents substantial fatigue.[15] A change in the FAS score of four points is considered to be clinically relevant (minimal clinically important difference).[25] The reliability and validity of the FAS appear to be good in sarcoidosis patients. The FAS has been validated in many languages and for various disorders. A PDF and digital version of a translation of the FAS in 20 languages, including an English version, can be found on the website of the World Association of Sarcoidosis and other Granulomatous Disorders (WASOG; www.wasog.org).[26]

Everyday Cognitive Failure

Consequences of cognitive failure for the patient can be discomfort, such as memory problems and problems of attention and concentration, and may affect self-management.[23,27] Giving patients with sarcoidosis insight into their cognitive functioning is of great importance to optimize their self-management skills. Indeed, cognitive deficits may lead to difficulties in managing their disease and negatively affect their treatment. Everyday cognitive failure and depressive symptoms have been found to be the most important predictors of high levels of fatigue,[21] whereas background variables (time since diagnosis, sex, and age) and social support appeared not to predict fatigue. Patients with high levels of cognitive failure also reported higher levels of fatigue than those with lower levels of cognitive failure.[27] Currently, however, no data are available on the extent of cognitive underperformance among sarcoidosis patients. Research among patients with multiple sclerosis found that memory complaints were not associated with memory performance but were associated with fatigue complaints.[28] It is hypothesized that functional cognitive impairment, if present, may lead to increased fatigue and low compliance with medical treatment. An alternative hypothesis is that patients who experience more cognitive failures are continuously putting extra cognitive effort into daily tasks (compensation) and consequently become more tired. It is tempting to speculate that this may also be the case in sarcoidosis patients. Although treatment should first focus on treating sarcoidosis and its activity, alternatives could be considered if this is not effective.[27] Elfferich et al. found that antitumor necrosis factor alpha (TNF-α) therapy had a positive effect on cognition, fatigue, and other symptoms of sarcoidosis.[27] Modafinil has been shown to have beneficial effects on cognitive function. Recently, Kaser et al. found that modafinil may have potential as a therapeutic agent to help remitted depressed patients with persistent cognitive difficulties by improving episodic memory and working memory performance.[29]

Depressive Symptoms and Anxiety

Depressive symptoms and anxiety in sarcoidosis are at least partly an expression of exhaustion owing to the ongoing disease, and these psychological symptoms indeed play an important role in sarcoidosis.[30] They have been reported in 17%–66% of patients with sarcoidosis. Bosse-Henck et al. found that depression and anxiety were predictors of the development of severe fatigue.[31] Depressive symptoms were negatively associated with patients' fatigue scores. In addition, the relationship between fatigue and depressive symptoms parallels the findings for other chronic illnesses, such as diabetes, chronic obstructive pulmonary disease, cardiac disease, and rheumatoid arthritis. Stepanski et al. examined fatigue in patients with cancer.[32] They also showed that depressive symptoms were related to fatigue. Moreover, anxiety and depressive and SFN-related symptoms in sarcoidosis are moderated by the severity and nature of fatigue. Fatigue and autonomic dysfunction are both dominant symptoms and risk factors for depression. Anxiety consists of physical or hyperarousal symptoms, such as increased heart rate, perspiration, and dizziness, which are inherent to the reaction of the sympathetic nervous system. In addition to a physical component, anxiety also has a cognitive component, that is, a thought (or chain of thoughts) that determines the emotion experienced. Anxiety is a major problem in sarcoidosis patients. Because fatigue is a symptom that is known to co-occur with anxiety, it is not surprising that anxiety in general and trait anxiety in particular were found to be related to fatigue. Trait anxiety predicted fatigue at follow-up.[21]

Neurobiological Abnormalities

The nature of fatigue moderates the relationships between fatigue and everyday cognitive failure, depressive symptoms, and anxiety in sarcoidosis. The symptoms may share several neurobiological abnormalities, such as an increase in TNF-α. The relationship between

TABLE 21.1
Fatigue Assessment Scale (FAS)

		Never	Sometimes	Regularly	Often	Always
1)	I am bothered by fatigue	1	2	3	4	5
2)	I get tired very quickly	1	2	3	4	5
3)	I don't do much during the day	1	2	3	4	5
4)	I have enough energy for everyday life	1	2	3	4	5
5)	Physically, I feel exhausted	1	2	3	4	5
6)	I have problems to start things	1	2	3	4	5
7)	I have problems to think clearly	1	2	3	4	5
8)	I feel no desire to do anything	1	2	3	4	5
9)	Mentally, I feel exhausted	1	2	3	4	5
10)	When I am doing something, I can concentrate quite well	1	2	3	4	5

For each statement, one out of five answer categories can be chosen, from never to always—1: never; 2: sometimes (about monthly or less); 3: regularly (about a few times a month); 4: often (about weekly); and 5: always (about every day). An answer to each question has to be given, even if the person does not have any complaints at the moment. Scores on questions 4 and 10 should be recoded (1 = 5, 2 = 4, 3 = 3, 4 = 2, 5 = 1). Subsequently, the total FAS score can be calculated by summing the scores on all questions (the recoded scores for questions 4 and 10). The sum of questions three and six to nine indicates mental fatigue, and the sum of questions 1, 2, 4, 5, and 10 indicates physical fatigue. Published with permission of the ild care foundation (www.ildcare.nl).

depressive symptoms and fatigue in sarcoidosis may also be based on a cytokine imbalance, induced by an inflammatory immune response. The cytokine balance of patients suffering from depression also appears to be disturbed. However, understanding the nature of the relationships between fatigue, depressive symptoms, and anxiety remains difficult. Recently, extrapyramidal signs in neurosarcoidosis have been associated with specific inflammatory pathways and specifically TNF-α.[33] To date, some studies demonstrated positive effect of anti–TNF-α treatment in pulmonary as well as extrapulmonary manifestations including fatigue and cognitive failure.[27,34,35]

SFN-Associated Symptoms

SFN was recognized as a symptom of sarcoidosis in 2002.[36] It is a disabling generalized sensory nerve disorder with a widespread spectrum of symptoms. The reported prevalence of SFN varies from 40% to 60% of patients with sarcoidosis and has been associated with poorer cognitive performance in a general sarcoidosis population.[27,37,38] Symptoms of SFN are disabling for patients and probably underrecognized.[3,39] Patients often feel misunderstood and are limited in their daily activities by the symptoms, which are moreover often difficult to treat.[40] Damage to or loss of small somatic nerve fibers results in pain, burning or tingling sensations, or numbness, typically affecting the limbs in a distal to proximal gradient. When autonomic fibers are affected, patients may experience restless legs, dry eyes, dry mouth, orthostatic dizziness, constipation, bladder incontinence, sexual dysfunction, and/or symptoms relating to autonomic cardiac dysfunction. Symptoms suggestive of SFN as assessed by the SFN Screening List were found to be related to fatigue.[41] Regarding the effect of the restless legs syndrome, the disturbance of sleep quality, i.e., sleep stages and sleep fragmentation, leads to daytime somnolence and fatigue. This may offer a partial explanation for the great burden of fatigue in patients with this syndrome.

Overall Impact on QoL

The impact of any disease depends on the way the patient perceives and experiences the disease and modifies his or her activities of daily living. Living with a long-term disease such as sarcoidosis significantly affects QoL, with negative consequences for general health and social and psychosocial well-being.[42,43] QoL is an important outcome measure of treatment, especially with regard to chronic diseases, including sarcoidosis (Fig. 21.1). It is a concept that concerns patients' evaluation of their functioning in a wide

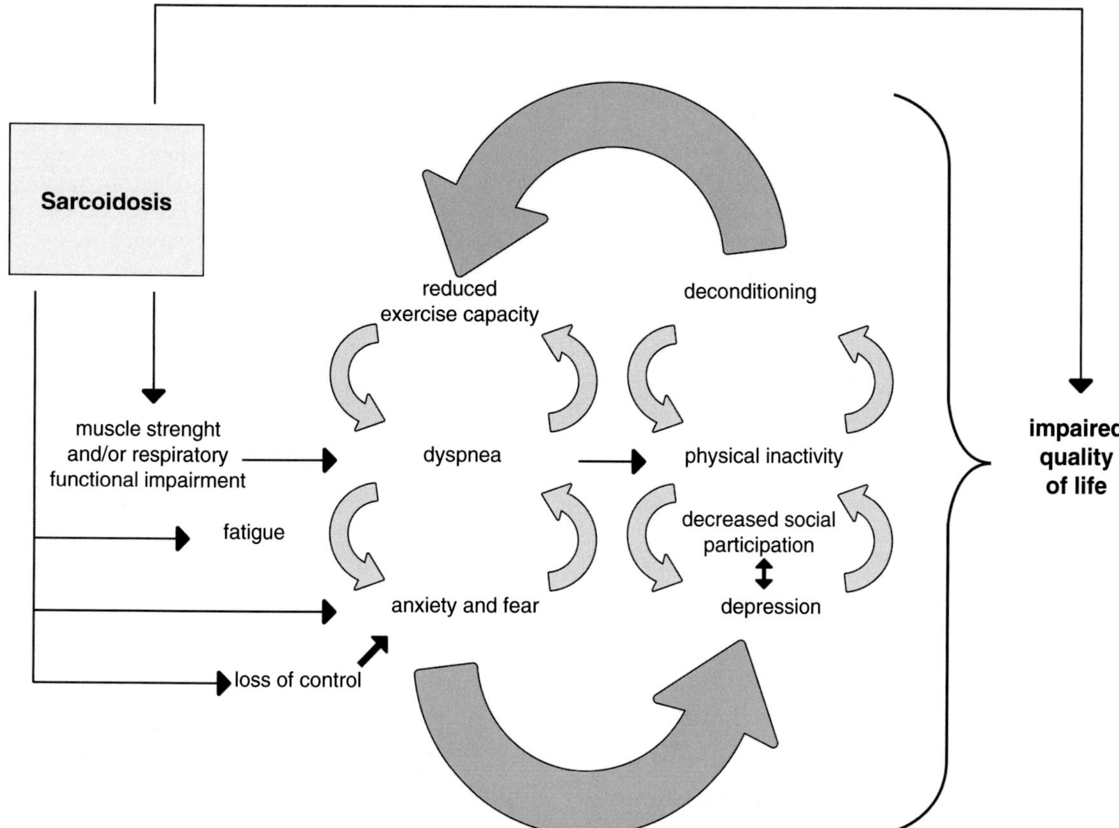

FIG. 21.1 Negative vicious circle of physical deconditioning. Disabling symptoms in sarcoidosis can reduce daily physical activities, resulting in general deconditioning and a reduced quality of life. (Adapted from Swigris JJ, Brown KK, Make BJ, et al. Pulmonary rehabilitation in idiopathic pulmonary fibrosis: a call for continued investigation. *Respir Med.* 2008;102(12):1675–1680. Published before in: Marcellis RG, Lenssen AF, De Vries J, et al. Reduced muscle strength, exercise intolerance and disabling symptoms in sarcoidosis. *Curr Opin Pulm Med.* 2013;19(5):528 and Drent M, Strookappe B, Hoitsma E, De Vries J. Consequences of sarcoidosis. *Clin Chest Med.* 2015;36:731.)

range of domains, but always including the physical, psychological, and social domains.[42] The assessment covering only these three domains is known as an assessment of health-related QoL.[42,43] QoL is often confused with health status, which concerns patients' physical, psychological, and social functioning.[42] QoL is influenced by psychological factors, such as burnout, emotional distress, and work-related social support.[44] Social support has been described as a buffer against pain and disability and also as being associated with greater activity levels among individuals with pain.[44,45] Support positively predicts return to work, and lack of social support at work is a well-known risk factor for developing pain.[46]

In sarcoidosis, there is poor agreement between physicians and patients with regard to the perceived symptoms attributable to the disease, with a particular failure of clinicians to recognize the impact of non–organ-specific features. For instance, pulmonary function test results do not always reflect changes in the severity of pulmonary sarcoidosis, which illustrates that the assessment of sarcoid activity and its clinical relevance remains an enigma. Assessment of inflammatory activity in sarcoidosis patients without deteriorating lung function or radiological deterioration, but with unexplained persistent disabling symptoms, is an important and often problematic issue. It has been proposed that assessment of QoL of sarcoidosis patients would help to bridge this gap, aiding communication and treatment and complementing existing clinical assessments.[47,48]

Disability Due to Sarcoidosis

Many sarcoidosis patients have to face disability due to disease-associated symptoms and are therefore unable to work or underemployed and incapable of achieving their full potential due to health-related issues.[49] Individuals affected by sarcoidosis usually appear completely healthy, so their symptoms are often not taken seriously by family, friends, health-care professionals, and employers. Consequently, some patients lose their desire and ability to effectively socialize with others, causing relationships and family dynamics to ultimately suffer. These combined factors have an impact on an individual's economic status, interpersonal relationships, and family dynamics, increase their stress levels, and induce depression.[3]

We are living in a world where people are increasingly expected to 'participate', for instance, at work and in managing their own care processes. In fact, everyone is now expected by society to 'take part' at all levels. But, is this a realistic expectation for sarcoidosis patients, considering the huge impact that sarcoidosis can have on their QoL, physical and mental capacities, and social life? Although sarcoidosis often causes severe fatigue and reduced exercise tolerance, other people usually do not notice this. Patients encounter problems due to their sarcoidosis, in their job, with their employer, and/or with various authorities, such as occupational health and safety services or benefits authorities. Moreover, sarcoidosis imposes a significant economic burden and health-care costs.[49]

In general, sarcoidosis patients are disabled by functional impairments due to sarcoidosis-associated symptoms. Functional impairments are defined as limitations in, or inability to perform, certain physical activities, such as walking and lifting, or mental activities such as concentrating and conflict handling.[50] Hence, functional impairments can be distinguished from symptoms (such as pain and fatigue), activity limitations (such as self-care tasks and gardening), and participation restrictions (such as leisure time activities and work). Usually, however, the course of sarcoidosis is only monitored using pulmonary function test results and imaging.

The most promising approach would appear to be to gather information using instruments such as questionnaires, performance tests, or interviews, interpreted and assessed by physicians.[51] This needs to be followed by a multidisciplinary meeting in which the patients themselves participate to achieve optimal shared decision-making.[52] There is an urgent need for more information and guidelines to assess the physical and mental capacities of patients with sarcoidosis, to ensure that lung function is not the only aspect taken into account. Obviously, because sarcoidosis requires a multidisciplinary approach in view of its wide range of symptoms, communication among the various health-care workers involved and the patients is of great importance.

Role of Self-Management?

The presence of depressive symptoms is a mediator of the relationship between trait anxiety and fatigue. Depressive symptoms may indirectly lead to increased symptoms as such symptoms are associated with poor self-care (diet, exercise, giving up smoking, medication regimens) in patients with chronic diseases.[21,30] However, physical symptoms, the resulting functional impairments and stress caused by complications of the medical illness, are also likely to impose a burden on the patient's life and to provoke depression.[20]

From this perspective, various researchers have rightly suggested that sarcoidosis patients may benefit from psychological interventions focusing on coping and appraisal, such as stress-reduction therapy.[53,54] In any case, the basis for the interventions should be a type of cognitive behavioral therapy. Successfully adapting to an illness enables people to work or to participate in social activities and accept their limitations.[55] This has been shown in evaluations of the Stanford chronic disease self-management program, in which extensively monitored patients with chronic illnesses, who learned to manage their life better and to cope with their disease, reported improved self-rated health, less distress, less fatigue, more energy, and fewer perceived disabilities and limitations in social activities after the training program. Even health-care costs fell.[56–58] It is interesting to speculate that this concept could also work in sarcoidosis, but this needs to be explored.

CONCLUSION/SUMMARY

In addition to specific organ-related symptoms with functional impairments, sarcoidosis patients tend to be disabled by less specific symptoms, including fatigue, everyday cognitive failure, symptoms suggestive of SFN, pain, and physical impairments. Therefore, the management of sarcoidosis patients should focus not only on organ-related symptoms but also on the increased burden of concomitant symptoms. Multidisciplinary care programs should focus on this burden and also teach patients how to cope with their disease. Because fatigue usually has a multifactorial cause, risk factors should also be examined and treated in combination. Future research involving more comprehensive neuropsychological batteries is warranted to investigate psychological functioning, SFN, and fatigue in sarcoidosis. A guideline to assess disability in sarcoidosis is also very much warranted.

ACKNOWLEDGMENTS

The authors wish to thank Petal Wijnen and Jan Klerkx for their help in preparing the chapter.

Conflict of interest

The authors declare that they do not have anything to disclose regarding funding or conflict of interest with respect to this chapter. All authors read and approved the final version.

REFERENCES

1. Culver DA, Baughman RP. It's time to evolve from Scadding: phenotyping sarcoidosis. *Eur Respir J*. 2018:51.
2. Valeyre D, Prasse A, Nunes H, et al. Sarcoidosis. *Lancet*. 2014;383:1155–1167.
3. Drent M, Strookappe B, Hoitsma E, et al. Consequences of sarcoidosis. *Clin Chest Med*. 2015;36:727–737.
4. Morgenthau AS, Iannuzzi MC. Recent advances in sarcoidosis. *Chest*. 2011;139:174–182.
5. Marcellis RG, Lenssen AF, Elfferich MD, et al. Exercise capacity, muscle strength and fatigue in sarcoidosis. *Eur Respir J*. 2011;38:628–634.
6. Fleischer M, Hinz A, Brahler E, et al. Factors associated with fatigue in sarcoidosis. *Respir Care*. 2014;59:1086–1094.
7. James DG. Complications of sarcoidosis. Chronic fatigue syndrome. *Sarcoidosis*. 1993;10:1–3.
8. Kouranos V, Jacob J, Wells AU. Severe sarcoidosis. *Clin Chest Med*. 2015;36:715–726.
9. Keijsers RG, van den Heuvel DA, Grutters JC. Imaging the inflammatory activity of sarcoidosis. *Eur Respir J*. 2013;41:743–751.
10. Mostard RL, Verschakelen JA, van Kroonenburgh MJ, et al. Severity of pulmonary involvement and (18)F-FDG PET activity in sarcoidosis. *Respir Med*. 2013;107:439–447.
11. Baughman RP, Nagai S, Balter M, et al. Defining the clinical outcome status (COS) in sarcoidosis: results of WASOG Task Force. *Sarcoidosis Vasc Diffuse Lung Dis*. 2011;28:56–64.
12. Gerke AK, Judson MA, Cozier YC, et al. Disease burden and variability in sarcoidosis. *Ann Am Thorac Soc*. 2017;14:S421–S428.
13. Schupp JC, Freitag-Wolf S, Bargagli E, et al. Phenotypes of organ involvement in sarcoidosis. *Eur Respir J*. 2018:51.
14. Gvozdenovic BS, Mihailovic-Vucinic V, Ilic-Dudvarski A, et al. Differences in symptom severity and health status impairment between patients with pulmonary and pulmonary plus extrapulmonary sarcoidosis. *Respir Med*. 2008;102:1636–1642.
15. Drent M, Lower EE, De Vries J. Sarcoidosis-associated fatigue. *Eur Respir J*. 2012;40:255–263.
16. Sharma OP. Fatigue and sarcoidosis. *Eur Respir J*. 1999;13:713–714.
17. de Kleijn WP, Drent M, Vermunt JK, et al. Types of fatigue in sarcoidosis patients. *J Psychosom Res*. 2011;71:416–422.
18. Korenromp IH, Heijnen CJ, Vogels OJ, et al. Characterization of chronic fatigue in patients with sarcoidosis in clinical remission. *Chest*. 2011;140:441–447.
19. Gvozdenovic BS, Mihailovic-Vucinic V, Vukovic M, et al. Effect of obesity on patient-reported outcomes in sarcoidosis. *Int J Tuberc Lung Dis*. 2013;17:559–564.
20. De Vries J, Drent M. Relationship between perceived stress and sarcoidosis in a Dutch patient population. *Sarcoidosis Vasc Diffuse Lung Dis*. 2004;21:57–63.
21. Hendriks C, Drent M, de Kleijn W, et al. Everyday cognitive failure and depressive symptoms predict fatigue in sarcoidosis: a prospective follow-up study. *Respir Med*. 2018;138S:S24–S30.
22. Strookappe B, De Vries J, Elfferich M, et al. Predictors of fatigue in sarcoidosis: the value of exercise testing. *Respir Med*. 2016;116:49–54.
23. McBride RL, Horsfield S, Sandler CX, et al. Cognitive remediation training improves performance in patients with chronic fatigue syndrome. *Psychiatry Res*. 2017;257:400–405.
24. Lower EE, Malhotra A, Surdulescu V, et al. Armodafinil for sarcoidosis-associated fatigue: a double-blind, placebo-controlled, crossover trial. *J Pain Symptom Manage*. 2013;45:159–169.
25. de Kleijn WP, De Vries J, Wijnen PA, et al. Minimal (clinically) important differences for the Fatigue Assessment Scale in sarcoidosis. *Respir Med*. 2011;105:1388–1395.
26. Hendriks C, Drent M, Elfferich M, De Vries J. The Fatigue Assessment Scale (FAS): quality and availability in sarcoidosis and other diseases. *Curr Opin Pulm Med*. 2018;24(5):495–503.
27. Elfferich MD, Nelemans PJ, Ponds RW, et al. Everyday cognitive failure in sarcoidosis: the prevalence and the effect of anti-TNF-alpha treatment. *Respiration*. 2010;80:212–219.
28. Jougleux-Vie C, Duhin E, Deken V, et al. Does fatigue complaint reflect memory impairment in multiple sclerosis? *Mult Scler Int*. 2014;2014:692468.
29. Kaser M, Deakin JB, Michael A, et al. Modafinil improves episodic memory and working memory cognition in patients with remitted depression: a double-blind, randomized, placebo-controlled study. *Biol Psychiatry Cogn Neurosci Neuroimag*. 2017;2:115–122.
30. Drent M, Wirnsberger RM, Breteler MH, et al. Quality of life and depressive symptoms in patients suffering from sarcoidosis. *Sarcoidosis Vasc Diffuse Lung Dis*. 1998;15:59–66.

31. Bosse-Henck A, Koch R, Wirtz H, et al. Fatigue and excessive daytime sleepiness in sarcoidosis: prevalence, predictors, and relationships between the two symptoms. *Respiration*. 2017;94:186–197.
32. Stepanski EJ, Walker MS, Schwartzberg LS, et al. The relation of trouble sleeping, depressed mood, pain, and fatigue in patients with cancer. *J Clin Sleep Med*. 2009;5:132–136.
33. Drori T, Givaty G, Chapman J, et al. Extrapyramidal signs in neurosarcoidosis versus multiple sclerosis: is TNF alpha the link? *Immunobiology*. 2017.
34. Judson MA, Baughman RP, Costabel U, et al. Efficacy of infliximab in extrapulmonary sarcoidosis: results from a randomised trial. *Eur Respir J*. 2008;31:1189–1196.
35. Baughman RP, Judson MA, Teirstein A, et al. Presenting characteristics as predictors of duration of treatment in sarcoidosis. *QJM*. 2006;99:307–315.
36. Hoitsma E, Marziniak M, Faber CG, et al. Small fibre neuropathy in sarcoidosis. *Lancet*. 2002;359:2085–2086.
37. Bakkers M, Merkies IS, Lauria G, et al. Intraepidermal nerve fiber density and its application in sarcoidosis. *Neurology*. 2009;73:1142–1148.
38. Hoitsma E, Drent M, Verstraete E, et al. Abnormal warm and cold sensation thresholds suggestive of small-fibre neuropathy in sarcoidosis. *Clin Neurophysiol*. 2003;114:2326–2333.
39. Tavee J, Culver D. Sarcoidosis and small-fiber neuropathy. *Curr Pain Headache Rep*. 2011;15:201–206.
40. Voortman M, Fritz D, Vogels OJM, et al. Small fiber neuropathy: a disabling and underrecognized syndrome. *Curr Opin Pulm Med*. 2017;23:447–457.
41. Hoitsma E, De Vries J, Drent M. The small fiber neuropathy screening list: construction and cross-validation in sarcoidosis. *Respir Med*. 2011;105:95–100.
42. De Vries J, Drent M. Quality of life and health status in sarcoidosis: a review of the literature. *Clin Chest Med*. 2008;29:525–532.
43. Patel AS, Siegert RJ, Creamer D, et al. The development and validation of the King's Sarcoidosis Questionnaire for the assessment of health status. *Thorax*. 2013;68:57–65.
44. Thomten J, Soares JJ, Sundin O. The influence of psychosocial factors on quality of life among women with pain: a prospective study in Sweden. *Qual Life Res*. 2011;20:1215–1225.
45. Holtzman S, Newth S, Delongis A. The role of social support in coping with daily pain among patients with rheumatoid arthritis. *J Health Psychol*. 2004;9:677–695.
46. Marhold C, Linton SJ, Melin L. Identification of obstacles for chronic pain patients to return to work: evaluation of a questionnaire. *J Occup Rehabil*. 2002;12:65–75.
47. Cox CE, Donohue JF, Brown CD, et al. Health-related quality of life of persons with sarcoidosis. *Chest*. 2004;125:997–1004.
48. Michielsen HJ, Peros-Golubicic T, Drent M, et al. Relationship between symptoms and quality of life in a sarcoidosis population. *Respiration*. 2007;74:401–405.
49. Rice JB, White A, Lopez A, et al. Economic burden of sarcoidosis in a commercially-insured population in the United States. *J Med Econ*. 2017;20:1048–1055.
50. Saketkoo LA, Escorpizo R, Keen KJ, et al. International Classification of Functioning, Disability and Health Core Set construction in systemic sclerosis and other rheumatic diseases: a EUSTAR initiative. *Rheumatology*. 2012;51:2170–2176.
51. Spanjer J, Groothoff JW, Brouwer S. Instruments used to assess functional limitations in workers applying for disability benefit: a systematic review. *Disabil Rehabil*. 2011;33:2143–2150.
52. Drent M, De Vries J, Lenters M, et al. Sarcoidosis: assessment of disease severity using HRCT. *Eur Radiol*. 2003;13:2462–2471.
53. Lorig KR, Sobel DS, Stewart AL, et al. Evidence suggesting that a chronic disease self-management program can improve health status while reducing hospitalization: a randomized trial. *Med Care*. 1999;37:5–14.
54. Smith ML, Wilson MG, DeJoy DM, et al. Chronic disease self-management program in the workplace: opportunities for health improvement. *Front Public Health*. 2014;2:179.
55. Huber M, Knottnerus JA, Green L, et al. How should we define health? *BMJ*. 2011;343:d4163.
56. de Lange FP, Koers A, Kalkman JS, et al. Increase in prefrontal cortical volume following cognitive behavioural therapy in patients with chronic fatigue syndrome. *Brain*. 2008;131:2172–2180.
57. Lorig KR, Ritter P, Stewart AL, et al. Chronic disease self-management program: 2-year health status and health care utilization outcomes. *Med Care*. 2001;39:1217–1223.
58. Lorig KR, Sobel DS, Ritter PL, et al. Effect of a self-management program on patients with chronic disease. *Eff Clin Pract*. 2001;4:256–262.

CHAPTER 22

Calcium Metabolism and Bone Health in Sarcoidosis

ELYSE E. LOWER, MD • NATHALIE SAIDENBERG-KERMANAC'H, MD, PHD

INTRODUCTION

Hypercalcemia, vitamin D deficiency, and bone fractures are interdependent problems faced by sarcoid patients. The first report of the sarcoid granulomatous reaction creating abnormal calcium metabolism was reported in the late 1939.[1] Hypercalcemia is a severe complication associated with disease activity due to an increased synthesis from 25-hydroxy vitamin D (25(OH)D) to calcitriol (1,25 dihydroxy vitamin D), which is the active form of vitamin D.[2] Thus, some experts recommend avoiding vitamin D supplementation in all patients. However, low vitamin D levels can increase bone fragility, especially in patients prescribed glucocorticosteroids to treat symptomatic disease and prevent danger from sarcoidosis. In most diseases where osteoporosis and impaired bone health occurs, calcium and vitamin D supplements are mainstays of primary prevention. However, additional calcium and vitamin D can be detrimental and potentially lead to hypercalcemia or even a granulomatous crisis. Moreover, the avoidance of vitamin D supplementation goes against general recommendations to prevent glucocorticosteroid-induced bone loss by prescribing calcium and vitamin D supplementation in conjunction with bisphosphonates. This chapter will focus on the epidemiology of hypercalcemia in sarcoidosis, explore the complex interaction between vitamin D and calcium homeostasis, and discuss evidence-based treatment strategies to maintain bone health in sarcoidosis patients.

Epidemiology

The incidence of hypercalcemia in sarcoidosis patients ranges from 5% to 25%.[3–6] Furthermore, up to 30% of sarcoidosis patients may develop hypercalciuria with or without nephrolithiasis.[7] Chronic disease, male sex, or Caucasian race is associated with increased calcium metabolism abnormalities. Similar to other conditions associated with elevated calcium, classic symptoms of hypercalcemia are often the presenting features. These symptoms range from fatigue, urinary frequency, dehydration, difficulty swallowing, and constipation to the development of calcium lithiasis affecting the gastrointestinal or genitourinary tract. Unfortunately, some of these complaints are relatively nonspecific and often attributed to other sarcoidosis-associated conditions such as diabetes mellitus, treatment side effects, or sarcoidosis itself. A history of unexplained nephrolithiasis may be the first tip-off suggesting altered calcium metabolism in a sarcoidosis patient.[8] Because of the nonspecificity of symptoms, the diagnosis may be unsuspected until a chemistry panel reveals elevated calcium.

Alterations in calcium remain one of the most common electrolyte problems encountered in both hospital and ambulatory setting.[1] The initial evaluation of hypercalcemia in sarcoidosis mirrors that of other causes of altered metabolism. The initial investigation includes serum testing, followed by 24-h urine collection for hypercalciuria (Fig. 22.1). Once hypercalcemia is confirmed, the usual causes of hypercalcemia, including primary hyperparathyroidism or malignancy, should be excluded. Because other granulomatous processes such as tuberculosis or fungal infections can lead to hypercalcemia, these infections need to be excluded. Increased 1-alpha hydroxylase activity in the granuloma leading to elevated 1,25 dihydroxy vitamin D is the mechanism of action responsible for hypercalcemia attributed to granulomatous diseases.[9,10] Exogeneous calcium supplementation remains extremely prevalent in our society, and a close ingestible history of both dietary and over-the-counter products may reveal high doses of thousands of milligrams of calcium consumed daily. This alone may lead to hypercalcemia in sarcoidosis patients.[11–13] This self-prescribed or health care–recommended exogeneous calcium supplementation is commonly encountered because of bone health concerns in sarcoidosis patients. Because primary

Sarcoidosis. https://doi.org/10.1016/B978-0-323-54429-0.00022-7

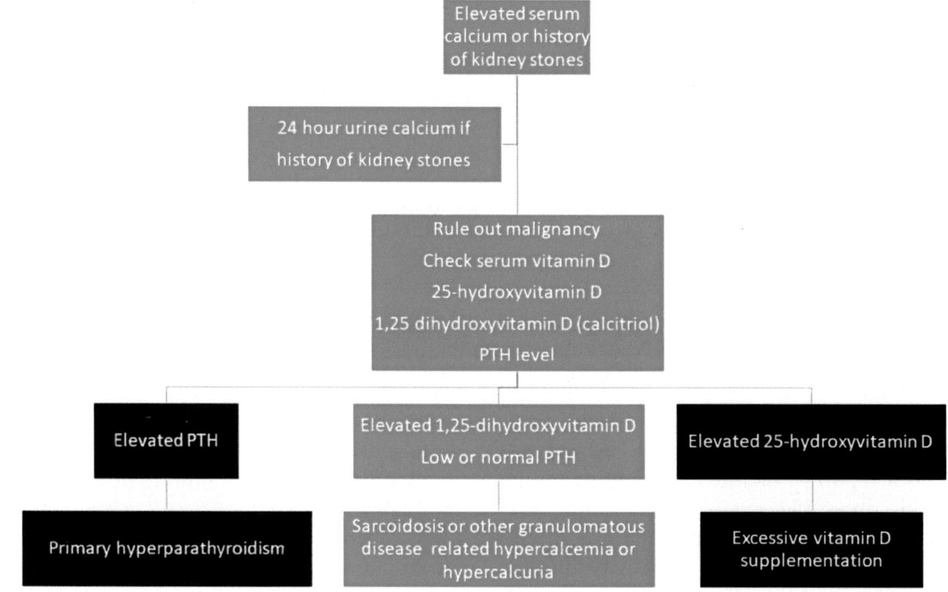

FIG. 22.1 Evaluation of hypercalcemia or hypercalciuria in sarcoidosis patient. *PTH*, parathyroid hormone.

hyperparathyroidism is the cause of 62% of elevated calcium levels reported in health care, an intact parathyroid hormone (PTH) or PTH-related peptide may aid in distinguishing this disorder.[14]

Perplexing Problem of Calcium and Vitamin D in Sarcoidosis

Multiple mechanisms are responsible for the altered calcium metabolism observed in sarcoidosis patients. The association of sarcoid granulomas synthesizing active 1,25 dihydroxy vitamin D was first reported more than 30 years ago. Sarcoid granulomas express high levels of 1-alpha hydroxylase, which is responsible for the extra-renal hydroxylation of 1 hydroxyvitamin D to 1,25 dihydroxy vitamin D. The conversion of 25(OH) D to 1,25(OH)2D normally occurs in the kidney proximal tubule cells, but sarcoidosis granulomas can autonomously increase this conversion.[15]

Natural vitamin D is inactive until hydroxylated by the hepatic CYP27A1 pathway into 25-hydroxy vitamin D which is the major form circulating in the blood. Subsequent 1-alpha hydroxylation by the renal CYP27B1 pathway converts the relatively inactive form into the active 1,25 dihydroxy vitamin D.[16] Maintaining calcium homeostasis is a major function of this activated vitamin D. However, this activated form is important not just in calcium metabolism but also in maintaining immune function in many disease states including malignancy, diabetes mellitus, autoimmune processes, infection, and so forth.

Unlike most vitamins, little vitamin D is available in food, and the major source of vitamin D remains sun exposure. This in part explains the higher incidence of kidney stones and hypercalcemia during the higher solar exposure in the summer months. Vitamin D3, cholecalciferol, is produced by the conversion of epidermal and dermal 7-dehydrocholesterol. Hence conversion to vitamin D3 is linked to sun exposure, race, and age. On the other hand, vitamin D2, which is contained in mushrooms and yeast, requires conversion to D3 to be efficacious in improving bone health. Increased skin pigmentation can reduce conversion to vitamin D3. Kidney alpha hydroxylation is regulated by both PTH and calcitriol. PTH increases in the setting of vitamin D metabolites and low levels of serum calcium. A negative feedback loop also exists with hypercalcemia and higher levels of D3 (calcitriol) inhibiting PTH release.[16]

Calcium Metabolism in Sarcoidosis Patients

In sarcoidosis, activated T cells and macrophages release increased amounts of interleukin 2 (IL-2) and gamma interferon (Fig. 22.2). Some investigators suggest that gamma interferon plays a major role in the pathogenesis of extra-renal synthesis of 1.25(OH)2D.[2] It remains unclear as to whether this mechanism is deleterious

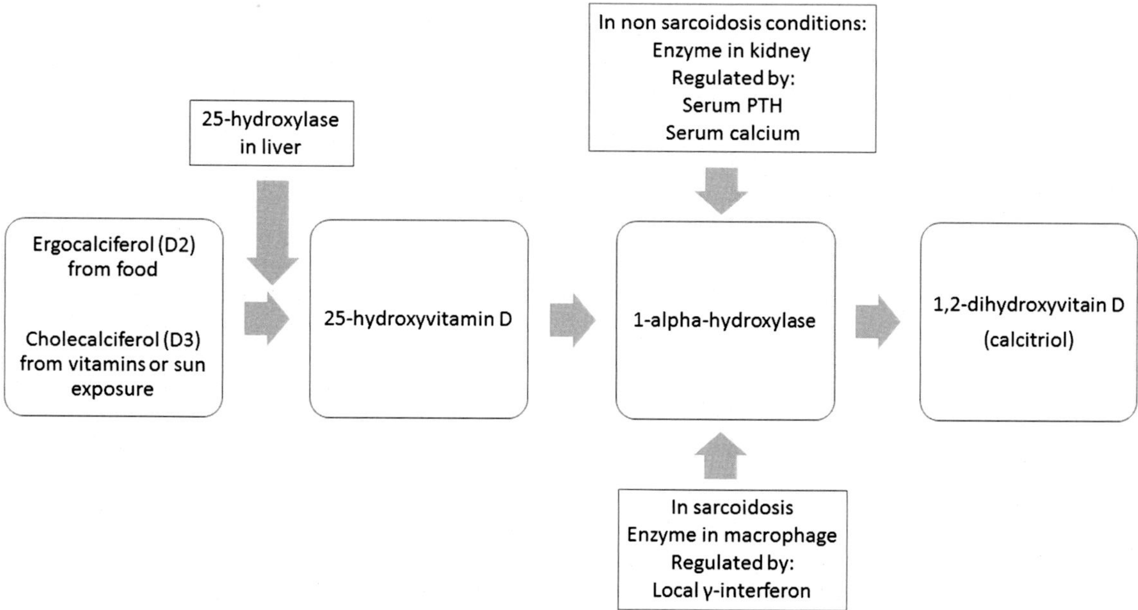

FIG. 22.2 Source and metabolism of vitamin D. The 1-alpha hydroxylase enzyme is crucial in production of calcitriol, the active form of vitamin D. Enzyme activity in the kidney is controlled by several factors, including parathyroid hormone (PTH) and serum calcium levels. In the granuloma, the production of 1-alpha hydroxylase is regulated by interferon gamma (γ-IFN). (From Baughman RP, Papanikolaou I. Current concepts regarding calcium metabolism and bone health in sarcoidosis. *Curr Opin Pulm Med.* 2017;23:476–481 with permission.[69])

or protective. Indeed, it is now established that high-affinity receptors for 1-alpha hydroxylase are present in macrophages, dendritic cells, and T cells along with the vitamin D receptor. In vitro, 1,25(OH)2D tends to exert beneficial effects with decreased production of Th1 proinflammatory cytokines by T cells,[17] probably through the inhibition of interferon gamma and IL-2 along with diminished antigen presentation by dendritic cells to lymphocytes.

Nevertheless, the feedback mechanisms that cause the dysregulation of calcitriol production are impaired in sarcoidosis. In contrast to the renal enzyme, the 1-alpha hydroxylase expressed by macrophages is not downregulated in response to high levels of 1.25(OH)2D. Furthermore, the stimulation of the 25(OH)D-24 hydroxylase which converts the 1.25(OH)2D into inactive 24.25(OH)2D requires higher levels of 1.25(OH)2D.[8,18] The resulting high level of calcitriol could contribute to increased intestinal absorption of calcium, which might explain, in part, the resulting hypercalcemia.

Moreover sarcoidosis patients are more sensitive than healthy subjects to vitamin D supplements. The rise in serum 1,25(OH)2D in response to calcium or vitamin D supplementation is greater in patients with sarcoidosis than that in healthy controls.[19] Similarly, calcium administration to sarcoidosis patients resulted in greater increases in 1.25(OH) 2D serum levels than in healthy subjects. Furthermore, via regulatory mechanisms, 1,25(OH)2D decreases in response to high-dose calcium in normal individuals but not in patients with sarcoidosis.[20]

Hypercalcemia has been associated with high levels of 1,25(OH)2D,[6,21] and elevated 1.25(OH)2D levels are usually associated with more active disease. Kavathia D et al. showed an association between high serum 1,25 (OH) 2 D levels in 59 patients with the need for chronic treatment.[22] In addition, Inui et al. correlated the expression of 1-alpha hydroxylase mRNA in alveolar macrophages, sarcoidosis activity, and ionized calcium serum levels in seven patients.[23]

Baughman et al. reported the prevalence of hypercalcemia in 1606 sarcoidosis patients who were followed up in one United States Sarcoidosis Clinic.[11] Information on 25-hydroxy and 1,25 dihydroxy vitamin D levels were available in 261 patients. Only 97 of 1601 (6%) patients had sarcoidosis-associated hypercalcemia, and hyperparathyroidism caused elevated calcium levels in nine additional patients. Approximately 90% of hypercalcemic patients improved with treatment. The withdrawal of exogeneous vitamin D supplementation as a sole treatment resulted in normalization of serum calcium in eight patients. Renal insufficiency, which was encountered in 41 (42%) patients, improved with treatment. Low levels of 25-hydroxy vitamin D were measured in 80% of sarcoidosis-associated hypercalcemic patients, whereas only one patient experienced a low 1,25 dihydroxy vitamin D level. In fact, 11% of patients developed elevated 1,25 levels. This suggests that a low level of 25 (OH)D may reflect an active disease especially if associated with a high level of 1.25 (OH)2D.

Diagnosis and Treatment of Hypercalcemia

Elevated serum calcium is a frequently encountered biochemical abnormality in clinical practice. Usually it is first identified as a test abnormality or part of a clinical evaluation for fatigue, dysphagia, nephrolithiasis, or unexplained bone thinning. Malignancy remains the number one etiology, followed by hyperparathyroidism[24,25]; however, abnormal vitamin D metabolism is frequently encountered in sarcoidosis patients.[16] Fifteen of 50 active sarcoidosis patients were found to have primary hyperparathyroidism and sarcoidosis.[26]

Patients with mild elevations in calcium (range, 10–11.5 mg/dL) are usually asymptomatic. However, those patients experiencing moderate (11.5–13.5 mg/dL) or severe hypercalcemia (>13.5 mg/dL) may develop weakness, fatigue, polyuria, polydipsia, dysphagia, nausea-vomiting, and abdominal pain. Hypercalcemia can lead to renal failure,[11,27] and if untreated, coma and death can occur. Changes in the electrocardiogram, including ST elevation and arrhythmias, can accompany severe hypercalcemia.

Hypercalciuria is three times more frequent than hypercalcemia in sarcoidosis.[28] This frequently encountered abnormality occurs due to increase in calcium absorption, impaired resorption, and/or increased osteoclast-activating factor.[29] Persistently elevated urinary calcium can create nephrolithiasis, collecting tubule obstruction, and renal failure. Rizzato et al. prospectively identified four of 110 patients with nephrolithiasis as a first manifestation of sarcoidosis in their Milano Sarcoidosis Clinic.[30] A Japanese report confirms that renal impairment and abnormal calcium metabolism predispose to nephrolithiasis.[31] Renal stones associated with sarcoidosis tend to be composed of calcium oxalate rather than the usual calcium phosphate stones associated with primary hyperparathyroidism.[31] This difference in stone composition may reflect differences in excretion of urinary phosphorous between sarcoidosis and hyperparathyroidism.

The initial treatment of sarcoidosis-associated hypercalcemia mimics that used for other causes of hypercalcemia. Patients with mild hypercalcemia do not require treatment; however, close monitoring is necessary as levels can fluctuate widely, particularly in the setting of dehydration or other abnormalities leading to impaired renal clearance. Hydration and corticosteroids remain the mainstay treatments of initial hypercalcemia management. After rehydration is achieved, a loop diuretic can be used to enhance calcium excretion. Patients are also encouraged to avoid calcium-containing food and supplements, as well as to avoid sunlight exposure. Prednisone and other corticosteroids do not affect 1-alpha hydroxylase function on the kidney, but they inhibit enzymatic macrophage conversion. Because corticosteroids may exacerbate hypercalciuria, controlling urinary calcium is important.

Scant data exist on the recommended doses of corticosteroids needed to control elevated calcium. Usual starting doses of prednisone range from 20 to 60 mg daily, and tapering of prednisone requires close monitoring of serum calcium.

Ketoconazole can be prescribed for some patients with refractory hypercalcemia or those unable to tolerate corticosteroids. This antifungal agent, which decreases calcitriol synthesis, has been most frequently prescribed in the setting of hyperparathyroidism. Isolated sarcoidosis case reports reveal some benefits when ketoconazole is administered with lower doses of corticosteroids.[32,33]

Treatment strategies that reduce the granulomatous burden can indirectly lower serum calcium. However, by inhibiting 25-hydroxy vitamin D conversion, only chloroquine and hydroxychloroquine appear to directly reduce serum calcium levels.[21]

Bisphosphonates are usually indicated in the treatment of nonparathyroid hypercalcemia. Gibbs et al. first reported the usage of the bisphosphonate pamidronic acid beneficial in treating sarcoidosis-associated hypercalcemia.[34] Subsequent small series have confirmed the use of zoledronic acid as a calcium-lowering agent in sarcoidosis patients[35] and demonstrate the glucocorticoid-sparing effect of zoledronic acid in sarcoidosis-associated hypercalcemia.

Bone Health in Sarcoidosis

Maintaining bone health in sarcoidosis patients can be particularly challenging. In clinical practice, concerns about hypercalcemia may limit vitamin D and calcium supplementation. This impairs adherence to osteoporosis treatment or corticosteroid-induced bone loss prevention strategies using combined bisphosphonates, calcium, and vitamin D supplements as recommended by international guidelines.[36] In vitamin D deficiency, bisphosphonate monotherapy increases the risk of secondary hyperparathyroidism and may be less effective in bone loss prevention.[16]

Impaired bone health in sarcoidosis occurs due to a variety of reasons.[37] As in autoimmune diseases, the inflammation observed in sarcoidosis may be responsible for bone loss without glucocorticoid treatment. Chronic inflammation has been recognized as an independent risk factor for osteoporosis and fragility fracture. Inflammatory cytokines have been found to play a role in accelerating bone resorption.[38] Several epidemiologic studies have demonstrated that patients with chronic inflammatory disorders, such as rheumatoid arthritis,[39] inflammatory bowel disease,[40] and systemic lupus erythematosus,[41] have a higher incidence of fragility fractures than the general population.

The vitamin D and calcium metabolism disorders responsible for hypercalcemia/hypercalciuria or the chronic vitamin D deficiency experienced in non-supplemented patients could have an impact on bone fragility. Finally, the prolonged prescribing of corticosteroids sometimes in high doses can have deleterious effects. Obviously balancing disease control with bone health is key.

Bone Mineral Density and Sarcoidosis

Patients with sarcoid granulomas may experience decreased bone mineral content even before corticosteroid institution. After assessing vertebral cancellous bone mineral content by quantitative computed tomography (QCT) in untreated sarcoidosis patients, Montemurro et al. found that sarcoidosis patients experience 1.1 + 0.3DS units lower levels than age- and sex-matched controls.[42] Although not entirely clear, the probable mechanism for this appears to be granuloma-derived osteoclast-stimulating factor or perhaps direct stimulation of osteoclasts by elevated levels of 1,25 (OH)2D.

The main culprit behind bone loss in sarcoidosis appears related to corticosteroid usage. The effects of prednisone on bone were first reported by Rizzato who found the vertebral cancellous bone mineral content score (QCT) of corticosteroid-treated patients to be 1.33 + 0.9 lower than age- and sex-matched controls.[43] A subsequent study by Montemurro revealed that this bone mineral decline occurs predominately within the first year of corticosteroid usage.[44]

However, more recent studies using bone densitometry (DEXA) report a decrease in bone mineral density (BMD) affecting only certain groups of sarcoidosis patients, especially postmenopausal women or corticosteroid-treated patients.[45,46] In a cross-sectional uncontrolled study, Heijckmann et al. observed a normal BMD in 124 patients with sarcoidosis despite an increased bone turnover.[47] At the 4-year follow-up time point, the BMD was unchanged in 66 patients, including approximately 50% treated with corticosteroids. The study patients were predominantly Caucasian with an average age of 43 years, and 50% were of female sex with 17% postmenopausal.

In another uncontrolled study of 64 patients with only 8% treated with glucocorticoids, no change in BMD was observed after 2 years.[48] In addition, Adler et al. noted no change in BMD after 1 year in a prospective study with a retrospective control cohort of chronic pulmonary disease patients.[45] This population consisted mainly of glucocorticoid-treated black American men with chronic disease duration averaging 20 years. However, 81% had T scores < −1 DS and among them, 37.8% experienced osteoporosis defined by a T score < −2.5 SD. In the cross-sectional study of Saidenberg et al., the mean BMD was normal in the 142 patients with 62% receiving glucocorticoids.[49] However, 34.8% of patients developed T scores < −1.5 DS, and 7.8% had osteoporosis. Using multivariate analysis, glucocorticoid therapy was not associated with increased risk of low BMD; however, low dietary calcium, fracture, age, gender, and menopause status were associated with increased risk. In addition, patients with 25(OH)D serum levels between 10 and 20 ng/mL were at lower risk of low BMD.

Bone Fracture Risk in Sarcoidosis

Fragility fracture is a common medical problem associated with significant morbidity and mortality. The risk of fracture in sarcoidosis patients is high and often directly related to corticosteroid usage. This prevalence is similar to that reported in young corticosteroid-treated patients with other chronic diseases.[50,51]

In a large retrospective cohort study of 5722 sarcoidosis patients and 28,704 matched controls, sarcoidosis patients compared with controls experienced an increased risk of clinical vertebral fractures. Furthermore, current glucocorticoid therapy users developed an increased risk of any fractures as well as osteoporotic fractures.[52]

To evaluate the rate of major osteoporotic fractures in patients with and without sarcoidosis, a case-control study was conducted between 1995 and 2011 using the Danish National Hospital Discharge Registry. Patients were stratified by average daily and cumulative dose exposures. In 124 sarcoidosis patients, current glucocorticoid use was associated with an increased risk of major osteoporotic fracture. However, fracture risk normalized after steroids were discontinued. In sarcoidosis patients, cumulative prednisone doses of 1.0–4.9 g were associated with increased risk of major osteoporotic fracture, whereas cumulative doses of <1.0 g were not associated with major osteoporotic fracture risk.[53]

Only one study did not confirm an association between glucocorticoid intake and fracture risk in sarcoidosis. Compared with age- and sex-matched controls, the incidence of fragility fracture in a population-based cohort of 345 sarcoidosis patients was increased (Hazards ratio (HR) = 2.18). However, in this cohort the use of glucocorticoids was not a significant predictor of fragility fracture even in a subgroup of patients receiving prednisone doses >10 mg daily for more than 3 months. The analysis may be limited by the lack of detailed information on glucocorticoid exposure and small event numbers of only 41 fragility fractures in 34 patients.[54]

As previously reported in corticosteroid-induced bone loss, BMD may underestimate bone fragility. In a cross-sectional study of younger sarcoidosis patients, half of whom were receiving glucocorticoids, vertebral abnormalities were identified by vertebral fracture assessment in 21% of patients. The prevalence of vertebral deformities persisted for 4 years in 66 (32%) patients. Low BMD in femoral neck and family history of hip fracture were predictive factors for subsequent fracture. However, the mean baseline BMD was normal in this group, and no significant change occurred during the follow-up period.[42] This confirms that in some settings the risk of fracture may be poorly estimated by BMD and that factors other than BMD should be considered when assessing global fracture risk in these patients.

Recently Saidenberg-Kermanach et al. evaluated the fracture risk in a cross-sectional study of 142 sarcoidosis patients.[49] Despite a young mean age of 51 years, approximately one quarter of patients experienced fractures. Greater glucocorticoid exposure, low calcium, along with serum 25-hydroxy D levels either low (<10 ng/mL) or too high (>20 ng/mL), were risk factors for higher fracture rates. However, in multivariate analysis, this increased risk was not associated with BMD.

BONE FRAGILITY TREATMENT

As in other corticosteroid-induced bone fragility, bisphosphonate therapy may be effective in the prevention and treatment of steroid-induced bone loss. Data are limited to one study by Gonnelli regarding the benefit of bisphosphonate therapy in sarcoidosis patients receiving prolonged steroids. In this study, 30 sarcoidosis patients receiving corticosteroids were randomized to either alendronate at an oral dose of 5 mg daily or placebo. After 1 year, less bone decline was reported in the alendronate-treated patients than in the placebo group ($P < .01$).[55]

In most osteoporosis clinical trials, bisphosphonate efficiency is evaluated in conjunction with vitamin D and calcium supplementation. The use of bisphosphonates alone can induce secondary hyperparathyroidism, which could create hypercalcemia in sarcoidosis patients.

Teriparatide is an alternative potential treatment for corticosteroid-induced osteoporosis. However, because PTH stimulates 1-alpha hydroxylase and increases serum calcium levels, caution should be used in sarcoidosis. Challal et al., 2016, reported that teriparatide was effective in halting the fracture cascade in four sarcoidosis patients with multiple vertebral fractures. This agent was beneficial in two patients who remained on long-term glucocorticoid therapy. Although no patient developed hypercalcemia, three of four patients developed adverse events including disease flare. Only the patient on stable glucocorticoid treatment did not develop any adverse reaction.[56]

Denosumab is also a therapeutic option for the treatment of steroid-induced bone loss[57] and can be an interesting option in patients with renal impairment. Unlike bisphosphonates, this biologic agent is not cleared by the kidney. By binding to RANKL, this fully humanized monoclonal antibody inhibits the ability of Receptor activator of nuclear factor kappa-B ligand (RANKL) to bind to osteoclast RANK receptors. Both RANKL and Receptor activator of nuclear factor κ B (RANK) are expressed in the bone and by cells of the immune system including activated T lymphocytes, B cells, and dendritic cells,[58] suggesting that RANKL inhibition might alter immune functions. In the pivotal study of denosumab in osteoporotic women, more cellulitis was observed in the treated population than that in the placebo group.[59] However, no overall increased incidence of infection was noted between the groups. No data are available on denosumab use in sarcoidosis patients receiving immunosuppressive treatment. However, other groups including rheumatoid arthritis patients and cancer patients receiving immunosuppressive agents did not experience increased serious infections with denosumab compared with zoledronic acid.[60]

Vitamin D with calcium supplement can be a primary prevention strategy to reduce osteoporotic fractures. Some experts are not convinced of the bone benefits of vitamin D and calcium supplementation. A meta-analysis found only a small increase of BMD in the femoral neck after vitamin D supplementation.[61] However, in subjects with risk factors for osteoporosis, studies argue for a beneficial effect of supplementation. A meta-analysis of eight randomized clinical trials revealed that the administration of >700–800 IU of daily vitamin D plus calcium reduced hip fracture and nonvertebral fractures in patients older than 65 years.[62] However, 45 and 27 patients were needed to treat or prevent one fracture, respectively. Chapuy et al. found a reduction in the risk of fractures after vitamin D and calcium supplementation in subjects with low 25 (OH) D serum levels and low calcium intake.[63] Furthermore, in the Women's Health Initiative, postmenopausal women receiving five or more years of vitamin D and calcium developed fewer hip fractures than placebo controls.[64]

Efficacy and Safety of Vitamin D Supplementation in Sarcoidosis

Low levels of vitamin D are associated with an increased risk of osteoporosis and subsequent bone fracture, as well as increased risks for malignancy, infection, heart disease, and diabetes mellitus.[65,66] Several observational studies and meta-analyses reveal positive effects of vitamin D supplementation on fragility fractures, cancer risk, mortality, and rheumatoid arthritis activity. Most of the vitamin D studies are based on measurements of the 25(OH)D level and not the 1,25(OH)2D form. However, in sarcoidosis patients, low 25(OH)D levels may reflect active disease, and decisions regarding vitamin D supplement may need to include assessments of both 25(OH)D and 1,25(OH)D2 levels as increases in 1,25(OH)D2 can be associated with active disease states.

Efficacy

The bone health benefit of vitamin D supplementation remains unknown in sarcoidosis. Early studies did show benefit for the use of vitamin D supplement for some groups.[62,67] However, even in nonsarcoidosis patients, the effect of such supplementation remains controversial and difficult to demonstrate. Adler et al. found no improvement in BMD after vitamin D and calcium supplementation in sarcoidosis patients with low 25-hydroxy levels.[45] Although the dose and duration of supplementation were unspecified, no cases of hypercalcemia developed, and only two patients experienced hypercalciuria. Only low body mass index was identified as a predictor for low bone mass density.

Using a randomized controlled design, Bolland et al. reported on the efficacy of vitamin D supplementation in 27 normal calcemic, non-osteoporotic sarcoidosis patients with 25(OH)D levels <50 nmol/L. Only 8% of patients were current users of glucocorticoids. Patients received either 50,000 IU of vitamin D weekly for 4 weeks then monthly for 11 times or placebo. No supplemental calcium was prescribed. Unfortunately, this aggressive supplementation regimen failed to improve surrogate markers of bone health, including no change in BMD after 1 year. The 25(OH)D serum levels were similar between supplemented and placebo-treated patients, and the initial mean BMD levels similar suggesting less effect of vitamin D supplementation alone.[12]

The cross-sectional study of 144 sarcoidosis patients by Saidenberg et al. linked serum 25-hydroxy D, calcium intake, and BMD. Results suggested that low BMD was associated with low calcium intake and serum 25-hydroxy D levels <10 or >20 ng/mL. These findings may suggest that optimal serum 25-hydroxy D levels in sarcoidosis may be lower than those recommended for the general population.[49]

Safety

The risk for developing hypercalcemia with vitamin D supplementation in sarcoidosis patients depends on whether patients are currently receiving glucocorticoids, renal function, past history of hypercalcemia, use of exogenous calcium, and granulomatous activity. In a retrospective study, hypercalcemia was noted in five of 104 calcium D–supplemented sarcoidosis patients. One patient had primary hyperparathyroidism, and three of the four remaining active sarcoidosis patients experienced vitamin D deficiency. A higher rate of hypercalcemia was observed in the nonsupplemented group, and patients treated with glucocorticoids rarely developed hypercalcemia.[68]

Bolland et al. did not observe any difference in serum calcium between his two studied groups of 27 normocalcemic patients and controls despite aggressive vitamin D supplementation. However, compared with placebo controls, 25(OH)D levels increased in the supplemented group from a baseline mean value of 35 mmol/L to 78 nmol/L at 12 months. One patient in the supplemented group developed asymptomatic hypercalciuria and hypercalcemia. This patient with active sarcoidosis was not receiving steroids. An additional patient experienced a severe hypercalcemic crisis after 6 weeks of supplementation.[12]

Between 2005 and 2011, investigators compared 196 sarcoidosis patients who received one treatment for 25(OH)D deficiency to 196 control patients.[13] The primary endpoint of this randomized trial was the incidence of hypercalcemia during the 2-year follow-up period. Dosage and duration of vitamin D supplementation were not specified. In 42.3% of the vitamin D–supplemented patients, hypercalcemia developed in contrast to only 18.3% of controls, $P < .0001$. Moderate to severe hypercalcemia was measured in 12.8% versus only 3.6%, $P = .001$. Unfortunately, 25(OH)D levels were measured in only 70% of patients, and 1,25 (OH)2D levels were available in only 23% of patients. In this retrospective study the authors highlight the risk of inappropriate supplementation more than supplementation itself. Renal impairment was a significant risk factor as well.

In a study by Saidenberg-Kermanac'h et al., vitamin D supplements increased serum 25(OH)D in a dose-dependent manner but had no effect on serum calcium level.[49] In two cohort populations of 1606[11] and 261,[27] hypercalcemia was more common in patients with renal impairment, and 1,25 (OH)2D levels were higher in patients with a history of hypercalcemia. Clinical cases reported in the literature suggest that untreated patients and renal failure are often risk factors for the development of hypercalcemia.

PREVENTION OF CORTICOSTEROID-INDUCED BONE LOSS

Routine supplementation with vitamin D and calcium is not warranted in sarcoidosis patients. However, in cases of prolonged corticosteroid therapy or identified bone fragility based on history of fracture or low BMD, physicians need to discuss with patients prevention strategies to maintain or improve bone health. A potential algorithm for bone health prevention and treatment is presented in Table 22.1.

Obviously, the risk for impaired bone health in sarcoidosis patients varies widely based on granulomatous disease activity, glucocorticoid usage, and other risk factors for osteoporosis. Bone density measurements must be used, but they may underestimate bone fragility in corticosteroid usage. Both glucocorticoid therapy and low serum 25(OH)D levels appear to be risk factors for bone fractures. Individualization of replacement therapies for primary prevention to maintain or improve bone health should be considered. Patients with active sarcoidosis requiring glucocorticoid therapy may be at higher risk for osteoporosis and subsequent fractures. However, this group may also be at higher risk for the development of hypercalcemia and its complications. Patients with glucocorticoid-controlled disease and low 25(OH)D levels could be considered for vitamin D supplementation only. Patients with inactive sarcoidosis either secondary to successful eradication of the granulomas or just natural "burn out" of the disease without renal impairment and a history of hypercalcemia may be at lower risk for developing hypercalcemia. However, as noted in the Baughman et al. study, 20% of their hypercalcemic patients were receiving corticosteroids.[11] Furthermore, low 25(OH)D serum levels could reflect granulomatous activity, and measurement of 1,25 (OH)2D should be considered. If elevated, caution is necessary as it may indicate active disease. Therefore, supplementation with vitamin D needs to be carefully monitored along with serum calcium levels.

TABLE 22.1
Proposed Approach to Monitoring Bone Health in Corticosteroid-Treated Sarcoidosis Patients

- Baseline evaluation of bone mineral density (BMD) scan and bone fracture history
    - Normal BMD and no history of bone fractures
        - Monitor bone density every 1 to 2 years
    - Normal BMD and no history of bone fractures. Reduced BMD and/or bone fractures
        - History of hypercalcemia or hypercalciuria
- Antiresorptive therapy only
    - No history of hypercalcemia or hypercalciuria
- Measure serum 25(OH)D and 1,25(OH)2D (calcitriol)
    - Normal BMD and no history of bone fractures. Elevated 1,25(OH)2D and/or normal 25(OH)D
        - Antiresorptive drug only
    - Normal BMD and no history of bone fractures. Low or normal 1,25(OH)2D and low 25(OH)D
        - Antiresorptive drug therapy plus vitamin D supplement
- Monitor serum and urine calcium and serum 25(OH)D and 1,25(OH)2D levels

Both glucocorticoids and bisphosphonates are used to treat sarcoidosis-related hypercalcemia, and they probably provide protective effects. Although incompletely studied, data from the Saidenberg-Kermanac'h study suggest that 25(OH)D levels of 15–20 ng/mL could be appropriate in sarcoidosis.[49] In their study, higher levels of vitamin D were associated with higher fracture risk. Dietary calcium intake of approximately 1000 mg daily also appears desirable. Because patients with a history of hypercalcemia or nephrolithiasis may be more sensitive to calcium and vitamin D supplements, these ingestible agents should be avoided. It is also important to remember that sarcoidosis patients can experience periods of disease exacerbation rendering them more sensitive to exogenous calcium and vitamin D. Close monitoring of electrolytes should be performed.

SUMMARY AND CONCLUSION

The management of bone health in sarcoidosis remains challenging. On the one hand, the risk of fracture may be high, and it is often directly related to corticosteroid usage, which may require bone prevention strategies. On the other hand, vitamin D and calcium supplements in addition to bisphosphonate therapy in this situation can increase the risk of hypercalcemia. The estimation of fracture risk in these patients is difficult as BMD may underestimate corticoid-induced fragility. However, in situations of prolonged corticosteroid therapy, bone prevention should be considered. Recent data suggest that in the setting of inactive corticosteroid-treated sarcoidosis without renal impairment or history of hypercalcemia, the risk of developing hypercalcemia with supplementation seems low. In addition, the prescribing of bisphosphonates could have additional protective effects. Because the dual action of bisphosphonates can reduce serum calcium and decrease corticosteroid-induced bone loss, combined bisphosphonates and vitamin D supplementation could reduce bone fragility. Continuous careful monitoring of calcium, 25(OH) D, and 1,25(OH)2D is needed because the balance between a positive benefit and a negative effect with supplementation may be slight.

REFERENCES

1. Harrell GT, Fisher S. Blood chemical changes in Boeck's sarcoid with particular reference to proein calcium and phosphatase levels. *J Clin Invest*. 1939;18:687–693.
2. Adams JS, Gacad MA. Characterization of 1 alpha-hydroxylation of vitamin D3 sterols by cultured alveolar macrophages from patients with sarcoidosis. *J Exp Med*. 1985;161:755–765.
3. Baughman RP, Teirstein AS, Judson MA, et al. Clinical characteristics of patients in a case control study of sarcoidosis. *Am J Respir Crit Care Med*. 2001;164:1885–1889.
4. Morimoto T, Azuma A, Abe S, et al. Epidemiology of sarcoidosis in Japan. *Eur Respir J*. 2008;31:372–379.
5. Kim DS. Sarcoidosis in Korea: report of the second nationwide survey. *Sarcoidosis Vasc Diffuse Lung Dis*. 2001;18:176–180.
6. Hamada K, Nagai S, Tsutsumi T, Izumi T. Ionized calcium and 1,25-dihydroxyvitamin D concentration in serum of patients with sarcoidosis. *Eur Respir J*. 1998;11:1015–1020.
7. Sharma OP. Hypercalcemia in granulomatous disorders: a clinical review. *Curr Opin Pulm Med*. 2000;6:442–447.
8. Rizzato G, Fraioli P, Montemurro L. Nephrolithiasis as a presenting feature of chronic sarcoidosis. *Thorax*. 1995;50:555–559.
9. Playford EG, Bansal AS, Looke DF, Whitby M, Hogan PG. Hypercalcaemia and elevated 1,25(OH)(2)D(3) levels associated with disseminated *Mycobacterium avium* infection in AIDS. *J Infect*. 2001;42:157–158.
10. Lavender TW, Martineau AR, Quinton R, Schwab U. Severe hypercalcaemia following vitamin D replacement for tuberculosis-associated hypovitaminosis D. *Int J Tubercul Lung Dis*. 2012;16:140.
11. Baughman RP, Janovcik J, Ray M, Sweiss N, Lower EE. Calcium and vitamin D metabolism in sarcoidosis. *Sarcoidosis Vasc Diffuse Lung Dis*. 2013;30:113–120.
12. Bolland MJ, Wilsher ML, Grey A, et al. Randomised controlled trial of vitamin D supplementation in sarcoidosis. *BMJ Open*. 2013;3:e003562.
13. Sodhi A, Aldrich T. Vitamin D supplementation: not so simple in sarcoidosis. *Am J Med Sci*. 2016;352:252–257.
14. Lafferty FW. Differential diagnosis of hypercalcemia. *J Bone Miner Res*. 1991;6(suppl 2):S51–S59. https://doi.org/10.1002/jbmr.5650061413; discussion S61.
15. Mason RS, Frankel T, Chan YL, Lissner D, Solomon P. Vitamin D conversion by sarcoid lymph node homogenate. *Ann Intern Med*. 1984;100:59–61.
16. Tebben PJ, Singh RJ, Kumar R. Vitamin D-mediated hypercalcemia: mechanisms, diagnosis, and treatment. *Endocr Rev*. 2016;37:521–547.
17. Helming L, Bose J, Ehrchen J, et al. 1alpha,25-Dihydroxyvitamin D3 is a potent suppressor of interferon gamma-mediated macrophage activation. *Blood*. 2005;106:4351–4358.
18. Reichel H, Koeffler HP, Barbers R, Norman AW. Regulation of 1,25-dihydroxyvitamin D3 production by cultured alveolar macrophages from normal human donors and from patients with pulmonary sarcoidosis. *J Clin Endocrinol Metab*. 1987;65:1201–1209.
19. Stern PH, De OJ, Bell NH. Evidence for abnormal regulation of circulating 1 alpha,25-dihydroxyvitamin D in patients with sarcoidosis and normal calcium metabolism. *J Clin Invest*. 1980;66:852–855.
20. Basile JN, Liel Y, Shary J, Bell NH. Increased calcium intake does not suppress circulating 1,25-dihydroxyvitamin

D in normocalcemic patients with sarcoidosis. *J Clin Invest*. 1993;91:1396–1398.

21. Adams JS, Diz MM, Sharma OP. Effective reduction in the serum 1,25-dihydroxyvitamin D and calcium concentration in sarcoidosis-associated hypercalcemia with short-course chloroquine therapy. *Ann Intern Med*. 1989;111:437–438.
22. Kavathia D, Buckley JD, Rao D, Rybicki B, Burke R. Elevated 1, 25-dihydroxyvitamin D levels are associated with protracted treatment in sarcoidosis. *Respir Med*. 2010;104:564–570.
23. Inui N, Murayama A, Sasaki S, et al. Correlation between 25-hydroxyvitamin D3 1 alpha-hydroxylase gene expression in alveolar macrophages and the activity of sarcoidosis. *Am J Med*. 2001;110:687–693.
24. Akirov A, Gorshtein A, Shraga-Slutzky I, Shimon I. Calcium levels on admission and before discharge are associated with mortality risk in hospitalized patients. *Endocrine*. 2017;57:344–351.
25. Soyfoo MS, Brenner K, Paesmans M, Body JJ. Non-malignant causes of hypercalcemia in cancer patients: a frequent and neglected occurrence. *Support Care Cancer*. 2013;21:1415–1419.
26. Lim V, Clarke BL. Coexisting primary hyperparathyroidism and sarcoidosis cause increased angiotensin-converting enzyme and decreased parathyroid hormone and phosphate levels. *J Clin Endocrinol Metab*. 2013;98:1939–1945.
27. Mahevas M, Lescure FX, Boffa JJ, et al. Renal sarcoidosis: clinical, laboratory, and histologic presentation and outcome in 47 patients. *Medicine (Baltim)*. 2009;88:98–106.
28. Sharma OP, Vucinic V. Sarcoidosis of the thyroid and kidneys and calcium metabolism. *Semin Respir Crit Care Med*. 2002;23:579–588.
29. ALBRIGHT F, CARROLL EL, DEMPSEY EF, HENNEMAN PH. The cause of hypercalcuria in sarcoid and its treatment with cortisone and sodium phytate. *J Clin Invest*. 1956;35:1229–1242.
30. Rizzato G, Colombo P. Nephrolithiasis as a presenting feature of chronic sarcoidosis: a prospective study. *Sarcoidosis*. 1996;13:167–172.
31. Kato Y, Taniguchi N, Okuyama M, Kakizaki H. Three cases of urolithiasis associated with sarcoidosis: a review of Japanese cases. *Int J Urol*. 2007;14:954–956.
32. Adams JS, Sharma OP, Diz M. Ketoconazole decreases the serum 1,25 dihydroxyvitamin D and calcium concentration in sarcoidosis associated hypercalcemia. *J Clin Endocrinol Metab*. 1990;70:1090–1095.
33. O'Leary TJ, Jones G, Yip A, Lohnes D, Cohanim M, Yendt ER. The effects of chloroquine on serum 1,25-dihydroxyvitamin D and calcium metabolism in sarcoidosis. *N Engl J Med*. 1986;315:727–730.
34. Gibbs CJ, Peacock M. Hypercalcaemia due to sarcoidosis corrects with bisphosphonate treatment. *Postgrad Med J*. 1986;62:937–938.
35. Kuchay MS, Mishra SK, Bansal B, Farooqui KJ, Sekhar L, Mithal A. Glucocorticoid sparing effect of zoledronic acid in sarcoid hypercalcemia. *Arch Osteoporos*. 2017;12:68–0360.
36. Adler RA, Hochberg MC. Suggested guidelines for evaluation and treatment of glucocorticoid-induced osteoporosis for the Department of Veterans Affairs. *Arch Intern Med*. 2003;163:2619–2624.
37. Sweiss NJ, Lower EE, Korsten P, Niewold TB, Favus MJ, Baughman RP. Bone health issues in sarcoidosis. *Curr Rheumatol Rep*. 2011.
38. Adamopoulos IE. Inflammation in bone physiology and pathology. *Curr Opin Rheumatol*. 2018;30:59–64.
39. Van Staa TP, Geusens P, Bijlsma JW, Leufkens HG, Cooper C. Clinical assessment of the long-term risk of fracture in patients with rheumatoid arthritis. *Arthritis Rheum*. 2006;54:3104–3112.
40. Van Staa TP, Cooper C, Brusse LS, Leufkens H, Javaid MK, Arden NK. Inflammatory bowel disease and the risk of fracture. *Gastroenterology*. 2003;125:1591–1597.
41. Almehed K, Hetenyi S, Ohlsson C, Carlsten H, Forsblad-d'Elia H. Prevalence and risk factors of vertebral compression fractures in female SLE patients. *Arthritis Res Ther*. 2010;12:R153.
42. Montemurro L, Fraioli P, Rizzato G. Bone loss in untreated longstanding sarcoidosis. *Sarcoidosis*. 1991;8:29–34.
43. Rizzato G, Tosi G, Mella C, Montemurro L, Zanni D, Sisti S. Prednisone-induced bone loss in sarcoidosis: a risk especially frequent in postmenopausal women. *Sarcoidosis*. 1988;5:93–98.
44. Montemurro L, Schiraldi G, Fraioli P, Tosi G, Riboldi A, Rizzato G. Prevention of corticosteroid-induced osteoporosis with salmon calcitonin in sarcoid patients. *Calcif Tissue Int*. 1991;49:71–76.
45. Adler RA, Funkhouser HL, Petkov VI, Berger MM. Glucocorticoid-induced osteoporosis in patients with sarcoidosis. *Am J Med Sci*. 2003;325:1–6.
46. Sipahi S, Tuzun S, Ozaras R, et al. Bone mineral density in women with sarcoidosis. *J Bone Miner Metabol*. 2004;22:48–52.
47. Heijckmann AC, Huijberts MS, De VJ, et al. Bone turnover and hip bone mineral density in patients with sarcoidosis. *Sarcoidosis Vasc Diffuse Lung Dis*. 2007;24:51–58.
48. Bolland MJ, Wilsher ML, Grey A, et al. Bone density is normal and does not change over 2 years in sarcoidosis. *Osteoporos Int*. 2015;26:611–616.
49. Saidenberg-Kermanac'h N, Semerano L, Nunes H, et al. Bone fragility in sarcoidosis and relationships with calcium metabolism disorders: a cross sectional study on 142 patients. *Arthritis Res Ther*. 2014;16:R78.
50. Siffledeen JS, Simonoski K, Ho J, Fedorak RN. Vertebral fractures and role of low bone mineral density in Crohn's disease. *Clin Gastroenterol Hepatol*. 2007;5:721–728.
51. Van Staa TP, Leufkens HG, Abenhaim L, Zhang B, Cooper C. Oral corticosteroids and fracture risk: relationship to daily and cumulative doses. *Rheumatology*. 2000;39:1383–1389.
52. Bours S, de VF, van den Bergh JPW, et al. Risk of vertebral and non-vertebral fractures in patients with sarcoidosis:

a population-based cohort. *Osteoporos Int*. 2016;27:1603–1610.

53. Oshagbemi OA, Driessen JHM, Pieffers A, et al. Use of systemic glucocorticoids and the risk of major osteoporotic fractures in patients with sarcoidosis. *Osteoporos Int*. 2017;28:2859–2866.
54. Ungprasert P, Crowson CS, Matteson EL. Risk of fragility fracture among patients with sarcoidosis: a population-based study 1976–2013. *Osteoporos Int*. 2017;28:1875–1879.
55. Gonnelli S, Rottoli P, Cepollaro C, et al. Prevention of corticosteroid-induced osteoporosis with alendronate in sarcoid patients. *Calcif Tissue Int*. 1997;61:382–385.
56. Challal S, Semerano L, Nunes H, Valeyre D, Boissier MC, Saidenberg-Kermanac'h N. Teriparatide for osteoporosis in patients with sarcoidosis: report on risk-benefit ratio in four cases. *Joint Bone Spine*. 2016;83:344–345.
57. Ishiguro S, Ito K, Nakagawa S, Hataji O, Sudo A. The clinical benefits of denosumab for prophylaxis of steroid-induced osteoporosis in patients with pulmonary disease. *Arch Osteoporos*. 2017;12:44–0336.
58. Narayanan P. Denosumab: a comprehensive review. *South Asian J Cancer*. 2013;2:272–277.
59. Watts NB, Roux C, Modlin JF, et al. Infections in postmenopausal women with osteoporosis treated with denosumab or placebo: coincidence or causal association? *Osteoporos Int*. 2012;23:327–337.
60. Curtis JR, Xie F, Yun H, Saag KG, Chen L, Delzell E. Risk of hospitalized infection among rheumatoid arthritis patients concurrently treated with a biologic agent and denosumab. *Arthritis Rheum*. 2015;67:1456–1464.
61. Reid IR, Bolland MJ, Grey A. Effects of vitamin D supplements on bone mineral density: a systematic review and meta-analysis. *Lancet*. 2014;383:146–155.
62. Bischoff-Ferrari HA, Willett WC, Orav EJ, et al. A pooled analysis of vitamin D dose requirements for fracture prevention. *N Engl J Med*. 2012;367:40–49.
63. Chapuy MC, Arlot ME, Duboeuf F, et al. Vitamin D3 and calcium to prevent hip fractures in elderly women. *N Engl J Med*. 1992;327:1637–1642.
64. Prentice RL, Pettinger MB, Jackson RD, et al. Health risks and benefits from calcium and vitamin D supplementation: women's Health Initiative clinical trial and cohort study. *Osteoporos Int*. 2013;24:567–580.
65. Lappe JM, Travers-Gustafson D, Davies KM, Recker RR, Heaney RP. Vitamin D and calcium supplementation reduces cancer risk: results of a randomized trial. *Am J Clin Nutr*. 2007;85:1586–1591.
66. Autier P, Gandini S. Vitamin D supplementation and total mortality: a meta-analysis of randomized controlled trials. *Arch Intern Med*. 2007;167:1730–1737.
67. Tang BM, Eslick GD, Nowson C, Smith C, Bensoussan A. Use of calcium or calcium in combination with vitamin D supplementation to prevent fractures and bone loss in people aged 50 years and older: a meta-analysis. *Lancet*. 2007;370:657–666.
68. Kamphuis LS, Bonte-Mineur F, van Laar JA, van Hagen PM, van Daele PL. Calcium and vitamin D in sarcoidosis: is supplementation safe? *J Bone Miner Res*. 2014;29:2498–2503.
69. Baughman RP, Papanikolaou I. Current concepts regarding calcium metabolism and bone health in sarcoidosis. *Curr Opin Pulm Med*. 2017;23:476–481.

CHAPTER 23

Nonpharmacological Therapy for Pulmonary Sarcoidosis

W. ENNIS JAMES, MD

INTRODUCTION

The management of pulmonary sarcoidosis in some patients requires consideration of nonpharmacological treatment options. This applies to the direct consequences of sarcoidosis inflammation in the airways, as well as pulmonary complications arising from architectural distortion of lung parenchyma. The purpose of this chapter is to review nonpharmacological therapeutic options for sarcoidosis patients with proximal airway involvement, mycetomas, and pulmonary hypertension (Table 23.1). The benefits of pulmonary rehabilitation for reduced quality of life (QOL) and fatigue, which are common in all levels of disease severity, will be discussed. Existing literature for solid organ transplantation as a last resort for pulmonary and extrapulmonary sarcoidosis will be reviewed in regard to transplant outcomes and considerations for transplant referral.

Proximal Airway Stenosis

Airflow obstruction from proximal airway stenosis occurs in up to 8% of pulmonary sarcoidosis patients (Fig. 23.1).[1] Treatment options may depend on the underlying etiology of airway narrowing, which can occur in airways as a result of endoluminal (endobronchial accumulation of granulomas in the airway) and extraluminal disease activity (extrinsic compression from enlarged lymph nodes). The majority of patients with endoluminal stenosis will have multiple areas of stenosis on bronchoscopy (defined as >50% narrowing) with visualized airways appearing erythematous, and granulomas will typically be seen on endobronchial biopsy.[2] Patients may present with wheezing, inspiratory "squeaks," and nonreversible obstruction on spirometry.[3] Chamberllan et al. found those patients treated within 3 months of symptom onset had resolution of stenosis, whereas patients with delayed treatment had persistent, severe stenosis.

Refractory airway stenosis can be managed with flexible bronchoscopy through ballooning or stenting. Owing to the diffuse mucosal involvement, there is no role for laser ablation, cryotherapy, or electrocautery.[4] Balloon dilation is well tolerated and effective in reducing symptoms after procedure, although long-term outcomes vary, with some patients requiring repeat dilation.[4,5] Case reports of adjunctive therapies such as mitomycin C also may have short-term improvement but no clear-lasting benefit.[6] Airway stenting is usually reserved for cases that are refractory to balloon dilation and are rarely pursued.[4] Case reports demonstrate improvement in forced expiratory volume 1 (FEV1) 6 months after procedure but can be complicated by formation of granulation tissue.[7]

Aspergilloma

Aspergillomas are observed in 1%–10% of patients with chronic pulmonary sarcoidosis and can occur in radiographic stage III or stage IV disease.[8,9] It is more common in blacks and is associated with increased mortality with a 73% 5-year survival.[8,10] Most patients will have poor lung function at presentation, and 90% will have positive aspergillus serology.[10] While there is no clear role for treatment of asymptomatic patients, current guidelines support the use of both itraconazole and voriconazole for those with symptoms, the most common being hemoptysis. In a large case series, 85%

TABLE 23.1
Potential Nonimmunosuppressive Therapies for Other Manifestations of Sarcoidosis

Condition	Therapy
Proximal airway stenosis	Bronchoscopic interventions • Balloon dilation • Stent placement
Aspergilloma/hemoptysis	Antifungal therapy • Oral • Intracavitary Bronchial artery embolization Surgical resection
Pulmonary hypertension	Angioplasty/stent placement
Reduced quality of life and fatigue	Pulmonary rehabilitation

Sarcoidosis. https://doi.org/10.1016/B978-0-323-54429-0.00023-9

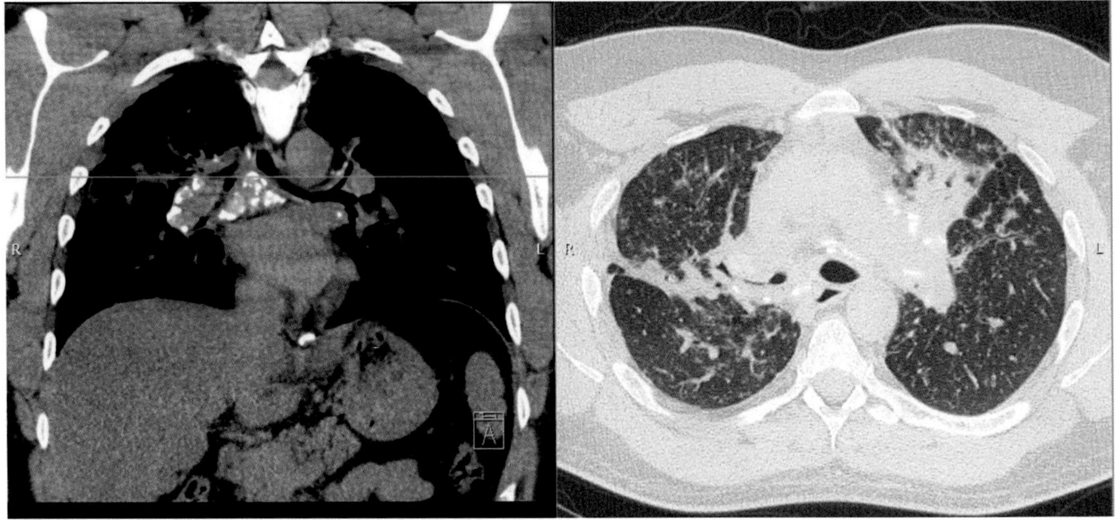

FIG. 23.1 Airway stenosis resulting from extraluminal compression.

of patients received antifungals for at least 6 weeks, but only those treated for more than 6 months showed improvement as evidenced by significant decrease in pleural and cavity wall thickness. Nonpharmacological therapy is primarily reserved for patients with radiographic progression or refractory hemoptysis and includes intracavitary/intrabronchial antifungals, bronchial artery embolism, and surgical resection.

Airway/cavity instillation of antifungals

Intracavitary amphotericin has been used for patients with refractory hemoptysis, who are not surgical candidates (Fig. 23.2A–C).[11] The procedure requires placement of a small bore chest tube into the cavity, and so is usually reserved for patients with larger cavities amenable to radiographic guided chest tube placement. In the case series reported by Kravitz, et al. 91% had successful chest tube placement. After 10 days of daily instillation of amphotericin B, 85% had resolution of hemoptysis by discharge (90% of the 10 sarcoidosis patients). Recurrence of minor and severe hemoptysis occurred in 60% and 30% of sarcoidosis patients after a mean interval of 8 and 36 months, respectively.[11] Intracavitary voriconazole has been used successfully in case reports for sarcoidosis-associated mycetomas.[12] Intracavitary chest tube placement requires expertise that is not readily available at most centers and is associated with a relatively high rate (26%) of pneumothorax, although none were associated with long-term complications.[11] Although retrospective data suggest intracavitary instillation of antifungals may have good outcomes in refractory nonsurgical patients, additional studies in larger cohorts are needed to clarify the long-term benefit.

Airway-directed antifungals including instillation with flexible bronchoscopy and using endobronchial ultrasound have been used successfully in nonsurgical patients to treat refractory hemoptysis secondary to aspergillomas.[13–15] However, their efficacy in sarcoidosis is unclear as such treatments have only been reported in nonsarcoidosis fibrotic/cavitary lung disease (idiopathic pulmonary fibrosis and posttubercular cavitary lung disease).

Bronchial artery embolization

Bronchial artery embolization (BAE) for hemoptysis in nonsarcoidosis aspergillomas is successful in alleviating hemoptysis in 67% of patients with recurrence rates around 33%, although success may vary by anatomic location.[16,17] Sarcoidosis patients undergoing BAE are more likely to rebleed after a shorter time interval than nonsarcoidosis patients (29 vs. 293 days, respectively), with lower survival rates (mean 3.6 months).[18] In the case series by Uzunhan et al. 36% of sarcoidosis patients undergoing BAE had nonlethal but severe complications including stroke, arterial dissection, and hemomediastinum.[10] Although BAE may be a viable option for short-term alleviation of severe, refractory hemoptysis, it is not a long-term solution and is associated with significant risk. The use of multidetector computed tomography angiogram before conventional angiography may reduce the failure rate of embolization in some patients.[19]

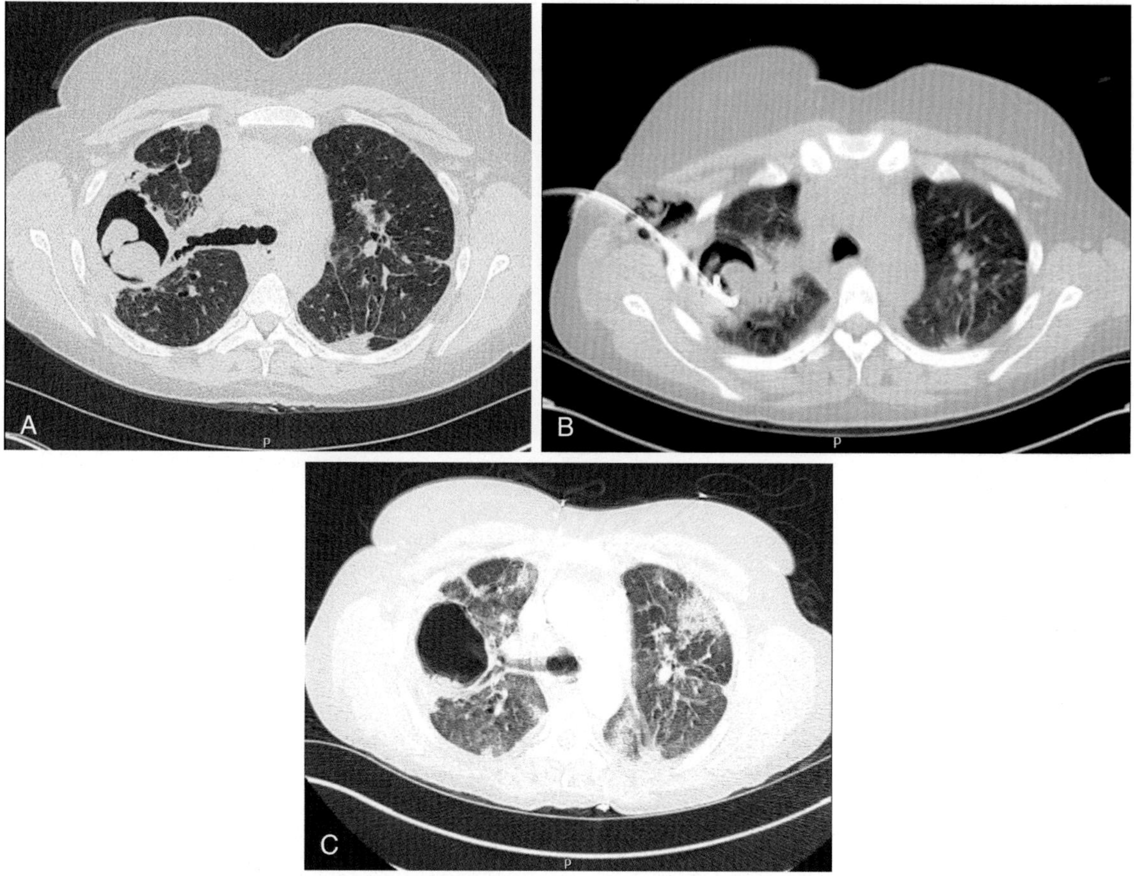

FIG. 23.2 **(A)** Aspergilloma in a 35-year-old female with fibrocystic pulmonary sarcoidosis and refractory hemoptysis. **(B)** Intracavitary placement of pigtail catheter. **(C)** Follow-up imaging 3 months after treatment with intracavitary amphotericin with complete resolution of hemoptysis.

Surgical resection

The success of surgical resection of aspergillomas in symptomatic sarcoidosis patients varies depending on the selection criteria of surgical candidates. Older studies that included patients with other cavitary lung disease have reported surgical mortality rates as high as 25%,[20] whereas more recent case series with more selective cases have mortality rates as low as 4.1%.[21] Surgical outcomes are generally worse in patients with complex aspergillomas, described as having thick walls, damage to surrounding lung tissue, or pleural involvement.[22] Postoperative complications are seen in 72% of patients with complex aspergillomas, compared with 25% of patients with simple aspergillomas, who are more likely to only require wedge resections or segementectomies.[22] A preoperative FEV1 >75% is predicted to be associated with good outcomes,[23] but the use of such selective criteria often eliminates surgical resection as an option for sarcoidosis patients who typically present with poor lung function.[10] Case series suggest that recurrence of pulmonary aspergillomas after surgical resection is more common in sarcoidosis than in other lung diseases.[10] Owing to the poor preoperative status of most sarcoidosis patients with aspergillomas, surgery is often not an option. However, successful aspergilloma resection is considered a definitive cure for hemoptysis and should be pursued if the patient is deemed a surgical candidate.[24] Postoperative management typically includes antifungal therapy, but there is little evidence to support the efficacy of this practice although data in sarcoidosis patients are limited.[25]

Pulmonary Hypertension

Nonpharmacological therapy for sarcoidosis-associated pulmonary hypertension (SAPH) is primarily directed at addressing vascular complications of the disease. Pulmonary hypertension due to narrowing of the pulmonary vasculature can be caused by granulomatous inflammation involving pulmonary arterial walls, extrinsic compression by enlarged hilar lymph nodes (Fig. 23.3), and fibrosing mediastinitis (FM).[26] The prevalence of pulmonary artery compression/stenosis in sarcoidosis varies,[27,28] with rates as high as 11% reported in one prospective case series.[29] Stent placement for external compression improves pulmonary artery pressure and WHO classification.[29] There are little data regarding recurrence rates, but one series reported recurrent stenosis in one of three patients who underwent stenting for external compression.[30] Angioplasty and stenting of pulmonary vasculature in FM also lead to increased pulmonary artery diameter and reduced pulmonary artery pressures.[31,32] Recurrence rates were found to be higher in FM patients undergoing pulmonary vein (25%) versus pulmonary artery (5%) stenting.[32] Pulmonary artery occlusion secondary to FM can also be managed surgically in appropriate patients, primarily through creation of a double-outlet right ventricle, although case series include relatively few patients and some patients may develop recurrent stenosis around the conduit.[33]

Transplant can be considered in SAPH. Long-term outcomes in double-lung and heart-lung transplant for pulmonary hypertension revealed similar survival rates in groups I, III, and IV compared with group V pulmonary hypertension (1- and 5-year survival, 68% and 41%, respectively).[34]

Chronic thromboembolic pulmonary hypertension (CTEPH) in sarcoidosis patients usually results from thromboembolic disease unrelated to sarcoidosis, although granulomatous inflammation within thrombi removed from sarcoidosis patients during thromboendarterectomy has been described.[35] Although there is an increased risk of pulmonary embolism in sarcoidosis patients,[36,37] very little data exist regarding outcomes after thromboendarterectomy in sarcoidosis patients with CTEPH.

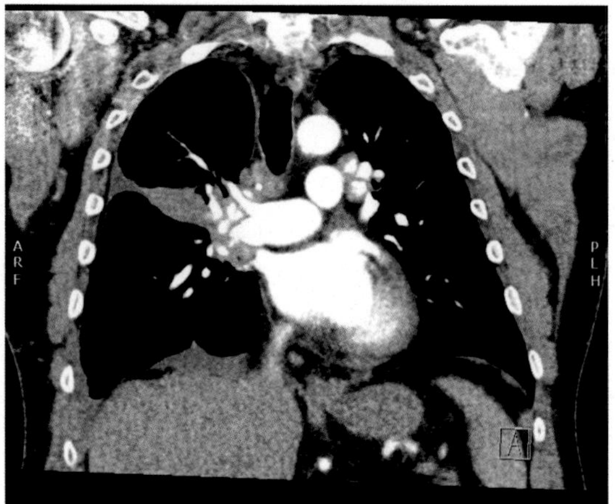

FIG. 23.3 Pulmonary artery stenosis.

Lung Transplant

Sarcoidosis patients account for approximately 3% of all lung transplants in the United States and are more likely to be female and black.[38,39] No specific recommendations exist regarding the timing of referral to transplant for sarcoidosis but are generally considered to be similar to those provided for patients with idiopathic pulmonary fibrosis (IPF).[40] One exception to this is the presence of pulmonary hypertension in sarcoidosis, which is associated with increased mortality[41,42] and is considered an indication for transplant referral.[43] Other predictors of increased mortality in sarcoidosis, including a forced vital capacity (FVC) less than 1.5 L[44] and the scoring system proposed by Walsh et al., may provide additional insight to assist in the decision for transplant referral. The presence of a mycetoma is associated with increased posttransplant mortality[45] and is generally considered a relative contraindication to transplant, especially in patients with complex mycetomas with pleural involvement.[43,46] Pretransplant assessment of extrapulmonary organ involvement is important to improve outcomes. Patients with cardiac sarcoidosis with left ventricular dysfunction may be more appropriate for a heart-lung transplant. Patients should be evaluated for hepatic sarcoidosis to ensure total bilirubin levels are not more than 2.0 mg/dL, which has been associated with worsened survival.[47]

Compared to IPF, sarcoidosis patients listed for transplant before implementation of the Lung Allocation Score (LAS) in 2005 had significantly worse lung function, had longer wait times (803 days vs. 555 days), and were less likely to undergo transplantation (30% vs. 37%). Despite these differences, survival rates before transplantation were similar.[48] In the LAS era, transplant wait times are similar although sarcoidosis patients are still less likely to receive a transplant.[38] This may result from sarcoidosis patients receiving lower LAS scores and having longer weight times than IPF patients with the same clinical features (Table 23.2).

TABLE 23.2
Lung Allocation Score of Sarcoidosis patient compared to idiopathic pulmonary fibrosis patients with the same clinical features

	Sarcoidosis	Idiopathic Pulmonary Fibrosis
Date of Birth	8/30/1955	8/30/1955
Height (cm)	160	160
Weight (kg)	76	76
Functional status	Performs activities of daily living with SOME assistance	Performs activities of daily living with SOME assistance
Diabetes	Not insulin dependent	Not insulin dependent
Assisted ventilation	No assisted ventilation needed	No assisted ventilation needed
Requires supplemental oxygen	At rest	At rest
Amount	4 l/min	4 l/min
Predicted FVC %	46	46
6-minute walk distance (feet)	150	150
Pulmonary artery systolic pressure (mm Hg)	60	60
Mean pulmonary artery pressure (mm Hg)	33	33
Cardiac index (L/min/m^2)	2.4	2.4
Central venous pressure (mm Hg)	5	5
PCO2 (mm Hg)		
Current	42	42
Highest	42	42
Lowest	42	42
Serum creatinine (mg/dL)		
Current	1.43	1.43
Highest	2.2	2.2
Lowest	1.4	1.4
Total bilirubin (mg/dL)		
Current	0.5	0.5
Highest	0.6	0.6
Lowest	0.4	0.4
Lung Allocation Score	**50.3**	**58.5**
Waitlist urgency measure (days)	**243**	**197**
Post-transplant survival measure (days)	**308**	**306**

Multiple studies have shown that posttransplant survival rates in sarcoidosis (median 69.7 months) are similar to other transplant indications, with 50% survival at 5 years.[38] Recently, survival after transplant has been shown to be similar between races,[49] an improvement over the pre-LAS era when black patients were nearly 50% more likely to die within 30 days of transplant.[39] Double-lung transplant is more common in sarcoidosis patients than in nonsarcoidosis patients (68.9% vs. 56.9%, respectively) and is associated with improved survival in sarcoidosis.[38]

Recurrence of disease in the transplanted lung occurs in 30% of patients[50] and is more commonly seen after single-lung transplant.[51] Recurrence occurs within the first year in the majority of patients on surveillance bronchoscopy but has no effect on overall survival,[50] suggesting the higher rate of double-lung transplants in sarcoidosis is more likely to be related to the tendency of fibrotic pulmonary sarcoidosis to have bilateral involvement. Recurrence rates are similar between race and sex, and the only variable predictive of recurrence is the presence of granulomas on the explanted lung.[52] Interestingly, episodes of acute cellular rejection are significantly less likely after disease recurrence.[52] There were minimal differences in the rate of airway inflammation score, in keeping with the observation that lung function remains similar between patients regardless of the presence of recurrent sarcoidosis.

PULMONARY REHABILITATION

It is well known that physical activity levels are lower in sarcoidosis patients than in healthy controls, and there are strong inverse associations between both fatigue and QOL with 6-minute walk distance (6MWD).[53] A large number of studies support the ability of pulmonary rehabilitation (PR) to improve exercise tolerance and QOL in patients with chronic obstructive pulmonary disease (COPD) and IPF. Despite comparatively less evidence, recent data support the benefit of PR for sarcoidosis and suggest its use should likely play a larger role in the management of the disease, regardless of severity.

A prospective, double-blind, randomized control trial showed that just 6 weeks of inspiratory muscle training results in significant improvements in 6MWD (mean difference 66.1 vs. 11.6 m, P = .001), severe fatigue (P=.002), and Borg dyspnea scale (P = .02) compared with controls.[54] Other studies to date have largely focused on the efficacy of structured inpatient or outpatient PR regimens. Multiple retrospective studies have demonstrated significant improvements in 6MWD, fatigue, and psychological health in those who participate in outpatient PR programs, as compared with no improvement in these outcomes in non-PR cohorts.[55,56] A prospective, observational study of a 3-week inpatient rehab program in Germany led to significant improvement in 6MWD as well as fatigue, QOL, anxiety, and depression.[57] Disease severity did have an impact on outcomes, with significantly greater improvement in fatigue scores (as measured by the Fatigue Assessment Scale) seen in patients with the poorest lung function and shortest walk distance at enrollment. A more recent randomized control trial of a twice-weekly 3-month outpatient PR program in patients with stage III and IV sarcoidosis also found significant improvements in 6MWD, perceived dyspnea (Borg scale and modified Medical Research Council Dyspnea Scale), QOL, and anxiety.[58] Interestingly, while there was no difference in FVC and diffusion capacity of carbon monoxide between groups, a significant improvement was seen in PaO_2 (11 mmHg vs. -2 mmHg, P=.009) and SaO_2 (1.8% vs. −1%, P = .007) in the intervention group compared with controls, although the clinical significance of this is unclear. The ability of mobile health and self-management programs to produce similar results is yet to be investigated in sarcoidosis but has the potential to benefit patients with greatest disease severity who often have limited access to healthcare in general.[59,60]

REFERENCES

1. Olsson T, Björnstad-Pettersen H, Stjernberg NL. Bronchostenosis due to sarcoidosis: a cause of atelectasis and airway obstruction simulating pulmonary neoplasm and chronic obstructive pulmonary disease. *Chest.* 1979;75(6):663–666.
2. Chambellan A, Turbie P, Nunes H, Brauner M, Battesti JP, Valeyre D. Endoluminal stenosis of proximal bronchi in sarcoidosis: bronchoscopy, function, and evolution. *Chest.* 2005;127(2):472–481.
3. Udwadia ZF, Pilling JR, Jenkins PF, Harrison BD. Bronchoscopic and bronchographic findings in 12 patients with sarcoidosis and severe or progressive airways obstruction. *Thorax.* 1990;45(4):272–275.
4. Chapman JT, Mehta AC. Bronchoscopy in sarcoidosis: diagnostic and therapeutic interventions. *Curr Opin Pulm Med.* 2003;9(5):402–407.
5. Fouty BW, Pomeranz M, Thigpen TP, Martin RJ. Dilatation of bronchial stenoses due to sarcoidosis using a flexible fiberoptic bronchoscope. *Chest.* 1994;106(3):677–680.
6. Teo F, Anantham D, Feller-Kopman D, Ernst A. Bronchoscopic management of sarcoidosis related bronchial stenosis with adjunctive topical mitomycin C. *Ann Thorac Surg.* 2010;89(6):2005–2007.
7. Fruchter O, Abed El Raouf B, Rosengarten D, Kramer MR. Long-term outcome of short metallic stents for lobar airway stenosis. *J Bronchology Interv Pulmonol.* 2017;24(3):211–215.
8. Wollschlager C, Khan F. Aspergillomas complicating sarcoidosis. A prospective study in 100 patients. *Chest.* 1984;86(4):585–588.
9. Panjabi C, Sahay S, Shah A. Aspergilloma formation in cavitary sarcoidosis. *J Bras Pneumol.* 2009;35(5):480–483.

10. Uzunhan Y, Nunes H, Jeny F, et al. Chronic pulmonary aspergillosis complicating sarcoidosis. *Eur Respir J.* 2017;49(6).
11. Kravitz JN, Berry MW, Schabel SI, Judson MA. A modern series of percutaneous intracavitary instillation of amphotericin B for the treatment of severe hemoptysis from pulmonary aspergilloma. *Chest.* 2013;143(5):1414–1421.
12. Kravitz JN, Steed LL, Judson MA. Intracavitary voriconazole for the treatment of hemoptysis complicating Pseudallescheria angusta pulmonary mycetomas in fibrocystic sarcoidosis. *Med Mycol.* 2011;49(2):198–201.
13. Takeda T, Itano H, Kakehashi R, Fukita S, Saitoh M, Takeda S. Direct transbronchial administration of liposomal amphotericin B into a pulmonary aspergilloma. *Respir Med Case Rep.* 2014;11:7–11.
14. Parikh MS, Seeley E, Nguyen-Tran E, Krishna G. Endobronchial ultrasound-guided transbronchial needle injection of liposomal amphotericin B for the treatment of symptomatic aspergilloma. *J Bronchology Interv Pulmonol.* 2017;24(4):330–333.
15. Mohan A, Tiwari P, Madan K, et al. Intrabronchial voriconazole is a safe and effective measure for hemoptysis control in pulmonary aspergilloma. *J Bronchology Interv Pulmonol.* 2017;24(1):29–34.
16. Shin B, Koh WJ, Shin SW, et al. Outcomes of bronchial artery embolization for life-threatening hemoptysis in patients with chronic pulmonary aspergillosis. *PLoS One.* 2016;11(12):e0168373.
17. Corr P. Management of severe hemoptysis from pulmonary aspergilloma using endovascular embolization. *Cardiovasc Intervent Radiol.* 2006;29(5):807–810.
18. Tom LM, Palevsky HI, Holsclaw DS, et al. Recurrent bleeding, survival, and longitudinal pulmonary function following bronchial artery embolization for hemoptysis in a U.S. Adult population. *J Vasc Interv Radiol.* 2015;26(12):1806–1813. e1801.
19. Subesinghe M, Pearce J, Hammond C, Robertson R, McPherson S. Pulmonary artery embolization for recurrent haemoptysis in cavitatory sarcoidosis. *Clin Radiol.* 2011;66(5):478–480.
20. Daly RC, Pairolero PC, Piehler JM, Trastek VF, Payne WS, Bernatz PE. Pulmonary aspergilloma. Results of surgical treatment. *J Thorac Cardiovasc Surg.* 1986;92(6):981–988.
21. Kasprzyk M, Pieczyński K, Mania K, Gabryel P, Piwkowski C, Dyszkiewicz W. Surgical treatment for pulmonary aspergilloma - early and long-term results. *Kardiochir Torakochirurgia Pol.* 2017;14(2):99–103.
22. Moodley L, Pillay J, Dheda K. Aspergilloma and the surgeon. *J Thorac Dis.* 2014;6(3):202–209.
23. Sagan D, Goździuk K, Korobowicz E. Predictive and prognostic value of preoperative symptoms in the surgical treatment of pulmonary aspergilloma. *J Surg Res.* 2010;163(2):e35–43.
24. Brik A, Salem AM, Kamal AR, et al. Surgical outcome of pulmonary aspergilloma. *Eur J Cardio Thorac Surg.* 2008;34(4):882–885.
25. Benhamed L, Woelffle D. Adjuvant antifungal therapy after pulmonary surgery for aspergilloma: is it useful? *Interact Cardiovasc Thorac Surg.* 2014;18(6):835–837.
26. Damuth TE, Bower JS, Cho K, Dantzker DR. Major pulmonary artery stenosis causing pulmonary hypertension in sarcoidosis. *Chest.* 1980;78(6):888–891.
27. Toonkel RL, Borczuk AC, Pearson GD, Horn EM, Thomashow BM. Sarcoidosis-associated fibrosing mediastinitis with resultant pulmonary hypertension: a case report and review of the literature. *Respiration.* 2010;79(4):341–345.
28. Hasegawa K, Ohno S, Takada M, et al. Sarcoidosis complicated with major pulmonary artery obstruction and stenosis. *Intern Med.* 2012;51(19):2775–2780.
29. Liu L, Xu J, Zhang Y, et al. Interventional therapy in sarcoidosis-associated pulmonary arterial stenosis and pulmonary hypertension. *Clin Respir J.* 2017;11(6):906–914.
30. Condado JF, Babaliaros V, Henry TS, Kaebnick B, Kim D, Staton GW. Pulmonary stenting for the treatment of sarcoid induced pulmonary vascular stenosis. *Sarcoidosis Vasc Diffuse Lung Dis.* 2016;33(3):281–287.
31. Hamilton-Craig CR, Slaughter R, McNeil K, Kermeen F, Walters DL. Improvement after angioplasty and stenting of pulmonary arteries due to sarcoid mediastinal fibrosis. *Heart Lung Circ.* 2009;18(3):222–225.
32. Albers EL, Pugh ME, Hill KD, Wang L, Loyd JE, Doyle TP. Percutaneous vascular stent implantation as treatment for central vascular obstruction due to fibrosing mediastinitis. *Circulation.* 2011;123(13):1391–1399.
33. Brown ML, Cedeño AR, Edell ES, Hagler DJ, Schaff HV. Operative strategies for pulmonary artery occlusion secondary to mediastinal fibrosis. *Ann Thorac Surg.* 2009;88(1):233–237.
34. Fadel E, Mercier O, Mussot S, et al. Long-term outcome of double-lung and heart-lung transplantation for pulmonary hypertension: a comparative retrospective study of 219 patients. *Eur J Cardio Thorac Surg.* 2010;38(3):277–284.
35. Bernard J, Yi ES. Pulmonary thromboendarterectomy: a clinicopathologic study of 200 consecutive pulmonary thromboendarterectomy cases in one institution. *Hum Pathol.* 2007;38(6):871–877.
36. Crawshaw AP, Wotton CJ, Yeates DG, Goldacre MJ, Ho LP. Evidence for association between sarcoidosis and pulmonary embolism from 35-year record linkage study. *Thorax.* 2011;66(5):447–448.
37. Swigris JJ, Olson AL, Huie TJ, et al. Increased risk of pulmonary embolism among US decedents with sarcoidosis from 1988 to 2007. *Chest.* 2011;140(5):1261–1266.
38. Taimeh Z, Hertz MI, Shumway S, Pritzker M. Lung transplantation for pulmonary sarcoidosis. Twenty-five years of experience in the USA. *Thorax.* 2016;71(4):378–379.
39. Shorr AF, Helman DL, Davies DB, Nathan SD. Sarcoidosis, race, and short-term outcomes following lung transplantation. *Chest.* 2004;125(3):990–996.

40. Weill D, Benden C, Corris PA, et al. A consensus document for the selection of lung transplant candidates: 2014–an update from the pulmonary transplantation Council of the international society for heart and lung transplantation. *J Heart Lung Transplant.* 2015;34(1):1–15.
41. Baughman RP, Engel PJ, Taylor L, Lower EE. Survival in sarcoidosis-associated pulmonary hypertension: the importance of hemodynamic evaluation. *Chest.* 2010;138(5):1078–1085.
42. Shorr AF, Davies DB, Nathan SD. Predicting mortality in patients with sarcoidosis awaiting lung transplantation. *Chest.* 2003;124(3):922–928.
43. Shah L. Lung transplantation in sarcoidosis. *Semin Respir Crit Care Med.* 2007;28(1):134–140.
44. Baughman RP, Winget DB, Bowen EH, Lower EE. Predicting respiratory failure in sarcoidosis patients. *Sarcoidosis Vasc Diffuse Lung Dis.* 1997;14(2):154–158.
45. Hadjiliadis D, Sporn TA, Perfect JR, Tapson VF, Davis RD, Palmer SM. Outcome of lung transplantation in patients with mycetomas. *Chest.* 2002;121(1):128–134.
46. Judson MA. Lung transplantation for pulmonary sarcoidosis. *Eur Respir J.* 1998;11(3):738–744.
47. Trulock EP, Edwards LB, Taylor DO, et al. Registry of the International Society for Heart and Lung Transplantation: twenty-third official adult lung and heart-lung transplantation report–2006. *J Heart Lung Transplant.* 2006;25(8):880–892.
48. Shorr AF, Davies DB, Nathan SD. Outcomes for patients with sarcoidosis awaiting lung transplantation. *Chest.* 2002;122(1):233–238.
49. Mooney J, Boyd J, Chhatwani L, Dhillon GS. Post lung transplant survival of recipients with sarcoidosis in LAS era. *J Heart Lung Transplant.* 2017;36(4):S307.
50. Schultz HH, Andersen CB, Steinbruuchel D, Perch M, Carlsen J, Iversen M. Recurrence of sarcoid granulomas in lung transplant recipients is common and does not affect overall survival. *Sarcoidosis Vasc Diffuse Lung Dis.* 2014;31(2):149–153.
51. Ionescu DN, Hunt JL, Lomago D, Yousem SA. Recurrent sarcoidosis in lung transplant allografts: granulomas are of recipient origin. *Diagn Mol Pathol.* 2005;14(3):140–145.
52. Banga A, Sahoo D, Lane CR, Farver CF, Budev MM. Disease recurrence and acute cellular rejection episodes during the first year after lung transplantation among patients with sarcoidosis. *Transplantation.* 2015;99(9):1940–1945.
53. Pilzak K, Żebrowska A, Sikora M, et al. Physical functioning and symptoms of chronic fatigue in sarcoidosis patients. *Adv Exp Med Biol.* 2017.
54. Karadalli M, Bosnak-Guclu M, Camcioglu B, Kokturk N, Turktas H. Effects of inspiratory muscle training in subjects with sarcoidosis: a randomized controlled clinical trial. *Respir Care.* 2016;61(4):483–494.
55. Strookappe B, Swigris J, De Vries J, Elfferich M, Knevel T, Drent M. Benefits of physical training in sarcoidosis. *Lung.* 2015;193(5):701–708.
56. Marcellis R, Van der Veeke M, Mesters I, et al. Does physical training reduce fatigue in sarcoidosis? *Sarcoidosis Vasc Diffuse Lung Dis.* 2015;32(1):53–62.
57. Lingner H, Buhr-Schinner H, Hummel S, et al. Short-term effects of a multimodal 3-week inpatient pulmonary rehabilitation programme for patients with sarcoidosis: the ProKaSaRe study. *Respiration.* 2018.
58. Naz I, Ozalevli S, Ozkan S, Sahin H. Efficacy of a structured exercise program for improving functional capacity and quality of life in patients with stage 3 and 4 sarcoidosis: a randomized controlled trial. *J Cardiopulm Rehabil Prev.* 2018;38(2):124–130.
59. Rabin DL, Richardson MS, Stein SR, Yeager Jr H. Sarcoidosis severity and socioeconomic status. *Eur Respir J.* 2001;18(3):499–506.
60. Rabin DL, Thompson B, Brown KM, et al. Sarcoidosis: social predictors of severity at presentation. *Eur Respir J.* 2004;24(4):601–608.

CHAPTER 24

Pulmonary Hypertension Associated With Sarcoidosis

HILARIO NUNES, MD, PHD • YURDAGÜL UZUNHAN, MD, PHD • MORGANE DIDIER, MD • PIERRE-YVES BRILLET, MD, PHD • MARIANNE KAMBOUCHNER, MD • DOMINIQUE VALEYRE, MD

Pulmonary hypertension (PH) is a serious complication of sarcoidosis (sarcoidosis PH), the frequency of which largely depends on the severity of pulmonary involvement. However, PH can occur at all stages of disease advancement, and its underlying mechanisms are various and incompletely elucidated. PH results in substantial morbidity and adversely impacts on the survival of affected sarcoidosis patients. Over the last years, PH has been the subject of growing attention in sarcoidosis, improving our understanding of its pathogenesis and providing a better appraisal of its prevalence, risk factors, and prognosis. In parallel, several studies have been conducted with agents approved for pulmonary arterial hypertension (PAH). This review examines the current literature regarding sarcoidosis PH, with an emphasis on the most recent insights, including therapeutic management.

CLASSIFICATION OF PH

PH is defined as an increase in mean pulmonary arterial pressure (mPAP) ≥ 25 mmHg at rest on right heart catheterization (RHC).[1] According to various combinations of mPAP, pulmonary arterial wedge pressure, cardiac index (CI), diastolic pressure gradient, and pulmonary vascular resistance (PVR), different hemodynamic profiles have been outlined (Table 24.1). In an attempt to assist physicians in their daily practice, the classification of PH categorizes multiple clinical conditions into five groups based on their similar clinical presentation, pathological features, hemodynamic characteristics, and treatment strategy. A task force under the aegis of the European Society of Cardiology (ESC) and the European Respiratory Society (ERS) has recently updated the guidelines for the diagnosis and treatment of PH (Table 24.2).[1]

Group three is "PH due to lung diseases and/or hypoxia", including interstitial lung diseases (ILDs).[1] In patients suffering from ILDs, PH is believed to result from the vascular ablation in fibrotic zones and hypoxic vasoconstriction, with mPAP rarely exceeding 35 mmHg.[1] Actually, a proportion of these patients sometimes exhibit a level of PH that seems insufficiently explained by lung mechanical disturbances. The terminology "out of proportion" PH, initially used to refer to these cases, has been abandoned for that of "severe" PH, which is defined as a mPAP > 35 mmHg or mPAP ≥ 25 mmHg together with a low CI (<2.5 L/min per m^2).[1] In such a context, it may be difficult to determine whether PH is due to lung disease or whether there is an underlying intrinsic vasculopathy or even two separate diseases, i.e., PAH and ILD.[1]

Group 5 is "PH with unclear and/or multifactorial mechanisms", including sarcoidosis.[1] This distinction from group 3 is justified by the pathogenesis of sarcoidosis PH, with complex interactions between the pulmonary vasculature and parenchymal, mediastinal, and cardiovascular compartments.

Another important point of the classification of PH is that pulmonary veno-occlusive disease (PVOD) and pulmonary capillary hemangiomatosis are individualized from PAH in a specific subgroup (group 1′).[1] Similarities in pathologic and clinical features and the risk of drug-induced pulmonary edema with PAH therapy suggest that these two conditions overlap. It has been proposed that pulmonary capillary hemangiomatosis could be a secondary angioproliferative process caused by postcapillary obstruction of PVOD rather than a distinct entity.[1]

FREQUENCY OF SARCOIDOSIS-ASSOCIATED PH

There is a wide distribution in published rates of the prevalence of PH complicating sarcoidosis, which is most likely due to the use of different measurement techniques, selection of diverse patient populations, or various stages of disease (Table 24.3). Overall, PH affects 1%–6% of sarcoidosis patients,[2–8] but it is much more frequent in advanced lung disease[9] and symptomatic cases.[10–12]

Sarcoidosis. https://doi.org/10.1016/B978-0-323-54429-0.00024-0

TABLE 24.1
Hemodynamic Definitions of PH[1]

Definition	Characteristics[a]	Clinical Groups[b]
PH	mPAP ≥ 25 mmHg	All
Precapillary PH	mPAP ≥ 25 mmHg PAWP ≤ 15 mmHg	1. PAH 3. PH due to lung diseases 4. CTEPH 5. PH with unclear and/or multifactorial mechanisms
Postcapillary PH *Isolated postcapillary PH* *Combined postcapillary and precapillary PH*	mPAP ≥ 25 mmHg PAWP > 15 mmHg *DPG < 7 mmHg and/or* *PVR ≤ 3 Wood units*[c] *DPG ≥ 7 mmHg and/or* *PVR > 3 Wood units*[c]	2. PH due to left heart disease 5. PH with unclear and/or multifactorial mechanisms

CTEPH, chronic thromboembolic PH; *DPG*, diastolic pressure gradient (diastolic PAP–mean PAWP); *mPAP*, mean pulmonary arterial pressure; *PAH*, pulmonary arterial hypertension; *PAWP*, pulmonary arterial wedge pressure; *PH*, pulmonary hypertension; *PVR*, pulmonary vascular resistance.
[a]All values measured at rest.
[b]According to Table 24.2.
[c]WU are preferred to dynes s cm^{-5}.

TABLE 24.2
Clinical Classification of PH[1]

1. PAH

1.1 Idiopathic
1.2 Heritable
  1.2.1 BMPR2 mutation
  1.2.2 Other mutations
1.3 Drugs and toxins induced
1.4 Associated with:
  1.4.1 Connective tissue diseases
  1.4.2 HIV infection
  1.4.3 Portal hypertension
  1.4.4 Congenital heart diseases
  1.4.5 Schistosomiasis

1′. PVOD AND/OR PULMONARY CAPILLARY HEMANGIOMATOSIS

1’.1 Idiopathic
1’.2 Heritable
  1’.2.1 EIF2AK4 mutation
  1’.2.2 Other mutations
1’.3 Drugs, toxins, and radiation induced
1’.4 Associated with:
  1’.4.1 Connective tissue diseases
  1’.4.2 HIV infection

1”. PERSISTENT PH OF THE NEWBORN

2. PH DUE TO LEFT HEART DISEASE

2.1 Left ventricular systolic dysfunction
2.2 Left ventricular diastolic dysfunction
2.3 Valvular disease
2.4 Congenital/acquired left heart inflow/outflow tract obstruction and congenital cardiomyopathies
2.5 Congenital/acquired pulmonary veins stenosis

3. PH DUE TO LUNG DISEASES AND/OR HYPOXIA

3.1 Chronic obstructive pulmonary disease
3.2 Interstitial lung disease
3.3 Other pulmonary diseases with mixed restrictive and obstructive pattern
3.4 Sleep-disordered breathing
3.5 Alveolar hypoventilation disorders
3.6 Chronic exposure to high altitude
3.7 Developmental lung diseases

4. CTEPH AND OTHER PULMONARY ARTERY OBSTRUCTIONS

4.1 CTEPH
4.2 Other pulmonary artery obstructions
  4.2.1 Angiosarcoma
  4.2.2 Other intravascular tumors
  4.2.3 Arteritis
  4.2.4 Congenital pulmonary arteries stenoses
  4.2.5 Parasites (hydatidosis)

5. PH WITH UNCLEAR AND/OR MULTIFACTORIAL MECHANISMS

5.1 Hematological disorders: chronic hemolytic anemia, myeloproliferative disorders, splenectomy
5.2 Systemic disorders: sarcoidosis, pulmonary histiocytosis, lymphangioleiomyomatosis, neurofibromatosis
5.3 Metabolic disorders: glycogen storage disease, Gaucher disease, thyroid disorders
5.4 Others: pulmonary tumoral thrombotic microangiopathy, fibrosing mediastinitis, chronic renal failure (with/without dialysis), segmental PH

BMPR2, bone morphogenetic protein receptor; *CTEPH*, chronic thromboembolic PH; *EIF2AK4*, eukaryotic translation initiation factor two alpha kinase four; *HIV*, human immunodeficiency virus; *PAH*, pulmonary arterial hypertension; *PH*, pulmonary hypertension; *type 2 PVOD*, pulmonary veno-occlusive disease.

TABLE 24.3
Main Studies on the Prevalence of PH in Sarcoidosis Patients

Design	Population	Diagnosis	Prevalence	Study
Not specified (n = 50)	Patients with various stages of disease (method of selection not specified)	RHC	Resting mPAP > 25 mmHg: 6%; exercise mPAP > 30 mmHg: 26.5%	3
Retrospective (n = 130)	Consecutive patients with persistent dyspnea despite systemic therapy	RHC	mPAP > 25 mmHg • with PAWP < 15 mmHg: 38.5% (mPAP ≥ 40 mmHg: 10.8%) • with PAWP ≥ 15 mmHg: 15.4%	11
Retrospective (n = 106)	Patients with various cardiorespiratory symptoms	TTE	sPAP ≥ 40 mmHg: 51%	12
Retrospective (n = 363)	US registry of patients listed for lung transplantation	RHC	mPAP > 25 mmHg: 73.8% (mPAP ≥ 40 mmHg: 36%)	9
Prospective (n = 212)	Consecutive patients with various stages of disease	TTE	sPAP ≥ 40 mmHg: 5.7%	4
Prospective (n = 111)	Consecutive patients with various stages of disease	TTE ± RHC	mPAP ≥ 25 mmHg: 3.6%	8
Cross-sectional (n = 313)	Consecutive patients with various stages of disease	TTE ± RHC	mPAP ≥ 25 mmHg: 2.9%	7
Prospective (n = 141)	Patients with available 6MWT	TTE ± RHC	mPAP ≥ 25 mmHg: 10.6%	13

mPAP, mean pulmonary arterial pressure on RHC; *PH*, pulmonary hypertension; *PWAP*, pulmonary arterial wedge pressure; *RHC*, right heart catheterization; *sPAP*, systolic pulmonary arterial estimated on TTE; *TTE*, transthoracic Doppler echocardiography; *6MWT*, 6-min walk test.

The prospective study by Handa et al. evaluated 212 consecutive sarcoidosis patients by transthoracic Doppler echocardiography (TTE).[4] An estimated systolic pulmonary arterial pressure (sPAP) > 40 mmHg was found in 5.7%, but regrettably, RHC was not performed to confirm the diagnosis of PH.[4] In the study by Pabst et al., 111 patients were prospectively screened for PH.[8] PH was assumed on TTE in 23 patients, of which 11 had left ventricular (LV) systolic or diastolic dysfunction or valvular disease. Of the 10 remaining patients undergoing RHC, four showed precapillary PH (3.6%), and one showed postcapillary PH.[8] Shorr et al. retrospectively reviewed the US cohort of 363 sarcoidosis patients listed for lung transplantation who had completed RHC.[9] PH was identified in 73.8% of cases, and mPAP was >40 mmHg in 36.1%.[9] In the retrospective study by Baughman et al., 130 patients with persistent dyspnea despite systemic therapy for their sarcoidosis were thoroughly investigated with RHC.[11] Seventy patients (53.9%) had evidence of PH, including 50 (38.5%) with precapillary PH and 20 (15.4%) with postcapillary PH. mPAP was over 35 and 40 mmHg in 46% and 28% of cases with precapillary PH, respectively.[11]

MECHANISMS OF SARCOIDOSIS PH

As indicated previously, sarcoidosis is classified in group 5 of the clinical classification of PH, but, essentially, the mechanisms of sarcoidosis PH may fit into all five categories.[1]

Precapillary PH

Destruction of the distal capillary bed and resultant hypoxia

The large majority of patients with sarcoidosis PH have advanced disease.[4,11–16] However, 28%–50% develop this complication in the absence of patent pulmonary fibrosis on chest radiography,[11,12,14,15] and a small subset of cases have no apparent underlying lung disease (radiographic stage 0 and I).[4,11,14,15,17] Moreover, hemodynamic measurements do not correlate well with spirometric parameters and PaO_2,[4,10,14,15,18] and mPAP is 9 mmHg higher in sarcoidosis candidates for lung transplantation than in those with idiopathic pulmonary fibrosis for equivalent respiratory impairment (34.4 versus 25.6 mmHg, $P < .0001$).[19] Finally, the degree of PH is sometimes disproportionate to functional abnormalities,[9,11,14,15,20] and PH may even be more severe when it occurs in patients without fibrotic disease.[14] For example, of the 156 patients with sarcoidosis PH collected from the French PH registry, 30 (19.2%) had mild PH, and 126 (87.8%) had severe PH, as defined as an mPAP > 35 mmHg or mPAP ≥ 25 mmHg plus CI < 2.5 L/min per m^2.[15] More than half of the cases with severe PH were under long-term oxygen therapy, but only 24% had a marked restrictive pattern with forced vital capacity (FVC) < 50% predicted.[15]

Taken together, these findings support the idea that other mechanisms may play a role in the development of sarcoidosis PH. These include specific pulmonary vasculopathy, locally increased vasoreactivity, extrinsic compression of pulmonary vessels, portal hypertension, and left heart dysfunction. Comorbidities associated with sarcoidosis can also cause PH.

Specific pulmonary vasculopathy

Vascular changes in pulmonary sarcoidosis. Granulomatous vascular involvement appears to be very common in the pulmonary circulation of sarcoidosis patients, as evidenced in 53% of transbronchial lung biopsy specimens,[21] 69% of open lung biopsies,[22] and 100% of autopsy cases.[23] This exists in whatever radiographic stage, and its extent is roughly linked to that of parenchymal granulomas. Although vascular involvement can be seen at all levels, from large branches of pulmonary arteries (PAs) to venules (Fig. 24.1), it clearly predominates in the venous side and in small vessels,

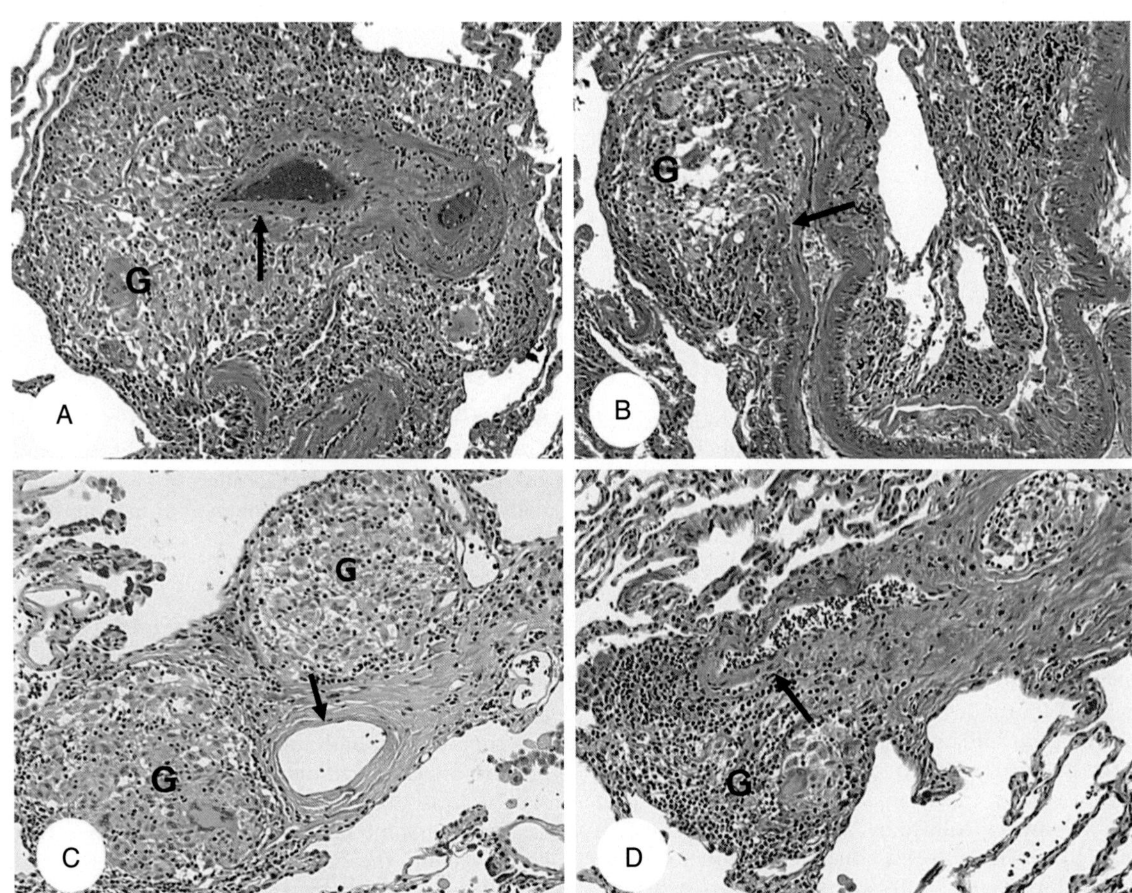

FIG. 24.1 Vascular involvement in sarcoidosis PH. **(A)** This medium-sized artery is totally engulfed *(arrow)* within a sarcoid granuloma (hematoxylin eosin staining × 100). **(B)** Nonnecrotizing sarcoid granuloma is seen *(arrow)*, partially replacing the wall of this pulmonary artery (hematoxylin eosin staining × 100). **(C)** This vein is altered by severe fibrosis *(arrow)*, with characteristic eccentric involvement of its outer wall by a couple of florid sarcoid granulomas (hematoxylin eosin staining × 100). **(D)** This vein is narrowed *(arrow)* by fibrosis nearby florid granulomas (hematoxylin eosin staining × 100). *PH*, pulmonary hypertension.

reflecting the lymphatic spreading of the granulomatous process.[21–24] Overall, there is evidence of venous involvement alone in 65%–67% of cases, both venous and arterial involvement in 24%–31%, and arterial involvement alone in 8%–11%.[21–24] Granulomas invade the vasculature of elastic PAs in 30% of cases, muscular PAs in 55%, arterioles in 60%, venules in 65%, and interlobular veins in 58%.

In both PAs and veins, the distribution of granulomas is segmental and preponderant at the bifurcation of the vessels.[21–24] Granulomas have a tropism for the outer wall of arteries and veins, being mainly localized in the adventitia and the outer section of the media, with focal dissociation of elastic fibers and destruction of the external elastic lamina, as well as around the vasa vasorum[21–24] (Fig. 24.1). In muscular arteries, granulomas commonly appear along the bronchovascular bundles. Arterioles and venules reveal focal disruption of lamina elastica with occasional obstruction (Fig. 24.1). In many cases, both granulomatous vascular involvement and its healed lesions coexist in the same lung at different stages[21–24] (Fig. 24.1). Destruction of vascular architecture can be noted, with loss of media and mural and adventitial fibrosis, contributing to luminal narrowing[21–24] (Fig. 24.1). Fibrosis in the venous walls has a tendency to extend into the interlobular space, whereas arterial granulomas evolve into fibrosis along the bronchovascular sheaths.[21–24]

Vascular changes in sarcoidosis PH. Despite extremely frequent granulomatous vascular involvement in sarcoidosis, clinically significant PH is intringuily rare. In the series of 40 cases studied by Takemura et al., all had vascular involvement, but only four had right heart overload.[23] The reasons why a proportion of sarcoidosis patients will eventually develop this complication remain obscure, with only few publications supplying pathologic description of sarcoidosis PH.

Obviously, nonspecific vascular remodeling secondary to the chronic lung disease can be seen, including intimal fibrosis and medial hypertrophy of PAs. Proliferative arteriopathy with plexiform lesions can exist but is exceedingly rare.[2,25–27] The complex changes detailed previously may result in obliterative vasculopathy and, when sufficiently extensive, ultimately incite PH. Reflecting the venous predilection of granulomatous vascular involvement, a PVOD-like disease is recognized as a cause of sarcoidosis PH.[28–30] The occlusive narrowing of venules and interlobular septal veins by widespread granulomas can mimic PVOD, which has been pathologically authenticated in a handful of cases with active sarcoidosis and PH.[28–30] Besides, Nunes et al. reported an intrinsic venopathy in explanted lungs from five patients with fibrotic sarcoidosis and severe PH. This venopathy consisted of salient occlusive intimal fibrosis and recanalization, together with chronic hemosiderosis and iron deposition in elastic lamina in all cases. In opposition, arterial changes were minor with no evidence of plexiform or thrombotic lesions.[14] Interestingly, a patient with sarcoidosis PH was recently reported displaying diffuse alveolar capillary multiplication and wall muscularization in macroscopically normal lung parenchyma, in addition to nonspecific vascular remodeling within fibrotic lesions.[31]

Pathogenesis of sarcoidosis pulmonary vasculopathy. These observations suggest that the intrinsic vasculopathy seen in sarcoidosis may be an indirect consequence of granulomatous process through the production of various vasoactive mediators, cytokines, or growth factors implicated in locally heightened vasoreactivity and vascular remodeling. No work has specifically explored these pathogenic pathways in sarcoidosis PH. Interestingly yet, a small study by Singla et al. used genome-wide peripheral blood gene expression analysis and identified an 18-gene signature capable of distinguishing sarcoidosis patients with PH from those without PH, with a very high discriminative accuracy.[32] Nine of these genes are linked to cellular proliferation, one of the central events of vascular remodeling. However, a major limitation of this study is the lack of reverse transcription polymerase chain reaction confirmation of the microarray findings and the absence of validation in an independent cohort.[32]

Mutations in several genes have been identified in familial or sporadic patients with PAH, the major being *BMPR2*, which encodes for a type 2 receptor for bone morphogenetic proteins involved in the control of vascular cell proliferation.[1] The extent to which gene polymorphism might contribute toward determining the severity of PH in other groups of PH remains unknown. Recently, a Spanish team reported 3 cases with sarcoidosis PH and genetic aberrations, including two with *BMPR2* gene mutations and one with KCNA5 (potassium voltage-gated channel, shaker-related subfamily, member 5) gene mutation.[33]

Extrinsic compression of pulmonary vessels

Sarcoidosis PH may be caused by extrinsic compression of the proximal PAs by enlarged lymph nodes or fibrosing mediastinitis (Figs. 24.2A and 24.3A).[14,15,34–36] Compression of the large pulmonary veins is much rarer and can provoke localized edema.[37] Although

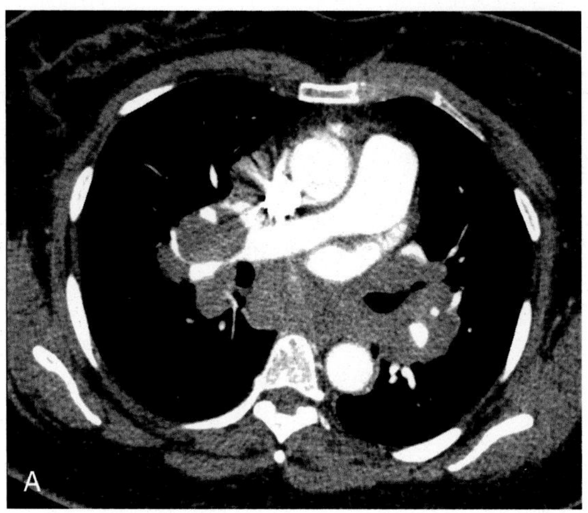
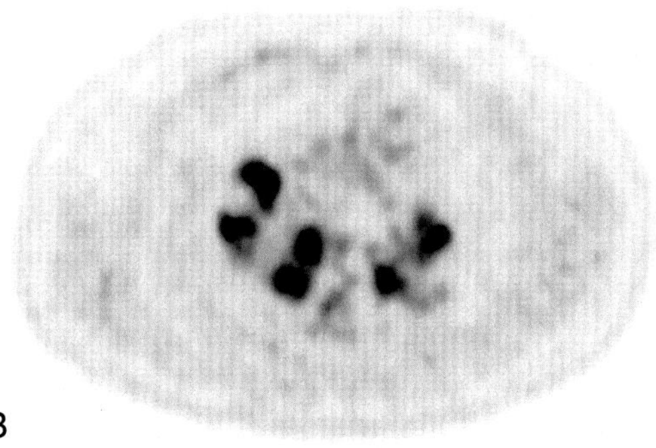

FIG. 24.2 A 50-year-old female patient presented with severe sarcoidosis PH due to extrinsic compression of pulmonary arteries by enlarged lymph nodes. The patient significantly improved after steroids. **(A)** Chest multidetector computed tomography angiography showing multiple bilateral lymph nodes with an extrinsic compression of the right main pulmonary artery. **(B)** ^{18}F-2-fluoro-2-deoxy-D-glucose positron emission tomography showing a significant uptake of the lymph nodes. *PH*, pulmonary hypertension.

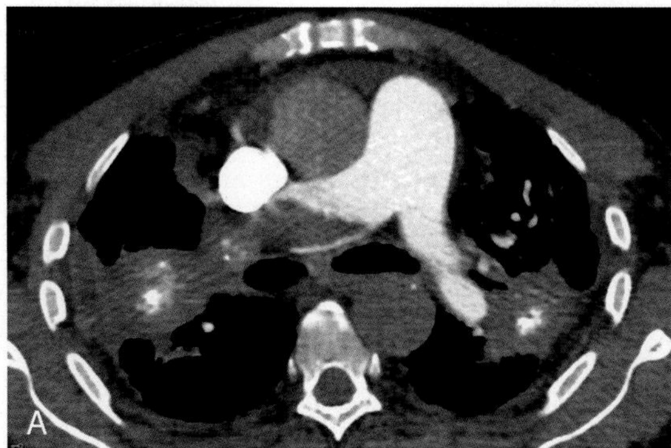
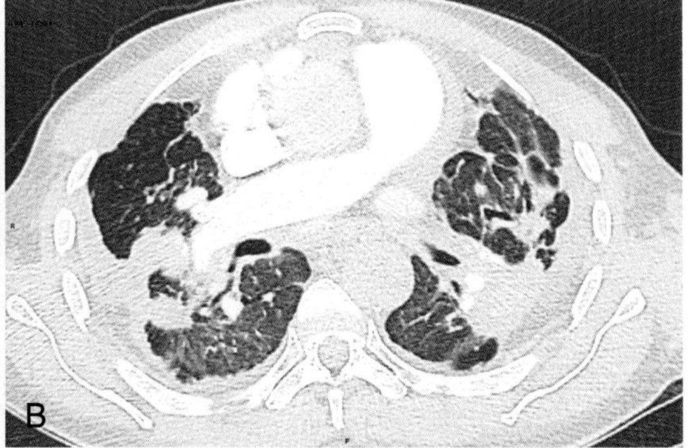

FIG. 24.3 Chest multidetector computed tomography angiography of a 69-year-old male patient with severe sarcoidosis PH due to both extrinsic compression of pulmonary arteries by fibrosing mediastinitis and extensive pulmonary fibrosis. The patient died of right heart failure despite immunosuppressive therapy. **(A)** The scan shows an aspect of fibrosing mediastinitis with an infiltration of the right pulmonary artery that mimics massive proximal pulmonary embolism. **(B)** The scan shows extensive bronchial distorsion and fibrotic calcified masses. *PH*, pulmonary hypertension.

occasionally described in early stages of sarcoidosis, vascular compression is much more frequent in patients with long-standing disease when lymph nodes become fibrotic and calcify. Sarcoidosis is one of the main causes of fibrosing mediastinitis, accounting for 11% of cases in an ancient review[38] and 48.1% in a recent original series.[39] Extrinsic compression of PAs represents 21.4% of patients with sarcoidosis PH and radiographic stage IV in the study of Nunes et al.[14] and 5% of all cases with severe sarcoidosis PH in that of Boucly et al.[15] Importantly, sarcoidosis-associated fibrosing mediastinitis with resultant PH can mimic chronic thromboembolic PH (CTEPH) (Fig. 24.3A).[40]

Portal hypertension

PH may also be the consequence of hepatic sarcoidosis, which can rarely lead to cirrhosis and portal hypertension.[41,42]

Postcapillary PH

Clinical myocardial involvement is observed in about 5% of sarcoidosis patients and can generate LV systolic or diastolic dysfunction, but occult involvement is much more frequently revealed at pathology. Several studies have pointed to a high prevalence of early myocardial damage with subclinical LV dysfunction in sarcoidosis patients, as evidenced by TTE, in particular using newer techniques of speckle tracking strain analysis,[43] cardiac magnetic resonance imaging (MRI),[44,45] and RHC.[11] However, the reliability of conventional TTE for the detection of heart failure with preserved LV ejection fraction is weak in sarcoidosis. In the study of Baughman et al., of 130 sarcoidosis patients with persistent dyspnea investigated by RHC, postcapillary PH was seen in 20 (15.4%),[11] which represented 28.6% of all cases with PH. Only seven of them (35%) had a reduced LV ejection fraction on TTE.[11]

Comorbidities

A link between sarcoidosis and venous thromboembolic events (VTEs) has recently been emphasized.[46–48] Crawshaw et al. analyzed a retrospective cohort using a well-established epidemiological data set, covering the period between 1963 and 1998, which recorded all hospital admissions to National Health Service hospitals and all deaths within Oxfordshire region.[46] A significant association was demonstrated between sarcoidosis and pulmonary embolism (PE), in comparison with a matched reference population (hazard ratio (HR): 1.92; 95% CI: 1.05–3.23, P = .01), but not deep vein thrombosis.[46] Using US death certificates from 1988 to 2007, Swigris et al. have shown that PE was declared in 2.54% of decedents with sarcoidosis compared with only 1.13% of the background population (HR: 2.3, 95% CI: 2.1–2.5, P<.0001).[47] The risk was significantly greater than that for decedents with COPD.[47] Last, Ungprasert et al. conducted another population-based study using a big database that allowed capture of nearly all the incident cases of sarcoidosis in the population of Olmsted County, Minnesota, from 1976 to 2013.[48] The risk of incident VTE adjusted for age, sex, and calendar year was significantly higher among sarcoidosis patients (HR: 3.04, 95% CI: 1.47–6.29), including for deep vein thrombosis (HR: 3.14, 95% CI: 1.32–7.48) and PE (HR: 4.29, 95% CI: 1.21–15.23).[48] However, to the best of our knowledge, CTEPH has been described in a unique sarcoidosis patients showing exuberant granulomas inside the thrombi at pathology.[49]

The factors conferring an increased risk for VTE in sarcoidosis remain to be clarified and may include chronic inflammation, the presence of antiphospholipid antibodies, and use of corticosteroids. The rate of either IgG or IgM antiphospholipid serum antibodies reaches 38% of sarcoidosis patients, which is significantly upper than that in healthy controls.[50] Several observations have described antiphospholipid syndrome occurring in sarcoidosis patients with[51] or without concomitant systemic lupus.[52,53] Also, sarcoidosis can co-exist with various auto-immune disorders known to facilitate VTE and/or PAH.[54–56] Last, a higher than expected prevalence of obstructive sleep apnea has been mentioned in sarcoidosis,[57,58] attaining 17% in one study.[58]

DIAGNOSIS OF SARCOIDOSIS PH

Clinical Presentation

In the largest cohort with severe sarcoidosis PH of Boucly et al., the median time between the diagnosis of sarcoidosis and that of PH was 17 years, the sex ratio was 1:1, and the mean age 57.5 years.[15] A study based on the US National Center for Health Statistics reported a two-folds higher prevalence of PH in African-American decedents than in Caucasians.[59] The clinical picture that should prompt diagnostic intervention include dyspnea more severe than one would expect from functional impairment, chest pain, palpitations, and near-syncope on exertion. Physical signs include a loud P2 component to the second heart sound, a fixed, split S2, a holosystolic murmur of tricuspid regurgitation, and a diastolic murmur of pulmonic regurgitation. More than two-thirds of patients with sarcoidosis PH present with NYHA functional class II or III and about one quarter with right ventricular (RV) failure.[12,14,15] ECG may show signs of RV strain, and chest radiography may show right cardiomegaly and PA enlargement.

Transthoracic Doppler Echocardiography

TTE is well known to be imperfect to detect PH in ILDs. The peak tricuspid regurgitation velocity (TRV) is measurable in only half of patients, and even if available, estimation of the sPAP is often inaccurate.[60] When considering estimated systolic PAP (sPAP)≥45 mm Hg as a determinant of PH, the positive and negative predictive values of TTE are 60% and 44%, respectively. RV abnormalities are valuable surrogates of PH, with a positive and negative predictive value of 57% and 74%, respectively.[60] There is little specific information for sarcoidosis PH.[11,13] In the study of Baughman et al., 80 patients had both echocardiographic and hemodynamic evaluation. Of these, only 70% had sufficient peak TRV identified so that sPAP could be estimated. For these cases, there was a significant correlation between estimated and measured sPAS, but sensitivity and specificity of TTE were not provided.[11] More recently, RV dysfunction detected by speckle tracking strain analysis has been associated with the presence of PH.[61]

Right Heart Catheterization

Although definite diagnosis relies on invasive measurements, not all sarcoidosis patients with suspected PH should undergo confirmatory RHC. The ESC/ERS guidelines do not give recommendations for group 5 PH but assert the following indications for RHC in group 3 PH: (1) proper diagnosis or exclusion of PH in candidates for lung transplantation; (2) suspected severe PH suggesting an associated PAH or CTEPH; (3) episodes of right heart failure; and (4) inconclusive TTE study in cases with a high index of clinical suspicion and potential therapeutic implications, including enrollment in a clinical trial.[1] In sarcoidosis, a wider adoption of RHC has however gained credit after the published experience of Baughman et al.[11] As discussed previously, LV dysfunction is not uncommon in sarcoidosis and probably underrated by TTE.[11] Furthermore, RHC also provides per se important information on prognosis: on the one hand, it allows assessment of severity of hemodynamic impairment; on the other, the pre capillary or postcapillary nature of PH has not only been therapeutic but also prognostic consequences.[11]

The hemodynamic severity of sarcoidosis PH is variable. In the study of Baughman et al., median mPAP was 33 mmHg (range: 25–75) and median PVR was 4.3 Wood units (range: 0.9–21.2).[11] Patients with precapillary PH had a similar mPAP but a significantly higher PVR than those with postcapillary PH.[11] As therapy with high doses of calcium channel blockers (CCBs) has no indication in group 5 PH, acute vasodilator challenge is not recommended in the majority of patients with sarcoidosis.[1]

Pulmonary Function Tests and Six-Minute Walk Test

Most of studies have shown statistically lower FVC, forced expiratory volume in 1 s (FEV1), total lung capacity (TLC), and diffusing capacity of the lung for carbon monoxide (DLCO) values in sarcoidosis patients with PH.[4,11–13,16,62] These patients are also more hypoxemic and/or require more frequently supplemental oxygen than those without PH.[4,9,11–13,16,62] Nonetheless, the contribution of pulmonary function tests (PFTs) alone for the identification of patients with PH is modest. In multivariate analysis, the need for oxygen remained the only predictor of PH in the transplant cohort of Shorr et al. (OR: 8.39, 95% CI: 3.44–20.47), with a specificity of 91.8% but a very low sensitivity of 32.6%.[9] Handa et al. demonstrated that only decreased TLC% was independently associated with echocardiographic PH in sarcoidosis patients (OR: 0.69, 95% CI: 0.48–0.99, $P < .05$), but its predictive power was mild.[4] Because the reduction of DLCO can be related to both interstitial and vascular involvement, it has been postulated that a high FVC%/DLCO% ratio (with a cutoff of 1.4–1.5), reflecting a disproportionately reduced DLCO for the degree of restriction, may be a better tool for gauging PH in ILDs. In sarcoidosis, FVC%/DLCO% ratio is significantly higher in patients with PH in two studies based on TTE[12,63] but not in another based on RHC.[16]

Patients with sarcoidosis PH accomplish a significantly shorter distance on six-minute walk test (6MWT) than those without PH.[63,64] The retrospective study of Bourbonnais et al. aimed to determine the clinical predictors of PH in 162 sarcoidosis patients.[13] The 22 patients with PH walked less (343 ± 116 m versus 426 ± 105 m, $P < .004$) and had a greater desaturation (8.85 ± 4.22% versus 2.99 ± 2.14%, $P < .001$) and Borg score at 6 min.[13] Multivariate analyses showed that the significant indicators of PH on TTE were $SaO_2 <$ 90% on 6MWT (HR: 12.1, 95% CI: 3.66–19.73) and DLCO < 60% predicted (HR: 7.3, 95% CI: 1.98–24.82). DLCO did no longer retain significance when PH was defined on RHC. The other variables tested, including marched distance, and all other PFT parameters failed to predict the presence of PH.[13] Interestingly, all seven patients being misdiagnosed as having no PH on TTE desaturated to <90% during 6MWT, suggesting that a composite model combining the results of SaO_2 on 6MWT with those of TTE would improve the pretest probability before performing RHC.[13] Although not properly evaluated, exercise testing may be interesting to identify PH in sarcoidosis patients.

Imaging

In PH, chest multidetector computed tomography angiography (MD-CTA) can show a raised caliber of PA (widest diameter of the main PA > 29 mm, PA diameter/ascending aorta diameter ratio > 1 or PA diameter indexed to body surface area) or enlarged right heart cavities (Figs. 24.4B and 24.5). Even so, the PA diameter and PA/aorta ratio are not reliable to predict the presence of PH in various ILDs,[65,66] possibly because the restrictive lung physiology may result in a traction effect on the mediastinal vascular structures, distending the PA independently of the underlying PAP. The ability of MD-CTA for predicting PH in sarcoidosis has been investigated by Huitema et al. in a unique retrospective study including 89 patients who were classified as

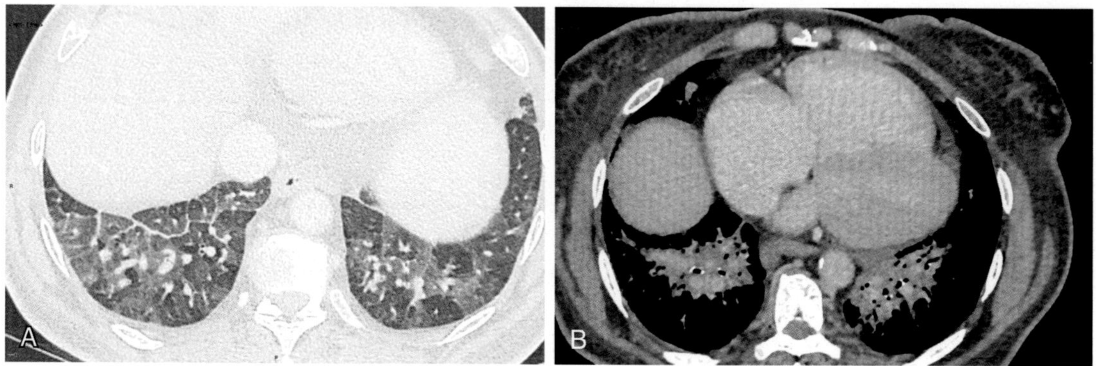

FIG. 24.4 High-resolution computed tomography of a 54-year-old female with severe sarcoidosis-associated PH and a suspicion of pulmonary veno-occlusive disease. The patient worsened despite immunosuppressive therapy and bosentan and was eventually transplanted. **(A)** The scan shows a network of septal reticulations in association with ground-glass opacities, raising the possibility of pulmonary veno-occlusive disease. **(B)** The scan shows right atrial and ventricular enlargement. *PH*, pulmonary hypertension.

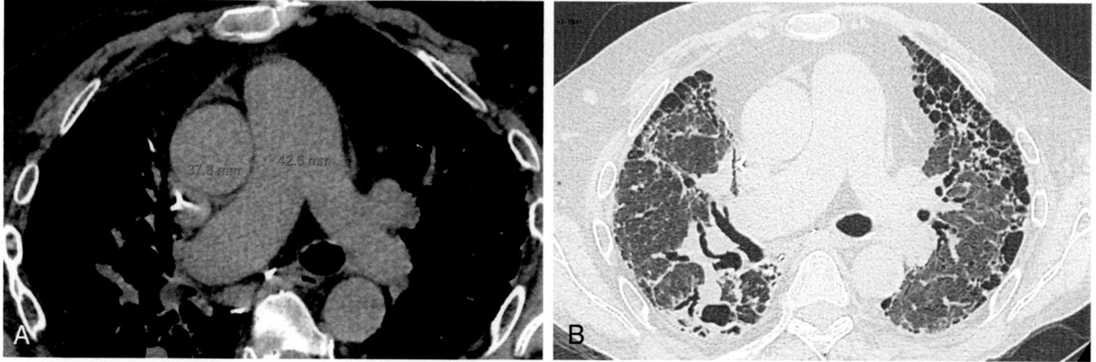

FIG. 24.5 High-resolution computed tomography of a 67-year-old male with severe sarcoidosis-associated PH and pulmonary fibrosis. After failure of immunosuppressive therapy, the patient received sildenafil and stabilized. **(A)** The scan shows a raised caliber of the main pulmonary artery, with a widest diameter >29 mm and a ratio over aorta diameter > 1. **(B)** The scan shows extensive pulmonary fibrosis with a predominant pattern of honeycombing. *PH*, pulmonary hypertension.

"PH likely", "PH possible", or "PH unlikely" according to TTE findings.[16] RHC, carried out if PH was likely or possible, confirmed PH in 25 cases. PA/aorta ratio and PA/body surface area ratio had a moderate correlation with invasive mPAP and a weak correlation with the extent of fibrosis. PA/body surface area ratio showed the best positive and negative predictive values for detecting PH (70% and 93.2%, respectively), followed by PA/aorta ratio (64.3% and 88.5%, respectively).[16] Only PA/body surface area ratio was able to discriminate between the presence and absence of PH in patients with possible PH on TTE with a high diagnostic accuracy using a cutoff of $15.2\,\mathrm{mm\,m^{-2}}$.[16]

In sarcoidosis, contrast-enhanced MD-CTA also aids to delineate the mechanisms of PH. First, it allows the diagnosis of extrinsic vascular compression (Figs. 24.2A and 24.3A). Second, several findings may hint to PVOD such as extensive ground-glass opacities and/or thickened interlobular septa (Fig. 24.4A).[14] The differentiation between extrinsic vascular compression and CTEPH is sometimes tricky (Fig. 24.3A). Mismatched segmental perfusion defects on the ventilation/perfusion lung scan can be observed in both the settings. The use of maximal intensity projection is helpful to recognize the process, but pulmonary angiography is required for the most difficult cases.[40]

TABLE 24.4
Probability of PH in Patients With a Suspicion of PH According to TTE (TVR and Additional Contributive Signs)[1]

TRV (m/s)	Presence of Other Signs of PH on TTE	Probability of PH
≤2.8 or not measurable	No	Low
≤2.8 or not measurable	Yes	Intermediate
2.9–3.4	No	
2.9–3.4	Yes	High
>3.4	Not required	
A. The Ventricles[a]	**B. PA[a]**	**C. IVC and Right Atrium[a]**
RV/LV basal diameter ratio >1.0	RV outflow Doppler acceleration time <105 ms and/or midsystolic notching	IVC diameter > 21 mm with decreased inspiratory collapse (<50% with a sniff or <20% with quiet inspiration)
Flattening of the interventricular septum (LV eccentricity index >1.1 in systole and/or diastole)	Early diastolic pulmonary regurgitation velocity >2.2 m/s	Right atrial area (end-systole) >18 cm^2
	PA diameter > 25 mm	

IVC, inferior vena cava; *PA*, pulmonary artery; *PH*, pulmonary hypertension; *LV*, left ventricular; *RV*, right ventricular; *TRV*, peak tricuspid regurgitation velocity; *TTE*, transthoracic Doppler echocardiography.
[a]Signs from at least two different categories (A/B/C) from the list should be present to alter the level of probability of PH on TTE.

In the presence of PH due to left heart disease, cardiac MRI and ^{18}F-2-fluoro-2-deoxy-D-glucose positron emission tomography (^{18}FDG-PET) are critical for the diagnosis of cardiac sarcoidosis. RV late gadolinium enhancement on cardiac MRI is associated with the presence of PH on TTE, but its diagnostic additional value is unknown.[67] ^{18}FDG-PET may be helpful to identify patients more likely to respond to immunosuppressive therapy (Fig. 24.2B).[15] Hepatic ultrasound is necessary to exclude porto-PH.[1]

Natriuretic Peptides

It has been suggested that plasma brain natriuretic peptide (BNP) or N-Terminal pro-BNP (NT-pro-BNP) may be helpful biomarkers for the detection of PH in patients with various ILDs, but specific data are rare in sarcoidosis.[16,63,68] Handa et al. performed a prospective study to evaluate the use of plasma NT-pro-BNP in the assessment of PH and cardiac involvement.[68] Among the 130 sarcoidosis subjects evaluable for PH status at TTE, 21 were diagnosed with PH, as defined by an sPAP > 35 mmHg. Patients with PH had significantly higher levels of NT-pro-BNP than those without, but the increase was milder than that in patients with cardiac involvement. Moreover, NT-pro-BNP had a poor discriminative capacity for PH, even when patients with cardiac sarcoidosis were excluded. The sensitivity and specificity were 75.0% and 60.9%, respectively, with a cutoff 103 pg/mL.[68]

SCREENING OF SARCOIDOSIS PH

As PH bears a severe prognosis in sarcoidosis, early diagnosis and consideration of treatment options may be key to improve patients' outcome. Nevertheless, the diagnosis of PH is difficult, and its recognition frequently delayed. Although several clinical and functional features may raise suspicion of PH, there is no consistent single criterion that can be used to adequately segregate sarcoidosis patients with a high or low risk. So far, conventional TTE remains the most appropriate modality for the noninvasive assessment of suspected PH. The ECS/ERS guidelines suggest grading the probability of PH as high, intermediate, or low based on TRV at rest and on the presence of additional prespecified echocardiographic variables that reinforce suspicion of PH (Table 24.4). However, owing to its limited accuracy in sarcoidosis, TTE should be interpreted in a clinical context and not serve as the only guide to decide who requires further invasive procedure.

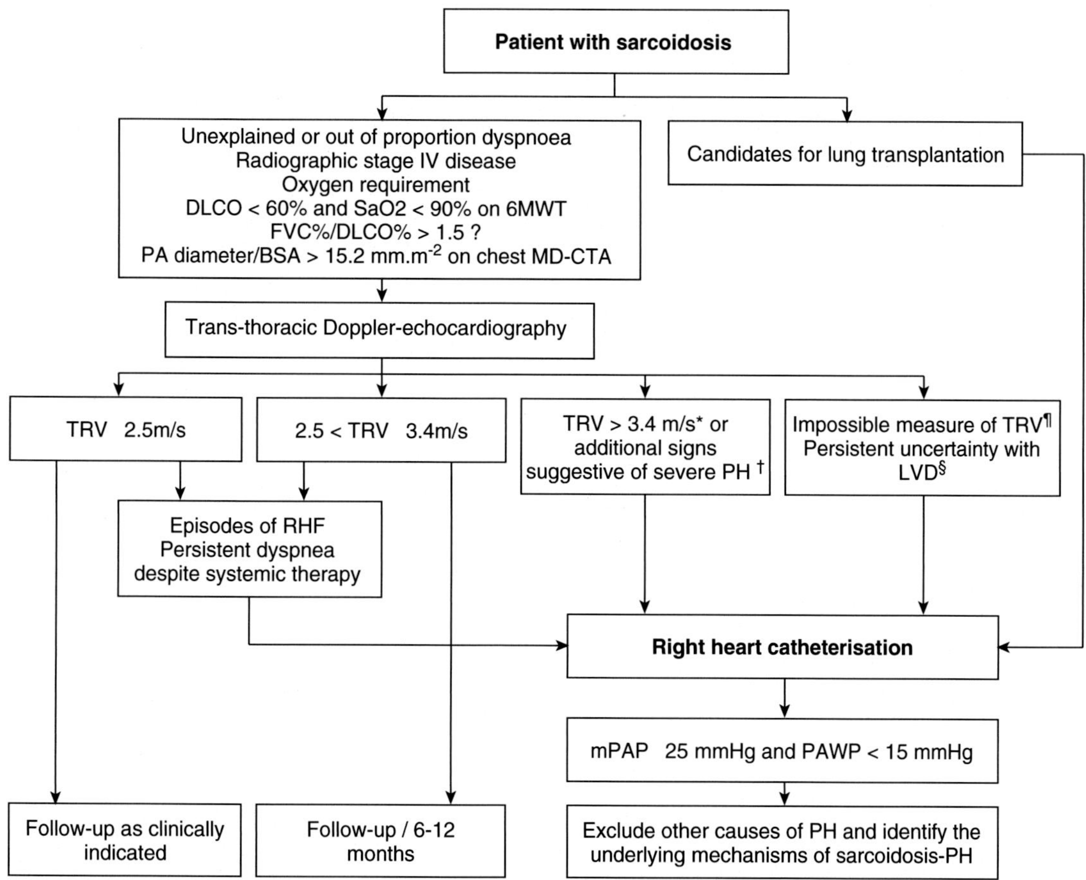

FIG. 24.6 Proposed algorithm for the screening of PH in sarcoidosis patients. *6MWT*, 6-minute walk test; *BSA*, body surface area; *DLCO*, single breath diffusing capacity for carbon monoxide; *FVC*, forced vital capacity; *LVD*, left ventricular dysfunction; *MD-CTA*, multidetector computed tomography angiography; *mPAP*, mean pulmonary arterial pressure; *PAWP*, pulmonary arterial wedge pressure; *PA*, main pulmonary artery; *RHF*, right heart failure; *TRV*, peak tricuspid regurgitation velocity. *Severe PH can be suspected on transthoracic Doppler echocardiography if TRV > 3.4 m/s (corresponding to an estimated systolic PAP > 55–60 mmHg). †Additional echocardiographic signs suggestive of PH are indicated in Table 24.4. ¶In cases with a high index of clinical suspicion and potential therapeutic implications. §In particular left ventricular diastolic dysfunction.

Conversely, one should keep in mind that the benefits of RHC need to be balanced against the risks so that it is justified only if clinical consequences are to be expected.[69] RHC seems reasonable in selected patients with persistant uncertainty regarding LV dysfunction, who endure unexplained dyspnea despite sarcoidosis treatment, or with severe PH potentially amenable to PAH therapy. Once PH is confirmed, a comprehensive workup is intended to scrupulously rule out the other classical causes of PH, chiefly CTEPH, but also portal hypertension, sleep apnea, autoimmune diseases, and human immunodeficiency virus infection. In cases with suspected heart sarcoidosis, several cardiac tests complement RHC. A screening algorithm for sarcoidosis PH is proposed in Fig. 24.6.

CLINICAL BURDEN AND PROGNOSIS OF SARCOIDOSIS PH

Compared with sarcoidosis patients without PH, those with sarcoidosis PH face more disabilities, including refractory dyspnea,[10] substantially reduced exercise capacity,[13,63,64] and functional status.[9] Candidates for lung transplantation with PH are more likely to need some or total assistance with their activities of daily living and to be unemployed due to disease.[9] Furthermore, PH is well known to portend a pejorative outcome.[11,14,15,17,19,62,70–72] PA/aorta ratio > 1 on MDCTA was strongly predictive of death in a large English cohort of unselected sarcoidosis patients,[73] but not in a similar American cohort where the only independent predictors of mortality were age, the extent of fibrosis, and the presence of PH confirmed by RHC (HR: 8.96; 95% CI: 3.85–20.87, P = .0484).[72] In the cohort of Nardi et al. on 142 stage IV patients originating from a nontransplant center, PH was the most robust correlate of mortality (HR: 8.1; 95% CI: 2.1–31.6, P = .002), and intractable right heart failure was the first cause of death (31.2%).[74]

Estimates of median survival of patients with sarcoidosis PH range between 4.2 and 6.8 years[11,15,75] with 2- and 5-year mortality rates of 26.5%–35% and 41%–63%,[14,15,75] respectively. The risk of death of precapillary PH is more than threefold higher than that of PH with LV dysfunction.[11] A level of PVR ≥ 3 Wood units was associated with worse prognosis in the study of Baughman et al. [11] but not in that of Boucly et al.[15] In this cohort focusing on patients with severe sarcoidosis PH, mortality was associated with NYHA functional class, 6MWT distance, and reduced FVC or DLCO, but with none of hemodynamic variables. In multivariate analysis, only 6MWT distance remained an independent predictor of poor survival.[15]

TREATMENT OF SARCOIDOSIS PH

According to the ECS/ERS guidelines, the axiom in patients with group 5 PH should be "Treat the lung not the pressure",[1] which may not apply to sarcoidosis. A pragmatic algorithm is proposed in Fig. 24.7. Obviously, supportive therapy is the cornerstone of management, including supplemental oxygen in patients who are hypoxemic at rest or during exercise and diuretics as needed. Iron deficiency and anemia, common in sarcoidosis patients,[76] should be monitored and corrected.[1]

The impact of therapy directed against sarcoidosis is still a matter of debate. PH can worsen despite corticosteroids as well as dramatically improve. Gluskowski et al. evaluated the effect of 12 months of corticosteroids on the hemodynamics of 24 patients with pulmonary sarcoidosis, of whom three had PH at rest and 18 had PH on exercise.[77] Whereas most patients were better on chest radiography and PFTs, only half demonstrated improved hemodynamics.[77] In the study of Nunes et al., 10 patients with sarcoidosis PH received high doses of oral prednisone. This was inefficient in the five patients with stage IV, but a sustained amelioration was obtained in 3 out of the 5 cases without pulmonary fibrosis.[14] Eleven patients with severe sarcoidosis PH of the cohort of Boucly et al. had an initiation or escalation of immunosuppressive therapy alone, including 5 cases with extrinsic compression of PAs.[15] Two patients with compressive lymph nodes improved (both with increased uptake on ^{18}FDG-PET), whereas none of the 3 with fibrosing mediastinitis did. Two of the six remaining cases improved with immunosuppressive therapy in terms of hemodynamics, but not NYHA functional class or 6MWT distance.[15]

There are four classes of agents accepted for PAH therapy: (1) CCB, which are reserved to a small subgroup of patients with a favorable response to acute vasoreactivity testing, (2) endothelin-1 receptor antagonists, (3) phosphodiesterase-5 inhibitors and guanylate cyclase stimulators, and (4) prostacyclin analogs and prostacyclin receptor agonists.[1] With respect to the use of these agents, there are no established recommendations for sarcoidosis PH. In the one hand, the possible role of specific vasculopathy makes this therapeutic approach appealing. In the other, there is some concern over systemic pulmonary vasodilators in sarcoidosis PH. First, they may lead to an aggravation of hypoxemia in patients with lung disease because of the inhibition of hypoxic pulmonary vasoconstriction with subsequent increased ventilation/perfusion mismatch and shunting. Second, the venous component that exists in a subset of patients may be at risk of drug-induced pulmonary edema.

Unfortunately though, available data on the long-term efficacy and safety of PAH-targeted medications in sarcoidosis PH are scarce, and results are inconsistent. Published studies comprise a majority of retrospective case series,[15,17,20,62,78–85] only three prospective uncontrolled open label trials,[78,86,87] and one double-blind randomized placebo-controlled trial (RPCT).[88] Diverse agents have been tested, including endothelin-1 receptor antagonists (Bosentan and Ambrisentan), phosphodiesterase-5 inhibitors (Sildenafil and Tadalafil), and prostacyclin analogs (inhaled Iloprost, Epoprostenol, and Treprostinil), in monotherapy or combination therapy. The main studies are summarized in Table 24.5.

Roughly, PAH therapy is beneficial in sarcoidosis PH in terms of hemodynamics, but this effect is generally not accompanied by an amelioration of exercise capacity, quality of life or survival. There is no definite advantage of one agent over the others in sarcoidosis H. These conflicting results are confusing for clinicians

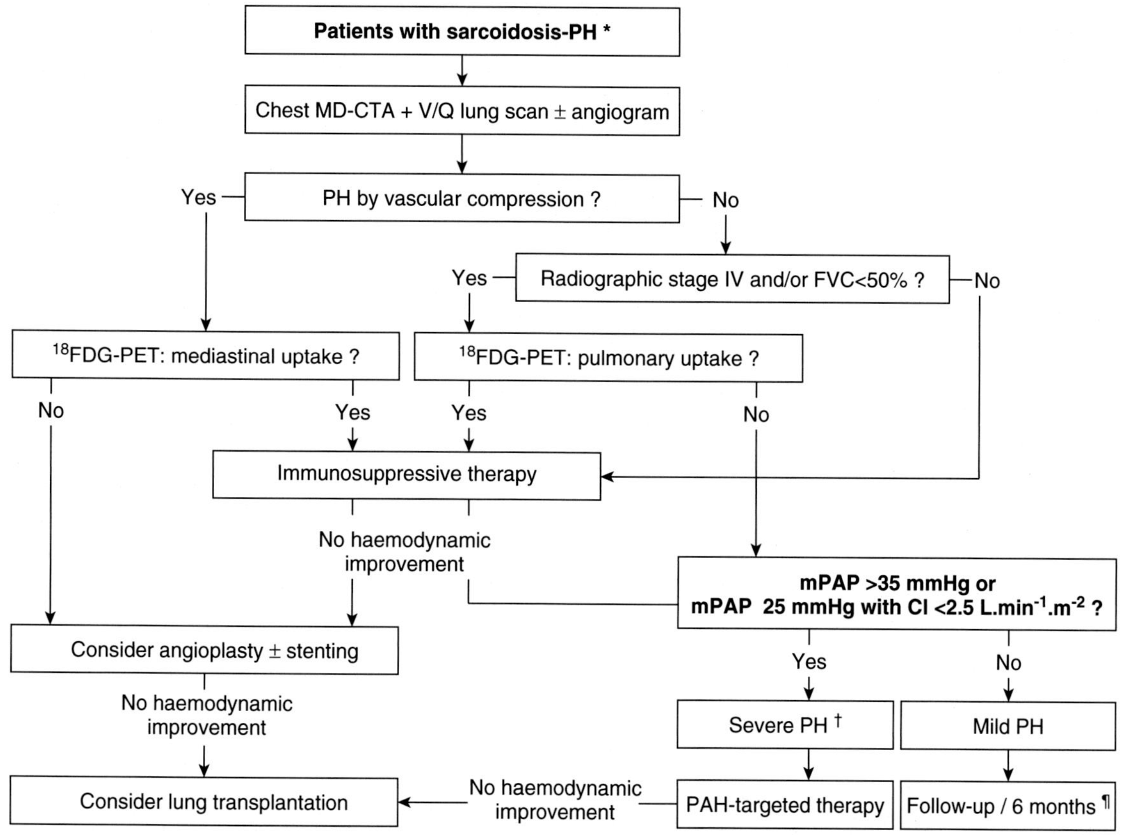

FIG. 24.7 Proposed therapeutic approach of sarcoidosis PH*. *PH*, pulmonary hypertension; *MD-CTA*, multidetector computed tomography angiography; *V/Q*, ventilation/perfusion; *18FDG-PET*, 18F-2-fluoro-2-deoxy-D-glucose positron emission tomography; *CI*, cardiac index; *mPAP*, mean pulmonary arterial pressure; *PAH*, pulmonary arterial hypertension. *All patients with sarcoidosis PH should receive symptomatic treatment, including supplemental oxygen in patients who are hypoxemic at rest or during exercise and diuretics as needed. †Severe PH suggests the presence of an intrinsic vasculopathy that may respond to PAH-targeted therapy. ¶Follow-up is essential to identify cases that will develop severe PH and may further benefit from PAH-targeted therapy.

and may be explained by several issues. The response to PAH therapy could be influenced by the prominent underlying mechanism of PH, the severity of functional alteration, the severity of PH, and the associated immunosuppressive therapy for sarcoidosis. The largest retrospective study of Boucly et al. had a rational therapeutic approach, with the prescription of PAH therapy only in patients with severe sarcoidosis PH.[15] Ninety-seven patients received various agents (including 22 with combined immunosuppressive treatment), as a single therapy in 83 cases and a double therapy in 14. In patients with repeat RHC, there were significant improvements in all hemodynamic variables from baseline to first follow-up visit (mPAP fell from 48 ± 9 to 42 ± 11 mmHg, $P<.00,001$ and PVR from 9.7 ± 4.4 to 6.9 ± 3.0 Wood units, $P<.00001$).[15] There was also an improvement of NYHA functional class but no significant change in 6MWT distance (324 ± 138 versus 311 ± 127, $P = .33$). Interestingly, in contrast to a previous study suggesting a better effect of PAH therapy in patients with more preserved FVC,[17] no difference was found in both 6MWT and hemodynamics on treatment according to the presence of radiological stage IV or severity of restrictive physiology (FVC > or ≤ 50%). Finally, treated and untreated patients had similar survival curves, provided that those under PAH therapy

TABLE 24.5
Main Studies on PAH-Targeted Therapy for Sarcoidosis PH

Number of Patients	Agent	Measurements	Results	Study
RETROSPECTIVE CASE SERIES INCLUDING MORE THAN 10 PATIENTS				
n=12	Sildenafil	After a median of 4–6 months: • RHC (n=9) • 6MWT (n=9)	Decrease in mPAP from 48 to 39 mmHg (*P*=.03) and in PVR from 10.7 to 5.6 (*P*<.01) No change in 6MWT distance	81
n=22	Initial monotherapy • Bosentan (n=12) • Sildenafil (n=9) • Epoprostenol (n=1) Combination therapy if inadequate response (n=8)	After a median of 11–15.2 months of the final PAH therapy: • RHC (n=12) • 6MWT (n=18) • NYHA FC (n=22)	Decrease in mPAP from 48.5 to 39.4 mmHg (*P*=.008) and in PVR from 11.1 to 6.7 (*P*=.011) Increase in 6MWT distance by 59 m (*P*=.032) Improvement in NYHA FC in 9 patients	17
n=33	Sildenafil (n=29) Sildenafil+Bosentan (n=4)	After 6 months: • TTE (n=25) • 6MWT (n=19) • Serum BNP (n=29) • WHO FC (n=33)	Imncrease in 6MWT distance by 13 m (*P*=.04) Improvement of BNP levels and TAPSE Improvement of WHO FC in 14 patients	85
n=13	Prostanoids as monotherapy or in combination therapy • Epoprostenol (n=7) • Treprostinil (n=6)	RHC after a mean of 12.7 months (n=10) Long-term follow-up at 3 years (n=7) • Serum NT-pro-BNP • WHO FC	Decrease in PVR from 11.6 to 5.9 Wood units (*P*=.037), but not in mPAP Improvement of WHO FC and NT-pro-BNP levels No difference in survival between patients receving prostanoids versus other oral agents alone	62
n=97 with severe PH	Monotherapy (n=83) • ERA (n=60) • PDE-5i (n=20) • Epoprostenol (n=2) • Inhaled Iloprost (n=1) Combination therapy (n=14) • ERA+PDE-5i (n=12) • ERA+Prostanoid (n=2)	After a median of 4.5 months (n=81) • RHC • 6MWT • NYHA FC Survival after a median follow-up of 28 months	Decrease in mPAP from 48 to 42 mmHg (*P*<.00001) and in PVR from 9.7 to 6.9 Wood units, (*P*<.00001) Improvement of NYHA FC No change in 6MWT distance No difference in survival between treated versus untreated patients	15
PROSPECTIVE OPEN-LABEL TRIAL				
n=15/22 completed trial	Inhaled iloprost	After 16 weeks • RHC • 6MWT • QOL: SF-36, SGRQ, SHQ, FAS	8/15 responders (either increased 6MWT distance≥30 m or decreased PVR≥20%) Overall significant improvement in SGRQ score	78
n=10/21 completed trial	Ambrisentan	After 24 weeks • 6MWT • Serum BNP • Dyspnea: WHO FC, Borg scale • QOL: SF-36, SGRQ	Improvement of WHO FC and SGRQ No change in 6MWT distance, BNP levels, Borg scale or SF-36 score	86

TABLE 24.5
Main Studies on PAH-Targeted Therapy for Sarcoidosis PH—cont'd

n=7/12 completed trial	Tadalafil	After 24 weeks • 6MWT (n=6/12) • Serum BNP • Dyspnea: WHO FC, Borg scale • QOL: SF-36, SGRQ	No change in 6MWT distance, dyspnea, BNP levels or QOL scores	87
RANDOMIZED PLACEBO-CONTROLLED TRIAL				
23/25 completed trial	Bosentan versus placebo	After 16 weeks • RHC (n=21/23) • 6MWT • Dyspnea: Borg scale dyspnea • QOL: SF-36, SGRQ, FAS	Decrease in mPAP from 36 to 32 mmHg (*P*=.0105) and in PVR from 5.9 to 4.4 Wood units (*P*=.0104) in the Bosentan group versus no change in the placebo group. No change in 6MWT distance, dyspnea, or QOL scores	88

6MWT, 6-min walk test; *BNP*, bone natriuretic peptide; *ERA*, endothelin-1 receptor antagonist; *FAS*, fatigue assessment scale; *FC*, functional class; *mPAP*, mean pulmonary arterial pressure; *NYHA*, New York heart Association; *PAH*, pulmonary arterial hypertension; *PDE-5i*, phosphodiesterase-5 inhibitors; *PH*, pulmonary hypertension; *PVR*, pulmonary vascular resistance; *QOL*, quality of life; *RHC*, right heart catherterization; *SF-36*, short form 36 questionnaire; *SGRQ*, Saint George respiratory questionnaire; *SGRQ*, St. Georges respiratory questionnaire; *TAPSE*, tricuspid annular plane systolic excursion; *TTE*, transthoracic echocardiography; *WHO*, World Health Organization.

had a worse condition at baseline.[15] The RPCT of Baughman et al. evaluated Bosentan in sarcoidosis PH with no restriction upon the severity of PH. Thirty-nine patients were randomized in a 2:1 ratio of drug to placebo, and 23 of 25 patients on Bosentan completed 16 weeks of treatment.[88] A significant improvement was demonstrated in both the mPAP (decrease of 4 ± 6.6 mm Hg, *P* = .0105) and PVR (decrease of 1.7 ± 2.75 Wood units, *P* = .0104) in Bosentan group, whereas there was no change in hemodynamics with placebo. There was no significant change in 6MWT for either group (distance declined by 23 ± 69.5 m on Bosentan) nor in quality of life. The change in hemodynamics and 6MWT distance on Bosentan did not differ according to FVC > or ≤50%.[88]

PAH therapy is generally well tolerated in sarcoidosis PH. One case of sudden death and one case of acute pulmonary edema have been reported after intravenous Epoprostenol supposedly because of underlying PVOD.[79] Although comprehensive data are missing, the hazard of PAH therapy on gas exchange seems marginal. In the RPCT of Baughman et al. the proportion of patients with worsening desaturation was similar between Bosentan and placebo, and only 2 of 23 patients on Bosentan required an increase in supplemental oxygen for more than 2 L/min.[88]

Endovascular procedures with angioplasty and stent placement have been proposed in highly selected patients with extrinsic compression of Pas, but these options are associated with high morbidity. The series by Liu et al. reported eight patients with sarcoidosis PH and proximal stenosis of PAs that did not respond to corticosteroids and underwent interventional therapy (balloon angioplasty in all cases plus stent implantation in 5).[36] Three months after interventional therapy, all patients evidenced improved hemodynamics (mPAP decreased from 42.5 ± 4.6 mmHg to 20.5 ± 3.2 mmHg, *P* = .035, and PVR from 12.3 ± 1.2 to 3.8 ± 0.3 Wood units, *P* = .004) and 6MWT (distance increased from 236.8 ± 36.7 to 456.4 ± 48.2 m, *P* = .028). Patients experienced several complications that were easily managed: one patient developed tachycardia, one thromboembolism, one hemoptysis, and one PA dissection.[36] Two additional cases of successful angioplasty and stenting have been described.[34] Given the high mortality rate of patients with sarcoidosis PH, referral for lung or heart-lung transplantation, when otherwise appropriate, should be considered.

CONCLUSION

PH is a challenging complication of sarcoidosis both from a diagnostic and therapeutic point of view. There are recent shreds of evidence suggesting that sarcoidosis PH may be more intricate than just being the result of parenchymal lung disease and hypoxemia. Various mechanisms are in place, of which intrinsic vasculopathy may play a critical role. The presence of PH signifies a grave prognosis in patients with sarcoidosis. There is a need for a better identification of patients with sarcoidosis PH who will respond to immunosuppressive treatment. PAH-targeted therapy is tempting. However, despite encouraging studies, the paucity of conclusive data leaves many uncertainties and questions in this area: (1) who to treat? (2) with which agent? and (3) for what objective? Although difficult to conduct in such a rare condition, RPCT are warranted. A currently enrolling RPCT on Riociguat, a direct and indirect nitric oxide potentiator, is underway for sarcoidosis PH in the United States (www.clinicaltrials.gov).

REFERENCES

1. Galiè N, Humbert M, Vachiery J-L, et al. 2015 ESC/ERS guidelines for the diagnosis and treatment of pulmonary hypertension. The Joint Task Force for the diagnosis and treatment of pulmonary hypertension of the European Society of Cardiology (ESC) and the European respiratory Society (ERS). *Eur Respir J*. 2015;46:903–975. https://doi.org/10.1183/13993003.51032-2015. *Eur Respir J*. 2015;46(6):1855–1856.
2. Battesti JP, Georges R, Basset F, Saumon G. Chronic cor pulmonale in pulmonary sarcoidosis. *Thorax*. 1978;33(1):76–84.
3. Głuskowski J, Hawryłkiewicz I, Zych D, Wojtczak A, Zieliński J. Pulmonary haemodynamics at rest and during exercise in patients with sarcoidosis. *Respir Int Rev Thorac Dis*. 1984;46(1):26–32. https://doi.org/10.1159/000194667.
4. Handa T, Nagai S, Miki S, et al. Incidence of pulmonary hypertension and its clinical relevance in patients with sarcoidosis. *Chest*. 2006;129(5):1246–1252. https://doi.org/10.1378/chest.129.5.1246.
5. Mayock RL, Bertrand P, Morrison CE, Scott JH. Manifestations of sarcoidosis. Analysis of 145 patients, with a review of nine series selected from the literature. *Am J Med*. 1963;35:67–89.
6. Rizzato G, Pezzano A, Sala G, et al. Right heart impairment in sarcoidosis: haemodynamic and echocardiographic study. *Eur J Respir Dis*. 1983;64(2):121–128.
7. Rapti A, Kouranos V, Gialafos E, et al. Elevated pulmonary arterial systolic pressure in patients with sarcoidosis: prevalence and risk factors. *Lung*. 2013;191(1):61–67. https://doi.org/10.1007/s00408-012-9442-4.
8. Pabst S, Hammerstingl C, Grau N, et al. Pulmonary arterial hypertension in patients with sarcoidosis: the Pulsar single center experience. *Adv Exp Med Biol*. 2013;755:299–305. https://doi.org/10.1007/978-94-007-4546-9_38.
9. Shorr AF, Helman DL, Davies DB, Nathan SD. Pulmonary hypertension in advanced sarcoidosis: epidemiology and clinical characteristics. *Eur Respir J*. 2005;25(5):783–788. https://doi.org/10.1183/09031936.05.00083404.
10. Baughman RP, Engel PJ, Meyer CA, Barrett AB, Lower EE. Pulmonary hypertension in sarcoidosis. *Sarcoidosis Vasc Diffuse Lung Dis Off J WASOG*. 2006;23(2):108–116.
11. Baughman RP, Engel PJ, Taylor L, Lower EE. Survival in sarcoidosis-associated pulmonary hypertension: the importance of hemodynamic evaluation. *Chest*. 2010;138(5):1078–1085. https://doi.org/10.1378/chest.09-2002.
12. Sulica R, Teirstein AS, Kakarla S, Nemani N, Behnegar A, Padilla ML. Distinctive clinical, radiographic, and functional characteristics of patients with sarcoidosis-related pulmonary hypertension. *Chest*. 2005;128(3):1483–1489. https://doi.org/10.1378/chest.128.3.1483.
13. Bourbonnais JM, Samavati L. Clinical predictors of pulmonary hypertension in sarcoidosis. *Eur Respir J*. 2008;32(2):296–302. https://doi.org/10.1183/09031936.00175907.
14. Nunes H, Humbert M, Capron F, et al. Pulmonary hypertension associated with sarcoidosis: mechanisms, haemodynamics and prognosis. *Thorax*. 2006;61(1):68–74. https://doi.org/10.1136/thx.2005.042838.
15. Boucly A, Cottin V, Nunes H, et al. Management and long-term outcomes of sarcoidosis-associated pulmonary hypertension. *Eur Respir J*. 2017;50(4). https://doi.org/10.1183/13993003.00465-2017.
16. Huitema MP, Spee M, Vorselaars VMM, et al. Pulmonary artery diameter to predict pulmonary hypertension in pulmonary sarcoidosis. *Eur Respir J*. 2016;47(2):673–676. https://doi.org/10.1183/13993003.01319-2015.
17. Barnett CF, Bonura EJ, Nathan SD, et al. Treatment of sarcoidosis-associated pulmonary hypertension. A two-center experience. *Chest*. 2009;135(6):1455–1461. https://doi.org/10.1378/chest.08-1881.
18. Emirgil C, Sobol BJ, Herbert WH, Trout K. The lesser circulation in pulmonary fibrosis secondary to sarcoidosis and its relationship to respiratory function. *Chest*. 1971;60(4):371–378.
19. Shorr AF, Davies DB, Nathan SD. Outcomes for patients with sarcoidosis awaiting lung transplantation. *Chest*. 2002;122(1):233–238.
20. Preston IR, Klinger JR, Landzberg MJ, Houtchens J, Nelson D, Hill NS. Vasoresponsiveness of sarcoidosis-associated pulmonary hypertension. *Chest*. 2001;120(3):866–872.
21. Takemura T, Matsui Y, Oritsu M, et al. Pulmonary vascular involvement in sarcoidosis: granulomatous angiitis and microangiopathy in transbronchial lung biopsies. *Virchows Arch a Pathol Anat Histopathol*. 1991;418(4):361–368.
22. Rosen Y, Moon S, Huang CT, Gourin A, Lyons HA. Granulomatous pulmonary angiitis in sarcoidosis. *Arch Pathol Lab Med*. 1977;101(4):170–174.
23. Takemura T, Matsui Y, Saiki S, Mikami R. Pulmonary vascular involvement in sarcoidosis: a report of 40 autopsy cases. *Hum Pathol*. 1992;23(11):1216–1223.
24. Kambouchner M, Pirici D, Uhl J-F, Mogoanta L, Valeyre D, Bernaudin J-F. Lymphatic and blood microvasculature organisation in pulmonary sarcoid granulomas. *Eur Respir J*. 2011;37(4):835–840. https://doi.org/10.1183/09031936.00086410.
25. Smith LJ, Lawrence JB, Katzenstein AA. Vascular sarcoidosis: a rare cause of pulmonary hypertension. *Am J Med Sci*. 1983;285(1):38–44.

26. Tayal S, Voelkel NF, Rai PR, Cool CD. Sarcoidois and pulmonary hypertension–a case report. *Eur J Med Res.* 2006;11(5):194–197.
27. Braam EAJE, Quanjel MJR, Van Haren-Willems JHGM, et al. Extensive pulmonary sarcoid reaction in a patient with BMPR-2 associated idiopathic pulmonary arterial hypertension. *Sarcoidosis Vasc Diffuse Lung Dis Off J WASOG.* 2016;33(2):182–185.
28. Hoffstein V, Ranganathan N, Mullen JB. Sarcoidosis simulating pulmonary veno-occlusive disease. *Am Rev Respir Dis.* 1986;134(4):809–811. https://doi.org/10.1164/arrd.1986.134.4.809.
29. Jones RM, Dawson A, Jenkins GH, Nicholson AG, Hansell DM, Harrison NK. Sarcoidosis-related pulmonary veno-occlusive disease presenting with recurrent haemoptysis. *Eur Respir J.* 2009;34(2):517–520. https://doi.org/10.1183/09031936.00044609.
30. Portier F, Lerebours-Pigeonniere G, Thiberville L, et al. Sarcoidosis simulating a pulmonary veno-occlusive disease. *Rev Mal Respir.* 1991;8(1):101–102.
31. Ota H, Sugino K, Uekusa T, Takemura T, Homma S. An autopsy case of refractory pulmonary hypertension with sarcoidosis. *Respir Investig.* 2016;54(6):490–493. https://doi.org/10.1016/j.resinv.2016.05.005.
32. Singla S, Zhou T, Javaid K, et al. Expression profiling elucidates a molecular gene signature for pulmonary hypertension in sarcoidosis. *Pulm Circ.* 2016;6(4):465–471. https://doi.org/10.1086/688316.
33. Baloira Villar A, Pousada Fernández G, Núñez Fernández M, Valverde Pérez D. Clinical and molecular study of 4 cases of pulmonary hypertension associated with sarcoidosis. *Arch Bronconeumol.* 2015;51(4):e19–e21. https://doi.org/10.1016/j.arbres.2014.03.022.
34. Hamilton-Craig CR, Slaughter R, McNeil K, Kermeen F, Walters DL. Improvement after angioplasty and stenting of pulmonary arteries due to sarcoid mediastinal fibrosis. *Heart Lung Circ.* 2009;18(3):222–225. https://doi.org/10.1016/j.hlc.2007.12.006.
35. Toonkel RL, Borczuk AC, Pearson GD, Horn EM, Thomashow BM. Sarcoidosis-associated fibrosing mediastinitis with resultant pulmonary hypertension: a case report and review of the literature. *Respir Int Rev Thorac Dis.* 2010;79(4):341–345. https://doi.org/10.1159/000243786.
36. Liu L, Xu J, Zhang Y, et al. Interventional therapy in sarcoidosis-associated pulmonary arterial stenosis and pulmonary hypertension. *Clin Respir J.* 2017;11(6):906–914. https://doi.org/10.1111/crj.12435.
37. Yangui F, Battesti J-P, Valeyre D, Kheder AB, Brillet P-Y. Fibrosing mediastinitis as a rare mechanism of pulmonary oedema in sarcoidosis. *Eur Respir J.* 2010;35(2):455–456. https://doi.org/10.1183/09031936.00132909.
38. Schowengerdt CG, Suyemoto R, Main FB. Granulomatous and fibrous mediastinitis. A review and analysis of 180 cases. *J Thorac Cardiovasc Surg.* 1969;57(3):365–379.
39. Seferian A, Steriade A, Jaïs X, et al. Pulmonary hypertension complicating fibrosing mediastinitis. *Medicine (Baltim).* 2015;94(44):e1800. https://doi.org/10.1097/MD.0000000000001800.
40. Bourlier D, O'Connell C, Montani D, et al. A rare case of sarcoidosis-associated pulmonary hypertension in a patient exposed to silica. *Eur Respir Rev Off J Eur Respir Soc.* 2016;25(139):93–96. https://doi.org/10.1183/16000617.0073-2015.
41. Salazar A, Mañá J, Sala J, Landoni BR, Manresa F. Combined portal and pulmonary hypertension in sarcoidosis. *Respir Int Rev Thorac Dis.* 1994;61(2):117–119. https://doi.org/10.1159/000196320.
42. Gupta S, Faughnan ME, Prud'homme GJ, Hwang DM, Munoz DG, Kopplin P. Sarcoidosis complicated by cirrhosis and hepatopulmonary syndrome. *Can Respir J.* 2008;15(3):124–126.
43. Joyce E, Ninaber MK, Katsanos S, et al. Subclinical left ventricular dysfunction by echocardiographic speckle-tracking strain analysis relates to outcome in sarcoidosis. *Eur J Heart Fail.* 2015;17(1):51–62. https://doi.org/10.1002/ejhf.205.
44. Patel AR, Klein MR, Chandra S, et al. Myocardial damage in patients with sarcoidosis and preserved left ventricular systolic function: an observational study. *Eur J Heart Fail.* 2011;13(11):1231–1237. https://doi.org/10.1093/eurjhf/hfr099.
45. Murtagh G, Laffin LJ, Beshai JF, et al. Prognosis of myocardial damage in sarcoidosis patients with preserved left ventricular ejection fraction: risk stratification using cardiovascular magnetic resonance. *Circ Cardiovasc Imaging.* 2016;9(1):e003738. https://doi.org/10.1161/CIRCIMAGING.115.003738.
46. Crawshaw AP, Wotton CJ, Yeates DGR, Goldacre MJ, Ho L-P. Evidence for association between sarcoidosis and pulmonary embolism from 35-year record linkage study. *Thorax.* 2011;66(5):447–448. https://doi.org/10.1136/thx.2010.134429.
47. Swigris JJ, Olson AL, Huie TJ, et al. Increased risk of pulmonary embolism among US decedents with sarcoidosis from 1988 to 2007. *Chest.* 2011;140(5):1261–1266. https://doi.org/10.1378/chest.11-0324.
48. Ungprasert P, Crowson CS, Matteson EL. Association of sarcoidosis with increased risk of VTE: a population-based study, 1976 to 2013. *Chest.* 2017;151(2):425–430. https://doi.org/10.1016/j.chest.2016.09.009.
49. Bernard J, Yi ES. Pulmonary thromboendarterectomy: a clinicopathologic study of 200 consecutive pulmonary thromboendarterectomy cases in one institution. *Hum Pathol.* 2007;38(6):871–877. https://doi.org/10.1016/j.humpath.2006.11.017.
50. Ina Y, Takada K, Yamamoto M, Sato T, Ito S, Sato S. Antiphospholipid antibodies. A prognostic factor in sarcoidosis? *Chest.* 1994;105(4):1179–1183.
51. Wesemann DR, Costenbader KH, Coblyn JS. Co-existing sarcoidosis, systemic lupus erythematosus and the antiphospholipid antibody syndrome: case reports and discussion from the Brigham and Women's Hospital Lupus Center. *Lupus.* 2009;18(3):202–205. https://doi.org/10.1177/0961203308100483.
52. Carragoso A, Silva JR, Capelo J, Faria B, Gaspar O. A patient with sarcoidosis and antiphospholipid syndrome. *Eur J Intern Med.* 2008;19(8):e80–e81. https://doi.org/10.1016/j.ejim.2008.01.020.

53. Takahashi F, Toba M, Takahashi K, et al. Pulmonary sarcoidosis and antiphospholipid syndrome. *Respirol Carlton Vic.* 2006;11(4):506–508. https://doi.org/10.1111/j.1440-1843.2006.00880.x.
54. Ishii A, Hoshii Y, Nakashima T, et al. Sarcoidosis with pulmonary hypertension exacerbated by Takayasu-like large vessel vasculitis. *Pathol Int.* 2011;61(9):546–550. https://doi.org/10.1111/j.1440-1827.2011.02703.x.
55. Senda S, Igawa K, Nishioka M, Murota H, Katayama I. Systemic sclerosis with sarcoidosis: case report and review of the published work. *J Dermatol.* 2014;41(5):421–423. https://doi.org/10.1111/1346-8138.12438.
56. Ocak S, Feoli F, Fastrez J, et al. Pulmonary arterial hypertension in a patient with stage II sarcoidosis and Hashitoxicosis. *Eur Respir Rev Off J Eur Respir Soc.* 2009;18(112):125–128. https://doi.org/10.1183/09031936.00000309.
57. Turner GA, Lower EE, Corser BC, Gunther KL, Baughman RP. Sleep apnea in sarcoidosis. *Sarcoidosis Vasc Diffuse Lung Dis Off J WASOG.* 1997;14(1):61–64.
58. Verbraecken J, Hoitsma E, van der Grinten CPM, Cobben NAM, Wouters EFM, Drent M. Sleep disturbances associated with periodic leg movements in chronic sarcoidosis. *Sarcoidosis Vasc Diffuse Lung Dis Off J WASOG.* 2004;21(2):137–146.
59. Mirsaeidi M, Machado RF, Schraufnagel D, Sweiss NJ, Baughman RP. Racial difference in sarcoidosis mortality in the United States. *Chest.* 2015;147(2):438–449. https://doi.org/10.1378/chest.14-1120.
60. Arcasoy SM, Christie JD, Ferrari VA, et al. Echocardiographic assessment of pulmonary hypertension in patients with advanced lung disease. *Am J Respir Crit Care Med.* 2003;167(5):735–740. https://doi.org/10.1164/rccm.200210-1130OC.
61. Patel MB, Mor-Avi V, Murtagh G, et al. Right heart involvement in patients with sarcoidosis. *Echocardiogr Mt Kisco N.* 2016;33(5):734–741. https://doi.org/10.1111/echo.13163.
62. Bonham CA, Oldham JM, Gomberg-Maitland M, Vij R. Prostacyclin and oral vasodilator therapy in sarcoidosis-associated pulmonary hypertension: a retrospective case series. *Chest.* 2015;148(4):1055–1062. https://doi.org/10.1378/chest.14-2546.
63. Mirsaeidi M, Omar HR, Baughman R, Machado R, Sweiss N. The association between BNP, 6MWD test, DLCO% and pulmonary hypertension in sarcoidosis. *Sarcoidosis Vasc Diffuse Lung Dis Off J WASOG.* 2016;33(4):317–320.
64. Baughman RP, Sparkman BK, Lower EE. Six-minute walk test and health status assessment in sarcoidosis. *Chest.* 2007;132(1):207–213. https://doi.org/10.1378/chest.06-2822.
65. Zisman DA, Karlamangla AS, Ross DJ, et al. High-resolution chest CT findings do not predict the presence of pulmonary hypertension in advanced idiopathic pulmonary fibrosis. *Chest.* 2007;132(3):773–779. https://doi.org/10.1378/chest.07-0116.
66. Devaraj A, Wells AU, Meister MG, Corte TJ, Hansell DM. The effect of diffuse pulmonary fibrosis on the reliability of CT signs of pulmonary hypertension. *Radiology.* 2008;249(3):1042–1049. https://doi.org/10.1148/radiol.2492080269.
67. Smedema J-P, van Geuns R-J, Ainslie G, Ector J, Heidbuchel H, Crijns HJGM. Right ventricular involvement in cardiac sarcoidosis demonstrated with cardiac magnetic resonance. *ESC Heart Fail.* 2017;4(4):535–544. https://doi.org/10.1002/ehf2.12166.
68. Handa T, Nagai S, Ueda S, et al. Significance of plasma NT-proBNP levels as a biomarker in the assessment of cardiac involvement and pulmonary hypertension in patients with sarcoidosis. *Sarcoidosis Vasc Diffuse Lung Dis Off J WASOG.* 2010;27(1):27–35.
69. Culver DA, Krasuski RA. Right-sided heart catheterization: de rigueur in sarcoidosis? *Chest.* 2010;138(5):1030–1032. https://doi.org/10.1378/chest.10-1241.
70. Arcasoy SM, Christie JD, Pochettino A, et al. Characteristics and outcomes of patients with sarcoidosis listed for lung transplantation. *Chest.* 2001;120(3):873–880.
71. Shorr AF, Davies DB, Nathan SD. Predicting mortality in patients with sarcoidosis awaiting lung transplantation. *Chest.* 2003;124(3):922–928.
72. Kirkil G, Lower EE, Baughman RP. Predictors of mortality in pulmonary sarcoidosis. *Chest.* 2018;153(1):105–113. https://doi.org/10.1016/j.chest.2017.07.008.
73. Walsh SL, Wells AU, Sverzellati N, et al. An integrated clinicoradiological staging system for pulmonary sarcoidosis: a case-cohort study. *Lancet Respir Med.* 2014;2(2):123–130. https://doi.org/10.1016/S2213-2600(13)70276-5.
74. Nardi A, Brillet P-Y, Letoumelin P, et al. Stage IV sarcoidosis: comparison of survival with the general population and causes of death. *Eur Respir J.* 2011;38(6):1368–1373. https://doi.org/10.1183/09031936.00187410.
75. Dobarro D, Schreiber BE, Handler C, Beynon H, Denton CP, Coghlan JG. Clinical characteristics, haemodynamics and treatment of pulmonary hypertension in sarcoidosis in a single centre, and meta-analysis of the published data. *Am J Cardiol.* 2013;111(2):278–285. https://doi.org/10.1016/j.amjcard.2012.09.031.
76. Lower EE, Smith JT, Martelo OJ, Baughman RP. The anemia of sarcoidosis. *Sarcoidosis.* 1988;5(1):51–55.
77. Gluskowski J, Hawrylkiewicz I, Zych D, Zieliński J. Effects of corticosteroid treatment on pulmonary haemodynamics in patients with sarcoidosis. *Eur Respir J.* 1990;3(4):403–407.
78. Baughman RP, Judson MA, Lower EE, et al. Inhaled iloprost for sarcoidosis associated pulmonary hypertension. *Sarcoidosis Vasc Diffuse Lung Dis Off J WASOG.* 2009;26(2):110–120.
79. Fisher KA, Serlin DM, Wilson KC, Walter RE, Berman JS, Farber HW. Sarcoidosis-associated pulmonary hypertension: outcome with long-term epoprostenol treatment. *Chest.* 2006;130(5):1481–1488. https://doi.org/10.1378/chest.130.5.1481.
80. Milman N, Svendsen CB, Iversen M, Videbaek R, Carlsen J. Sarcoidosis-associated pulmonary hypertension: acute vasoresponsiveness to inhaled nitric oxide and the relation to long-term effect of sildenafil. *Clin Respir J.* 2009;3(4):207–213. https://doi.org/10.1111/j.1752-699X.2008.00120.x.

81. Milman N, Burton CM, Iversen M, Videbaek R, Jensen CV, Carlsen J. Pulmonary hypertension in end-stage pulmonary sarcoidosis: therapeutic effect of sildenafil? *J Heart Lung Transplant Off Publ Int Soc Heart Transplant*. 2008;27(3):329–334. https://doi.org/10.1016/j.healun.2007.11.576.
82. Minai OA, Sahoo D, Chapman JT, Mehta AC. Vaso-active therapy can improve 6-min walk distance in patients with pulmonary hypertension and fibrotic interstitial lung disease. *Respir Med*. 2008;102(7):1015–1020. https://doi.org/10.1016/j.rmed.2008.02.002.
83. Corte TJ, Gatzoulis MA, Parfitt L, Harries C, Wells AU, Wort SJ. The use of sildenafil to treat pulmonary hypertension associated with interstitial lung disease. *Respirol Carlton Vic*. 2010;15(8):1226–1232. https://doi.org/10.1111/j.1440-1843.2010.01860.x.
84. Foley RJ, Metersky ML. Successful treatment of sarcoidosis-associated pulmonary hypertension with bosentan. *Respir Int Rev Thorac Dis*. 2008;75(2):211–214. https://doi.org/10.1159/000089815.
85. Keir GJ, Walsh SLF, Gatzoulis MA, et al. Treatment of sarcoidosis-associated pulmonary hypertension: a single centre retrospective experience using targeted therapies. *Sarcoidosis Vasc Diffuse Lung Dis Off J WASOG*. 2014;31(2):82–90.
86. Judson MA, Highland KB, Kwon S, et al. Ambrisentan for sarcoidosis associated pulmonary hypertension. *Sarcoidosis Vasc Diffuse Lung Dis Off J WASOG*. 2011;28(2):139–145.
87. Ford HJ, Baughman RP, Aris R, Engel P, Donohue JF. Tadalafil therapy for sarcoidosis-associated pulmonary hypertension. *Pulm Circ*. 2016;6(4):557–562. https://doi.org/10.1086/688775.
88. Baughman RP, Culver DA, Cordova FC, et al. Bosentan for sarcoidosis-associated pulmonary hypertension: a double-blind placebo controlled randomized trial. *Chest*. 2014;145(4):810–817. https://doi.org/10.1378/chest.13-1766.

CHAPTER 25

Mortality in Sarcoidosis

ATHOL WELLS, MD • KOURANOS V, MD

INTRODUCTION

Sarcoidosis is often viewed as a relatively benign chronic disease, especially by those clinicians who also manage other progressive diseases with a poor outcome. The perception of a good outcome in sarcoidosis includes patients with clinically significant pulmonary involvement, the most prevalent major organ involvement in that disease. For example, respirologists specializing in interstitial lung diseases are confronted by outcomes in idiopathic pulmonary fibrosis with a 3-year survival of 50% before the advent of disease-modifying antifibrotic agents. In other interstitial lung diseases such as hypersensitivity pneumonitis, idiopathic nonspecific interstitial pneumonia, and connective tissue disease–associated lung disease, a large subset of patients progresses inexorably or insidiously despite treatment. In contrast, in sarcoidosis, the majority of patients with lung disease stabilize with time or with therapy. Cardiac sarcoidosis and neurosarcoidosis tend to be viewed as "special cases" in which poor outcomes may be more frequent: exceptions to a generally benign outcome, applying to a small proportion of cases. The large number of sarcoidosis patients without major organ involvement, characterized by a good long-term outcome, reinforces the view that a low key approach in sarcoidosis management is appropriate in most cases.

In this chapter we review and discuss outcomes in sarcoidosis with particular regard to mortality, scrutinizing whether, in truth, sarcoidosis should be regarded as essentially benign. Causes of death are highlighted with an overview of the identification of "dangerous disease", in which a higher mortality must be expected with or without intervention.

PREVALENCE AND CAUSES OF SARCOIDOSIS-RELATED DEATHS

The view that sarcoidosis-related mortality is low comes from two main sources. It reflects, in part, the major heterogeneity in disease presentation and course. In many cases, sarcoidosis is asymptomatic or incidentally detected on chest imaging. Indeed, it is known, from radiographic screening studies, that in many asymptomatic cases, the diagnosis is never made, reinforcing a perceived benign outcome. In other cases there may be prominent systemic symptoms such as fatigue and disabling arthralgia, without evidence of major organ involvement. Thus an important subgroup of patients with a more malignant disease course are disenfranchised by "whole-population statements" of the likelihood of sarcoidosis-related deaths. Clinicians managing sarcoidosis at large sometimes view such cases as "exceptions that prove the rule".

A superficial review of current data appears to support this impression. Death certificate data are notoriously imprecise, but conclusions reached from this source are concordant with recent case-cohort studies. In general, taking into account estimates made in many countries using a variety of methodologies, sarcoidosis-related mortality is considered to exceed 5% and is probably approximately 6%–8%.[1–8] As discussed later, a focus on mortality directly due to sarcoidosis progression almost certainly understates the true mortality associated with sarcoidosis. However, data emerging from selected recent studies serve as a useful starting point in the discussion that follows.

In an outcome analysis of the Swedish National Patient Register, containing data from 8207 patients with sarcoidosis, the mortality rate was 11.0 per 1000 person-years in sarcoidosis patients compared with 6.7 per 1000 person-years in matched subjects in the general population.[2] Although exact causes of death were not reported, sarcoidosis was the most frequent underlying and/or contributing cause of a fatal outcome. Mortality was not associated with age or gender, but there was a highly significant increase in mortality (hazard ratio [HR] 2.34 [95% CI 1.99–2.75]) in patients requiring sarcoidosis-specific treatment in the first 3 months. Based on these data, expected mortality from sarcoidosis in this patient subgroup may be up to threefold higher than in the general population. Thus perceptions of sarcoidosis-related mortality drawn from the general sarcoidosis population may be very misleading when applied to easily recognized patient subgroups.

In another important recent study, a French group evaluated sarcoidosis-related mortality in their country, exploring the underlying causes of death among French

Sarcoidosis. https://doi.org/10.1016/B978-0-323-54429-0.00025-2

decedents with sarcoidosis between 2002 and 2011. The age-adjusted sarcoidosis mortality rate of 3.6 per million was higher than the general population mortality rate, and an increase in sarcoidosis mortality during the study period was observed.[4] The mean age of death in sarcoidosis patients was 70.4 years, compared with 76.2 years in the general population. Compared with the general population, sarcoidosis-related deaths were more frequent in males aged <65 years and in females aged ≥65 years, with most deaths (53%) occurring between the ages of 60 and 79 years. Mortality associated with sarcoidosis rose with increasing age, a trend that applied equally to cases in which sarcoidosis was considered to be the underlying cause of death and in the remaining sarcoidosis decedents. Sarcoidosis was the commonest cause of deaths associated with the disease, usually due to chronic respiratory or cardiovascular disease. Although mortality rates were, as expected, much lower below the age of 40 years, both in sarcoidosis patients and in the general population, the disease was the underlying cause of death in 59% of fatal sarcoidosis outcomes in that age group. In essence, these data establish that there is major adult mortality caused by sarcoidosis, irrespective of age.

Sarcoidosis mortality rates in Sweden and France are broadly consistent with earlier UK data of 1019 sarcoidosis patients.[8] In that study, mortality was even higher (14 per 1000 person-years) than in the Swedish report although, in contrast to Swedish observations, male gender and increased age were associated with increased mortality. A similar message emerges from all three studies discussed previously, with little to gain from a focus on minor differences between the three countries. Sarcoidosis severity was not documented (e.g., by Scadding chest radiographic criteria), and thus the impact of baseline severity on ultimate mortality cannot be captured in such a way to allow severity-adjusted mortality comparisons between countries.

Equally importantly the influence of genetic factors on population outcomes cannot be dissected in the three cosmopolitan countries where these population analyses were conducted. The potential importance of genetic differences is highlighted by findings in the United States. Based on two reports, it can be concluded that in the United States, sarcoidosis mortality was linked to both race and gender. Individuals of African American origin and female gender had a worse prognosis, with more extrapulmonary organ involvement, a longer duration of disease, and a higher prevalence of sarcoidosis-related hospitalization.[6,7] It is unclear whether socioeconomic factors contributed to these observations: it is possible that cultural differences exist in the detection of sarcoidosis, with a diagnosis of sarcoidosis made later in the disease course or made selectively in more severe disease in some racial or socioeconomic groups.

IS SARCOIDOSIS-RELATED MORTALITY SIGNIFICANTLY UNDERRECOGNIZED?

It is usual, in studies of the mortality of chronic diseases, to identify the studied disease as the underlying cause of death when a fatal outcome is primarily due to major organ involvement. However, this analytic strategy does not take into account disease comorbidities that may have a greater prevalence or impact in sarcoidosis patients than in the general population, especially when comorbidities are in part ascribable to long-term sarcoidosis therapies. Causes of death directly or indirectly ascribable to sarcoidosis are summarized in Table 25.1.

In sarcoidosis, comorbidities and multimorbidity have a major effect on a patient's quality of life, health care, and health economics and are associated with increased mortality.[9–15] Sarcoidosis patients have a higher risk of developing concomitant chronic conditions than age-/sex-matched individuals in the general population. Although this observation may arise in part from the persistence of inflammatory organ damage (which may be an important cofactor in the initiation of other chronic disorders), it appears likely that side effects caused by antiinflammatory treatment are at least equally important.[12–15]

In a comparison between 345 sarcoidosis patients and an age-/sex-matched control group from the general population, sarcoidosis was associated with a higher cumulative incidence of coronary artery disease,

TABLE 25.1
Causes of Death Directly or Indirectly Ascribable to Sarcoidosis

- Progressive pulmonary fibrosis
- Pulmonary hypertension
- Cardiac sarcoidosis
- Other organ involvements: neurosarcoidosis, renal disease, hepatic disease, and hypercalcemia
- Comorbidities resulting from prolonged sarcoid-specific treatment, especially infection, diabetes, and hypertension
- Isolated undiagnosed cardiac sarcoidosis

congestive heart failure, arrhythmia, stroke or transient ischemic attacks, arthritis, depression, diabetes, and major osteoporotic fractures.[12] Similar findings have been reported in other studies.[13,15] In a recent cohort of 218 sarcoidosis patients, mortality was linked to the comorbidity burden, as shown by an association between a higher Charlson Comorbidity Index and a higher mortality rate ($P<.001$).[13] The association of mortality with higher numbers of comorbidities (>2) was also evident in a study of 557 sarcoidosis patients.[14] However, this observation must be interpreted with caution as the death rate was low (2.9%) and thyroid disease was the only individual comorbid disease that was significantly more prevalent in decedent cases than in the general sarcoidosis population.

Sarcoidosis has been linked with a higher frequency of subsequent malignant disease, but whether this association makes an important contribution to sarcoidosis-related mortality is uncertain.[13,16] Similar associations exist in other autoimmune inflammatory conditions such as the connective tissue diseases, possibly reflecting universal effects of persistent inflammatory process and/or antiinflammatory medication.[17,18]

The linkage between prolonged corticosteroid therapy and the development of hypertension and diabetes is universally recognized. Infectious disease due to immunosuppressive therapies is a major cause in many autoimmune disorders, such as the vasculitides. In individual sarcoidosis patients, it is often impossible to ascertain whether these comorbidities arise due to the deleterious effects of sarcoidosis-specific treatments, and thus fatalities due to diabetes, hypertension, and infectious disease are not generally viewed as deaths caused by sarcoidosis in cohort studies. However, it is difficult to argue, given the combined contribution of these diseases to sarcoidosis-associated mortality, that mortality ascribable to sarcoidosis-specific treatments (and thus ascribable to sarcoidosis) is not seriously underestimated.

One important implication is that statements of change in sarcoidosis-ascribable mortality with time need to be interpreted with great caution. For example, the significance of observations of a decline in mortality due to sarcoidosis in recent years is uncertain. In principle, this finding might have resulted from improved sarcoidosis management. However, it is equally possible that it reflects a shift from deaths due to sarcoidosis to deaths related to sarcoidosis therapy, with the use of more aggressive and prolonged interventional strategies in patients at higher risk due to major organ involvement.

In a recent United States report, approximately 50% of patients newly diagnosed with sarcoidosis-received therapy, with this figure inflated by more frequent treatment in the in the African American population.[11] Thus the possibility exists that the excess African American mortality in sarcoidosis results, in part, from treatment-related deaths. The exact influence of the dose and duration of maintenance therapy on the development of comorbidities has not been delineated. However, the adverse effects of corticosteroids were underlined in the study summarized previously of 105 newly diagnosed sarcoidosis patients. Patients receiving corticosteroids were at higher risk of reaching a composite comorbidity end-point that included diabetes, hypertension, weight gain, hyperlipidemia, and osteoporosis, all known to be associated with more frequent hospitalization.

The underestimation of sarcoidosis-ascribable mortality includes the underrecognition of fatal cardiac sarcoidosis, a problem that applies especially to fatal cardiomyopathy and arrhythmias in isolated cardiac sarcoidosis. The high prevalence of unrecognized cardiac involvement emerging from autopsy studies in patients with a known diagnosis of sarcoidosis is well recognized. With the recent advent of advanced cardiac imaging modalities, there are numerous anecdotal reports of the existence of underlying cardiac sarcoidosis in many patients previously considered to have idiopathic cardiac disease. It is too soon to make population statements about this phenomenon as the use of advanced imaging is still in its infancy. However, it is possible that with the correct attribution of mortality in this subset of patients, the prevalence of sarcoidosis-ascribable mortality will increase significantly. Research in this area should be prioritized.

MORTALITY DATA AND THE PERCEPTION THAT SARCOIDOSIS IS A BENIGN DISEASE

From a superficial review of broad cohort statements, it can be concluded that sarcoidosis is usually a benign disorder, leading to an underinvestment in urgently needed interventional studies. Plainly the exclusion of treatment-related fatal comorbidities and mortality due to undiagnosed isolated cardiac sarcoidosis from population-based statements of sarcoidosis-ascribable mortality, discussed previously, can only have resulted in a major understatement of the dangers associated with a diagnosis of sarcoidosis. However, the ultimately fatal impact of comorbidities and the existence of patients with major cardiac disease due to undiagnosed sarcoidosis cannot be taken into account in the identification of newly or recently diagnosed patients at high risk of death. The broad population statements reviewed earlier in this chapter may have contributed to misplaced complacency with regard to this important question. In reality, complacency is wholly inappropriate.

The statement that a reduction in life expectancy due to sarcoidosis exists in only 5%–8% of patients with sarcoidosis is not helpful as it understates the dangers of major organ involvement. Integrating data from many sources, it can be concluded that 50%–70% of deaths directly ascribable to sarcoidosis in cohort studies are due to interstitial lung disease or pulmonary vasculopathy. Deaths attributable to cardiac sarcoidosis make up approximately 15%–20%% of fatalities. The remaining causes of death include neurosarcoidosis, hepatic disease, renal disease, hypercalcemia, and other rare fatal outcomes. Major racial differences in the pattern of fatal organ involvement are not captured by global average statements. For example, in Japanese cohorts a fatal outcome is most often due to cardiac involvement.[19] However, accepting that preventative strategies must be nuanced according to the nature of the population to which they are applied, the need for an algorithm to identify patients at high risk of death is amply justified.

In this regard, the mathematics are stark. An overall mortality due to sarcoidosis of 7% occurs almost exclusively in patients with major organ involvement. In a highly influential review of sarcoidosis, widely cited throughout the world, it was estimated that 30% of sarcoidosis patients have clinically significant major organ involvement.[20] Thus it would appear that sarcoidosis-ascribable mortality approximates 20%–25% (7/30) in this patient subgroup. This figure rises further, perhaps to 35%, if cases with early spontaneous regression of disease and those with complete resolution with treatment are excluded. In this large patient subset, in a disease that is not rare, complacency about the risk of death needs to be resisted. Nihilism on this point would be easier to accept if major organ involvement was difficult to identify. However, significant pulmonary interstitial involvement is obvious based on symptoms and routine baseline tests recommended in an expert group statement.[21] Pulmonary vasculopathy may be more difficult to identify but will be largely contained within patients found to have clinically significant "lung involvement". Major hepatic and renal involvement is also very evident at baseline testing or will become obvious during routine monitoring. Neurosarcoidosis is usually clinically overt. It must be acknowledged that cardiac sarcoidosis does pose special problems in risk stratification due to underdetection, as discussed briefly later. However, given the very considerable mortality associated with readily identifiable major organ involvement, it can be argued that organ-based risk stratification is urgently required in sarcoidosis, especially in patients with interstitial lung disease, pulmonary vascular disease, or cardiac involvement.

ORGAN-BASED MORTALITY RISK STRATIFICATION

In patients with sarcoidosis a pragmatic definition of severe disease is needed, based on studies in which markers of severe disease are examined against mortality. Ideally, symptoms should be integrated with results from functional and imaging modalities and observed disease behavior in the definition of severe sarcoidosis.[22] Key variables that can usefully be applied to risk stratification are summarized in Table 25.2.

In patients with *pulmonary sarcoidosis*, progressive interstitial lung disease results in major pulmonary fibrosis in 20%–30% of cases.[20] Advanced pulmonary sarcoidosis with evidence of fibrosis on high-resolution computed tomography (HRCT) has been an important predictor of mortality in several series[23–25] with pulmonary fibrosis, either on chest radiography or HRCT, a predictor of mortality (independently of the presence

TABLE 25.2
Key Variables in Organ-Specific Sarcoidosis Risk Stratification

PULMONARY DISEASE
• Extensive fibrotic disease on HRCT
• Severe reduction in pulmonary function tests, especially DLCO levels
• Composite physiologic index >40 units
• Presence of pulmonary hypertension
(Presence of chronic pulmonary aspergillosis)[a]
CARDIAC DISEASE
• Left ventricular ejection fraction <50%
• Ventricular tachycardia
• Extensive late gadolinium enhancement on CMR
• Prominent cardiac inflammation on PET

CMR, cardiac magnetic resonance; *DLCO*, diffusion capacity for carbon monoxide; *HRCT*, high-resolution computed tomography; *PET*, positron emission tomography.

[a]Chronic pulmonary aspergillosis adds to risk only in patients with major hemoptysis but is associated with advanced pulmonary disease and should prompt risk stratification.

of pulmonary hypertension) in a cohort of 452 sarcoidosis patients from Cincinnati.[23]

Recent data suggest that the integration of pulmonary function parameters and HRCT findings may provide more accurate risk stratification. Walsh et al. reported a user-friendly staging system, developed using split-sample testing in more than 500 patients evaluated at a referral center.[25] In this system, patients were stratified into low- and high-risk groups based on the extent of pulmonary involvement (as judged by the composite physiologic index [CPI] and the extent of fibrosis on HRCT) and, in patients with lesser pulmonary involvement, HRCT evidence of pulmonary vasculopathy (i.e., an increase in the ratio of the main pulmonary artery diameter to ascending aorta diameter to >1.0). In the validation cohort the high-risk patient group had a substantially increased mortality (HR 5.89, $P < .0001$).

In a subsequent study of sarcoidosis patients with chronic pulmonary aspergillosis, a significant increase in mortality was observed in patients meeting criteria in the Walsh algorithm for high-risk disease.[26] Individual risk components in the Walsh algorithm (CPI > 40, extent of fibrosis on HRCT >20%, pulmonary artery diameter/ascending aorta diameter >1.0) and the presence of pulmonary hypertension were also associated with increased mortality. In a general sarcoidosis population the Walsh system was predictive of mortality on univariate analysis, although age was the most malignant prognostic determinant on multivariate analysis.[23]

It is currently uncertain whether a CPI threshold offers advantages over a diffusion capacity for carbon monoxide (DLCO) threshold in pulmonary fibrosis risk stratification. The two variables are influenced both by the severity of interstitial lung disease and by the severity of pulmonary vasculopathy. However, impairment of DLco can be deconstructed into interstitial and vasculopathic profiles (depending on whether reduction in DLco is disproportionate to reduction lung volumes), information that may be invaluable in guiding management.

Pulmonary hypertension (PH) in sarcoidosis is an independent determinant of morbidity and mortality[23,27] and is present in approximately 75% of sarcoidosis patients listed for lung transplantation.[27] In a series of 125 patients with sarcoidosis-related PH, the 5-year survival of 55% illustrates the importance of PH as a malignant prognostic determinant.[28] In this cohort a prevalence of stage IV disease of 72% reflects the fact that in this cohort of 72% PH is most commonly associated with major pulmonary fibrosis, although there was a poor correlation between the severity of interstitial lung disease and pulmonary hemodynamic variables at right heart catheterization. However, PH may result from a multiplicity of underlying pathophysiologic mechanisms, including granulomatous vascular inflammation, extrinsic compression from lymphadenopathy, and/or mediastinal fibrosis, pulmonary veno-occlusive disease, and left heart disease. In a series of sarcoidosis patients with proven PH, there was no evidence of pulmonary fibrosis on HRCT in 32% of cases.[29]

Thus effective risk stratification requires the identification of PH, irrespective of the presence or absence of severe pulmonary fibrosis. Unfortunately, no single noninvasive test has been reliable in identifying patients who should undergo right heart catheterization. Echocardiography is the most widely used screening tool, despite significant discrepancies between the echocardiographic systolic pulmonary artery pressure and right heart catheterization data.[30] There is a need to validate the integration of a number of noninvasive variables associated with PH in a PH-screening algorithm, including enlargement of the pulmonary artery on HRCT,[25,31] increased serum brain natriuretic peptide (BNP) levels, disproportionate reductions in gas transfer (against lung volumes), resting hypoxia, and striking oxygen desaturation during a 6-min walking test.

Chronic pulmonary aspergillosis (CPA) is associated with increased mortality in pulmonary sarcoidosis and should also be taken into account in sarcoidosis risk stratification. CPA is a well-recognized complication of fibrotic pulmonary sarcoidosis, usually associated with immunosuppressive treatment in patients with extensive fibrotic lung disease.[32,33] Mycetomas manifest on HRCT as a mass of soft tissue density within the lung cavity, usually located in the upper lobes and separated from the cavity itself by an air crescent.[34] Erosion of the fungal ball into a hypervascular cavity wall results in hemoptysis, which is life threatening in approximately 5% of patients. However, mortality associated with CPA often reflects the severity of underlying pulmonary sarcoidosis, rather than fatal hemoptysis. In a recent case series of patients with sarcoidosis and CPA, severe fibrotic pulmonary sarcoidosis was present in 64 of 65 (98.5%) patients, with PH present in 31%.[26] A proportion of 41.5% of patients died at a mean age of 55.8 years. Death seldom resulted from hemoptysis but was usually due to progression of advanced sarcoidosis. Thus the presence of CPA should alert the clinician to the likelihood of high risk from advanced pulmonary disease but adds risk only in those patients with recurrent major hemoptysis.

The presence of cardiac sarcoidosis has historically been considered as indicative of "dangerous sarcoidosis", based on the considerable morbidity and mortality associated with this form of disease. In a Japanese cohort of 95 cardiac sarcoidosis patients, patients with clinically overt cardiac sarcoidosis (a presentation with sustained ventricular tachycardia and a left ventricular ejection fraction [LVEF] < 50%) had a worse outcome with sudden cardiac death in 27% of cases. The 5-year survival of 60% was significantly higher in patients treated with steroids and/or preserved cardiac function (LVEF >50%).[35] The adverse outcomes associated with cardiac dysfunction and rhythm disturbances (particularly sustained ventricular tachycardia) was confirmed in a cohort of 73 cardiac sarcoidosis patients, with age greater than 46 years being an independent predictor of mortality.[36]

General statements of outcomes associated with cardiac sarcoidosis in historical series were to some extent skewed by the difficulty in identifying milder forms of cardiac sarcoidosis before the advent of advanced imaging modalities. One of the main challenges in evaluating risks associated with cardiac involvement in the general sarcoidosis population is the lack of a gold standard for the diagnosis of cardiac sarcoidosis. A histological diagnosis is seldom pursued as the diagnostic yield of cardiac biopsy is reduced by the patchy nature of the disease, and the procedure is not without risk. Application of the Japanese Ministry and Welfare diagnostic criteria suggests a prevalence of 5%–10% of clinically overt cardiac sarcoidosis.

However, these criteria do not identify subclinical disease, detectable only by advanced imaging modalities (cardiac resonance magnetic [CMR] imaging and positron emission tomography [PET]).[37–39] Recent data indicate that CMR and PET provide important prognostic information in identifying sarcoidosis patients at higher risk of mortality and life-threatening cardiac complications.[37–40] Based on these findings, CMR and PET were recently highlighted as recommended noninvasive diagnostic tests in suspected cardiac sarcoidosis in an expert consensus statement.[41] In the Heart Rhythm Society consensus statement, patients with biopsy-proven extracardiac sarcoidosis are considered to have a highly probable diagnosis of cardiac sarcoidosis if there is otherwise unexplained advanced atrioventricular block, sustained ventricular tachycardia, new onset heart failure (LVEF <40%), or a suggestive pattern of myocardial fibrosis or inflammation on CMR and/or PET. With the use of these criteria, the prevalence of cardiac sarcoidosis in the general sarcoidosis population increases to 25%–30%, increasing further in patients with suspected cardiac sarcoidosis. In a study of 321 patients with biopsy-proven sarcoidosis, screening with CMR revealed evidence of cardiac involvement in 29% of cases.[38]

However, although the use of advanced imaging modalities has identified a large subgroup of sarcoidosis patients with subclinical cardiac disease, the optimal use of these tests in risk stratification remains uncertain. In the study discussed previously, adverse cardiac outcomes were present in patients with evidence of cardiac involvement on CMR only when it was associated with cardiac symptoms and/or electrocardiogram (ECG) abnormalities.[38] Preliminary data indicate that the integration of advanced imaging findings is likely to have an important future role in risk stratification, with the severity of cardiac dysfunction and the presence of late gadolinium enhancement (LGE) on CMR-independent determinants of mortality. In a recent cohort an extent of LGE >20% of the myocardial mass was associated with a worse outcome, even after adjustment for the degree of left ventricular impairment.[42] Evidence of cardiac inflammation as judged by PET signal has also been associated with increased mortality in suspected cardiac sarcoidosis, but it is unclear whether this remains the case if PET signal is viewed as an indication for antiinflammatory/immunosuppressive therapy. Currently it would seem that prominent cardiac abnormalities on advanced imaging can reasonably be viewed as indicative of an increased risk of mortality to be integrated with LVEF <50% and ventricular tachycardia as a means of enhancing risk stratification in cardiac sarcoidosis. However, much work remains to be carried out to define exact thresholds indicative of a higher risk of mortality when advanced imaging abnormalities are less extensive.

CONCLUSION

In this chapter we have emphasized that sarcoidosis should not be viewed as a benign disease in patients with major organ involvement, despite apparently reassuring statements that in the general sarcoidosis populations, deaths directly ascribable to sarcoidosis occur in only 5%–8% of cases. Deaths due to comorbidities associated with sarcoidosis-specific therapies are not included in such estimates. Importantly it is possible to stratify risk in patients with interstitial lung disease, pulmonary vascular disease, and cardiac involvement which, taken together, accounts for more than 80% of deaths caused by sarcoidosis.

It should be emphasized that treatment algorithms aimed at reducing mortality are yet to be validated in those patients believed to have dangerous sarcoidosis. Severe major organ involvement may identify patients who have increased mortality despite treatment. However, it is not logical to introduce therapies for potentially dangerous disease only when excess mortality is unavoidable. Ideally, risk stratification should also identify those patients at higher risk of mortality if disease continues to progress, with a view to therapeutic intervention before "the train has left the station".

REFERENCES

1. Park JE, Kim YS, Kang MJ, et al. Prevalence, incidence, and mortality of sarcoidosis in Korea, 2003–2015: a nationwide population-based study. *Respir Med.* 2018;18:30100-30108. pii: S0954-6111.
2. Rossides M, Kullberg S, Askling J, et al. Sarcoidosis mortality in Sweden: a population-based cohort study. *Eur Respir J.* 2018;51. pii: 1701815.
3. Hu X, Carmona EM, Yi ES, et al. Causes of death in patients with chronic sarcoidosis. *Sarcoidosis Vasc Diffuse Lung Dis.* 2016;33:275–280.
4. Jamilloux Y, Maucort-Boulch D, Kerever S, et al. Sarcoidosis-related mortality in France: a multiple-cause-of-death analysis. *Eur Respir J.* 2016;48:1700–1709.
5. Ungprasert P, Carmona EM, Utz JP, et al. Epidemiology of sarcoidosis 1946-2013: a population-based study. *Mayo Clin Proc.* 2016;91:183–188.
6. Mirsaeidi M, Machado RF, Schraufnagel D, et al. Racial difference in sarcoidosis mortality in the United States. *Chest.* 2015;147:438–449.
7. Tukey MH, Berman JS, Boggs DA, et al. Mortality among African American women with sarcoidosis: data from the black women's health study. *Sarcoidosis Vasc Diffuse Lung Dis.* 2013;30:128–133.
8. Gribbin J, Hubbard RB, Le Jeune I, et al. Incidence and mortality of idiopathic pulmonary fibrosis and sarcoidosis in the UK. *Thorax.* 2006;61:980–985.
9. Bargagli E, Rosi E, Pistolesi M, et al. Increased risk of atherosclerosis in patients with sarcoidosis. *Pathobiology.* 2017;84:258–263.
10. Ungprasert P, Crowson CS, Matteson EL. Risk of cardiovascular disease among patients with sarcoidosis: a population-based retrospective cohort study, 1976–2013. *Eur Respir J.* 2017;49:1602396.
11. Khan NA, Donatelli CV, Tonelli AR, et al. Toxicity risk from glucocorticoids in sarcoidosis patients. *Respir Med.* 2017;132:9–14.
12. Ungprasert P, Matteson EL, Crowson CS. Increased risk of multimorbidity in patients with sarcoidosis: a population-based cohort study 1976 to 2013. *Mayo Clin Proc.* 2017;92:1791–1799.
13. Brito-Zerón P, Acar-Denizli N, Sisó-Almirall A, et al. The burden of comorbidity and complexity in sarcoidosis: impact of associated chronic diseases. *Lung.* 2018;196:239-248.
14. Nowiński A, Puścińska E, Goljan A, et al. The influence of comorbidities on mortality in sarcoidosis: an observational prospective cohort study. *Clin Respir J.* 2017;11:648-656.
15. Martusewicz-Boros MM, Boros PW, Wiatr E, Roszkowski-Śliż K. What comorbidities accompany sarcoidosis? A large cohort (n=1779) patients analysis. *Sarcoidosis Vasc Diffuse Lung Dis.* 2015;32:115–120.
16. Bonifazi M, Bravi F, Gasparini S, et al. Sarcoidosis and cancer risk: systematic review and meta-analysis of observational studies. *Chest.* 2015;147:778–791.
17. Zöller B, Li X, Sunquist J, Sundquist K. Risk of subsequent coronary heart disease in patients hospitalized for immune mediated diseases: a nationwide follow-up study from Sweden. *PLoS One.* 2012;7(3):e33442.
18. Ungprasert P, Suksaranjit P, Spanuchart I, Leeaphorn N, Permpalung N. Risk of coronary artery disease in patients with idiopathic inflammatory myopathies: a systematic review and meta-analysis of observational studies. *Semin Arthritis Rheum.* 2014;44:63–77.
19. Morimoto T, Azuma A, Abe S, et al. Epidemiology of sarcoidosis in Japan. *Eur Respir J.* 2008;31:372–379.
20. Iannuzzi MC, Rybicki BA, Teirstein AS. Sarcoidosis. *N Engl J Med.* 2007;357:2153–2165.
21. Statement on sarcoidosis. Joint statement of the American Thoracic Society (ATS), the European Respiratory Society (ERS) and the world association of sarcoidosis and other granulomatous disorders (WASOG) adopted by the ATS board of directors and by the ERS Executive Committee, February 1999. *Am J Respir Crit Care Med.* 1999;160:736-755.
22. Kouranos V, Jacob J, Wells AU. Severe sarcoidosis. *Clin Chest Med.* 2015;36:715–726.
23. Kirkil G, Lower EE, Baughman RP. Predictors of mortality in pulmonary sarcoidosis. *Chest.* 2018;153:105–113.
24. Handa T, Nagai S, Fushimi Y, et al. Clinical and radiographic indices associated with airflow limitation in patients with sarcoidosis. *Chest.* 2006;130:1851–1856.
25. Walsh SL, Wells AU, Sverzellati N, et al. An integrated clinicoradiological staging system for pulmonary sarcoidosis: a case-cohort study. *Lancet Respir Med.* 2014;2:123–130.
26. Uzunhan Y, Nunes H, Jeny F, et al. Chronic pulmonary aspergillosis complicating sarcoidosis. *Eur Respir J.* 2017;49. pii: 1602396.
27. Shorr AF, Davies DB, Nathan SD. Predicting mortality in patients with sarcoidosis awaiting lung transplantation. *Chest.* 2003;124:922–928.
28. Boucly A, Cottin V, Nunes H, et al. Management and long-term outcomes of sarcoidosis-associated pulmonary hypertension. *Eur Respir J.* 2017;50. pii: 1700465.
29. Nunes H, Humbert M, Capron F, et al. Pulmonary hypertension associated with sarcoidosis: mechanisms, haemodynamics and prognosis. *Thorax.* 2006;61:68–74.
30. Janda S, Shahidi N, Gin K, et al. Diagnostic accuracy of echocardiography for pulmonary hypertension: a systematic review and meta-analysis. *Heart.* 2011;97:612–622.

31. Devaraj A, Wells AU, Meister MG, et al. Detection of pulmonary hypertension with multidetector CT and echocardiography alone and in combination. *Radiology*. 2010;254:609–616.
32. Denning DW, Cadranel J, Beigelman-Aubry C, et al. Chronic pulmonary aspergillosis: rationale and clinical guidelines for diagnosis and management. *Eur Respir J*. 2016;47:45–68.
33. Denning DW, Pleuvry A, Cole DC. Global burden of chronic pulmonary aspergillosis complicating sarcoidosis. *Eur Respir J*. 2013;41:621–626.
34. Kouranos V, Hansell DM, Sharma R, Wells AU. Advances in imaging of cardiopulmonary involvement in sarcoidosis. *Curr Opin Pulm Med*. 2015;21:538–545.
35. Yazaki Y, Isobe M, Hiroe M, et al. Prognostic determinants of long-term survival in Japanese patients with cardiac sarcoidosis treated with prednisone. *Am J Cardiol*. 2001;88:1006–1010.
36. Zhou Y, Lower EE, Li HP, et al. Cardiac sarcoidosis: the impact of age and implanted devices on survival. *Chest*. 2017;151:139–148.
37. Patel MR, Cawley PJ, Heitner JF, et al. Detection of myocardial damage in patients with sarcoidosis. *Circulation*. 2009;120:1969–1977.
38. Kouranos V, Tzelepis GE, Rapti A, et al. Complementary role of CMR to conventional screening in the diagnosis and prognosis of cardiac sarcoidosis. *JACC Cardiovasc Imaging*. 2017;10:1437–1447.
39. Blankstein R, Osborne M, Naya M, et al. Cardiac positron emission tomography enhances prognostic assessments of patients with suspected cardiac sarcoidosis. *J Am Coll Cardiol*. 2014;63:329–336.
40. Hulten E, Agarwal V, Cahill M, et al. Presence of late gadolinium enhancement by cardiac magnetic resonance among patients with suspected cardiac sarcoidosis is associated with adverse cardiovascular prognosis: a systematic review and meta-analysis. *Circ Cardiovasc Imaging*. 2016;9:e005001.
41. Birnie DH, Sauer WH, Bogun F, et al. HRS expert consensus statement on the diagnosis and management of arrhythmias associated with cardiac sarcoidosis. *Heart Rhythm*. 2014;11:1305–1323.
42. Osborne MT, Hulten EA, Singh A, et al. Reduction in ^{18}F-fluorodeoxyglucose uptake on serial cardiac positron emission tomography is associated with improved left ventricular ejection fraction in patients with cardiac sarcoidosis. *J Nucl Cardiol*. 2014;21:166–174.

Index

Note: Page numbers followed by "f" indicate figures, "t" indicate tables.

Printed in the United States
By Bookmasters